W9-ADC-897

Professional Nursing
Concepts & Challenges

NWTC Library
2740 W. Mason St.
Green Bay, WI 54307

Professional Nursing
Concepts & Challenges

Ninth Edition

Beth Perry Black, PhD, RN, FAAN

Associate Professor
University of North Carolina at Chapel Hill
School of Nursing
Chapel Hill, North Carolina

ELSEVIER

3251 Riverport Lane
St. Louis, Missouri 63043

PROFESSIONAL NURSING: CONCEPTS & CHALLENGES,
NINE EDITION

ISBN: 978-0-323-55113-7

Copyright © 2020, Elsevier Inc. All Rights Reserved.

No part of this publication may be reproduced or transmitted in any form or by any means, electronic or mechanical, including photocopying, recording, or any information storage and retrieval system, without permission in writing from the publisher. Details on how to seek permission, further information about the Publisher's permissions policies and our arrangements with organizations such as the Copyright Clearance Center and the Copyright Licensing Agency, can be found at our website: www.elsevier.com/permissions.

This book and the individual contributions contained in it are protected under copyright by the Publisher (other than as may be noted herein).

Notice

Practitioners and researchers must always rely on their own experience and knowledge in evaluating and using any information, methods, compounds, or experiments described herein. Because of rapid advances in the medical sciences—in particular, independent verification of diagnoses and drug dosages—should be made. To the fullest extent of the law, no responsibility is assumed by Elsevier, authors, editors, or contributors for any injury and/or damage to persons or property as a matter of products liability, negligence or otherwise, or from any use or operation of any methods, products, instructions, or ideas contained in the material herein.

Library of Congress Control Number: 2019939335

Senior Content Strategist: Sandra Clark
Senior Content Development Manager: Luke Held
Senior Content Development Specialist: Jennifer Wade
Publishing Services Manager: Deepthi Unni
Senior Project Manager: Manchu Mohan
Designer: Ryan Cook

Printed in China

Last digit is the print number: 9   8   7   6   5   4   3   2   1

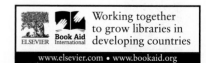

I dedicate this edition to my smart, funny, and spirited daughters, Amanda and Kylie,
who, like their mom, chose their life partners well. Thank you,
Hudson and Pierce, for becoming family.

—BPB

CONTRIBUTORS

Maureen J. Baker, BSN, MSN, PhD
Clinical Associate Professor
University of North Carolina at Chapel Hill
Chapel Hill, North Carolina

Josie K. Christian, DNP, MSN, BSN, RN, PHN
Chair and Associate Professor
Nursing Department
Concordia University Saint Paul
St. Paul, Minnesota

Janna Louise Dieckmann, BA, BSN, MSN, PhD
Clinical Associate Professor
School of Nursing
University of North Carolina at Chapel Hill
Chapel Hill, North Carolina

Maxine Fearrington, MS, RN-BC
Level III RN
Strong Surgical Center
University of Rochester Medical Center
Rochester, New York

Kimberly Fenstermacher, PhD
Chair, Department of Nursing
Associate Professor
School of Science, Engineering and Health
Messiah College
Mechanicsburg, PA

Beverly Brown Foster, MN, MPH, PhD, RN
Clinical Professor
School of Nursing
University of North Carolina at Chapel Hill
Chapel Hill, North Carolina

Heather Moulzolf, DNP, MA-N, BA-N, ARNP-BC, CNP-BC
Assistant Professor
Nursing - RN to BSN
Concordia University
Saint Paul, Minnesota;
Associate Professor
Nursing - DNP
St. Catherine University
Saint Paul, Minnesota

Anita Tesh, BSN, MSN, PhD, CNE, ANEF, RN
Assistant Dean
Undergraduate Division, School of Nursing
University of North Carolina at Chapel Hill
Chapel Hill, North Carolina; Adjunct Professor
School of Nursing
University of North Carolina at Greensboro
Greensboro, North Carolina

Amy Holland, RN, MSN
Clinical Instructor
School of Nursing
University of Texas
Austin, Texas

Josie K. Christian, DNP, MSN, BSN, RN, PHN
Chair and Associate Professor
Nursing Department
Concordiau University Saint Paul
St. Paul, Minnesota

Gina M. Oliver, PhD, APRN, FNP-BC, CNE
Associate Teaching Professor
Sinclair School of Nursing
University of Missouri
Columbia, Missouri

Linda Jean Porter-Wenzlaff, RN, LPC-S, PhD, MSN, MA, CENP, NEA-BC, CNE, NCC
Lillie Cranz Cullen Endowed Professorship in Nursing, Distinguished Teaching Professor, Clinical
Office of Faculty Affairs and Diversity
School of Nursing
UT Health San Antonio
San Antonio, Texas

Lynnann Baumann Murphy, MN, BSN, RN
Faculty Instructor
Leach College of Nursing
University of St. Francis
Joliet, Illinois

PREFACE

Nursing is evolving, as is health care, in the United States. With the debates and discussions, lawsuits, and legislation that surround the Affordable Care Act (ACA), health care has become a flashpoint in American political and social discourse. With the increasing response to calls to advance their education and with their strong record of safety and quality care, nurses are well situated to be leaders in the provision of health care in the United States.

To be effective leaders, nurses must master knowledge about health and illness and human responses to each, think critically and creatively, participate in robust interprofessional education and collaborations, be both caring and professional, and grapple with complex ethical dilemmas that challenge providers in a time when health care resources are strained. As leaders, nurses should understand their history because the past informs the present; vision for the future builds on the lessons of today.

The ninth edition of *Professional Nursing: Concepts & Challenges* reflects my commitment to present current and relevant information. Since the last edition, the ACA has been subject to attempts to defund it, destabilize the insurance markets, and change key components of this important legislation, including doing away with protections of persons with preexisting conditions. By the time this edition is published, the 2018 midterm elections will have taken place and some of the questions that now trouble the ACA and health care in general are likely to have been resolved in one way or another. Although at the time of this writing the future of the ACA is unclear, what is clear is that questions of health care as a human right and how health care is best delivered and paid for will continue to spark lively debate in America.

In this edition, the order of the chapters has remained the same as in the eighth edition, based on generous feedback from faculty that this order provides a cohesive view of nursing; its history, education, and conceptual and theoretical bases; and the place of nursing in the U.S. health care system. Faculty are encouraged, however, to use the chapters in any order that reflects their own pedagogic and theoretical approaches. By using contributors with content expertise, this edition remains fresh and up-to-date. The effects of social media on nursing are addressed extensively regarding the legal and ethical implications of their use by nurses and their role in professional socialization and communication. With the easy and free availability of health-related statistics from .gov and other websites, I and the contributors decided to continue with the plan that was successful in the eighth edition: more narrative and fewer statistics. I have rarely met an engaged nurse who didn't start a story with, "I had a patient once who…" These narratives teach us about what is important in nursing.

Throughout the book, we have been very careful to be inclusive, to avoid heteronormative and ethnocentric language, to use examples that avoid stereotypes of all types, and to include photographs that capture the wonderful diversity of American nursing.

A note about references: older references refer to classic papers or texts. There are a few references that do not reach the level of "classic" texts, but the author turned a phrase in a clever or elegant way that needed to be cited. No manner of updated paper could replace these interesting comments or points of view. Research and clinical works are relevant and contemporary.

As with the last four editions, the ninth edition is written at a level appropriate for use in early courses in baccalaureate curricula, in RN-to-BSN and RN-to-MSN courses, and as a resource for practicing nurses and graduate students. An increasing number of students in nursing programs are seeking second undergraduate degrees, such as midlife adults seeking a career change and others who bring considerable experience to the learning situation. Accordingly, every effort has been made to present material that is comprehensive enough to challenge users at all levels without overwhelming beginning students. The text has been written to be engaging and interesting, and care has been taken to minimize jargon so prevalent in health care. A comprehensive glossary is provided to assist in developing and refining a professional vocabulary. As in previous editions, key terms are highlighted in the text itself. All terms in color print are in the Glossary. The Glossary also contains basic terms that are not necessarily used in the text but may be unfamiliar to students new to nursing.

I hope that the ninth edition continues to meet the high standards set forth by Kay Chitty, who edited the first four editions of this book. I hope that students and faculty will find this edition readable, informative, and thought provoking. More than anything, I hope that

Professional Nursing: Concepts & Challenges, Ninth Edition, will contribute to the continuing evolution of the profession of nursing and, ultimately, to the excellent care of patients, their families, and their communities.

Beth Perry Black

ACKNOWLEDGMENTS

With each new edition of *Professional Nursing: Concepts & Challenges,* I find myself increasingly in awe of the intelligence, creativity, humility, and work ethic of the nurses who continue to inspire me.

I am grateful to the many people whose support and assistance have made this book possible, each in different ways:

- To faculty who used earlier editions and shared their helpful suggestions to make this book better.
- To students who sent e-mails, expressing their gratitude for an interesting and readable textbook while offering ideas for improvement.
- To the contributors in this edition—Anita, Bev, Maureen, Janna, Kimberly, Maxine, Heather, Josie—whose expertise and commitment to excellence has made working on this edition particularly enjoyable.
- To my colleagues in the School of Nursing at the University of North Carolina at Chapel Hill, and to our extraordinary nursing students and alumni, who make us proud.
- To the faculty and students at Guangzhou (PRC) University School of Nursing and Traditional Chinese Medicine, especially Jiagen Xiang, whom I am proud to have as my colleague and friend.
- To Claudia Christy, my friend and traveling companion across the years, whose common sense and keen intelligence are a formidable combination.
- To Bonnie Barbour, whose friendship in our childhood and now again as (not-quite!) seniors is a treasure.
- To my brothers Dennis, David, and Mike Perry, because I would be lost without my bros.
- To my nieces Kelsey and Olivia. You are lights in my life, girls.

I am so lucky to have each of you grace my life with your unique gifts. I can't thank you enough.

CONTENTS

CONTENTS

Nursing in Today's Evolving Health Care Environment

Heather Moulzolf, DNP, MA-N, BA-N, ARNP-BC, CNP-BC,
Josie K. Christian, DNP, MSN, BSN, RN, PHN

ⓔ To enhance your understanding of this chapter, try the Student Exercises on the Evolve site at
http://evolve.elsevier.com/Black/professional.

LEARNING OUTCOMES

After studying this chapter, students will be able to:
- Describe the demographic profile of registered nurses today.
- Recognize the wide range of settings and roles in which today's registered nurses practice.

- Identify evolving practice opportunities for nurses.
- Consider nursing roles in various practice settings.
- Explain the roles and education of advanced practice nurses.

Nurses comprise the largest segment of the health care workforce in the United States and have increasing opportunities to practice in a wide variety of settings. In fact, nurses specialize in 104 areas: 34 specialties are outside the hospital, 68 are research oriented, 37 are managerial, and 92 are patient facing (see the Campaign for Nursing Explore Specialties at https://www.discovernursing.com/explore-specialties#.WhXOF0qnE2w). More than ever, the profession requires a well-trained, flexible, and knowledgeable workforce of nurses who can practice in today's evolving health care environment. Recent legislation, demands of patients as consumers of health care, and the need to control costs while optimizing outcomes have had a great influence on the way that health care is delivered in the United States. Nursing is evolving to meet these demands.

One of the most notable influences on today's health care environment is the Affordable Care Act (ACA), passed in 2010 by the 111th Congress and signed into law by President Barack Obama. The ACA is actually two laws—the Patient Protection and Affordable Care

Act (PL 111-148) and the Health Care and Education Affordability Reconciliation Act (PL 111-152). These laws provide for incremental but progressive change to the way that Americans gain access to and pay for their health care. Although likely to be revised to some extent by Congress, the ACA has nonetheless provided increased opportunities for nurses: the Committee on the Robert Wood Johnson Foundation (RWJF) Initiative on the Future of Nursing at the National Academy of Medicine (formerly the Institute of Medicine [IOM]) noted, "Nurses have a considerable opportunity to act as full partners with other health professionals and to lead in the improvement and redesign of the health care system and its practice environment" (Institute of Medicine, 2010, pp. 1–2). This important initiative continues to have a profound influence on the evolution of nursing and nursing education since its publication.

Writing about "nursing today" poses a challenge, because what is current today may have already changed by the time you read this. What does not change, however, is the commitment of nurses to what

Rosenberg (1995) referred to as "the care of strangers"—professional caring, learned through focused education and deliberate socialization (Storr, 2010). In other words, you will be taught to think like a nurse and to do well those things that nurses do. You will become a nurse. Importantly, some of you are already nurses and are returning to school to further your education. Thank you for your commitment to the profession and to your own professional development! You have experienced firsthand the shifting needs of the profession in response to an evolving health care system in a changing world and are poised to move nursing forward with your knowledge from both your education and your wide variety of experiences.

In this chapter you will learn some basic information about today's nursing workforce: who nurses are, the settings where they practice, and the patients for whom they are providing care. You will also be introduced to some nurses who have had intriguing experiences and opportunities that you may not know are even possible. Your nursing education will provide you with a flexible set of skills and opens to you a wide variety of experiences that await you as you begin—or continue—your career as a professional registered nurse (RN).

NURSING IN THE UNITED STATES TODAY

High-quality, culturally competent nursing care depends on a culturally diverse nursing workforce (American Association of Colleges of Nursing [AACN], 2014a). The need to enhance diversity in nursing through the recruitment of underrepresented groups into the profession is a priority (AACN, 2014b). Understanding the composition of the nursing workforce is necessary to identify underrepresented groups and to recognize workforce trends such as the age of nurses in practice and the percentage of licensed nurses holding jobs in nursing.

The U.S. Department of Health and Human Services responded to this need by conducting a comprehensive survey of the nursing workforce every 4 years, beginning in 1977. Known as the National Sample Survey of Registered Nurses (NSSRN), this effort gave policymakers, educators, and other nurse leaders data about the workforce, allowing them to make informed decisions about allocation of resources, development of programs, and recruitment of nurses. The final NSSRN was conducted in 2008, and results were published in 2010. The federal government has since discontinued this very

useful survey. The final version of the 2008 federal nursing workforce survey, *The Registered Nurse Population: Findings from the 2008 National Sample Survey of Registered Nurses* (U.S. Department of Health and Human Services, 2010), is available as a .pdf file in a direct link: https://bhw.hrsa.gov/sites/default/files/bhw/nchwa/rnsurveyfinal.pdf.

In response to the discontinuation of the NSSRN and the ongoing need to understand the nursing workforce, in 2013 the National Council of State Boards of Nursing (NCSBN) and the Forum of State Nursing Workforce Centers (FSNWC) combined efforts to conduct a comprehensive national survey of RNs (Budden et al., 2013). In this chapter, data from the 2015 NCSBN and FSNWC survey are presented in conjunction with other sources of workforce data, including the final 2008 NSSRN data, to provide you with a thumbnail sketch of nursing, specifically focusing on the number of nurses in the workforce, as well as their gender, age, race, ethnicity, and educational levels.

Nurses in the Workforce

RNs are the largest group of health care providers in the United States and in the 2000s grew by 24.1% (Health Resources and Services Administration, 2013). More than 4 million individuals held licenses as RNs in 2016 (National Council of State Boards of Nursing, 2016). In 2013 approximately 2.8 million nurses were currently working (Health Resources and Services Administration, 2013). In the 2015 NCSBN and FSNWC National Workforce Survey of RNs, the majority (91%) of nurses younger than age 50 are employed in nursing. A significant number of survey respondents (82%) were actively employed in nursing, with 63% reporting working full time. Respondents worked an average of 36.6 hours per week (one position), and RNs with two or more positions worked an average of 42.2 hours per week.

Gender

Nursing remains a profession dominated by women; however, the percentage of men in nursing increased by 50% between 2000 and 2008 (U.S. Department of Health and Human Services, 2010). Among NCSBN/FSNWC 2015 survey respondents, 8% were men compared with 7% in the 2013 survey. In 2014 men comprised 15% of students in entry-level bachelor of science in nursing (BSN) programs (National League for Nursing [NLN], 2014). According to the AACN (2015a), data obtained from nurses in practice showed that male and female RNs were equally likely to have a bachelor's or higher degree in nursing or nursing-related fields (49.9% and 50.3%, respectively). Men, however, were more likely than women to have a bachelor's or higher degree in nursing and any nonnursing field (62% vs. 55%). A higher percentage of the men work in hospitals (76% vs. 62%). At 41%, men are overrepresented in the advanced practice role of certified registered nurse anesthetists. Among all other job titles held by men, staff nurse and administration have proportional representation, with about 7% of these positions held by men. Nurse practitioners and positions designated as "other" (e.g., consultant, clinical nurse leader, informatics, researcher) are slightly less proportional, with 6% of these positions held by men. Men hold only about 3.8% of faculty positions.

Age

The future of any profession depends on the infusion of youth, and the steady increase in the age of the nursing workforce has been a concern. Earlier data indicated that the rate of aging has slowed in the nursing workforce as a result of the increased number of working RNs younger than age 30, which offsets the increasing number of nurses aged 60 or older who continue to work (U.S. Department of Health and Human Services, 2010). The rise in the number of nurses younger than age 30 is attributed to the increased number of BSN graduates, who tend to be younger than graduates from other types of nursing programs. Since 2005, the average age of graduates from all nursing programs has been 31 years old. BSN graduates, at an average age of 28 years old, are 5 years younger than graduates of associate degree and diploma (hospital-based) programs, who are on average 33 years old.

The median age is that point at which half of the nurses are older and half are younger, and it provides a more useful metric of the workforce than does calculating a mean age. Since 1988, when the median age was 38, the median age of nurses rose by 2 years between each survey, so that by 2004, the median age was 46, a worrisome figure that meant the nursing workforce was continuing to age. The increasing number of nurses aged 60 and older who are still in the workforce may reflect economic conditions requiring older nurses to remain employed rather than retiring. Nursing is reasonably protected from the layoffs and downsizing experienced in other professions.

This stabilization of the aging pattern seen in the final NSSRN survey is an optimistic sign that nursing is seen as an option for younger people entering the workforce and that nursing will not face a shortage as older nurses age out of the workforce in a few years. However, with approximately one-third of the current nursing workforce older than age 50 (Health Resources and Services Administration, 2013), the profession of nursing must continue to recruit and educate younger nurses to prevent a nursing shortage as older nurses move toward retirement.

Race and Ethnicity

Racial and ethnic minorities comprise 37% of the U.S. population today but only 19% of the RN population, an underrepresentation by about 50% in 2013 (Budden et al., 2013). This is similar to the findings in 2008 in the NSSRN (Fig. 1.1). Although troublesome, the number is an improvement from 2004, when only 12.2% of RNs had racial/ethnic minority backgrounds. Detailed data from the NSSRN showed that the largest disparity between the U.S. general population and the RN population is seen with Hispanics/Latinos of any race. Although this group forms about 15.4% of the U.S. population, they make up only 3.6% of RNs. Black/African American, non-Hispanics also have a significant disparity; now constituting 12.2% of the U.S. population, this group makes up just 5.4% of RNs. The only group that exceeds its representational percentage in the general population is the Asian or Native Hawaiian/Pacific Islander, non-Hispanic group. Comprising 4.5% of the general population, this group makes up 5.8% of the RN population, possibly because a substantial number of RNs practicing in the United States received their nursing education in India or the Philippines, thus contributing to their overrepresentation (U.S. Department of Health and Human Services, 2010). In 2014 a biennial survey of nursing schools by the NLN demonstrated promise that the diversity of the profession is improving. In 1995 fewer than 18% of students enrolled in a professional nursing program were from underrepresented racial or ethnic minority groups, in contrast to more than 35% in 2014 (NLN, 2014).

Despite efforts to recruit and retain racial/ethnic minority women and men to the profession, nursing still has a long way to go before the racial/ethnic composition of the profession more accurately reflects that of the United States as a whole. This situation is improving,

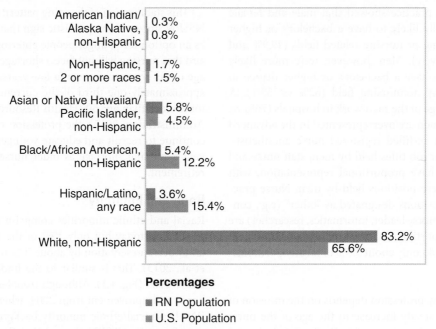

Fig. 1.1 Registered nurse (RN) and U.S. populations by race/ethnicity, 2008. The proportion of nurses who are White, non-Hispanic is greater than their proportion in the U.S. population. (Data from U.S. Department of Health and Human Services, Health Resources and Services Administration: *The Registered Nurse Population: Findings from the 2008 National Sample Survey of Registered Nurses,* Washington, DC, 2010, U.S. Government Printing Office, p. 7-7.)

however. In a recent report on enrollment and graduation in bachelor's and graduate programs in nursing, the AACN (2015a) found that 30.1% of nursing students in entry-level BSN programs were from underrepresented backgrounds.

Education

The basic education to become a nurse is referred to as the *entry level* into practice. Successful completion of your basic education, however, does not qualify you to become a nurse. Once you have graduated from a school of nursing approved by your state, you are qualified to take the National Council Licensure Examination for Registered Nurses, known as the NCLEX-RN®. Once you have passed the NCLEX-RN®, you can be licensed as an RN if you meet other requirements by your state board of nursing, such as passing a background check.

Nursing has three mechanisms by which you can get basic nursing education to qualify to take the NCLEX®: (1) a 4-year education at a college or university conferring a BSN degree; (2) a 2-year education at a community college or technical school conferring an

associate degree in nursing (ADN); and (3) a diploma in nursing, awarded after the successful completion of a hospital-based program that typically takes 3 years to complete, including prerequisite courses that may be taken at another school.

According to the National League for Nursing (NLN), the number of diploma programs educated only 3% to 4% of all new RNs in between 2003 and 2014 (NLN, 2014) as nursing education has shifted to colleges and universities (AACN, 2011). The majority of nurses (53%) in the United States get their initial nursing education in ADN programs (RWJF, 2013); in the NCSBN/FSNWC (2013) survey, 39% of the 41,823 respondents reported having an ADN as their first degree or credential, and 36% reported having a BSN as their first degree or credential.

Many ADN-prepared RNs eventually return to school to complete a BSN degree. Between 2004 and 2012, the number of RNs enrolled in BSN programs almost tripled, from 35,000 to slightly fewer than 105,000 (RWJF, 2013). Currently, approximately 55% of RNs have BSN or higher degrees (Health Resources and Services

Administration, 2013). Many colleges and universities offer BSN programs, often online, to accommodate RNs in practice who want to work toward a BSN degree as a supplement to their basic nursing education at the ADN or diploma level. Nursing education is discussed in greater detail in Chapter 4.

Globalization and the international migration of nurses have increased internationally educated nurses (IENs) practicing in the United States by 40% between 2006 and 2015, and in 2016 approximately 15% of all RNs in the United States were educated in other countries (World Education Service, 2018). The recruitment of IENs to the United States has been a strategy to expand the nursing workforce in response to the recent nursing shortage. This strategy, however, may result in nursing shortages in their own countries. IENs face challenges as they join the workforce in the United States, including English as a second language and problems with their peers who may not perceive them as knowledgeable (Thekdi et al., 2011). Deep cultural differences may further separate the IENs from their American peers. Thekdi and colleagues (2011) noted that IENs might have views of gender, authority, power, and age that vary from those of Americans, and which may affect their communication styles.

Sigma Theta Tau International (STTI) published a position paper on international nurse migration. Although this paper was published in 2005, it reflects STTI's current, ongoing position regarding international nurse migration (STTI, 2005). STTI recognizes the autonomy of nurses in making decisions for themselves about where to live and work, noting that "push/pull" factors shape nurse migration. Push factors include poor compensation and working conditions, political instability, and lack of opportunities for career development that drive (push) a nurse to seek employment in another country. Factors that pull nurses to emigrate include opportunities for a better quality of life, personal safety, and professional incentives such as increased pay, better working conditions, and career development. STTI calls for further exploration of the issue with a focus on identifying "solutions that do not promote one nation's health at the expense of another's" (p. 2). Furthermore, STTI endorsed the International Council of Nurses position in calling for a regulated recruitment process based on ethical principles that deter exploitation of foreign-educated nurses and reinforce sound employment policies (p. 4).

Practice Settings for Professional Nurses

As members of the largest health care profession in the United States, nurses practice in a wide variety of settings. The most common setting is the hospital, and many new nurses seek employment there to strengthen their clinical and assessment skills. Nurses practice in clinics, community-based facilities, medical offices, skilled nursing facilities (SNFs), and other long-term settings. Nurses also provide care in places where people spend much of their time: homes, schools, and workplaces. In communities, nurses work in the military, community and senior centers, children's camps, homeless shelters, and, recently, in retail clinics found in some pharmacies. Nurses also provide palliative care (i.e., symptom management to improve quality of life) and end-of-life care, often in the homes of patients who are terminally ill or in inpatient hospice homes or facilities. Increasingly, nurses with advanced degrees, training, and certification are working in their own private practices or in partnership with physicians or other providers. This expansion of practice holds promise for nurses to widen their roles in health care, especially as the American health care system continues to evolve.

Hospitals remained the primary work site for RNs, with 63.2% of nurses employed by hospitals in either inpatient or outpatient settings, an increase of 25% in the past decade (Health Resources and Services Administration, 2013). Most of these nurses (39.6%) work in inpatient units in community hospitals, whereas others work in specialty hospitals, long-term care hospitals, and psychiatric units. The federal government employs nurses, generally in the U.S. Department of Veterans Affairs (VA) hospitals, where 1.1% of RNs work.

Ambulatory care settings, such as nurse-based practices, physician-based practices, and free-standing emergency and surgical centers, accounted for 10.5%, the second largest segment of the nurse workforce. Public and community health accounted for 7.8% of employed nurses, and an additional 6.4% worked in home health. Skilled nursing facilities (SNFs), or extended care facilities, employed 5.3% of nurses in the workforce. The remainder of employed RNs worked in settings such as schools of nursing; nursing associations; local, state, or federal governmental agencies; state boards of nursing; or insurance companies (U.S. Department of Health and Human Services, 2010, pp. 3–9).

Not all nurses provide direct patient care as their primary role. A small but important group of nurses spend the majority of their time conducting research, teaching undergraduate and graduate students in the classroom and in clinical settings, managing companies as chief executives, and consulting with health care organizations. Nurses with advanced levels of education, such as master's and doctoral degrees, are prepared to become researchers, educators, and administrators. Nurses can practice as advanced practice nurses (APNs), including a variety of types of nurse practitioners (NPs), clinical nurse specialists (CNSs), certified nurse-midwives (CNMs), and certified registered nurse anesthetists (CRNAs). These advanced practice roles are described later in this chapter.

Nurses have much to consider in deciding where to practice. Some settings will not be immediately open to new nurses because they require additional educational preparation or work experience. Importantly, nurses entering the workforce need to consider their special talents, likes, and dislikes—neither the nurse nor patients benefit when a nurse is working with a population for which he or she has little affinity. A nurse who enjoys working with children may not feel at ease in caring for elderly patients; on the other hand, a nurse who loves children may find that caring for sick children is emotionally stressful. A nurse with excellent communication skills may find that a postanesthesia care unit (PACU) does not allow the formation of professional relationships with patients that this nurse might appreciate in a psychiatric setting. Nursing school offers the chance to experience a wide variety of settings with diverse patient populations. At the end of your studies, you may be surprised by the skills you have developed and populations that appeal to you (Fig. 1.2).

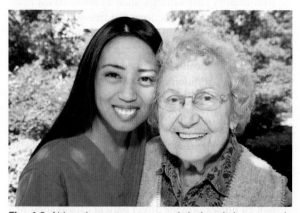

Fig. 1.2 Although most nurses work in hospitals, nurses in home health settings often enjoy long-term relationships with their patients. (Photo used with permission from iStockphoto.)

Health care reform and the push to transform the health care system are moving nurses into new territory. Numerous new opportunities and roles are being developed that use nurses' skills in innovative and exciting ways. In the following section, you will be introduced to a range of settings in which nurses practice. These areas are only a sample of the growing variety of opportunities available to nurses entering practice today.

Nursing in Hospitals

Nursing care originated and was practiced informally in home and community settings and moved into hospitals only within the past 150 years. Hospitals vary widely in size and services. Certain hospitals are referred to as medical centers and offer comprehensive specialty services, such as cancer centers, maternal-fetal medicine services, and heart centers. Medical centers are usually associated with university medical schools and have a complex array of providers. Medical centers can have 1000 or more beds and have a huge nursing workforce. Medical centers are often designated as level 1 trauma centers because they offer highly specialized surgical and supportive care for the most severely injured patients. The patients at community-based hospitals usually are less severely ill than those needing comprehensive care or trauma care at a medical center. However, if a patient becomes unstable or if the patient's condition warrants, he or she can be transported to a larger hospital or a medical center. Nurses play an important role in identifying very ill patients, assisting in stabilizing their conditions, and preparing them for transport.

In general, nurses in hospitals care for patients who have medical or surgical conditions (e.g., those with cancer or diabetes, those in need of postoperative care), children and their families on pediatric units, women and their newborns, and patients who have had severe trauma or burns. Specialty areas are referred to as "units," such as operating suites or emergency departments, intensive care units (e.g., cardiac, neurology, medical), and step-down or progressive care units, among others. In addition to providing direct patient care, nurses are educators, managers, and administrators who teach or supervise others and establish the direction of nursing on a hospital-wide basis.

Various generalist and specialist certification opportunities are appropriate for hospital-based nurses, including medical-surgical nursing, pediatric nursing, pain management nursing, informatics nursing, genetics nursing–advanced, psychiatric–mental health nursing,

nursing executive, nursing executive–advanced, hemostasis nursing, and cardiovascular nursing, among others. *Certification* means that nurses have demonstrated their expertise in a particular area of care and have passed rigorous credentialing testing offered by the American Nurses Credentialing Center (ANCC), one of three entities comprising the ANA Enterprise. No other health care facility offers such variety of opportunities for practice as hospitals offer.

The educational credentials required of RNs practicing in hospitals can range from associate degrees and diplomas to doctoral degrees. In general, entry-level positions require only RN licensure. Many hospitals require nurses to hold bachelor's degrees to advance on the clinical ladder or to assume management positions. A **clinical ladder** is a multiple-step program that begins with entry-level staff nurse positions. As nurses gain experience, participate in continuing education (CE), demonstrate clinical competence, pursue formal education, and become certified, they become eligible to move up the clinical ladder. There is no single model for clinical advancement for nurses across hospitals and other health care agencies. When exploring work settings, nurses as prospective employees should ask about the clinical ladder and opportunities for career advancement.

Most new nurses choose to work in hospitals as staff nurses initially to gain experience in organizing and delivering care to multiple patients. For many, staff nursing is extremely gratifying, and nurses continue in this role across their careers. Others pursue additional education, sometimes provided by the hospital, to work in specialty units such as neonatal intensive care or cardiac care. Although specialty units often require clinical experience and additional training, some hospitals allow new graduates to work in these units.

Some nurses find that management is their strength. **Nurse managers** are in charge of all activities on their units, including patient care, continuous quality improvement (CQI), personnel hiring and evaluation, and resource management, including the unit budget. Being a nurse manager in a hospital today requires business acumen and knowledge of business and financial principles to be most effective in this role. Nurse managers typically assume 24-hour accountability for the units they manage and are often required to have earned a master's degree.

Most nurses in hospitals provide direct patient care, sometimes referred to as bedside nursing. In the past,

becoming administrators or managers was often necessary for nurses to be promoted or receive salary increases, which removed them from bedside care. Today, in hospitals with clinical ladder programs, nurses no longer must make that choice; clinical ladder programs allow nurses to progress professionally while staying in direct patient care roles.

At the top of most clinical ladders are **clinical nurse specialists** (CNS), who are APNs with master's, post-master's, or doctoral degrees in specialized areas of nursing, such as oncology (cancer) or diabetes care. The CNS role varies but generally includes responsibility for serving as a clinical mentor and role model for other nurses, as well as setting standards for nursing care on one or more particular units. The oncology clinical specialist, for example, works with the nurses on the oncology unit to help them stay informed regarding the latest research and skills useful in the care of patients with cancer. The clinical specialist is a resource person for the unit and may provide direct care to patients or families with particularly difficult or complex problems, establish nursing protocols, and ensure that nursing practice on the unit is evidence based. **Evidence-based practice (EBP)** refers to nursing care that is based on the best available research evidence, clinical expertise, and patient preference. More details about EBP are found in Chapter 10.

Salaries and responsibilities increase at the upper levels of the clinical ladder. The clinical ladder concept benefits nurses by allowing them to advance while still working directly with patients. Hospitals also benefit by retaining experienced clinical nurses in direct patient care, thus improving the quality of nursing care throughout the hospital. Research has demonstrated that patient outcomes are more positive for patients cared for by RNs with a bachelor's or higher degree. Linda Aiken, PhD, RN, FAAN, is a leader in nursing who has conducted important research documenting the positive impact of adequate RN staffing on patient outcomes. More than a decade ago, Aiken and colleagues (2003) published a groundbreaking study in which they found that patients on surgical units with more BSN-prepared nurses had fewer complications than patients on units with fewer BSN nurses. Aiken has published widely on nurse staffing and safety since publishing this landmark study. In 2010 Aiken and colleagues reported on a comparison of nurse and patient outcomes among hospitals in California, which has state-mandated nurse-to-patient ratios, and in Pennsylvania and New Jersey, neither of which has state-mandated nurse-to-patient ratios. Furthermore, concern about patient quality and safety is an international issue. In 2012 Aiken and colleagues led a very large team in examining nurse and patient satisfaction, hospital environments, quality of care, and patient safety across 12 European countries and the United States. Again in 2014, Aiken et al. conducted a retrospective observational study of nine European countries analyzing 422,730 patient records. They found the proportion of nurses with a baccalaureate education is associated with significantly fewer deaths after surgery: Every 10% increase in baccalaureate-prepared nurses is associated with a 7% reduction in mortality. See Evidence-Based Practice Box 1.1 for a description of these landmark studies.

Rigid work scheduling was one of the greatest drawbacks to hospital nursing in the past. These schedules usually included evenings, nights, weekends, and holidays. Although hospital units must be staffed around the clock,

EVIDENCE-BASED PRACTICE BOX 1.1

The Evidence: Better Professional Nurse Staffing Improves Quality and Safety of Patient Care

Linda Aiken, PhD, RN, FAAN, Professor of Nursing and Professor of Sociology at the University of Pennsylvania School of Nursing, is the director of the Center for Health Outcomes and Policy Research. She is an authority on causes, consequences, and solutions for nursing shortages both in the United States and worldwide. Dr. Aiken has published extensively. She and her colleagues noted growing evidence suggesting "that nurse staffing affects the quality of care in hospitals, but little is known about whether the educational composition of registered nurses (RNs) in hospitals is related to patient outcomes" (Aiken et al., 2003). They wondered whether the proportion of a hospital's staff of bachelor's or higher degree–prepared RNs contributed to improved patient outcomes. To answer this question, they undertook a large analysis of outcome data for 232,342 general, orthopedic, and vascular surgery patients discharged from 168 Pennsylvania hospitals over a 19-month period. They used statistical methods to control for risk factors such as age, gender, emergency or routine surgeries, type of surgery, preexisting conditions, surgeon qualifications, size of hospital, and other factors. Their findings were very important:

To our knowledge, this study provides the first empirical evidence that hospitals' employment of nurses with BSN and higher degrees is associated with improved patient outcomes. Our findings indicate that surgical patients cared for in hospitals in which higher proportions of direct-care RNs held bachelor's degrees experienced a substantial survival advantage over those treated in hospitals in which fewer staff nurses had BSN [bachelor of science in nursing] or higher degrees. Similarly, surgical patients experiencing serious complications during hospitalization were significantly more likely to survive in hospitals with a higher proportion of nurses with baccalaureate education (p. 1621).

Noting that fewer than half of all hospital staff nurses nationally are prepared at the bachelor's or higher level, and citing a shortage of nurses as a complicating factor, this group of researchers recommended "placing greater emphasis in national nurse workforce planning on policies to alter the educational composition of the future nurse workforce toward a greater proportion with bachelor's or higher education as well as ensuring the adequacy of the overall supply" (p. 1623). They concluded that improved public financing of nursing education and increased employers' efforts to recruit and retain highly prepared bedside nurses could lead to substantial improvements in quality of care.

More recently, California became the first state to enforce state-mandated minimum nurse-to-patient ratios. Much commentary about the pros and cons of these types of mandates has been generated. To determine whether nurse and patient outcomes were different in California than in two states without mandated staffing, Aiken and colleagues (2010) analyzed survey data from 22,336 hospital staff nurses in California, Pennsylvania, and New Jersey, as well as state hospital discharge databases. From this highly complex analysis they determined the following:

When we use the predicted probabilities of dying from our adjusted models to estimate how many fewer deaths would have occurred in New Jersey and Pennsylvania hospitals if the average patient-to-nurse ratios in those hospitals had been equivalent to the average ratio across the California hospitals, we get 13.9% (222/1598) fewer surgical deaths in New Jersey and 10.6% (264/2479) fewer surgical deaths in Pennsylvania (p. 917).

In addition, the nurses in California experienced lower levels of burnout (a condition associated with intense and prolonged stress in work settings) and were less likely to report being dissatisfied with their jobs. These important findings can inform ongoing debates in other states regarding legislation regulating nurse-patient ratio or mandatory reporting of nurse staffing. Aiken and colleagues (2010) concluded, "Improved nurse staffing, however it is achieved, is associated with better outcomes for nurses and patients" (p. 918).

EVIDENCE-BASED PRACTICE BOX 1.1—cont'd

The Evidence: Better Professional Nurse Staffing Improves Quality and Safety of Patient Care

Quality and safety of patient care are of international concern. In 2012 Aiken and a team of researchers from the United States and Europe published findings from a very large, cross-sectional study of 488 general acute care hospitals in 12 European countries and 617 similar hospitals in the United States. Despite deficits in the quality of care present in all countries, Aiken and colleagues found that hospitals providing good work environments and better staffing by professional nurses had nurses and patients who were more satisfied with care. Furthermore, their findings suggested that good work environments and better professional nurse staffing resulted in improving quality and safety of care. The implication of these findings is that improvement of hospital work environments could be an affordable strategy to improve both patient outcomes and retention of professional nurses who provide high-quality care.

In 2014 Aiken et al. published seminal research assessing the impact of nursing patient ratios and educational qualifications in 300 hospitals in nine European countries. They reviewed more than 422,730 patient records of patients who underwent common surgeries and surveyed 26,516 nurses practicing in the study hospitals to gather data on nurse staffing and education. The researchers identified that an increase of 10% of nurses holding a baccalaureate degree in the hospital setting is associated with a 7% reduction in mortality. Also, an increase of a nurse's patient load by one patient increased the likelihood of an inpatient dying within 30 days of admission by 7%. In other words, cutting nurse staff to reduce the nursing budget may adversely affect patient outcomes. Also, increasing the number of baccalaureate-prepared nurses may prevent hospital deaths.

In 2018 New York became the first state to require that new RNs obtain their baccalaureate degree within 10 years of graduation. Much of the evidence presented to back this legislative bill came from the pivotal work done by Aiken and colleagues. The bill is located here: https://www.nysenate.gov/legislation/bills/2017/s6768.

Resources

Aiken LH, Clarke SP, Cheung RB, Sloane D, Silber JH: Educational levels of hospital nurses and surgical patient mortality, Journal of the American Medical Association 290(12):1617–1623, 2003.

Aiken LH, Sermeus W, Van den Heede K, Sloane DM, Busse R, McKee M, Kutney-Lee A: Patient safety, satisfaction, and quality of hospital care: cross sectional survey of nurses and patients in 12 countries in Europe and the United States, British Medical Journal 344:1717, 2012.

Aiken LH, Sloane DM, Bruyneel L, Van den Heede K, Griffiths P, Busse R, Sermeu W: Nurse staffing and education and the hospital mortiality in nine European countries: a retrospective observational study, Lancet 383(9931):1824–1830, 2014.

Aiken LH, Sloane DM, Cimiotti JP, Clarke SP, Flynn L, Seago JA, Spetz J, Smith HK: Implications of the California nurse staffing mandate for other states, Health Services Research 45(4):904–921, 2010.

flexible staffing is more common now, a process by which nurses on a particular unit negotiate with one another and establish their own schedules to meet personal and family responsibilities while ensuring that appropriate staffing for high-quality patient care is provided. Staffing needs may be predictable, such as in the emergency department or surgical units when times of high use can be anticipated. Accordingly, some units may decrease staffing over major holidays because numbers of admissions are known to be low during certain days of the year when elective procedures are not routinely scheduled.

Each hospital nursing role has its own unique characteristics. In the following profile, an RN discusses his role as a nurse in a neonatal intensive care unit (NICU):

Many people are surprised when I tell them that I work in a NICU. They don't seem to expect that a man might enjoy working with the tiniest patients in the hospital.

But I appreciate the technical challenges of providing care for an infant born very prematurely or that has a serious congenital condition. The biggest challenge for me though is working with a full-term baby that had some kind of unexpected trauma at birth. These babies can be very, very sick, and their parents need a lot of support and information. I take care of my little patients the same way I would want someone to take care of my own child. I can only imagine how terrifying it is for the parents for their baby to be so sick. I know that some of the procedures that I have to do are painful, so I make sure that I talk to a baby while I am doing a procedure and try to provide comfort the best I can. Sometimes, when it is possible, I'll wrap a baby in a blanket and rock him or her for a while when things are quiet in the unit. The only thing better than that is the day the parents take the baby home.

When the "fit" between nurses and their role requirements is good, being a nurse is particularly gratifying, as an oncology nurse demonstrates in discussing her role:

Being an oncology nurse and working with people with cancer that may shorten their lives brings you close to patients and their families. The family room for our patients and their families is much like someone's home. Families bring in food and have dinner with their loved one right here. Working with terminally ill patients is a tall order. I look for ways to help families determine what they hope for as their loved one nears the end of life. It varies. Sometimes they hope for a peaceful death, or hope to make amends with an estranged family member or friend or hope to go to a favorite place one more time. The diagnosis of cancer is traumatic, and patients may struggle to cope, especially if their cancer is very advanced or untreatable. I love getting to know my patients and their families and feel that I can be helpful to them as they face death, sometimes by simply being with them. They cry, I cry—it is part of nursing for me, and I would have it no other way.

These are only two of the many possible roles nurses in hospital settings may choose. Although brief, these descriptions convey the flavor of the responsibility, complexity, and fulfillment to be found in hospital-based nursing (Fig. 1.3).

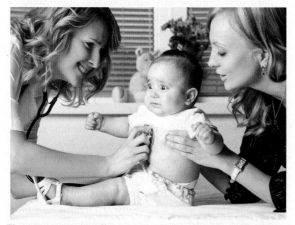

Fig. 1.3 Hospital staff nurses work closely with the families of patients, as well as with the patients themselves. (Photo used with permission from Photos.com.)

Nursing in Communities

Lillian Wald (1867–1940) is credited with initiating community health nursing when she established the Henry Street Settlement in New York City in 1895. Community health nursing today is a broad field, encompassing areas formerly known as public health nursing. Community health nurses work in ambulatory clinics, health departments, hospices, homes, and a variety of other community-based settings.

Community health nurses may work for either the government or private agencies. Those working for public health departments provide care in clinics, schools, retirement communities, and other community settings. They focus on improving the overall health of communities by planning and implementing health programs, as well as delivering care for individuals with chronic health problems. Community health nurses provide educational programs in health maintenance, disease prevention, nutrition, and child care, among others. They conduct immunization clinics and health screenings and work with teachers, parents, physicians, and community leaders toward a healthier community.

Many health departments also have a home health component. Over the past several decades an increasing number of public and private agencies provides home health services, a form of community health nursing. In fact, home health care is a growing segment of the health care industry.

Home health care is a natural fit for nursing. Home health nurses across the United States provide quality care in the most cost-effective and, for patients, most comfortable setting possible. Patients cared for at home may face significant health challenges because of management of chronic illnesses or early hospital discharges in efforts to control costs. As a result, technological devices such as ventilators and intravenous pumps, and significant interventions such as administration of chemotherapy and total parenteral nutrition, are encountered in home health care. Wound care is another domain of home health nursing. Wounds managed in the patient's home can be extensive, and home health nurses providing wound care can assess the patient's home environment for factors that help or hinder healing.

Home health nurses must possess up-to-date nursing knowledge and be secure in their own nursing skills because they do not have the expertise of more experienced nurses quickly available, as they would have in a hospital setting. Strong assessment and communication skills are essential in home health nursing. These nurses must make independent judgments and be able to recognize patients' and families' learning needs. Home health nurses must also recognize the limits of their education and experience and seek help when the patient's needs are beyond the scope of their abilities. An RN working in home health care relates her experience:

> I have always found home care to be very rewarding. I get to know patients in a way I could never have if I had continued to work in a hospital. One of my favorite success stories involved a man with a long history of osteomyelitis—an infection in the bone—resulting from a car wreck 18 years earlier. He had a new central line and was going to get 6 months of intravenous antibiotics. If this treatment didn't work, he was facing an above-the-knee amputation. I taught his wife how to assess the dressing and site, how to change the dressing, and how to infuse the antibiotics twice a day. At my once-a-week visits to draw blood, I counseled the patient about losing weight and quitting smoking because these measures would help in his healing. He lost 80 pounds, quit smoking completely, and at the end of 6 months, he had no signs of infection. He described himself as "a new man." I was so happy for him and his wife. Holistic nursing care in his own home made a huge difference for the rest of his life.

Some nurses are certified as community health or home health nurses by the ANCC. The examinations for these two specialties have now been retired, but nurses certified before this can have their credentials renewed. The ANCC does have an examination for certification as a public health nurse–advanced. The demand for nurses to work in a variety of community settings is expected to continue to increase as care moves from hospitals to homes and other community sites.

Nursing in Medical Offices

Nurses who are employed in medical office settings work in collaboration with physicians, NPs, and their patients. Office-based nursing activities include performing health assessments, reviewing medications, drawing blood, giving immunizations, administering medications, and providing health teaching. Nurses in office settings also act as liaisons between patients and physicians or NPs. They expand on and clarify recommendations for patients, as well as provide emotional support to anxious patients. They may visit hospitalized patients, and some assist in surgery. Often, RNs in office practices supervise other care providers, such as licensed practical/vocational nurses, nurse aides, and, depending on the size of the practice, other employees of the practice such as assistants who schedule patient appointments and manage patient records.

An RN who works for a nephrology practice with three nephrologists describes a typical day:

> I first make rounds independently on patients in the dialysis center, making sure they are tolerating the dialysis procedure and answering questions about their treatments and diets. I then make rounds with one of the physicians in the hospital as she visits patients and prescribes new treatments. The afternoon is spent in the office assessing patients as they come for their physician's visit. I might draw blood for a diagnostic test on one patient and do patient teaching regarding diet with another. No two days are alike, and that is what I love about this position. I have a sense of independence but still have daily patient contact.

RNs considering employment in office settings need good communication skills because many of their responsibilities involve communicating with patients, families, employers, pharmacists, and hospital admissions offices. Nurses should be careful to ask prospective employers the specifics of the position because nursing roles in office practices can range from routine tasks to challenging responsibilities requiring expertise in a particular practice setting, such as that described by the nurse in the nephrology practice. Educational requirements, hours of work, and specific responsibilities vary, depending on the preferences of the employer. Some nurses find a predictable daily schedule with weekends and holidays off to be an advantage in working in an office practice. An important advantage of employment in an office setting is that over time, nurses get to know their patients well, including several members of a family, depending on the type of practice.

Nursing in the Workplace

Many companies today employ occupational and environmental health nurses to provide basic health care services, health education, screenings, and emergency treatment to employees in the workplace. Corporate executives have long known that good employee health reduces absenteeism, insurance costs, and worker errors, thereby improving company profitability. Occupational health nurses (OHNs) represent an important investment by companies in the health and safety of their employees.

They are often asked to serve as consultants on health matters within the company. OHNs may participate in health-related decisions, such as policies affecting health insurance benefits, family leaves, and acquisition and placement of automatic external defibrillators. Depending on the size of the company, the OHN may be the only health professional employed in a company and therefore may have a good deal of autonomy.

Being licensed is generally the minimum requirement for nurses in occupational health roles. The American Association of Occupational Health Nurses (AAOHN) recommends that OHNs have a bachelor's degree. OHNs must possess knowledge and skills that enable them to perform routine physical assessments (e.g., vision and hearing screenings) for all employees. Good interpersonal skills to provide counseling and referrals for lifestyle problems, such as stress or substance abuse, are a bonus for these nurses. At a minimum, they must know first aid and basic life support. If employed in a heavy industrial setting where the risk of burns or trauma is present, OHNs must have special training to manage those types of medical emergencies.

OHNs also have responsibilities for identifying health risks in the entire work environment. They must be able to assess the environment for potential safety hazards and work with management to eliminate or reduce them. They need in-depth knowledge of governmental regulations, such as those of the Occupational Safety and Health Administration (OSHA) and must ensure the company complies. They may instruct new workers in the effective use of protective devices such as safety glasses and noise-canceling earphones. OHNs also understand workers' compensation regulations and coordinate the care of injured workers with the facilities and providers who provide care for an employee with a work-related injury. Some injuries may be life threatening; others may be chronic but clearly related to work, such as musculoskeletal injuries from repetitive motion or poorly designed workspaces.

Nurses in occupational settings have to be confident in their nursing skills, be effective communicators with both employees and managers, be able to motivate employees to adopt healthier habits, and be able to function independently in providing care. The AAOHN is the professional organization for OHNs. The AAOHN provides conferences, webcasts, a newsletter, a journal, and other resources to help OHNs stay up-to-date (website: www.aaohn.org). Certification for OHNs is available through the American Board for Occupational Health Nurses (ABOHN).

Nursing in the Armed Services

Nurses practice in both peacetime and wartime settings in the armed services. Nurses serving in the military ("military nurses") may serve on active duty or in military reserve units, which means that they will be called to duty in the case of an emergency. They serve as staff nurses and supervisors in all major medical specialties. Both general and advanced practice opportunities are available in military nursing, and the settings in which these nurses practice use state-of-the-art technology.

Military nurses often find themselves with broader responsibilities and scope of practice than do civilian nurses because of the demands of nursing in the field, on aircraft, or onboard ship. Previous critical care, surgery, or trauma care experience is desirable but not required. Military nurses are required to have a BSN degree for active duty. They enter active duty as officers and must be between the ages of 21 and 46½ years when they begin active duty. Professional Profile Box 1.1 is a profile of the work of Lt. Joseph Biddix, BSN, RN, a nurse in the Navy who was stationed on a hospital ship.

A major benefit of military nursing is the opportunity for advanced education. Military nurses are encouraged to seek advanced degrees, and support is provided during schooling. The U.S. Department of Defense pays for tuition, books, moving expenses, and even salary for nurses obtaining advanced degrees. This allows the student to focus on his or her studies. Nurses with advanced degrees are eligible for promotion in rank at an accelerated pace.

Travel and change are integral to military nursing, so these nurses must be flexible. Military nurses in the reserves must be committed to readiness; they must be ready to go at a moment's notice. All military nurses may be called on for active wartime duty anywhere in the world.

In 2011 Lieutenant General (Lt. Gen.) Patricia Horoho was nominated and confirmed to become the Army Surgeon General, the first nurse and the first woman to serve in this capacity. Horoho had previously commanded the Walter Reed Health Care System and was serving in the Pentagon on September 11, 2001, where she cared for the wounded after terrorists crashed a plane into the building. Lt. Gen. Horoho is an experienced clinical trauma nurse (*National Journal*, 2011).

PROFESSIONAL PROFILE BOX 1.1 MILITARY NURSE

My nursing path was untraditional. I graduated from college in 2005 with an Arts degree in Media Studies and Production and immediately began an internship with the entertainment industry in Los Angeles. I eventually worked for a top talent management firm, yet after 4 successful years in the business, something was missing. I kept asking myself, "Why doesn't this feel more rewarding?"

I began exploring other options in search of professional gratification, and the idea of military service kept popping into my head. I questioned what the military would do with a film major whose only job experience was working in Hollywood. While deciding options, a close friend told me that he was planning to return to school for a second-degree nursing program. It didn't sound like a bad idea and this would be a perfect career for the military. My internal wheels were spinning, so I called my mom for advice about what I should do, because she was a nurse of 30 years. She said, "I've always thought you would make an excellent nurse, but I never wanted to push it. I figured I would let you find your path on your own."

That was all the encouragement I needed. Once accepted into a nursing program, I contacted the local Navy recruiter. After a rigorous application process, I was accepted into a program to become a Nurse Corps Officer, and on graduation, I was commissioned as an ensign in the United States Navy.

Nearly 3 years later, I have found military nursing to be a phenomenal experience. I have the opportunity to provide nursing care to active duty and retired service members and their families. Additionally, it is my responsibility to train our hospital corpsmen who regularly care for our forward deployed sailors and marines. These young men and women carry a heavy responsibility to provide first responder care to our warfighters. As a Navy nurse, I have a direct role in mentoring them. There is no greater reward than training newly enlisted corpsmen and seeing their faces light up when they "get it." Whether we're discussing the physiology of hypertension or how to treat for shock after a blast injury, you know when the light-bulb turns on and your sailor has added another layer to his or her knowledge base.

Earlier in my career, I was stationed aboard the USNS Comfort (T-AH 20) hospital ship for 6 months in support of Continuing Promise 2015. This mission allowed me to provide humanitarian assistance alongside partner nation and civilian experts to patients in 11 countries in Central and South America and the Caribbean. As a Navy nurse, I spent 10 days in Belize providing nursing care and education to patients and helped provide nursing assistance to our Seabees construction crew while painting buildings in Panama. In between providing care to thousands of patients in other nations, I was a postoperative nurse on a hospital ship. This all is a world away from my old life in Hollywood, but I wouldn't trade anything for my time at sea with my fellow Navy nurses and corpsmen and helping those in need.

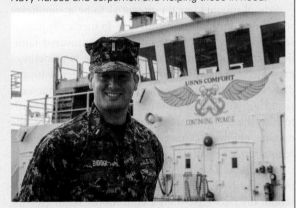

Lt. Joseph Biddix, USN
U.S. Navy Medical Center, Camp Lejeune, NC

Note: The views expressed in this article are those of the author and do not necessarily reflect the official policy or position of the Department of the Navy, the Department of Defense, or the United States government.
Reference: Courtesy Lt. Joseph Biddix.

Nursing in Schools

School nursing is an interesting, specialized practice of professional nursing. In 2017 the National Association of School Nurses (NASN) defined school nursing as "a specialized practice of nursing [that] protects and promotes student health, facilitates optimal development, and advances academic success. School nurses, grounded in ethical and evidence-based practice, are the leaders who bridge health care and education, provide care coordination, advocate for quality student-centered care, and collaborate to design systems that allow individuals and communities to develop their full potential" (NASN, 2017). To that end, school nurses facilitate positive student responses to normal development; promote health and safety, including a healthy environment; intervene with actual and potential health problems; provide case management services; and actively collaborate with others to build student and family capacity for adaptation, self-management, self-advocacy, and learning.

School nurses are in short supply. Very few states achieve the federally recommended ratio of 1:750 (a recommended minimum number of 1 school nurse for every 750 students). In 2016 only 8 states had set a nurse-to-student ratio; however, these ratios were not necessarily consistent with the guidelines set by the Centers for Disease Control and Prevention (CDC) and NASN. For instance, Pennsylvania's ratio was set at 1 nurse per 1500 students, twice the prescribed ratio (Camera, 2016). This poses a serious problem for children with disabilities, for those with chronic illnesses in need of occasional management at school, and for children who become ill or are injured at school. With higher than recommended ratios of students per RN, children may lack the substantial health benefits of having a school nurse available to them during the school day.

School nursing has the potential to be a significant source of communities' health care. In medically underserved areas and with the number of uninsured families increasing, the role of school nurse is sometimes expanded to include members of the student's immediate family. This requires many more school nurses—requiring willingness of state and local school boards to hire them. Without adequate qualified staffing, the nation's children cannot receive the full benefits of school nurse programs.

Most school systems require nurses to have a minimum of a bachelor's degree in nursing, whereas some school districts have higher educational requirements. Prior experience working with children is also usually required. School health has become a specialty in its own right, and in states where school health is a priority, graduate programs in school health nursing have been established. The National Board for Certification of School Nurses (NBCSN) is the official certifying body for school nurses.

School nurses need a working knowledge of human growth and development to detect developmental problems early and refer children to appropriate therapists. Counseling skills are important because many children turn to the school nurse as a counselor. School nurses keep records of children's required immunizations and are responsible for ensuring that immunizations are current. When an outbreak of a childhood communicable illness occurs, school nurses educate parents, teachers, and students about treatment and prevention of transmission. For children with special needs, school nurses must work closely with families, teachers, and the students' primary providers to care for these children while at school—and these needs can be significant. Management of the health of children with diabetes and serious allergies is important in the daily life of school nurses.

School nurses work closely with teachers to incorporate health concepts into the curriculum. They endorse the teaching of basic health practices, such as handwashing and caring for teeth. School nurses encourage the inclusion of age-appropriate nutritional information in school curricula and work with children to make healthful food choices in the cafeteria and when choosing snacks. They conduct vision and hearing screenings and make referrals to physicians or other health care providers when routine screenings identify problems outside the nurses' scopes of practice.

School nurses must be prepared to handle both routine illnesses of children and adolescents and emergencies. One of their major concerns is safety. Accidents are the leading cause of death in children of all ages, yet some accidents are preventable. Prevention includes both protection from obvious hazards and education of teachers, parents, and students about how to avoid accidents. School nurses work with teachers, school bus drivers, cafeteria workers, and other school employees to provide the safest possible environment. When accidents occur, first aid for minor injuries and emergency care for more severe ones are additional skills school nurses use (Fig. 1.4). Detection of evidence of child neglect and abuse is a sensitive but essential aspect of school nursing. School violence or bullying can also result in injury, absenteeism, and anxiety. In the wake of school violence involving guns and the possibility of experiencing a natural disaster, the NASN has made disaster preparedness a priority.

The mission of NASN is "advancing school nurse practice to keep students healthy, safe, and ready to learn" (www.nasn.org). This underscores their commitment to both the health and education of schoolchildren across the United States. The NASN 2013–2014 annual report noted that sensitivity to the cultural needs of students is important in assisting with a child's health and to that end created a section on their website focusing on cultural competence. An important recent initiative by the NASN has been to address the epidemic of childhood obesity, creating a CE program for school nurses to provide them with resources and skills to address the

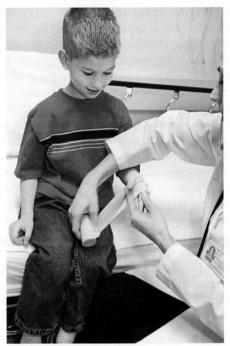

Fig. 1.4 School nurses manage a variety of students' health problems, from playground injuries to chronic illnesses such as asthma and diabetes. (Photo used with permission from iStockphoto.)

problems and challenges of overweight and obese children (NASN Annual Report, 2014).

Nursing in Palliative Care and End-of-Life Settings

Hospice and palliative care nursing is a nursing specialty dedicated to improving the quality of life of patients who are seriously or terminally ill and their families. The World Health Organization (WHO) defines *palliative care* as "an approach that improves the quality of life of patients and their families facing the problem associated with life-threatening illness, through the prevention and relief of suffering by means of early identification and impeccable assessment and treatment of pain and other problems, physical, psychosocial and spiritual" (WHO, 2018). Hospice care is "the model for quality, compassionate care for people facing a life-limiting illness or injury" and involves an interdisciplinary approach to symptom management, including pain management and emotional and spiritual support shaped to the specific needs of the patient and family as the patient approaches the end of his or her life (National Hospice and Palliative Care Organization, 2018).

In the past decade, schools of nursing and other nursing organizations have increased attention to this important realm of care. According to the American Nurses Association (ANA) document *Hospice and Palliative Care Nursing: Scope and Standards of Practice,* "Hospice and palliative care nursing reflects a holistic philosophy of care implemented across the lifespan and across diverse health settings. The goal of hospice and palliative nursing is to promote and improve the patient's quality of life through the relief of suffering along the course of the illness, through the death of the patient, and into the bereavement period of the family" (ANA, 2007, p. 1). Three major concepts are foundational to end-of-life care (ANA, 2007):

1. Persons are living until the moment of death.
2. Coordinated care should be offered by a variety of professionals, with attention to the physical, psychological, social, and spiritual needs of patients and their families.
3. Care should be sensitive to patient and family diversity (or cultural beliefs).

In 1986 the Hospice and Palliative Nurses Association (HPNA) was established, and it is now the largest and oldest professional nursing organization dedicated to the practice of hospice and palliative care. HPNA has a journal, *JHPN—Journal of Hospice and Palliative Nursing,* a peer-reviewed publication that promotes excellence in end-of-life care, which is published six times each year and can be followed on Twitter at @JHPN_online. HPNA's website is https://advancingexpertcare.org/ and can be followed on Twitter at @HPNAinfo. In addition to HPNA, two other organizations are central to supporting this domain of nursing: the Hospice and Palliative Nurses Foundation (HPNF) and the Hospice and Palliative Credentialing Center (HPCC). In 2014 these three organizations adopted shared mission and vision statements, in addition to pillars of excellence held in common. The shared mission is "advancing expert care in serious illness" and the shared vision is "transforming the care and culture of serious illness." The pillars on which these organizations base their work are education, competence, advocacy, leadership, and research (HPNA, 2015).

Because nursing curricula traditionally have not included extensive content to prepare nurses to deal effectively with dying patients and their families, the AACN developed *CARES: Competencies and Recommendations for Educating Undergraduate Nursing Students Preparing*

Nurses to Care for the Seriously Ill and Their Families. This document provides palliative care competencies for the undergraduate nursing student and may be viewed online at http://www.aacnnursing.org/Portals/42/EL-NEC/PDF/New-Palliative-Care-Competencies.pdf.

In 2000 End-of-Life Nursing Education Consortium (ELNEC) was funded by the Robert Wood Johnson Foundation, and it has since received additional funding by a variety of organizations. The foundation for the ELNEC project reflects the core areas identified by the AACN in the *CARES* document. As of 2015, more than 19,500 nurses and other providers had received ELNEC education in "train the trainer" symposia. These new ELNEC trainers then returned to their communities and institutions and have educated more than 600,000 other nurses and providers in end-of-life care. Currently there are seven available curricula: core, pediatric palliative care, critical care, geriatric, advance practice registered nurse, international, and veterans (AACN, 2018). To expand the reach of *CARES* and ELNEC, AACN launched six interactive online modules for undergraduate nursing students. The online ELNEC modules had more than 200 schools and more than 7000 users enrolled in its first year. For more information see http://elnec.academy.reliaslearning.com.

Hospice and palliative care nurses work in a variety of settings, including inpatient palliative/hospice units, free-standing residential hospices, community-based or home hospice programs, ambulatory palliative care programs, teams of consultants in palliative care, and SNFs. Both generalists and APNs work in palliative care.

Information Technologies in Nursing: Telehealth and Informatics

Telehealth is the delivery of health care services and related health care activities through telecommunication technologies. **Telehealth nursing** (also known as *telenursing* or *nursing telepractice*) is not a separate nursing specialty, because few nurses use telehealth systems exclusively in their practices. Rather, it is most often found as a part of other nursing roles. Current technology includes bedside computers, interactive audio and video links, teleconferencing, real-time (synchronous) transmission of patients' diagnostic and clinical data, and more. The fastest growing applications of these technologies are phone triage, remote monitoring, and home care. Some aspects of patient health can be monitored from a distance via remote patient monitoring (RPM) and include physiologic data (e.g., blood pressure, blood glucose, oxygen levels) (healthit.gov, 2017). The use of telehealth devices expands access to health care for underserved populations and individuals in both urban and rural areas. Telehealth can also reduce the sense of professional isolation experienced by those who work in such areas and may assist in attracting and retaining health care professionals in remote areas.

Technologies available for telehealth nurses include remote access to laboratory reports and digitalized imaging; counseling patients on medications, diet, activity, or other therapy on mobile phones or by voice-over-Internet (VOI) protocol services (e.g., Skype; FaceTime); or participating in interactive video sessions, such as an interdisciplinary team consultation about a complex patient issue. Although the fundamentals of basic nursing practice do not change because of the nurse's use of telehealth technologies, their use may require adaptation or modification of usual procedures. In addition, telehealth nurses must develop competence in the use of each new type of telehealth technology, which changes rapidly.

Numerous legal and regulatory issues surround nursing care delivered through telehealth technologies; for instance, care of patients across state lines may require licensing in the state not only where the nurse is employed but also where the patients reside. The Robert J. Waters Center for Telehealth and e-Health Law (www.ctel.org) (2018) is a clearinghouse organization for information about legal and regulatory issues related to telehealth, including nurse licensure, credentialing, Medicare and Medicaid reimbursement, and other issues related to the provision of health care from a distance. You can learn more about telehealth, an area of growing interest in nursing and other health professions, as well as some controversy, from the Association of Telehealth Service Providers (www.atsp.org), from the American Telemedicine Association (www.americantelemed.org), and from the American Academy of Ambulatory Care Nursing (www.aaacn.org).

Nursing informatics (NI) is a rapidly evolving specialty area defined by the Nursing Informatics Nursing Group as "the science and practice [integrating] nursing, its information and knowledge, with management of information and communication technologies to promote the health of people, families, and communities worldwide" (American Medical Informatics Association, 2015). **Informatics nurses** (also known as *nurse informaticians*) were well positioned to assist in the implementation of the 2009 American Recovery and

Reinvestment Act and the Health Information Technology Act. This legislation contained federal incentives for the adoption of electronic health records (EHRs) with criteria known as meaningful use. To qualify for Centers for Medicare and Medicaid Services (CMS) incentive payments, health care organizations had to select, implement, enhance, and/or measure the impact of EHRs on patient care. **Meaningful Use (MU)** was a three-stage initiative implemented in 2011–2016. MU focused on the use of technology to improve patient outcomes through the engagement of patients and families, improved care coordination, and increased privacy and security of patient information. MU is now included as part of the Medicare Access and Chip Reauthorization Act, which focuses on merit-based incentives and the use of EHR technology for multiple purposes, including quality care (HealthIT.gov, 2017).

Because they are nurses themselves, nurse informaticians are best able to understand the needs of nurses who use the systems and can customize or design them with the needs, skills, and time constraints of those nurses in mind. In contrast to computer science systems analysts, nurse informaticians must clearly understand the information they handle and how other nurses will use it. According to the 2017 Healthcare Information and Management Systems Society Nursing Informatics Work Survey, nurses in this field were overall satisfied with their work. Their two main job responsibilities included systems implementation and utilization/optimization, suggesting that their role is imperative in the effective use of electronic medical and health records (EMR/EHR) (2018).

As health care organizations continue to adopt and implement EHRs, nurse informaticians will be in increasing demand.

At a minimum, nurses specializing in informatics should have a BSN and additional knowledge and experience in the field of informatics. An increasing number of nurse informaticians have advanced degrees, including doctorates. Certification as an informatics nurse is available through the ANCC. The American Medical Informatics Association (AMIA; www.amia.org) and the Health Information and Management Systems Society (HIMSS; www.himss.org) sponsor the Alliance for Nursing Informatics (ANI), whose mission is to "advance nursing informatics practice, education, policy and research through a unified voice of nursing informatics organizations" (ANI, 2015). The ANI website is www.allianceni.org.

Thede (2012) published an interesting retrospective on NI, describing the developments that she has seen in this field over the past 30 years, reporting that basic computer skills, informatics knowledge, and information literacy are three "threads" of importance to nursing. She noted that one of the failures of "early dreamers" in informatics was not considering the cultural changes that would be required to move into a multidisciplinary perspective regarding the use of information in health care settings, including "abandonment of the paper chart mentality." With the incentives from CMS driving the widespread adoption of EHR, nurse informaticians will be instrumental in moving the development of these technologies into clinical usefulness with the goal of improving the population's health.

Nursing in a Faith Community

Interest in spirituality and its relation to wellness and healing in recent years prompted the development of the rapidly growing practice specialty of **faith community nursing (FCN)**, previously known as *parish nursing*. "FCN is a nursing practice specialty that focuses on the intentional care of the spirit, promotion of an integrative model of health, and prevention and minimization of illness within the context of a faith community" (ANA, 2017). FCN takes a holistic approach to healing that involves partnerships among congregations, their pastoral staffs, and health care providers. Since its development in the Chicago area in the 1980s by a hospital chaplain, Dr. Granger E. Westberg, FCN has spread rapidly and now includes more than 15,000 nurses in paid and volunteer positions in a variety of religious faiths, cultures, and countries.

The FCN reclaims the historical custom of health and healing found in many faith traditions. The spiritual dimension is central to FCN practice with a focus on the intentional care of the spirit while assisting individuals and faith-based communities to regain wholeness in body, mind, and spirit (Westberg Institute for Faith Community Nursing, 2018). FCNs are instrumental in connecting individuals disconnected from the health care system with preventative services and local health care resources, can clarify provider orders, and identify and recommend needed medical care (Schroepfer, 2016). Research with small FCN projects and partnerships demonstrates the benefits of the combined health and spiritual ministry; however, follow-up research that can more broadly address the impact of the FCN is needed (Schroepfer, 2016).

Since 1997 the ANA (2017) has recognized FCM as a specialty nursing practice within diverse faith communities. The Health Ministries Association Inc. and the ANA in their third edition of *Faith Community Nursing: Scope and Standards of Practice* collaboratively define six standards of practice for FCN and 11 standards of professional performance (ANA, 2017). Faith community nurses serve as members of the pastoral team in a faith community. The practice of FCN is governed by the nurse's state nurse practice act, *Nursing: Scopes and Standards of Practice* (ANA, 2015a), *Faith Community Nursing: Scope and Standards* (ANA, 2017), and the *Code of Ethics for Nurses with Interpretive Statements* (ANA, 2015b). FCNs work as health educators and counselors, advocates for health services, referral agents, and coordinators of volunteer health ministers. Faith community nurses often sponsor health screenings and facilitate support groups while integrating the concepts of health and spirituality.

Many FCNs work independently and benefit from networking with other FCNs. Throughout the United States, many local and regional FCN organizations support FCN networking and collaboration, providing grant opportunities and even specialized training in the ministry of FCN practice. Nurses interested in FCN may pursue specialized training with a local or regional FCN organization. According to the Westberg Institute for Faith Community Nursing (2018), an FCN should (1) maintain an active nursing license in the state of practice; (2) have a baccalaureate degree in nursing with experience in community nursing; (3) have completed an educational course to prepare for FCN practice; (4) have specialized knowledge of the spiritual beliefs and practices of the faith community; (5) reflect personal spiritual maturity in his or her practice; and (6) be organized, flexible, a self-starter, and an excellent communicator.

Nurses in Business: Entrepreneurs

Some nurses are highly creative and are challenged by the risks of starting a new enterprise. Such nurses may make good nurse entrepreneurs.

Similar to an entrepreneur in any field, a **nurse entrepreneur** identifies a need and creates a service to meet the identified need. Nurse entrepreneurs enjoy the **autonomy** derived from owning and operating their own health-related businesses. Groups of nurses, some of whom are faculty members in schools of nursing, have opened nurse-managed centers to provide direct care to clients. Nurse entrepreneurs are self-employed as consultants to hospitals, nursing homes, and schools of nursing. Others have started nurse-based practices and carry their own caseloads of patients with physical or emotional needs. They are sometimes involved in presenting educational workshops and seminars. Some nurses establish their own apparel businesses, manufacturing clothing for premature babies or for persons with physical challenges. Others own and operate their own health equipment companies, health insurance agencies, and home health agencies. Still others invent products such as stethoscope covers that can be changed between patients to prevent the spread of infection. Here are a few comments from one such entrepreneur, the chief executive officer of a privately owned home health agency:

I enjoy working for myself. I know that my success or failure in my business is up to me. Having your own home health agency is a lot of work. You have to be very organized, manage other people effectively, and have excellent communication skills. You cannot be afraid to say no to the people. There is nothing better than the feeling I get when a family calls to say our nurses have made a difference in their loved one's life, but I also have to take the calls of complaint about my agency. Those are tough.

Increasingly, nurses are entering the business of health care, finding increasing opportunities to create their own companies. One such company offers nursing care for mothers, babies, and children. This company's emphasis is the care of women whose pregnancies may be complicated by diabetes, hypertension, or multiple births. The RN who founded this company described the services offered by her company:

Our main specialty is managing high-risk pregnancies and high-risk newborns. Home care for these individuals is a boon not only to the patients themselves but also to hospitals, insurance companies, and doctors. Now with shorter hospital stays, risks are minimized if skilled maternity nurses are on hand to provide patients with specialty care in their homes.

As with almost any endeavor, disadvantages come with owning a business, such as the risk of losing your financial investment if the business is unsuccessful. Fluctuations in income are common, especially in the early months, and regular paychecks may be somewhat rare, at least in the beginning. A certain amount of pressure is created because of the total responsibility for meeting deadlines and paying bills, salaries, and taxes, but there is great opportunity as well.

In addition to financial incentives, there are also intangible rewards in entrepreneurship. For some people, the autonomy and freedom to control their own practice are more than enough to compensate for the increased pressure and initial uncertainty.

With rapid changes occurring daily in the health care system, new and exciting possibilities abound. Alert nurses who possess creativity, initiative, and business savvy have tremendous opportunities as entrepreneurs. The website www.nursingentrepreneurs.com provides a long list of categories of businesses operated by nurse entrepreneurs, the variety of which is extensive (e.g., movie set nurses, holistic life change strategists, medical bill auditing, nurse poet, nursing business startup coaching). In Professional Profile Box 1.2, you can read a description of the career of Kay Wagoner, PhD, RN,

---

PROFESSIONAL PROFILE BOX 1.2   NURSE ENTREPRENEUR

It is my belief that everyone should go to nursing school, because it prepares one for diverse professional opportunities and life in general. My life has taken several tumbles and turns, careening forward, backward, up, and down. At each point along the way, there were reasons to be forever grateful to nursing. Nursing taught me to look in more detail at incongruences, to seek the essence of each dilemma, while keeping a holistic perspective. I have been a consistent collector of data, be it from direct patient experience, from educational endeavors, or from scientific experimentation. Although the data always molded my thinking, final decisions were based on a desire to do something that made a difference in health and health care.

I cherished my time in intensive care nursing, one of my first careers, because it was there that I began to appreciate the need to better understand organ systems and cellular interactions to intervene with the critically ill on a moment-to-moment basis. My desire to learn more about how one responds to a variety of health challenges and life crises propelled me to advance my nursing education at the master's level.

With my newly minted master's degree and a specialty in cardiovascular nursing, I was challenged to teach undergraduate nursing students that which I strove hardest to understand: how organ systems and the cells that comprised them functioned and malfunctioned. While learning through teaching, my nursing practice shifted to cardiovascular disease prevention and rehabilitation. I founded my first company, which provided a new treatment paradigm for individuals attempting to stave off or repair from cardiovascular disease. This combination of teaching and practice provided great growth opportunities for me, including the confidence to delve deeper into the science of health and disease.

I went back to the classroom and completed doctoral and postdoctoral studies in physiology and pharmacology. I gained a more complete understanding of how cells, organ systems, and the human body works and fails. I also came to realize that many of the available treatments were too little too late and many of the available medications woefully inadequate in terms of efficacy and safety.

Thus for the next 20 years, I explored the discovery and development of new treatments and medications by founding the science-based drug discovery company Icagen, Inc., which was sold to Pfizer, Inc., in 2011. As the CEO and president of Icagen, I used my nursing background to provide focus on truly unmet medical needs such as new treatments for sickle cell disease, arrhythmias, epilepsy, and pain. We sought to make data-driven decisions by asking and answering the question, "What are the most efficacious and safe mechanisms to target for new treatments to improve patient outcomes?"

Today I am working with nurse educators and entrepreneurs and can be often heard asking, "How can we innovate to make a difference?" Our great nursing profession can lead us down many different career paths, some clearly more direct than mine. Along the way we can let nursing help drive evidence-based decision making to make a positive difference in health and health care.

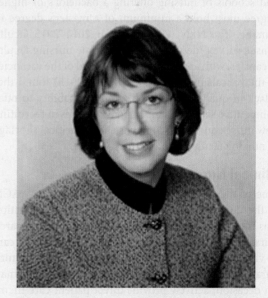

Kay Wagoner, PhD, RN
(Cardiovascular Nurse Specialist)

Reference: Courtesy Kay Wagoner.

whose career in nursing gave her expertise in cardiovascular nursing; using her knowledge from nursing, she founded her own drug development company.

NURSING OPPORTUNITIES REQUIRING ADVANCED DEGREES

Many RNs choose to pursue careers that require a master's degree, doctoral degree, or specialized education in a specific area. These roles include clinical nurse leaders, nurse managers, nurse executives in hospital settings, nurse educators (whether in clinical or academic settings), nurse anesthetists, nurse-midwives, clinical nurse specialists, and advanced practice nursing in a variety of settings. Some of these careers are described next.

Nurse Educators

In 2008, 98,268 RNs reported working in academic education programs (U.S. Department of Health and Human Services, 2010). Since 2005, more than 5300 nurse educators have achieved specialty certification as certified nurse educators through the National League of Nursing (Simmons, 2017). Nurse educators teach in licensed practical nurse/licensed vocational nurse programs, diploma programs, associate degree programs, bachelor's and higher degree programs, and programs preparing nursing assistants. Nurse educators in accredited schools of nursing offering a bachelor's or higher degree must hold a minimum of a master's degree in nursing. The NLN (2015) in their 2014–2015 faculty census survey identified 1072 full-time nursing faculty vacancies, with approximately one-third of the vacancies at the baccalaureate level. The NLN (2015) found that a lack of qualified candidates and an inability to offer competitive salaries as the main difficulties in recruiting new nurse educators. Concerns about a critical shortage of nursing faculty in the future continue.

Clinical Nurse Leaders

One of the newer credentials approved by the AACN is the **clinical nurse leader** (CNL). This designation was intended as a means of allowing master's-prepared nurses to oversee and manage care at the point of care in various settings. CNLs are not intended to be administrators or managers but are clinical experts who may, on occasion, actively provide direct patient care themselves. The CNL is a generalist providing and managing care at the point of care to patients, individuals, families,

and communities and is prepared to facilitate a culture of safety for specific groups of patients with the goal of improving patient outcomes (Rankin, 2015).

The role of CNL was not without controversy and objections from CNSs, who are APNs and who saw the proposed role as duplicating and potentially disenfranchising CNSs. Currently, 117 schools affiliated with AACN offer CNL programs. More information can be found on the AACN's website: http://www.aacnnursing.org/CNL/About.

Advanced Practice Nursing

Advanced practice nursing is a general term applied to an RN who has met advanced educational and clinical practice requirements beyond the 2 to 4 years of basic nursing education required of all RNs. Advanced practice nursing has grown since it evolved more than 40 years ago. The 2017 workforce data reports that more than 250,000 nurses are practicing in advanced practice roles, and the projected demand for these roles will increase by over 30% in the next 10 years (Bureau of Labor Statistics, 2018; National Association of Clinical Nurse Specialists, 2018). Increased demand for primary care coupled with increased specialization of physicians and heightened demand for efficient and cost-effective treatment mean that advanced practice poses excellent career opportunities for nurses. The implementation of the Affordable Care Act stimulated even greater interest and growth in the numbers of APNs. Patient acceptance of APNs is high, and the evidence consistently demonstrates that APNs provide high-quality, cost-effective care that can reduce the burden of the growing shortage of primary care providers (Swan et al., 2015). There are four categories of APNs: nurse practitioner, clinical nurse specialist, certified nurse-midwife, and certified registered nurse anesthetist.

Nurse Practitioner

Opportunities for nurses in expanded roles in health care have created a demand in **nurse practitioner** (NP) education. These programs grant master's degrees or post-master's certificates and prepare nurses to sit for national certification examinations as NPs. The length of the programs varies, depending on the student's prior education. Programs of study leading to the doctor of nursing practice (DNP) degree have been implemented in schools of nursing across the country in response to the AACN member institution's endorsement of a clinical doctorate for advanced practice. The DNP is consistent with other health professions that offer practice doctorates, including medicine (MD), dentistry (DDS), pharmacy (PharmD), physical therapy (DPT), and psychology (PsyD), among others. There are currently 303 DNP programs actively enrolling students across all 50 states, and another 124 programs in the planning stages, which demonstrates the rapid growth of this degree path (AACN, 2017).

States vary in the level of practice autonomy accorded to NPs. NPs beginning practice in a new state should check the status of the advanced practice laws in that state before making firm commitments, because some states still place limitations on NP independence. These barriers to practice include the variation of scope of practice across states (with implications for practice opportunities); lack of physician understanding of NP scope of practice (limits successful collaboration); and payer policies that are linked to state practice regulations (Hain and Fleck, 2014).

NPs work in clinics, nursing homes, their own offices, or physicians' offices. Others work for hospitals, health maintenance organizations, or private industry. Most NPs choose a specialty area such as adult–gerontology, psychiatric–mental health, family, or pediatric care. They are qualified to handle a wide range of health problems in primary or acute care settings. These nurses can perform physical examinations, take medical histories, diagnose and treat common acute and chronic illnesses and injuries, order and interpret laboratory tests and x-ray films, and counsel and educate patients. Despite the restrictions on practice in some states, in other states, NPs are independent practitioners with full prescriptive authority and can be directly reimbursed by Medicare, Medicaid, and military and private insurers for their work.

In Professional Profile Box 1.3, Sebastian White, MSN, FNP, BC-ADM, RN, describes his work as an NP providing diabetes care in partnership with a physician in Bozeman, Montana.

Clinical Nurse Specialist

Clinical nurse specialists (CNSs) are APNs who work in a variety of settings, including hospitals, clinics, nursing homes, their own offices, industry, home care, and health maintenance organizations. These nurses hold master's or doctoral degrees and are qualified to handle a wide range of physical and mental health problems. They are experts in a particular field of clinical practice, such as mental health, gerontology, cardiac care, cancer

care, community health, or neonatal health, and they perform health assessments, make diagnoses, deliver treatment, and develop quality control methods. In addition, CNSs work in consultation, research, education, and administration. Direct reimbursement to some CNSs is possible through Medicare, Medicaid, and military and private insurers.

Certified Nurse-Midwife

Certified nurse-midwives (CNMs) provide well-woman care and attend or assist in childbirth in various settings, including hospitals, birthing centers, private practice, and home birthing services. By 2010 all CNM training programs were required to award a master's of science in nursing (MSN) degree. CNM programs require an average of 1.5 years of specialized education beyond basic nursing education and must be accredited by the Accreditation Commission for Midwifery Education (ACME).

CNMs are licensed, independent health care providers who can prescribe medications in all 50 states, the District of Columbia, and most U.S. territories. Federal law designates CNMs as primary care providers. More than half of CNMs identify reproductive care as their main responsibility rather than attending births. According to the National Center for Health Statistics, CNMs attended 332,107 births in 2014, representing more than 8% of the total births in the United States in 2014 (American College of Nurse-Midwives, 2016). Historically, births attended by CNMs have had half the national average rates for cesarean sections and higher rates of successful vaginal births after a previous cesarean, both considered measures of high-quality obstetric care. Karen Sheffield, MSN, CNM, describes her work as a certified nurse-midwife in Professional Profile Box 1.4.

Certified Registered Nurse Anesthetist

In 2015 there were approximately 48,000 certified registered nurse anesthetists (CRNAs) and CRNA students in the United States (American Association of Nurse Anesthetists [AANA], 2015). Nurse anesthetists administer approximately 43 million anesthetics each year and are the only anesthesia providers in nearly one-third of U.S. hospitals (AANA, 2016). Collaborating with physician anesthesiologists or working independently, they are found in a variety of settings, including operating suites; obstetric delivery rooms; the offices of dentists,

PROFESSIONAL PROFILE BOX 1.3　DIABETES NURSE PRACTITIONER

I am a nurse practitioner who specializes in the care of persons with diabetes. I am also a father, a husband, and an endurance athlete. My path to nursing started as a young boy being raised by my mother, Angela Willett-Calnan, RN, and later, my maternal grandparents. My mother's mother is also a nurse, Mary Grace Willett, RN. Several other family members are health care professionals.

As an undergraduate student, I graduated with a bachelor of science degree in biology and a minor in psychology while leading my college's soccer team as captain for 2 years. After college I moved to Bozeman, Montana, falling in love with the high peaks of the Rocky Mountains. My original intent was to spend a summer in Montana and then attend physical therapy school. That summer ended much too quickly! After 2 years of trying my best to be a ski bum, I realized that I didn't have much bum in me, so I attended an emergency medical technician training course and became a member of the Big Sky Professional Ski Patrol. There I was back in my element: helping people.

My search for the next step began. I volunteered at our local community health center, asking many questions of the providers there. I knew I wanted a role in primary care, so medical or nursing school would be my next step. The final decision was inspired by my uncle, Dr. Michael Willett, who said to me, "Sebastian, I have worked with and trained many nurse practitioners and physicians. You are meant to be a nurse." At that point, I really had no idea what he meant—I was just relieved to have a plan.

Energized, I enrolled in a nursing school offering an accelerated bachelor of science in nursing for students who already had a college degree. In my first nursing position, I became interested in diabetes. After completing my master of science in nursing degree, I was recruited back to Montana by a large multispecialty clinic—the Billings Clinic—where I was welcomed into their department of endocrinology. I was integral in the establishment of a comprehensive inpatient diabetes management program. Soon I was recruited by the hospital in Bozeman to start a diabetes center with an internist who is now my partner in practice. Back to the mountains I love! I am now the only National Committee for Quality Assurance diabetes nurse practitioner in the Pacific Northwest.

Nursing is the greatest gift we can offer patients. Our health care system in the United States is broken—costs spiraling and measures of health worsening every year. As a nurse, I am trained to focus on the missing element in our health care system: the patient. I am trained to treat my patients, not their disease; I am trained to listen to their concerns and focus my interventions on helping them improve their lives. I am a nurse.

To my wife, my mother, my grandmother, my uncle, and the high mountains of Montana: All the credit belongs to you. Thank you.

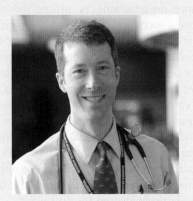

Sebastian White, MSN, FNP, BC-ADM, RN

Reference: Courtesy Sebastian White.

podiatrists, ophthalmologists, and plastic surgeons; ambulatory surgical facilities; and military and governmental health services (AANA, 2015).

To become a CRNA, nurses must complete 2 to 3 years of specialized education in a master's program beyond the required bachelor's degree; 32 nurse anesthesia programs are approved to award doctoral degrees for entry into CRNA practice, which is likely to be the requirement in the near future (AANA, 2015). In 2014 there were 114 accredited nurse anesthesia programs in the United States, ranging from 24 to 36 months in length. Nurse anesthetists must also meet national certification and recertification requirements. The safety of care delivered by CRNAs is well established. Anesthesia care today is safer than in the past, and numerous outcome studies have demonstrated that there is "no difference in the quality of care provided by CRNAs and their physician counterparts" (AANA, 2015).

PROFESSIONAL PROFILE BOX 1.4 CERTIFIED NURSE-MIDWIFE

Being a nurse-midwife is at the core of who I am, not just what I do. I decided to become a nurse-midwife after working as a chemist for many years and recognizing that my true passion resided in all aspects of women's health care. After the birth of two of my children, one by a physician and one by a nurse-midwife, I realized that I was "called" to the profession of nurse-midwifery and the philosophy of care that nurse-midwives provide. Delivering comprehensive, holistic wellness care to women throughout their life span is one of the most rewarding and inspirational aspects of my profession. I feel privileged and honored to share in the important and often life-changing decisions that women make during the many transitions that occur during the years between puberty and menopause and beyond.

I have a bachelor of arts in physics and received a master's degree in nursing from Yale University in 2005 with a specialty in nurse-midwifery. Additionally, I am certified in nurse-midwifery by the American Midwifery Certification Board (AMCB). Certification by the AMCB is considered the gold standard in midwifery and is recognized in all 50 states. As a nurse-midwife, I must also complete the requirements of the Certification Maintenance Program through AMCB by completing continuing education units every 5-year certification cycle. Maintaining competence in evidence-based, up-to-date management and treatment for women's health is critical to being an effective clinician.

Although the professional work environment for nurse-midwives varies, a typical day as a nurse-midwife with a full scope of practice involves providing gynecologic, antepartum, intrapartum, and postpartum care, which includes hospital rounds on patients who have given birth, as well as seeing patients in the office. Evidence-based care in the office setting includes contraceptive management, family planning, primary care, gynecologic care, and sick visits, among others. In addition to gynecologic care, nurse-midwives provide obstetric care that is grounded in our belief that childbirth is a normal, healthy human event. However, we are educated in how and when to collaborate with physician colleagues for emergent care that necessitates a physician's specific expertise.

I strongly believe that my role as a nurse-midwife is to be "with a woman" and to honor her journey toward health and wellness, as well as respecting her wishes for her birth within the limits of safety. When I reflect on my journey as a nurse-midwife for the past decade, I know that I am truly carrying out my purpose in providing holistic women's health care to the highest standard of excellence.

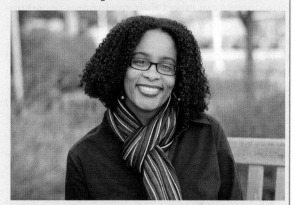

Karen Sheffield, MSN, CNM
Yale University, 2005

Reference: Courtesy Karen Sheffield, MSN, CNM.

Issues in Advanced Practice Nursing

Each year in January, *The Nurse Practitioner: The American Journal of Primary Health Care* publishes an update on legislation affecting advanced practice nursing. Over the years, advances have been made toward removing the barriers to autonomous practice for APNs in many, but not all, states.

In the past, substantial barriers to APN autonomy existed because of the overlap between traditional medical and nursing functions. A decade ago, the picture was considerably less optimistic than it is now. The issue of APNs practicing autonomously was a politically charged arena, with organized medicine positioned firmly against all efforts of nurses to be recognized as independent health care providers receiving direct reimbursement for their services. Organized nursing, however, persevered. Nurses, through their professional associations, continued their efforts to change laws that limit the scope of nursing practice. Their efforts were aided by the fact that numerous published studies validated the safety, cost efficiency, and high patient acceptance of advanced practice nursing care.

Both the public and legislators at state and national levels have begun to appreciate the role that APNs have played in increasing the efficiency and availability of primary health care delivery while reducing costs; however, opposition to APN autonomy persists. Roadblocks to full practice autonomy continue, primarily because of the resistance of organized physician groups despite data indicating positive patient outcomes. Although progress has been made, there remains the need for APNs to continue to work with their professional organizations to promote legislation mandating full autonomy.

EMPLOYMENT OUTLOOK IN NURSING

The Bureau of Labor Statistics, a division of the U.S. Department of Labor, is confident about nursing's overall employment prospects in the near and distant future. According to the bureau (U.S. Department of Labor, 2016), nurses can expect their employment opportunities to grow "15% from 2016 to 2026, much faster than average for all occupations." The bureau estimates that, during this time, 438,100 new RN jobs will be created to meet growing patient needs and to replace retiring nurses (U.S. Department of Labor, 2016). Several factors are fueling this growth, including technological advances and the increasing emphasis on primary care. The aging of the nation's population also has a significant impact, because older people are more likely to require medical care. As aging nurses retire, many additional job openings will result.

Opportunities in hospitals, traditionally the largest employers of nurses, will grow more slowly than those in community-based sectors. The most rapid hospital-based growth is projected to occur in outpatient facilities, such as same-day surgery centers, rehabilitation programs, and outpatient cancer centers. Home health positions are expected to increase the fastest of all. This is in response to the expanding elderly population's needs and the preference for and cost effectiveness of home care. Furthermore, technological advances are making it possible to bring increasingly complex treatments into the home.

Another expected area of high growth is in assisted living and nursing home care; this is primarily in response to the larger number of frail elderly in their 80s and 90s requiring long-term care. As hospitals come under greater pressure to decrease the average patient length of stay, nursing home admissions will increase, as will growth in long-term rehabilitation units (U.S. Department of Labor, 2016).

An additional factor influencing employment patterns for RNs is the tendency for sophisticated medical procedures to be performed in physicians' offices, clinics, ambulatory surgical centers, and other outpatient settings. RNs' expertise will be needed to care for patients undergoing procedures formerly performed only in hospital settings. APNs can also expect to be in higher demand for the foreseeable future. The evolution of integrated health care networks focusing on primary care and health maintenance and pressure for cost-effective care are ideal conditions for advanced practice nursing.

Salaries in the nursing profession vary widely according to practice setting, level of preparation, credentials, experience, and region of the country. According to the U.S. Board of Labor Statistics, in 2016, median annual salary for nurses was $68,450 (as a comparison, the median salary for all workers was $37,040). The lowest paid 10% earned less than $47,120, and the highest paid 10% earned more than $102,990. Salaries were the highest with government and hospital employers and lowest in educational services. About 21% of RNs are members of unions or are covered by union contracts. Interestingly, California has the highest nursing salaries in the United States and has a vigorous union in the California Nurses Association/National Nurses United. Salaries in nursing vary by region, as do salaries in other professions and occupations.

APNs have higher salaries than do staff nurses; CRNAs average the highest salary of any advanced practice specialty group. Clearly, in nursing as in most other professions, additional preparation and responsibility increase earning potential.

Most of the wage growth for nurses occurs early in their careers and tapers off as nurses near the top of the salary scale. This leads to a flattening of salaries for more experienced nurses in a phenomenon known as *wage compression*. Wage compression may account for nurses leaving patient care for additional education or other careers in nursing or outside the profession, an issue that must be addressed to improve retention of the most experienced nurses in the profession.

CONCEPTS AND CHALLENGES

- *Concept:* Nursing is the largest workforce in health care in the United States.

  Challenge: The influence of nursing is not as powerful as it could be because the large majority of nurses do not belong to professional organizations such as the ANA, a federation of state nurses associations that is the voice of nursing.

- *Concept:* More than half of working nurses are employed in hospitals, a traditional setting for nursing practice.

  Challenge: As health care becomes increasingly based in the community, more nurses will be working outside of the hospital. Nursing must consider the impact of this migration from hospital to community.

- *Concept:* The Affordable Care Act and other changes in health care will create more opportunities for practice

for nurses. Increased use of APNs as providers of primary care may be part of the solution to the American health care crisis as the "baby boom" generation ages, the numbers of elderly increase, and the need for health care cost containment becomes critical.

Challenge: APNs are capable of delivering high-quality care to many segments of the population who do not have adequate care; however, educating adequate numbers of advanced practice nurses is essential to meet the demands on the health care system.

- *Concept:* Nursing will continue to be a profession in high demand in the foreseeable future.

  Challenge: Nursing faculty shortages at all levels of nursing education pose an ongoing challenge to educate enough professional nurses to meet the health needs of the population.

IDEAS FOR FURTHER EXPLORATION

1. Think of the areas of nursing that interest you most. How do your personal interests and nursing education compare with the characteristics needed in the roles presented in this chapter?

2. As you continue your nursing education, ask questions of nurses in various practice settings to learn how they prepared for their positions, what their work life is like, and what they find most challenging and rewarding about their work.

3. Call the nurse recruiter or personnel office of a nearby hospital to inquire about education, experience,

and salaries and other benefits for entry-level and advanced practice nursing. Is there a clinical ladder program? How does it work?

4. Ask an advanced practice RN in your community about his or her practice. What are the advantages and major barriers to practice that this advanced practice RN encounters?

5. Contact your state nurses association to find out what legislative initiatives are being undertaken to remove barriers to full advanced practice nursing in your state.

REFERENCES

Aiken LH, Clarke SP, Cheung RB, et al.: Educational levels of hospital nurses and surgical patient mortality, *JAMA* 290(12):1617–1623, 2003.

Aiken LH, Sermeus W, Van den Heede K, et al.: Patient safety, satisfaction, and quality of hospital care: cross sectional survey of nurses and patients in 12 countries in Europe and the United States, *BMJ* 344:1717, 2012.

Aiken LH, Sloane DM, Bruyneel L, et al.: Nurse staffing and education and the hospital mortality in nine European countries: a retrospective observational study, *Lancet* 383(9931):1824–1830, 2014.

Aiken LH, Sloane DM, Cimiotti JP, et al.: Implications of the California nurse staffing mandate for other states, *Health Serv Res* 45(4):904–921, 2010.

Alliance for Nursing Informatics (ANI) (website): *Our mission,* 2015. Available at: www.allianceni.org.

American Association of Colleges of Nursing (AACN): *Nursing fact sheet,* 2011. Available at: www.aacn.nche.edu/media-relations/fact-sheets/nursing-fact-sheet.

American Association of Colleges of Nursing (AACN): *DNP fact sheet,* 2017. Retrieved from: http://www.aacnnursing.org/DNP/Fact-Sheet.

American Association of Colleges of Nursing (AACN): *Creating a more qualified nursing workforce* (website), 2014. Available at: www.aacn.nche.edu/media-relations/diversityFS.pdf.

American Association of Colleges of Nursing (AACN): *Fact sheet: Enhancing diversity in the nursing workforce* (website), 2014. Available at: www.aacn.nche.edu/media-relations/fact-sheets/nursing-workforce.

NWTC Library
2740 W. Mason St.
Green Bay, WI 54307

American Association of Colleges of Nursing (AACN): *New AACN data confirm enrollment surge in schools of nursing* (website), 2015. Available at: www.aacn.nche.edu/news/articles/2015/enrollment.

American Association of Colleges of Nursing (AACN): *End-of-life nursing education consortium* (website), 2018. Available at: http://www.aacnnursing.org/ELNEC/About/ELNEC-Curricula.

American Nurses Association: *Nursing: scope and standards of practice*, Silver Spring, MD, 2015a, American Nurses Association.

American Nurses Association: *Code of ethics for nurses with interpretive statements*, Silver Spring, MD, 2015b, American Nurses Association.

American Nurses Association: *Faith community nursing, scope and standards of practice*, 3rd ed, Silver Spring, D, 2017, Nursing Knowledge Center.

American Association of Nurse Anesthetists (AANA). *Certified registered nurse anesthetists at a glance* (website). Available at: www.aana.com.

American Association of Nurse Anesthetists (AANA): *Certified registered nurse anesthesists fact sheet* (website), 2016. Available at: https://www.aana.com/patients/certified-registered-nurse-anesthetists-fact-sheet.

American College of Nurse Midwives: *Fact sheet CNM/CM attended birth statistics in the United States* (website), 2016, March. Retrieved from: http://www.midwife.org/acnm/files/ccLibraryFiles/Filename/000000005950/CNM-CM-AttendedBirths-2014-031416FINAL.pdf.

American Association of Colleges of Nursing: *DNP fact sheet*, 2017, June. Retrieved from: http://www.aacnnursing.org/DNP/Fact-Sheet.

American College of Nurse Midwives: *Fact sheet CNM/CM attended birth statistics in the United States* (website), 2016, March. Available at: http://www.midwife.org/acnm/files/ccLibraryFiles/Filename/000000005950/CNM-CM-AttendedBirths-2014-031416FINAL.pdf.

American Medical Informatics Association: 2015 (website). Available at: www.amia.org/programs/working-groups/nursing-informatics.

American Nurses Association (ANA): *Position statement on pain management and control of distressing symptoms in dying patients*, Washington, DC, 2003, The Association.

American Nurses Association (ANA): *Hospice and palliative care nursing: scope and standards of practice*, Silver Spring, MD, 2007, The Association.

American Nurses Association (ANA): *News release: ANA and Health Ministries Association to co-publish faith community nursing: scope and standards of practice*, ed 2 (website), 2012. Available at: http://nursingworld.org/FunctionalMenuCategories/MediaResources/PressReleases/2012-PR/ANA-and-Health-Ministries-Association-Co-Publish-Faith-Community-Nursing-Scope-Standards.pdf.

American Nurses Association (ANA): *News release: ANA and Health Ministries Association to co-publish faith community nursing: scope and standards of practice*, ed 2 (website), 2012. Available at: http://nursingworld.org.

American Telemedicine Association: *Telehealth nursing fact sheet* (website), 2015. Retrieved from: www.americantelemed.org/docs/default-document-library/fact_sheet_final.pdf?sfvrsn=2.

American Telemedicine Association, Congress keeps pushing out proposals to promote telemedicine, 2015 (website). Retrieved from: www.americantelemed.org/news-landing/2015/05/27/congress-keeps-pushing-out-proposals-to-promote-telemedicine#.

Bauer JC: Nurse practitioners as an underutilized resource for health reform: evidence-based demonstrations of cost-effectiveness, *JAANP* 22(4):228–231, 2010.

Budden JW, Zhong EH, Moulton P, Cimiotti JP: Highlights of the national workforce survey of registered nurses, *J Nurs Regulation* 4(2):5–14, 2013.

Bureau of Labor Statistics: *U.S. Department of labor, occupational outlook handbook, nurse anesthetists, nurse midwives, and nurse practitioners*, 2018, June 13. Retrieved from: https://www.bls.gov/ooh/healthcare/nurse-anesthetists-nurse-midwives-and-nurse-practitioners.htm.

Camera L: *Many school districts don't have enough school nurses*, 2016. Available at: https://www.usnews.com/news/articles/2016-03-23/the-school-nurse-scourge.

Hain D, Fleck L: Barriers to nurse practitioner practice that impact healthcare redesign, *OJIN Online J Issues Nurs* 19(2):5–31, 2014.

HealthIT.gov: *Meaningful use and the shift to merit-based incentive payment system* (website), 2017. Available at: https://www.healthit.gov/topic/federal-incentive-programs/meaningful-use.

Healthcare Information and Management Systems Society Nursing Informatics: *2017 Nursing informatics work survey*, 2018. Retrieved from: www.himss.org/sites/himssorg/files/2017-nursing-informatics-workforce-executive-summary.pdf HealthIT.gov.

Health Resources and Services Administration: *National center for health workforce analysis: The U.S. nursing workforce: trends in supply and education*, 2013. Washington, DC. Retrieved from: http://bhpr.hrsa.gov/healthworkforce.

Hospice and Palliative Nurses Association (HPNA): *Shared Mission, Vision & Pillars*, 2015 (website). Available at: www.advancingexpertcare.org.

Institute of Medicine: *The future of nursing: leading change*, Washington, DC, 2010, Advancing Health, National Academy of Sciences.

Murphy J: The nursing informatics workforce: who are they and what do they do? *Nurs Econ* 29(3):150–152, 2011.

National Association of School Nurses (NASN): *Transforming school health* (website), 2014. Available at: www.joomag.com/magazine/annual-report-2013-2014/0147811001426704218?short.

National Association of School Nurses (NASN): *FAQ: about school nursing: the definition of school nursing* (website). Available at: https://www.nasn.org/faq.

National Council of State Boards of Nursing: *Active RN licenses*, 2016. Retrieved from: https://www.ncsbn.org/6161.htm.

National Council of State Boards of Nursing and the Forum of State Nursing Workforce Centers: *2015 national workforce survey of RNs*, 2015. Retrieved from: https://www.ncsbn.org/2015ExecutiveSummary.pdf.

National Hospice and Palliative Care Organization: *Hospice care* (website), 2018. Available at: www.nhpco.org/about/hospice-care.

National League for Nursing: *Percentage of basic RN programs by program type*, 2014. Retrieved from: http://www.nln.org/docs/default-source/newsroom/nursing-education-statistics/percentage-of-basic-rn-programs-by-program-type-1994-to-1995-and-2003-to-2012-and-2014-%28pdf%29.pdf?sfvrsn=0.

National League for Nursing: *Nursing student demographics*, 2014. Retrieved from: http://www.nln.org/newsroom/nursing-education-statistics/nursing-student-demographics.

National League for Nursing: *NON faculty census survey 2014-15*, 2015. Retrieved from: http://www.nln.org/newsroom/nursing-education-statistics/annual-survey-of-schools-of-nursing-academic-year-2015-2016.

National Journal: *First nurse nominated as Army Surgeon General*, 2011. Retrieved from: www.nationaljournal.com/nationalsecurity/first-nurse-nominated-as-army-surgeon-general-20110505.

National Association of Clinical Nurse Specialists: *2016-2018 public policy agenda*, 2018. Retrieved from: https://nacns.org/advocacy-policy/public-policy-agenda/.

Rankin V: Clinical nurse leader: a role for the 21st century, *MEDSURG Nursing* 24(3):199–201, 2015.

Reid K, Dennison P: The clinical nurse leader (CNL)®: point-of-care safety clinician, *Online J Issues Nurs* 16(3):4, 2011.

Robert J: *Waters center for telehealth and e-health law: our mission* (website), 2018. Available at: http://ctel.org/about-2/our-mission/.

Robert Wood Johnson Foundation: *Charting nursing's future: the case for academic progression* (website), 2013. Retrieved from: www.rwjf.org/content/dam/farm/reports/issue_briefs/2013/rwjf407597.

Rosenberg CE: *The care of strangers: the rise of America's hospital system*, Baltimore, MD, 1995, Johns Hopkins University Press.

Schroepfer E: A renewed look at faith community nursing, *MEDSURGNursing* 25(1):62–66, 2016.

Sigma Theta Tau International (STTI): *Policy/position statement: International nurse migration* (website), 2005. Retrieved from: www.nursingsociety.org/aboutus/PositionPapers/Documents/policy_migration.pdf.

Storr GB: Learning how to effectively connect with patients through low-tech simulation scenarios, *Int J Hum Caring* 14(2):36–40, 2010.

Swan M, Ferguson S, Chang A, Larson E, Smaldone A: Quality of primary care by advanced practice nurses: a systematic review, *Intern J Qual Health Care* 27(5):396–404, 2015.

Telemedicine and Telehealth, 2017 (website). Available at: https://www.healthit.gov/topic/health-it-initiatives/telemedicine-and-telehealth.

Thede L: Informatics: where is it? *Online J Issues Nurs* 17(1):10, 2012.

Thekdi P, Wilson BL, Xu Y: Understanding post-hire transitional challenges of foreign-educated nurses, *Nurs Manage* 42(9):8–14, 2011.

U.S. Department of Health and Human Services, Health Resources and Services Administration: *The registered nurse population: findings from the 2008 national sample survey of registered nurses*, Washington, DC, 2010, U.S. Government Printing Office. Retrieved from: http://bhpr.hrsa.gov/healthworkforce/rnsurveys/rnsurveyfinal.pdf.

U.S. Department of Labor Bureau of Labor Statistics: *Occupational outlook handbook: Registered Nurses*, 2016. Retrieved from: https://www.bls.gov/ooh/healthcare/registered-nurses.htm.

Westberg Institute for Faith Community Nurses: *What is faith community nursing?* 2018. Retrieved from: https://westberginstitute.org/faith-community-nursing/.

World Education Service, 2018. Available at: https://wenr.wes.org/2018/03/how-well-do-foreign-educated-nurses-integrate-into-the-u-s-and-canada#_edn6.

World Health Organization: *WHO definition of palliative care*, 2018. Available at: www.who.int/cancer/palliative/definition/en/.

2

The History and Social Context of Nursing

Janna Louise Dieckmann, BA, BSN, MSN, PhD

e To enhance your understanding of this chapter, try the Student Exercises on the Evolve site at http://evolve.elsevier.com/Black/professional.

LEARNING OUTCOMES

After studying this chapter, students will be able to:

- Identify the social, political, and economic factors and trends that influenced the development of professional nursing in the United States.
- Describe the influence of Florence Nightingale on the development of the nursing profession.
- Identify nursing leaders and explain their significance to nursing.
- Describe the development of schools of nursing.
- Explain the role that the military and wars have had on the development of the nursing profession.

- Describe the struggles and contributions of minorities and men in nursing.
- Describe nursing's efforts to manage and improve its image in the media.
- Evaluate the implications for nursing in a technologically driven era.
- Describe how nursing has reacted to nursing shortages.
- Explain how nursing shortages affect patient outcomes.

HISTORICAL CONTEXT OF NURSING

From the work of Florence Nightingale in the Crimea in the mid-1800s to the present, the profession of nursing has been influenced by the social, political, and economic climate of the times, as well as by technological advances and theoretical shifts in medicine and science. This chapter presents an overview of some of the highlights of nursing's history and its early leaders, as well as a discussion of current and past social forces that have shaped the profession's course of development.

Mid–19th-Century Nursing in England

Nursing's most notable early figure, Florence Nightingale, was born into the aristocratic social sphere of Victorian England in 1820. As a young woman, Nightingale (Fig. 2.1) often felt stifled by her privileged and protected social position. As was customary at the time, aristocratic women visited the sick and poor to deliver food, care for the sick, and provide religious outreach. Young Florence often accompanied her mother on these visits. Yet her parents were surprised and opposed her announcement when, at age 30, Nightingale entered the 3-year nurse training program at Kaiserswerth, Germany, where she learned the basics of nursing under the guidance of the Protestant deaconesses. Later, she continued her nursing education when she studied with the Sisters of Charity in Paris. Care of the sick was often in the purview of women and men in religious orders, within both Roman Catholic and Protestant religious traditions.

Having secured her education and training in nursing practice, Nightingale sought the means to communicate her emerging ideas about health and sickness. On

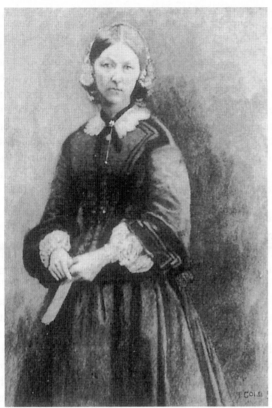

Fig. 2.1 Florence Nightingale (1820–1910), founder of modern nursing. (T. Cole, wood engraving, National Library of Medicine, Bethesda, MD.)

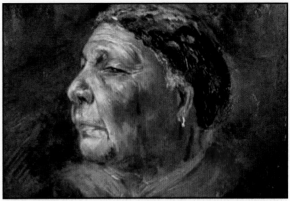

Fig. 2.2 Mary Seacole (1805–1881). Seacole's contributions in the Crimea and elsewhere are often overlooked. A beloved figure, she was voted as the "Greatest Black Briton" in history in 2003. (Albert Charles Challen, oil on panel, National Portrait Gallery, London.)

hearing of the terrible conditions suffered by the sick and wounded British soldiers in Turkey during the Crimean War (1853–1856), Nightingale lobbied British decision makers to support her travel and interventions to aid the sick and wounded. Nightingale took 38 nurses to the British hospital in Scutari, Turkey. With great compassion, and despite the opposition of military officers, Nightingale and the other nurses organized and cleaned the hospital and provided care to the wounded soldiers. Armed with an excellent education in statistics, Nightingale collected very detailed data on morbidity and mortality of the soldiers in Scutari. Using this dramatic supporting evidence, she effectively argued the case for reform of the entire British Army medical system. Gill and Gill (2005) claimed that "Nightingale's influence today extends beyond her undeniable impact on the field of modern nursing to the areas of infection control, hospital epidemiology, and hospice care" (p. 1799).

On her return to England after the Crimean War, Nightingale founded the first English training school for nurses at St. Thomas' Hospital in London in 1860. St. Thomas' Hospital became the model for nursing education in nurse training schools in the United States. Nightingale's most famous publication was *Notes on Nursing: What It Is and What It Is Not* (1859). In this document Nightingale stated clearly for the first time that mastering a unique body of knowledge was required of those wishing to practice professional nursing (Nightingale, 1859/1946). Her publications, dedication to hospital reform, commitment to upgrading conditions for the sick and wounded in the military, and establishment of training schools for nurses influenced the development of nursing in the United States, especially after the Civil War, as well as in her native England.

Mary Seacole (1805–1881) was an interesting Black woman who made significant contributions to the health of soldiers in the Crimean War. Although she and Nightingale were in proximity during the war, they did not work together. Described as a Jamaican nurse and businesswoman, Seacole (Fig. 2.2) was voted as "the greatest Black Briton" in history in a 2003 poll and campaign to raise the profile of contributions of Blacks to Britain over the past 1000 years (100 Great Black Britons, 2015). Although historical accounts of Seacole's life and contributions refer to her as a nurse, Seacole did not refer to herself as a nurse despite her desire to be part of Nightingale's team of nurses going to the Crimea. Her request to be part of the team was refused.

An independent woman with some wealth, Seacole funded her own travel to the Crimea, where her offer to be of service at the British hospital run by Nightingale was again refused. Seacole later reflected in her 1857 autobiography, *Wonderful Adventures of Mrs. Seacole,* "Once again I tried, and had an interview this time with one of Miss Nightingale's companions. She gave me the same reply, and I read in her face the fact that, had there been a vacancy, I should not have been chosen to fill it.... Was it possible that American prejudices against colour had some root here? Did these ladies shrink from accepting my aid because my blood flowed beneath a somewhat duskier skin than theirs?" (Spartacus Educational, 2014). Not only did Seacole face the challenge of racial bias when she sought to be of assistance, but she also faced the bias and the minimization directed toward "colonials," the residents of the widely dispersed countries of the British Empire, which included Seacole's home of Jamaica.

Undeterred by her opposition, Seacole then gathered resources to an establishment she referred to as a "hotel," where injured soldiers received care. Seacole visited the battlefield to tend to the injured and sick and brought many to her hotel. Seacole had a great deal of experience in the management of cholera because of an outbreak in Panama while she was visiting her brother; cholera and other infectious diseases were the cause of a huge percentage of deaths of soldiers in the Crimea. In her autobiography, Seacole described performing an autopsy on a small child who had died of cholera in Panama, the results of which she did not make public but which shaped her understanding of the effects of cholera and how it should be managed. Criticism of Seacole surrounded her entrepreneurship—she sold food and drinks during the war to officers and spectators (Spartacus Educational, 2014).

Called "Mother Seacole" by British soldiers, news accounts of the day described her as a heroine, compassionate, fearless, and determined. Many referred to her as a physician or "doctress"; however, an article in 2012 published in the London newspaper *The Daily Mail* referred to Seacole as "our greatest Black Briton, a woman who did more to advance the cause of nursing and race relations than almost any other individual.... she is said to have saved the lives of countless wounded soldiers and nursed them to health in a clinic paid for out of her own pocket" (Spartacus Educational, 2014). When Seacole filed for bankruptcy soon after her return to England, 80,000 persons attended a 4-day fundraising event organized in her honor.

She was a beloved figure in England, described in 2013 by writer Hugh Muir for *The Guardian* as not a threat to the legacy of Nightingale but as a woman who "reigned on the battlefield." The context for Muir's remarks is an ongoing controversy among politicians and historians about whether Seacole's story will continue to be taught to schoolchildren in a national curriculum and whether to erect a monument to Seacole that is larger than the one honoring Nightingale (Spartacus Educational, 2014).

1861–1873: The American Civil War—An Impetus for Training for Nursing

At the onset of the American Civil War, no professional nurses were available to care for the wounded, and no organized system of medical care existed in either the Union or the Confederacy. Conditions on the battlefield and in military hospitals were unimaginable, with wounded and dying men lying in agony in squalor and filth. Military leadership made appeals for nurses, and the women of both the North and the South responded. Most significant perhaps was the response by the Roman Catholic orders, particularly the Sisters of Charity, the Sisters of Mercy, and the Sisters of the Holy Cross, who had a long history of providing care for the sick (Wall, 1995). Likely the most skilled and devoted of the women who provided nursing care in the Civil War, these Catholic sisters were highly disciplined, organized, and efficient.

On both the Union and the Confederate sides of the war, as well as on the war's Western Front, women responded to meet the needs of the sick and wounded. A number of leaders emerged, including Dorothea L. Dix, a longtime advocate for the mentally ill in prewar years. She was appointed Superintendent of Women Nurses by the Union Army. In that position she was instrumental in creating a month-long training program at two New York hospitals for women who wanted to serve. Thousands of women volunteered and gained nursing skills that made them employable in the postwar era. The lives of countless Union soldiers were saved through Dix's efforts. Several African American women took care of injured Union soldiers, including the famous abolitionist Sojourner Truth and Harriet Tubman, a former field slave who established the Underground Railroad and led slaves to freedom in the North. Another former slave, Susie King Taylor, first worked as a laundress but was called on to assist as a nurse. She is noted for teaching soldiers, African American and White, how to read and write.

Mary Ann ("Mother") Bickerdyke, who attended Oberlin College in Ohio, was a widow who moved to Illinois and worked as an herbalist, creating alternative treatments with plants and herbs. An active member of her Congregationalist Church, she learned of the squalid conditions of the battlefield hospitals through a letter sent to the church by her friend, a surgeon with the 22nd Illinois infantry. She was selected by her congregation to deliver supplies to troops on the Western Front and to investigate the situation in the hospital camp at Cairo, Illinois, where conditions were as bad as described. Bickerdyke had no official authority and was opposed by the camp surgeons, but this did not deter her efforts to bring order out of chaos and create cleaner conditions. She set up field hospitals as she accompanied Ulysses S. Grant and his troops down the Mississippi River, making cleanliness a priority. She hired escaped and former slaves to work with her. Even though she was not a formally trained nurse, she provided much-needed nursing services and deserves her place in history.

Clara Barton is another well-known nursing pioneer. Barton, a Massachusetts woman who worked as a copyist in the U.S. Patent Office, began an independent campaign to provide relief for the soldiers. Appealing to the nation for supplies of woolen shirts, blankets, towels, lanterns, camp kettles, and other necessities (Barton, 1862), she established her own system of distribution, refusing to enlist in the military nurse corps headed by Dorothea Dix (Oates, 1994). Barton took a leave of absence from her patent job and traveled to Culpeper, Virginia. Because of Culpeper's strategically important location, many battles occurred there, including Cedar Mountain, Kelly's Ford, and Brandy Station. The latter was the largest cavalry battle in the Western Hemisphere, with more than 20,000 soldiers in combat. Barton set up a makeshift field hospital and cared for the wounded and dying. During her time at Culpeper, Barton gained her famous title, "Angel of the Battlefield." In 1881, Barton founded the American Red Cross, an organization whose name continues to be synonymous with compassionate service.

The women of the South also responded with an outpouring of support for their Confederate soldiers. Until late 1861 and early 1862, female volunteers or wounded soldiers staffed Confederate hospitals. When the Confederate government assumed control, several women were appointed as superintendents of hospitals. Superintendent Sallie Thompkins, who had earlier established a private hospital in Richmond, Virginia, was commissioned a "captain of Cavalry, unassigned" by Confederate President Jefferson Davis and was the only woman in the Confederacy to hold military rank. Women living near battlefields in both the North and South brought men wounded in battle into their homes to care for them.

Although thousands of women supported the war effort, only a few were appointed as hospital matrons. One of the earliest was Phoebe Pember, whose initial assignment in 1862 to Chimborazo Hospital in Richmond, Virginia, put her in charge of a sprawling government-run institution crowded with "sick or wounded men, convalescing and placed in that position, however ignorant they might be until strong enough for field duty" (Pember, 1959, p. 18).

The Civil War, for all of its destruction and horror, set the stage to advance professional nursing practice because the leaders, although largely untrained, had achieved dramatic improvements in care during the conflict. The successful reforms in military hospitals served as models for reform of civilian hospitals nationwide.

After the Civil War: Moving toward Education and Licensure under the Challenges of Segregation

The move toward formal education and training for nurses grew after the Civil War. Support was garnered from physicians as well as the U.S. Sanitary Commission, the private relief agency created by the federal government in 1861 to provide, coordinate, and support sick and wounded soldiers during the Civil War. After the war, the Sanitary Commission raised massive resources—the equivalent of an estimated $385 million today. At the 1869 American Medical Association meeting, Dr. Samuel Gross, Chair of the Committee on the Training of Nurses, presented three proposals. The most significant was the recommendation that large hospitals begin the process of developing nurse training schools. At the same time, members of the influential U.S. Sanitary Commission, who had seen the effectiveness of nursing care during the Civil War, also lobbied for the creation of nursing schools (Donahue, 1996). Support for their efforts gained momentum as advocates of social reform reported the shockingly inadequate conditions that existed in many hospitals.

The First Training Schools for Nurses and the Feminizing of Nursing

In 1872 the New England Hospital expanded its "nursing course" into "the first general training school for nurses in America" (Kalisch and Kalisch, 2004, p. 65–66). The first diploma was earned by Linda Richards, who is considered to be America's first professionally trained nurse.

The first three American training schools based on the Nightingale model were the Bellevue Training School for Nurses in New York City, the Connecticut Training School for Nurses in New Haven, and the Boston Training School for Nurses at Massachusetts General Hospital in Boston. Opening in 1873, these schools were modeled after Nightingale's school at St. Thomas' Hospital in London. Although these schools were American, they were called *Nightingale Schools*.

The Victorian belief in women's innate sensitivity and high morals led to the early requirement that applicants to these programs be women, for it was thought that these feminine qualities were useful qualities in a nurse. Sensitivity, intelligence, and characteristics of "ladylike" behavior, including submission to authority, were highly desired personal characteristics for applicants. Conversely, men were generally prevented from entering the profession, except among Roman Catholics orders, such as the Alexian Brothers. The number of training schools increased steadily during the last decades of the 19th century, and by 1900 these schools provided hospitals with a steady, albeit subservient, female workforce, as hospitals came to be staffed primarily by students (Fig. 2.3).

Some schools in the North admitted a small number of African American students to their programs. The training school at the New England Hospital for Women and Children in Boston agreed to admit one African American and one Jewish student in each of their classes if they met all entrance qualifications. Mary Eliza Mahoney (Fig. 2.4), the first African American professionally educated nurse, received her training there. Historical Note 2.1 gives some details about Mahoney.

The development of separate nursing schools for African Americans reflected the segregated American society. African Americans received care at separate hospitals from Whites and were cared for by African American nurses. The first program established exclusively for training of African American women in nursing was established at the Atlanta Baptist Female Seminary (later Spelman Seminary, now Spelman College) in Atlanta, Georgia, in 1886. This program was 2 years long and

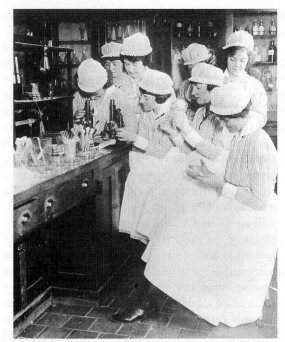

Fig. 2.3 Nurses training in the bacteriologic laboratory at Bellevue Hospital, New York City, circa 1900. (Bettman/Corbis Images.)

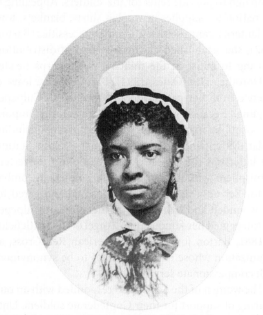

Fig. 2.4 Mary Eliza Mahoney (1845–1926), the first trained African American nurse in the United States.

HISTORICAL NOTE 2.1

Mary Eliza Mahoney (1845–1926) is known as the first educated, professionally trained African American nurse (Miller, 1986). She began her nursing training at the New England Hospital for Women and Children at age 33. An inscription in records from the New England Hospital reads "Mary E. Mahoney, first coloured girl admitted" (Miller, p. 19). The course of study was rigorous, and admission was highly competitive. When Ms. Mahoney applied, there were 40 applicants; 18 were accepted for a probationary period; only 9 were kept after probation, and only 3 earned the diploma. Mahoney was among those 3. As was common in her day, her practice mainly consisted of private duty nursing with families in the Boston area. To celebrate her accomplishments and her status as the first African American professional nurse, the Mary Mahoney Award was established by the National Association of Colored Graduate Nurses in 1935, with the first award given in 1936. This organization was later combined with the ANA.

Miller HS: *America's first black professional nurse,* Atlanta, 1986, Wright Publishing.

led to a diploma in nursing. Although Spelman closed its nursing program in 1928 after graduating 117 nurses (Carnegie, 1995), it remains a global leader in the education of women of African descent today.

Male students were not allowed in the early nursing schools that enrolled women. The earliest school established exclusively for the training of men in nursing was the School for Male Nurses at the New York City Training School, established in 1886. The Mills College of Nursing at Bellevue Hospital was the second school for men, founded in 1888. In 1898 the Alexian Brothers Hospital in Chicago established a nursing school to train men. They opened a second school in 1928 in St. Louis. The Alexian Brothers ministry dates back to the Middle Ages in Europe, where they tended to the sick and hungry and, in the mid-1300s, cared for victims of the Black Plague that devastated the continent. The Alexian Brothers Health System still exists today.

Professionalization through Organization

The 1893 Chicago World's Fair was an unlikely setting for a turning point in nursing's history. Several influential nursing leaders of the century, including Isabel Hampton Robb, Lavinia Lloyd Dock, and Bedford Fenwick of Great Britain, gathered to share ideas and discuss issues pertaining to nursing education. Isabel Hampton Robb

presented a paper in which she protested the lack of uniformity across nursing schools, which led to inadequate curriculum development and nursing education. A paper by Florence Nightingale on the need for scientific training of nurses was presented at this same meeting. Also at this event the precursor to the National League for Nursing, the American Society of Superintendents of Training Schools for Nurses, was formed to address issues in nursing education. The society changed its name in 1912 to the National League of Nursing Education (NLNE), and in 1952 it became the National League for Nursing (NLN). This event held during the Chicago World's Fair became a pivotal point in nursing history.

Three years later, in 1896, Isabel Hampton Robb founded the group that eventually became the American Nurses Association (ANA) in 1911. Originally known as the Nurses' Associated Alumnae of the United States and Canada, the initial mission of this group was to enhance collaboration among practicing nurses and educators.

At the close of the century, in 1899, this same group of energetic American nursing leaders, along with nursing leaders from abroad, collaborated with Bedford Fenwick of Britain to found the International Council of Nurses (ICN). The ICN was and remains dedicated to uniting nursing organizations of all nations; fittingly, its first meeting was held in 1901 at the Pan-American Exposition in Buffalo, New York. At that meeting, a major topic of discussion was one that would dramatically change the practice of nursing: state registration of nurses.

Early nursing professional organizations reflected the segregation that characterized post–Civil War America. Initially nurses from minority groups were excluded from the ANA. After 1916, African American nurses were admitted to membership, but only through their constituent or state associations. In the parts of the United States that remained segregated, including the southern states and the District of Columbia, African American nurses lacked a pathway to membership.

African American nurses recognized the need for their own professional organization to represent and manage their specific challenges. Martha Franklin sent 1500 letters to African American nurses and nursing schools across the country to gather support for this idea (Carnegie, 1995). In response, the National Association of Colored Graduate Nurses (NACGN) was formed in 1908 in New York with the objectives of achieving higher professional standards, breaking down discriminatory practices faced by African Americans in schools of nursing and nursing organizations, and developing

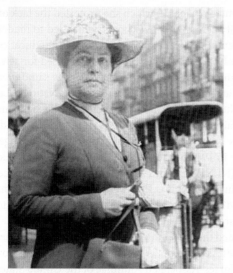

Fig. 2.5 Lillian Wald (1867–1940), nurse and social activist. Wald founded the Henry Street Settlement, which is still in operation today, and was one of the founders of the National Association for the Advancement of Colored People (NAACP).

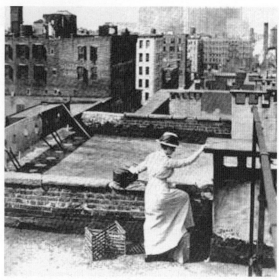

Fig. 2.6 The Henry Street Settlement nurses were undeterred from their daily visits to their patients in New York's Lower East Side.

leadership among African American nurses. Believing they had met their objectives, and with declining funding for the NACGN, in 1949 the group accepted a proposed merger with the ANA, which was finalized in 1951.The ANA had by that time committed full support to minority groups, as well as abolishment of discrimination in all aspects of the profession.

Nursing's Focus on Social Justice: The Henry Street Settlement

From the late 1800s into the 20th century, the young profession of nursing addressed the serious health conditions related to the arrival of European immigrants who sought work in the urban and rural factories of the northeastern United States. Infectious diseases were easily spread in the overcrowded living conditions of inner city tenement housing. In response to these primitive conditions and the lack of sufficient medical services, the Henry Street Settlement was established on New York's Lower East Side in 1893. Its founders, Lillian Wald (Fig. 2.5) and her colleague Mary Brewster, obtained financial assistance from local philanthropists and began the first formalized public health nursing practice established in a settlement house. The Henry Street Settlement continues to serve its immediate community in the 21st century. Social activist and reformer Lavinia Dock and others worked with Wald to provide services through visiting nurse home visits and

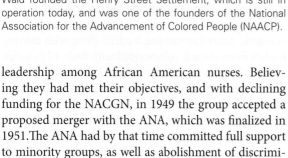

HISTORICAL NOTE 2.2

Margaret Sanger, a nurse who worked on the Lower East Side of New York City in 1912, was struck by the lack of knowledge of immigrant women about pregnancy and contraception. After witnessing the death of Sadie Sachs from a self-attempted abortion, Sanger was inspired to action by this tragedy and became determined to teach women about birth control. A radical activist in her early years, Sanger devoted the remainder of her life to the birth control movement and became a national figure in that cause (Kennedy, 1970).

clinic services that cared for well babies, treated minor illnesses, prevented disease transmission, and provided health education to the neighborhood (Cherry and Jacob, 2005). Through the Henry Street Settlement, in 1902 Lina Rogers became the first school nurse in the United States. The public health nurses of the Henry Street Settlement were relentless in establishing and achieving broad goals to improve the health of the immigrants who were seeking better lives in America (Fig. 2.6). Historical Note 2.2 describes another pioneering nurse, Margaret Sanger, whose work was inspired by the plight of immigrant women on the Lower East Side (Kennedy, 1970). Sanger became the face of the battle for safe contraception and family planning for women. Her work was sometimes dangerous and always controversial, yet she persisted

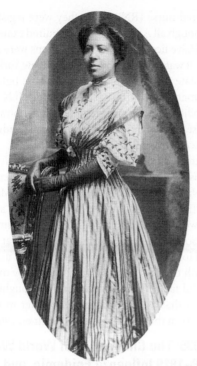

Fig. 2.7 Jessie Sleet Scales, a visionary African American nurse, was among the first to bring community health nursing principles to the tenements of New York City around 1900. (Courtesy Hampton University Archives.)

in her work to preserve reproductive and contraceptive rights for women. The Henry Street Settlement still provides services to fight urban poverty in New York's Lower East Side, serving all ages with a variety of health services, social services, and the arts. A more comprehensive view of the remarkable history and work of the Henry Street Settlement is available at www.henrystreet.org.

A Common Cause, but Still Segregated

Tuberculosis was a major health problem in the tenements of America's crowded industrial cities. Dr. Edward T. Devine, president of the Charity Organization Society, noted the high incidence of tuberculosis among New York City's African American population. Aware of racial barriers to receiving health care and the related cultural resistance to seeking medical care, Dr. Devine determined that a Black district nurse should be hired to conduct outreach into the African American community to persuade local residents to accept health services, screen for tuberculosis, and provide treatment if needed. Jessie Sleet Scales (Fig. 2.7), an African American nurse trained at Providence Hospital in Chicago, was hired as

a district nurse and soon earned a permanent position. Her report to New York's Charity Organization Society, published in the *American Journal of Nursing* in 1901, was titled "A Successful Experiment":

> *I beg to render to you a report of the work done by me as a district nurse among the colored people of New York City during the months of October and November. I have visited forty-one families and made 156 calls in connection with these families, caring for nine cases of consumption, four cases of peritonitis, two cases of chickenpox, two cases of cancer, one case of diphtheria, two cases of heart disease, two cases of tumor, one case of gastric catarrh, two cases of pneumonia, four cases of rheumatism, and two cases of scalp wound. I have given baths, applied poultices, dressed wounds, washed and dressed newborn babies, cared for mothers.*
>
> ***(Sleet, 1901, p. 729)***

Jessie Sleet Scales later recommended to Lillian Wald that Elizabeth Tyler, a graduate of Freedmen's Hospital Training School for Nurses in Washington, D.C., work with African American patients through the Henry Street Settlement. Working within the confines of segregation, Scales and Tyler established the Stillman House, a branch of the Henry Street Settlement that served Black persons in a small store on New York's West 61st Street. For community health nursing, the addition of these pioneer African American nurses to the ranks of the Henry Street Settlement signified activism, expansion, and growth. Despite the persistent racial barriers and squalid living and health conditions, Scales and Tyler succeeded in providing excellent nursing care to underserved families with increasing but manageable health problems. Their common focus on prevention of disease and management of illness bound these visionary nurses of the Henry Street Settlement across the deep racial divide.

War Again Creates the Need for Nurses: The Spanish-American War

In 1898 the U.S. Congress declared war on Spain, and once again nursing had a major role in the care of those soldiers sick and injured in war. Anita M. McGee, MD, was appointed head of the Hospital Corps, a group formed to recruit nurses. Encouraged by Isabel Hampton Robb and the fledgling Nurses' Associated Alumnae of the United States and Canada, McGee initially wanted only graduates of nurse training schools in the Hospital Corps (Wall, 1995); however, it soon became clear

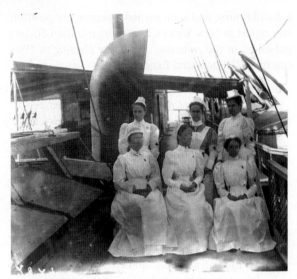

Fig. 2.8 Red Cross nursing in the Spanish-American War, circa 1898. Nurses on deck of the hospital ship Relief near Cuba. (National Library of Medicine, Bethesda, MD.)

that this requirement could not be met. A widespread epidemic of typhoid fever created a greater need than anticipated, and as a result others, including the Sisters of the Holy Cross (whose order had served during the Civil War) and untrained African American nurses who had had typhoid fever in the past, were accepted for service (Wall, 1995). Namahyoke Curtis was employed as a contract nurse by the War Department during the Spanish-American War, making her the first trained African American nurse in this capacity. Although McGee and Robb had to enlist untrained persons to care for the sick and wounded during the Spanish-American War, their efforts set the stage for the development of a permanent Army Nurse Corps (1901) and Navy Nurse Corps (1908) (Fig. 2.8).

Professionalization and Standardization of Nursing through Licensure

The institution of state licensure for nurses was a huge milestone for nursing in the early 20th century, although early efforts to establish licensure were not well received. After an educational campaign, the ICN passed a resolution asking each country and each American state to provide for licensure of the nurses working there. As a result, state legislatures in New Jersey, New York, North Carolina, and Virginia passed what were known as permissive licensure laws for nursing in 1903. Nurses did not have to be registered to practice but could not use the title

of registered nurse (RN) unless they were registered. By 1923, although all American states required examinations for permissive licensure, the examinations were not standardized. It was not until the 1930s that New York became the first state to have mandatory licensure, but this was not fully mandated until 1947. In 1950 the NLN assumed responsibility for administering the first nationwide State Board Test Pool Examination, meaning all candidates for nursing licensure took the same examination.

The first edition of the *American Journal of Nursing*, published in October 1900, was a key event of this decade. Nurse leaders Isabel Hampton Robb, Mary Adelaide Nutting, Lavinia L. Dock, Sophia Palmer, and Mary E. Davis were heavily involved in the development of the journal. Sophia Palmer, director of nursing at Rochester City Hospital, New York, was appointed as the first editor, with the goal of presenting "month by month the most useful facts, the most progressive thought and the latest news that the profession has to offer in the most attractive form that can be secured" (Palmer, 1900, p. 64).

1917–1935: The Challenges of World War I, the 1918–1919 Influenza Epidemic, and the 1930s Depression Era

The significant events of 1917–1918 combined to challenge nursing resources and organized responses. The United States entered World War I. The utility of trained female nurses to provide care for soldiers during warfare had been demonstrated successfully in previous military campaigns and wars. When the United States entered the war in Europe in early April 1917, the National Committee on Nursing was formed (Dock and Stewart, 1920). This committee was chaired by Mary Adelaide Nutting, professor of Nursing and Health at Columbia University, with membership including Jane A. Delano, Director of Nursing for the American Red Cross, and other prominent nursing leaders. Charged with supplying an adequate number of trained nurses to U.S. Army hospitals abroad, the National Committee on Nursing initiated a national publicity campaign to enhance recruitment of young women to enter nurse training (Fig. 2.9), established the Army School of Nursing with Annie Goodrich as its dean, and introduced college women to nursing through participation in the Vassar Training Camp for Nurses.

From September 1918 to August 1919, an influenza pandemic swept the nation and eventually the world, infecting a staggering one-third of the world's population. The influenza pandemic spurred widespread public

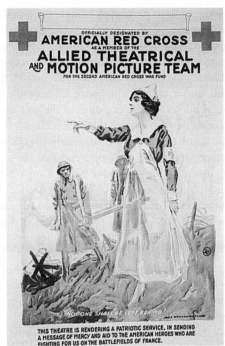

OFFICIALLY DESIGNATED BY
AMERICAN RED CROSS
AS A MEMBER OF THE
ALLIED THEATRICAL
AND MOTION PICTURE TEAM
FOR THE SECOND AMERICAN RED CROSS WAR FUND

"NOT ONE SHALL BE LEFT BEHIND!"

THIS THEATRE IS RENDERING A PATRIOTIC SERVICE, IN SENDING A MESSAGE OF MERCY AND AID TO THE AMERICAN HEROES WHO ARE FIGHTING FOR US ON THE BATTLEFIELDS OF FRANCE.

Fig. 2.9 A World War I Red Cross nursing poster, 1918. "Not one shall be left behind!" by James Montgomery Flagg is typical of World War I recruitment posters. Nurses answered the call in record numbers. (Collection of the Library of Congress.)

education in home care and hygiene through Red Cross nursing. Historical Note 2.3 describes the impact of the influenza pandemic on the nation and the profession.

By the time World War I ended, the nursing profession had demonstrated its ability both to provide care to wounded soldiers and to respond effectively to the influenza pandemic. In 1920 Congress passed a bill that provided nurses with military rank (Dock and Stewart, 1920). The 1920s also saw increased use of hospitals and an acceptance of the scientific basis of medicine.

Two other noteworthy events of the decade included the publication of the 1923 Goldmark Report, a study of nursing education (discussed further in Chapter 4) that advocated for the establishment of schools of nursing associated with colleges and universities, rather than hospital-based diploma programs, and encouraged the establishment of rural programs in midwifery, and the establishment of the Frontier Nursing Service (FNS) in 1925.

The FNS was established in 1925 by Mary Breckinridge, a nurse and midwife. Originally established as the Kentucky Committee for Mothers and Babies, this

HISTORICAL NOTE 2.3

The influenza pandemic of 1918–1919 increased the public's awareness of the necessity of public health nursing. A pandemic is an epidemic over a very large geographic area—a continent or even the world, crossing international boundaries—and simultaneously affects a large proportion of the population. Across the United States, the U.S. Public Health Service, American Red Cross, and local Visiting Nurse and Public Health Nursing agencies mobilized to provide care for the hundreds of thousands who contracted influenza, known as "La Grippe" or "Spanish flu." One-third of the world's population (approximately 500,000,000 persons) was affected, and in the United States, 28% of all Americans became infected, killing an estimated 675,000 citizens. The influenza was most deadly to persons 20 to 40 years of age. This age group is typically least susceptible to death by infectious disease, whereas infants, children, and the elderly are usually most affected—but this was no ordinary seasonal influenza. Approximately half of the fatalities among U.S. soldiers in Europe were due to influenza, not war injuries, and in total, an estimated 43,000 servicemen mobilized during World War I died of influenza. In Spring 1919 the second wave of the flu epidemic struck the U.S. East Coast and swept across the country. Although not as lethal as the first epidemic wave, the 1919 flu epidemic closed businesses, schools, and churches. The demand for nursing services increased across these two waves of influenza.

service provided the first organized nurse-midwifery program in the United States. Nurses of the FNS worked in isolated rural areas in the Appalachian Mountains, traveling by horseback to serve the health needs of the poverty-stricken mountain people (Fig. 2.10). FNS nurses delivered babies, provided prenatal and postnatal care, educated mothers and their families about nutrition and hygiene, and cared for the sick. Through this rural midwifery service, Breckinridge demonstrated that nurses could play a significant role in providing primary rural health care.

1931–1945: Challenges of the Great Depression and World War II

With hospitals largely staffed by nursing students, most nurses who had completed their training worked as private duty nurses in patients' homes. The Great Depression, however, meant that many families could no longer afford private duty nurses, forcing many nurses into

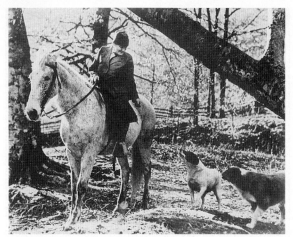

Fig. 2.10 Mary Breckinridge, founder of the FNS, on her way to visit patients in rural Kentucky. (Used with permission of the Frontier Nursing Service, Wendover, KY.)

unemployment. In 1933 President Franklin D. Roosevelt established the Civil Works Administration (CWA) in which nurses participated by providing rural and school health services. They also took part in specific projects such as conducting health surveys on communicable disease and nutrition of children. Hospitals, as a result of the severe economic conditions of the Depression, were forced to close their schools of nursing. Consequently, hospitals no longer had a reliable, inexpensive student workforce at the time when there was a significant increase in the number of patients needing charity care. The solution soon became apparent: unemployed graduate nurses, willing to work for minimum pay, were recruited to work in the hospitals rather than doing private duty for wealthy families. This had a lasting effect on the staffing of hospitals.

The Social Security Act (SSA) of 1935, a significant part of President Roosevelt's plans to bring the nation out of the Depression, enhanced the practice of public health nursing. One of the purposes of the SSA was to strengthen public health services and to provide medical care for children with disabilities and blind persons. Public health nursing was supported by the SSA and became the major avenue of care to dependent mothers and children, the blind, and children with disabilities.

World War II: Challenges and Opportunities for Nursing

During World War II, the nation's military once again found itself without an adequate supply of nurses. In response to the need for nurses, Congress enacted legislation to provide substantial financial support for nursing education. The military and collegiate programs of nursing formed the Cadet Nurse Corps, an alliance to train student nurses. Students received tuition, books, a stipend, and a uniform in return for a commitment to serve as nurses for the duration of the war in either civilian or military hospitals, the Indian Health Service, or public health facilities. Approximately 124,000 nurses volunteered, graduated, and were certified for military services in the Army and Navy Nurse Corps between 1943 and 1948. As a result of lobbying by U.S. Congresswoman Frances Payne Bolton, First Lady Eleanor Roosevelt, and the National Organization of Colored Graduate Nurses, for the first time, America's African American nurses were permitted to provide nursing services to injured soldiers in foreign countries. At home, despite ongoing racial segregation, African American collegiate programs, as well as the NACGN, were active participants in the Cadet Nurse Corps.

Historical Note 2.4 describes the courage of nurses in the Philippines at Corregidor and Bataan during World War II, who were held in captivity for 3 years in an internment camp.

1945–1960: The Rise of Hospitals— Bureaucracy, Science, and Shortages

The professionalization of nursing continued after the end of World War II. In 1947 military nurses were awarded full commissioned officer status in both the Army and the Navy Nurse Corps, and segregation of African American nurses was ended. Julie O. Flikke was the first nurse to be promoted to the rank of colonel in the U.S. Army. In 1954 men were allowed to enter the military nursing corps.

In 1946 the Hill-Burton Act was enacted, providing funds to construct hospitals, which led to a surge in the growth of new facilities. This rapid expansion in the number of hospital beds resulted in an acute shortage of nurses and increasingly difficult working conditions. Long hours, inadequate salaries, and increasing patient loads made many nurses unhappy with their jobs, and threats of strikes and collective bargaining ensued.

In response to the shortages, "team nursing" was introduced. Team nursing involved the provision of care to a group of patients by a group of care providers. Although efficient, the method fragmented patient care and removed the RN from the bedside. Another

HISTORICAL NOTE 2.4

Hours after Pearl Harbor was attacked on December 7, 1941, a successful surprise attack on U.S. installations in the Philippines crippled the air force in the South Pacific. At that time, more than 100 nurses were enlisted with the U.S. Army and Navy units in the Philippines. Some of the most dramatic stories in nursing's history played out over the next weeks and months during the Japanese takeover of the Bataan peninsula, a large land mass at the northern tip of the Philippines, and then Corregidor, a small island (about 6 square miles) in a strategically advantageous location at the opening on the Manila Bay. Nurses proved their ingenuity, commitment, courage, and intelligence during the first months of 1942 as they were forced to provide care under the most extreme conditions. The two field hospitals that were built to handle 1000 patients each had 11,000 patients by the end of March 1942. One month later, there were 24,000 sick and wounded. The field hospitals themselves were bombed twice. With the imminent fall of the Bataan to Japanese control, the nurses were evacuated to Corregidor.

Corregidor contained a huge bomb-proof tunnel system, a complex of a main tunnel (the Malinta Tunnel, 1400 feet long and 30 feet wide) and numerous lateral tunnels with electricity and ventilation, and a hospital. At first, the conditions deep in the tunnel were a stark contrast to the horrors of Bataan, until conditions deteriorated over the next few weeks as Corregidor continued to be under relentless air attack by the Japanese. The number of wounded soldiers increased, until finally 1000 young men were being cared for by the nurses in a space where power outages, poor ventilation, oppressive heat, and vermin were common.

Although many nurses were evacuated from Corregidor before the final takeover of the island fortress by the Japanese military, about 85 American and Filipino nurses remained in the tunnel hospital to attend to the wounded.

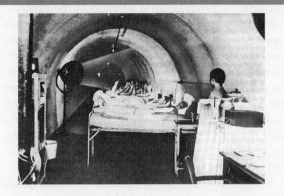

On May 4, 1942, the American forces on Corregidor surrendered. The nurses remaining on Corregidor were confined to the tunnel hospital, were not allowed to go outside for fresh air, and were given only two small meals a day, and yet they continued to provide effective nursing care for 1000 sick and injured soldiers. This continued for 6 weeks until they were moved to the old hospital site outside the tunnel. One week later, they were bound for Manila, not knowing that they were soon to be providing care at an internment camp, where they would also be interned for the next 33 months. On February 3, 1945, U.S. troops liberated the internment camp.

For more details of the nurses' work during their ordeal at Bataan, Corregidor, and the internment camp, consult these excellent resources:

Kalisch PA, Kalisch BJ: Nurses under fire: the World War II experiences of nurses on Bataan and Corregidor, *Nurs Res* 44(5):260–271, 1995.

Norman E: *We band of angels: the untold story of American nurses trapped on Bataan by the Japanese,* New York, 1999, Random House.

---

response to the shortage was the institution of the associate degree in nursing (ADN), discussed in more detail in Chapter 4. As nursing continued to search for its identity, it focused on the scientific basis for nursing practice. Clinical nursing research began in earnest, and the *Journal of Nursing Research* was first published in 1952.

1961–1982: The Great Society, Vietnam, and the Change in Women's Role

Two 1965 amendments to the Social Security Act, designed to ensure access to health care for elderly, poor,

and disabled Americans, resulted in the establishment of Medicare and Medicaid. Soon after, hospitals began to rely heavily on reimbursements from Medicare and Medicaid. Because most of the care for the sick was taking place in hospitals rather than homes, the hospital setting became the preferred place of employment for nurses, giving rise to new opportunities and roles for nurses.

The 1960s were the era of specialty care and clinical specialization for nurses. The successful development of the clinical specialist role in psychiatric nursing—combined with the proliferation of intensive care units and technological advances of the period—fostered the growth of clinical specialization in many areas, including cardiac-thoracic surgery and coronary care. The increase in medical specialization, along with the concurrent shortage of primary care physicians and the public demand for improved access to health care that grew out of President Lyndon B. Johnson's "Great Society" reforms, fostered the emergence of the nurse practitioner (NP) in primary care. In 1971 Idaho became the first state to recognize diagnosis and treatment as part of the legal scope of practice for NPs.

Again, war—this time in Vietnam—provided nurses with opportunities to stretch the boundaries of the discipline. The Vietnam War occurred in jungles not easily accessed by rescue workers or medics and without clearly drawn lines of combat. Mobile hospital units were set up in the jungles, where nurses often worked without the direct supervision of physicians as they fought to save the lives of the wounded. They performed advanced emergency procedures such as tracheotomies and chest tube insertions, never before executed by nurses. They also had to deal with the lack of support at home, where the Vietnam War was controversial and widely protested. The trauma of the battlefield was intensified by this lack of support at home, and many nurses suffered posttraumatic stress disorder, as did the returning soldiers. In 1993 the Vietnam Women's Memorial statue was dedicated, which featured two nurses—one White, one Black—tending to the prostrate figure of an injured soldier. Most of the American women who served in Vietnam were nurses. This memorial captured the difficult and crucial role of nurses in the Vietnam War, and it stands in sharp contrast to the days of segregation from earlier decades. The Vietnam Women's Memorial statue is featured on the title page of this chapter.

1983–2000: Challenges for Nursing—HIV/AIDS and Life Support Technologies

The early 1980s was marked by the recognition of the rapid spread of a retrovirus that later became known as the human immunodeficiency virus (HIV). This virus was isolated from a person with acquired immunodeficiency syndrome (AIDS) and ultimately resulted in a change in health care globally. At first believed to be confined to the gay community, in 1983 the first incidence of the spread of HIV was noted in hemophiliacs as a result of HIV-contaminated blood products. It became

clear that all persons were susceptible to HIV. Although much is known about HIV and its transmission now, 30 years ago the questions that surrounded HIV were frightening and resulted in massive changes to the daily routines in health care, including the implementation of universal precautions. The development of antiretroviral treatments proved to be useful in prolonging the time from infection with HIV to the development of AIDS, and the use of antiretroviral drugs during pregnancy reduced the incidence of mother-to-child transmission from 30% to 3%. Very quickly, the HIV/AIDS epidemic changed the landscape of health care, affecting everything from materials such as needles, intravenous catheters, and gloves to global AIDS initiatives in resource-poor nations, particularly in Africa.

The 1980s and 1990s were also marked by an enormous increase in the use of medical technologies, including the wide use of life support. Many ethical questions were raised during these years regarding the use of life support technologies and when they are appropriate. A prominent case involved the decision of the parents of Karen Ann Quinlan to discontinue ventilatory support after she lapsed into a drug- and alcohol-induced coma in 1975. The phrase "persistent vegetative state" became well known, if not entirely understood, by the public. Ms. Quinlan lived for a decade after the discontinuation of the ventilator, never regaining consciousness. Another case involving a young woman, Nancy Cruzan, raised questions of "right to die" and what the patient would have wanted. Ms. Cruzan was in a persistent vegetative state, and her parents asked for her feeding tube to be removed, eventually taking their fight to the U.S. Supreme Court, which upheld a ruling by the Missouri court that prevented them from discontinuing her nutritional support. They eventually won a court order under the Due Process Clause that supports a person's right to refuse medical treatment. The Cruzans provided evidence that their daughter would have wanted her life support terminated, and they were allowed to have nutritional support discontinued. These prominent cases moved forward support for advance directives that would provide evidence of a patient's wishes while still competent.

2001–2018: The Post–9/11 Era, Natural Disasters, and Health Care Reform

The United States underwent a sudden and cataclysmic social and cultural shift in the aftermath of the September 11, 2001, attacks. Almost all areas of American life were touched by the events of that day, including nursing. Disaster management became a focus of nursing efforts to be better prepared for mass casualties, and disaster drills have become part of the routine in hospitals to ensure that nurses and other personnel can respond effectively and efficiently, with a focus on saving as many lives as possible during a wide-scale disaster.

In 2005 Hurricane Katrina created a disaster along the Gulf Coast of Louisiana, Mississippi, and beyond. Parts of the city of New Orleans were underwater, and the images of people sitting on housetops and propped in wheelchairs along the walls of the Superdome became part of the story of Katrina. In hospitals filled with floodwaters in their lower floors, nurses, physicians, and other providers sought to protect and comfort patients under horrendous conditions. In 2006, in response to the arrest of two nurses for administering lethal doses of morphine and midazolam to four terminally ill patients in the aftermath of Hurricane Katrina, the ANA published comments on nursing care during disasters, citing the "unfamiliar and unusual conditions with the health care environment that may necessitate adaptations to recognized standards of nursing practice"; the comments, however, did not address the specific details of these nurses' situations. The ANA comments can be found at www.nursingworld.org/DocumentVault/Ethics/ANAonKatrina.html. What was clear from both the World Trade Center attacks and the aftermath of Hurricane Katrina is that nurses were called on to act in conditions that had been previously unimaginable and unaddressed. Nursing as a profession has responded by increasing preparedness for human catastrophes and natural disasters that are certain to occur in the future.

Another marker of the current social context of nursing was the passage of the Affordable Care Act (ACA), signed into law by President Barack Obama in March 2010. This legislation was and continues to be debated vigorously. This legislation was often referred to as "health care reform." The ANA supported the passage of this Act and in 2011 affirmed its continuing support for the Act in the face of efforts by subsequent sessions of Congress to repeal it. Provisions of the ACA were implemented over time. Early provisions banned lifetime limits on insurance coverage by insurers so that patients with extreme medical costs can be assured of continuing benefits over the course of their illness and lifetime. Young adults up to age 26 were allowed coverage on their parents' insurance plan unless they had insurance coverage at work. The ACA also prevented insurance companies from denying coverage to children and teens younger than age 19 because of a preexisting condition. An estimated 162,000 children benefitted from these two provisions. Later provisions included coverage of recommended preventive services with no out-of-pocket expenses for insurance holders, the right to appeal coverage decisions, and having a choice of primary care providers. By 2015, more than 16 million Americans had a health care plan under the ACA, meaning that only 10.1% were without health coverage, a decrease of more than 4% since the first ACA open enrollment in 2013. The Congressional Budget Office, a nonpartisan department of the federal government, estimated a cost savings of more than $1.7 trillion over two decades. Interestingly, the ACA has improved patient safety and prevented an estimated 50,000 deaths between 2010 and 2013 from health care–related harm. An important provision of the ACA was that persons with a preexisting health condition could not be denied health insurance coverage. This provision affected 129 million Americans.

Another major development in the health care field that affects the nursing profession has been the rapid development of informational and medical technologies. Electronic health records have become common as the U.S. health care system is moving toward becoming paperless. Digitalized health records allow for access across disciplines and across distance, with the goal to improve continuity of health care no matter where a person may require medical treatment. In many institutions, nurses enter patient data into computers at the bedside. Life-sustaining medical technologies have created new ethical challenges for nurses, who continue to be the first line of defense on behalf of their vulnerable patients. This role has never changed for nurses, even though technologies have altered the terrain of health care over time.

Many of the issues that confronted nurses of the past still confront nurses today. War, infectious disease, poverty, and immigration still pose challenges to public health. With an increasing interest in global health, nurses are finding that, although many infectious diseases have been managed, HIV/AIDS and malaria still threaten the health of people in Africa and other underdeveloped parts of the world. Nurses are increasingly aware of the need for cultural competence in providing care to others with whom nurses share little in common demographically. Monsivais (2011) noted that, although cultural markers such as age, gender, education, and socioeconomic class all create a certain cultural experience, the intersection of an illness along any or all of these markers may create an entirely different set of circumstances that nurses are challenged to identify and address. More simply, the shared experience of a particular illness may create a subgroup with more cultural significance than an individual's age, gender, or ethnic identity. For example, there is a sizable online community of parents who vary greatly across demographic indicators but who are connected through their children who have heart disease. These parents often refer to their children as "cardiac kids," a signal of both their children's serious health struggles and the lifestyle changes that are created around these conditions. Other illnesses such as cancer or genetic conditions have resulted in similar patient and family communities that reach beyond cultural markers.

Significant language barriers exist as nurses manage the care of large numbers of Latinos who have immigrated into the United States in recent years, and for whom Spanish is their primary language. Even among patients of any language who speak English fluently as a second language, the stresses and distresses associated with illness, hospitalization, and entry into the health care system can diminish language skills, resulting in an increased dependence on their native language.

In addition, with the simultaneous wars in Iraq and Afghanistan, many soldiers returned to the United States with significant injuries that will require lifelong management. Improved initial care in the field prevented many deaths of soldiers immediately after their injuries.

Profound lower extremity injuries among Middle East veterans are common and are related to encounters with improvised explosive devices (IEDs), also known as roadside bombs. The changing nature of health care in one arena (e.g., rapid responses in the field) has implications for care in another arena (e.g., long-term rehabilitation of veterans with missing limbs).

SOCIAL CONTEXT OF NURSING

No endeavor functions separately from its social and historical context. Nursing is no exception. The influences on nursing in several contexts are identified and discussed in the remaining pages of this chapter. The social context also influences who chooses nursing as a career.

As you read this section, think about what drew you into the profession of nursing. What is the story of your own journey into nursing? One nurse's story is found in Thinking Critically Box 2.1. As you read his story, identify the factors that influenced his choice of career and the challenges that he faced as he became a nurse. Then think of your own story, and identify the social forces that have influenced your career choice.

Several social factors that have influenced the development of professional nursing will be explored in this section, including the following:
- Gender
- The image of nursing
- National population trends
- Technology
- The shortage of nurses

 THINKING CRITICALLY BOX 2.1

Challenging Gender Norms: One Nurse's Journey Into Nursing

Analyze the following story, and determine some of the factors that influenced this nurse's choice of a career. What assumptions did he make about the profession before entering it? Were his assumptions accurate or inaccurate? How would his assumptions hold up today?

"I never wanted to be anything but a nurse. As a child, I loved to bandage my sister's dolls and stuffed animals, and later as a teen, I volunteered at the animal shelter and took care of sick and wounded animals. As soon as I was old enough, I volunteered at a local skilled nursing facility taking care of the elderly, helping feed them and reading to them, and sometimes writing letters for them. When I was 18, I was hired as an 'orderly' (a male assistant) at a small local hospital and provided care to male

patients who were being prepared for surgery. One of the doctors there asked me if I was going to go to medical school, and I told him that I was saving my money to go to nursing school. He told me, 'What a waste. You have a great mind. And how is a man going to provide for a family on a nurse's salary?' Needless to say, I was very upset by his response, and didn't feel like I could defend my career choice very well at the time. I have now completed my bachelor of science in nursing (BSN) and am working as an RN in a large, busy emergency department, and am planning to return to graduate school. I sometimes think about that conversation with that doctor, and wish that I could go back in time and answer him better than I did then."

Gender

Gender is a social construction of behaviors, roles, beliefs, and values that are specific to women or men. Gender is not the same as sex, which is a biologic entity. A fundamental example has to do with asking a pregnant woman whether she is having a girl or a boy. This is a question of biology: is the fetus a female (XX) or a male (XY)? If the woman responds, "It's a girl—she's so graceful, she just moves so gently, and we can see in her ultrasound pictures that she has long legs and arms. I can tell that she is going to be a ballerina someday!" she has assigned a gender role to the biologic entity of a female fetus. Because the fetus is gentle and has long limbs, the pregnant woman has interpreted these attributes in light of the fetus's sex—she is going to be a ballerina.

Assignment of gender roles starts early (even before birth in some cases) and is part of *socialization,* the process through which values and expectations are transmitted from generation to generation. Parents and others in a child's sphere of influence teach lessons about gender roles and behavior, both intentionally and unintentionally. A consequence of this is that gender-role stereotyping occurs. Stereotypes are also social constructions that portray how men and women "should" behave in society or within their cultural group. Gender-role stereotyping can be subtle but begins early with cues as commonplace as pink clothing for baby girls and blue for boys; dolls for girls and trucks for boys; and comments such as "big boys don't cry" and "girls shouldn't get dirty when they play."

Gender-specific stereotypes have affected nursing for 160 years. When nursing as a modern profession began in the mid-1800s, the most common roles assumed by women were within their families and involved caring for others, maintaining a household, and taking care of their husbands and children. Women did not work outside the home for money but rather relied on their husbands or families for support. The first formal schools of nursing in the United States were developed to attract "respectable" women into nursing, a criterion that was designed to increase the value society put on nursing. Stereotyping of women also included the notion that women were intellectually inferior to men and hence women were not called on to make decisions or think for themselves. This type of stereotyping shaped the type of training that nurses received, which was fundamentally task oriented, and this form of instruction persisted for many years.

Men are not new to the profession of nursing. During the 11th, 12th, and 13th centuries in Europe,

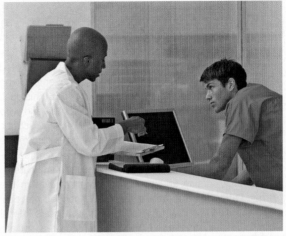

Fig. 2.11 Attracting men to nursing continues to be a priority for the profession. (Photo used with permission from Photos.com.)

men provided much of the nursing care, often under the authority of military or religious orders. Florence Nightingale worked hard to establish nursing as a worthy career for women and largely ignored the historical contributions of men. The male role in her estimation was confined to supplying physical strength, such as lifting, moving, or controlling patients when needed. Early schools of nursing in the United States did not admit men, establishing an early tradition of discrimination in the profession. An exception was psychiatric nursing, which often required physical stamina and strength and was therefore considered an appropriate setting for men in nursing. Now women and men in nursing have the same choices of settings available to them (Fig. 2.11). (The editor of this textbook recalls with fondness her first male nurse colleague in the neonatal intensive care unit. He was an exceptionally caring nurse with an extraordinary way of reassuring worried parents.)

Today about 11% of students enrolled in undergraduate programs are men. Men in nursing, compared with women in nursing, are likely to be younger, to be employed full time in nursing, to have more non-nursing education, and to have chosen nursing as a second career. Their motivations for entering nursing, however, are similar to those of their female counterparts. The top three reasons identified by men for becoming nurses are (1) a desire to help people, (2) the perception that nursing is a growth profession with many career paths, and (3) the desire to have a stable

PROFESSIONAL PROFILE BOX 2.1
FROM FLIGHT MEDIC TO FLIGHT NURSE: ONE MAN'S STORY

I was on active duty in the Army when I decided to become a nurse. I was a flight medic at the time and wanted to be more involved in caring for critically ill patients. Going to nursing school seemed to be the way to reach this goal. I had a couple of nurse mentors who were men and who were instrumental in my decision to go to nursing school. They really enjoyed the profession and encouraged me to give it a try. The Army was a good place to be a nurse because the rank structure is equal for physicians and nurses.

My initial nursing education began while I was in the Army. I attended the Army's version of licensed practical nurse (LPN) school. After I left the Army 3 years later, I wanted to become an RN, so I first earned an associate degree and then went back to school and earned an associate degree in nursing so I could sit for the NCLEX® examination and begin work as an RN. Although I am currently working full time, I am also taking courses toward a bachelor of science in nursing (BSN) degree. Then I plan to pursue a master's degree.

Like many of my male colleagues, I am interested in emergency nursing, and that has driven my career path. Being a flight medic in the service really sparked my interest to return to that job as an RN. I have worked in a postanesthesia care unit, a telemetry unit, an emergency department, and an intensive care unit and have done both ground and air transport of critically ill and trauma patients. It took several years to get the work experience as an RN to get a flight nurse job. You have to be an experienced nurse to even apply for a flight nurse position.

I now have my dream job as a flight nurse for a major medical center. I get to take care of the sickest, most badly injured patients you can imagine. I know that I really get to make a difference on a daily basis in the lives of the patients who I help care for.

One of the best aspects of my job is that not only do I do air transport, but I get to do research as well. I have been the principal investigator for two studies, the first of which has been published in a peer-reviewed journal. I also am the outreach coordinator for our program. This affords me the opportunity to interact with emergency medical services, fire departments, and referring hospitals.

Nursing is an occupation where you can find your love in your job. I look forward to going to work every day. I am glad that I had mentors who guided me into nursing as a career. I have never regretted that decision.

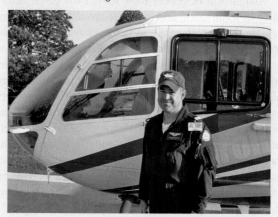

Christopher McGrath, RN
Reference: Courtesy Christopher McGrath.

career. Professional Profile Box 2.1 contains the story of Christopher McGrath, RN, who was encouraged to become a nurse, and how his career and educational paths have developed.

In 1974 the American Assembly for Men in Nursing (AAMN) was organized to address, discuss, and influence factors that affect men in nursing. Open to men and women, this national organization has local chapters. The goals for AAMN organization are as follows:

- Encourage men of all ages to become nurses and join together with all nurses in strengthening and humanizing health care.
- Support men who are nurses to grow professionally and demonstrate to each other and to society the increasing contributions being made by men within the nursing profession.

- Advocate for continued research, education, and dissemination of information about men's health issues, men in nursing, and nursing knowledge at the local and national levels.
- Support members' full participation in the nursing profession and its organizations, and use this Assembly for the limited objectives stated earlier (AAMN, 2015).

Social change in the 1960s had a profound effect on society and has both hurt and helped the nursing profession. Women began to recognize that they had career opportunities beyond the traditional and stereotypical "female" ones such as teaching and nursing. Gifted women who might have otherwise become nurses pursued careers in a variety of other fields. This meant that nursing faced more competition for students than it once did because of the heightened interest in other careers by young women. Women sought opportunities that offered higher salaries, better working conditions, and schedules more accommodating of family life.

An interesting recent phenomenon has occurred, however. Across the United States, nursing programs are seeing an increasing number of applicants who have degrees in other areas or who have had careers in other disciplines such as teachers, attorneys, engineers, information technology (IT) specialists, and entrepreneurs. The current appeal of nursing seems to be related to the fact that a career in nursing can provide economic and job security. A more significant reason for this trend is that, in spite of the wide array of career choices, nursing's appeal is strong to individuals who want to make a difference in the lives of others.

The women's movement benefited nursing in numerous ways. First, economic inequities and poor working conditions were exposed. The movement provoked a conscious awareness that equality and autonomy for women were inherent rights, not privileges, and stimulated the passage of legislation to ensure those rights. Unfortunately, however, results of a study of published in 2015 showed that male RNs earn more than female RNs across settings, specialty areas, and positions over time, with no evidence that the gap in pay has narrowed over time; men earned an estimated $5148 more per year than their female colleagues (Muench et al., 2015).

Nursing also benefited from the women's movement in more subtle ways. As nursing students were increasingly educated in colleges and universities, they were exposed to campus activism, protests, and organizations that were trying to change the status of women. Learning informal lessons about influence and power and how to foster change had a positive effect on students, who later used this knowledge to improve the status of nursing. With the firm commitment of all of its practitioners, the profession of nursing can give voice to all its members and ultimately contribute to the advancement of society at large.

Image of Nursing

A quick search of images available on a popular search engine using the word "nurse" recently resulted in 15 million results. Of the first 25 images returned in the search, all 25 were stock photos (professional copyrighted photographs for purchase) of young women and men wearing scrubs with their stethoscopes around their necks. This search—in stark contrast to those reported on in previous editions of this text—is remarkably representative of nursing now, with the exception of the youthfulness of those posing as nurses in the photos. The photos show ethnic diversity and a slight overrepresentation of men in nursing. Nurses older than around 30 years are not represented, despite the "graying" problem of the profession as many highly experienced nurses are nearing retirement. Importantly, the highly sexualized images that have plagued the representation of nursing were notably absent among the first 300 images. In the previous edition of this text, published in 2015, the same search returned two cartoon images of White females wearing nurse's caps and white dresses among the first 25 images, and further down the page was a photo of a tired, distressed woman with her hand to her forehead, eyes closed, with the words "nursing crisis" and "JOB" in large capital letters superimposed on her image. One image was of a young Asian woman in a highly sexualized image, wearing a very short, white, fake nursing uniform, complete with a plunging neckline and a large red cross on her chest; the same red cross was on her nursing cap. One was a photo of a nurse in a 1950s-era uniform and cap with a large syringe, smiling into the camera; her words in a text balloon are, "I have no idea what I'm injecting into your child." The author noted: "Finally, gratefully, there is an image of a nurse who appears to be talking to an elderly man in his hospital bed. If this was a representative sample of nursing, it is no wonder that we have a shortage. If this is a representative sample of the public's image of nursing, we have an image problem." The difference between results of the 2015 search and the 2018 search are greatly encouraging in the lack of attention to sexist stereotypes and cartoonish images of nurses and, importantly, the increased attention to diversity and the seriousness of the profession. This is progress.

Images are powerful. They surround us, and we become saturated by images. The images of nurses seen in advertisements and on television shows may be the first and lasting impression that people have of nursing. These impressions based on media images affect public attitudes toward the profession. Although the public's view of nursing has changed over time, most people still do not appreciate the complexity and range of today's professional nursing role.

Nurses are not so identifiable in health care settings as they once were. Once worn by nurses everywhere, caps were for decades a symbol of the profession. In the United States, each school had a unique cap that was instantly recognizable. Nursing schools held capping ceremonies during which they presented caps to students as a symbol of their progress toward graduation. The cap saw its demise by the late 1970s; many, if not most, nurses were glad to forgo wearing a cap, believing it was part of the stereotypical image of nursing. With many different providers involved in the care of patients, there is no distinct way of determining who is an RN. Identification (ID) badges carry titles but may be difficult to read. Interestingly, in the interest of safety, some personnel on certain units, such as urban emergency departments, are no longer putting their last names on their badges or have them in a font so small as to be unreadable in usual emergency department lighting. Some medical centers and hospitals have recently made some movement toward reestablishing identifiable dress norms across health care disciplines. This is often accomplished by having staff of various professions wear attire or scrubs that are distinct in color or style. Others identify registered nurses by "RN" printed in large red letters on ID badges.

The manner in which health professionals address one another is a matter of image. Nurses in most agencies refer to themselves by first name, for example: "Good morning, my name is David, and I'm going to be your nurse for this shift." Physicians usually introduce themselves by title and last name, for example: "I am Dr. Roberts." Nurses rarely refer to each other by last name such as "Ms. Kyle" or "Mr. Pierce," and it is even rarer to hear them refer to each other as "Nurse Kyle" or "Nurse Pierce." Moreover, physicians often refer to nurses by their first names, whereas nurses typically refer to physicians by their title and last name. Nurses have reported being uncomfortable introducing themselves by last name, thinking that it establishes a formality that could interfere with the nurse-patient relationship. Gordon (2005), in an informal survey of approximately 30 laypeople, found that the respondents did not think it would be odd for nurses to refer to themselves more formally. One of the most damaging—and lingering—images of nursing was the portrayal by Louise Fletcher of a cold, sadistic, and controlling psychiatric nurse in the 1975 movie *One Flew Over the Cuckoo's Nest*. Fletcher won an Academy Award for her role as Nurse Ratched, a name that has become synonymous for a cold, uncaring nurse.

In spite of the challenges facing the nursing profession, nurses are well respected by the public and enjoy a generally positive image. In a report released by Gallup in late 2017, for the 16th consecutive year, nurses were rated the highest among a number of professions and occupations on honesty and ethics. Nurses also ranked highest in 1999 and 2000; in 2001, nursing ranked second to firefighters in the wake of the September 11 attacks, at a time when a great deal of positive media coverage focused on firefighters. The full report can be found at https://news.gallup.com/poll/224639/nurses-keep-healthy-lead-honest-ethical-profession.aspx.

Foundations and corporations, as well as nursing groups, have undertaken initiatives to analyze and/or improve nursing's image. Three major initiatives are discussed here.

The Woodhull Study on Nursing and the Media

The Woodhull Study on Nursing and the Media was a comprehensive study of nursing in the print media conducted in September 1997 by 17 students and 3 faculty coordinators from the University of Rochester (New York) School of Nursing (URSN). In this study, sponsored by Sigma Theta Tau International (STTI) and URSN, students examined approximately 20,000 articles from 16 newspapers, magazines, and trade publications. The study was named in memory of Nancy Woodhull, a founding editor of *USA Today*. Woodhull became an advocate of nursing after her diagnosis of lung cancer, when she was impressed with the comprehensive nursing care she received. She suggested the study and assisted in the design of the survey after she became concerned about the absence of media attention to nurses and nursing.

In December 1997 the students presented their findings and recommendations to a mixed audience of nurses and national media representatives at the STTI Biennial Convention. The key finding was that "Nurses and the nursing profession are essentially invisible to the media and, consequently, to the American public" (STTI, 1998, p. 8). The purpose of the Woodhull Study, its major findings, and strategies to guide the nursing profession's collective response are found in Box 2.1.

The Johnson & Johnson Campaign

Johnson & Johnson, the giant health care corporation, began a multimillion-dollar campaign, the Campaign for Nursing's Future, in 2002, "to enhance the image of the nursing profession, recruit new nurses and educators, and to retain nurses currently in the system" (Donelan et al., 2005). This campaign included initiatives in print media, television advertising, student scholarships, fundraising, and research.

BOX 2.1   The Woodhull Study at a Glance

Purpose, Findings, and Recommendations

Purpose of the Study

The Woodhull Study was designed to survey and analyze the portrayal of health care and nursing in U.S. newspapers, news magazines, and health care industry trade publications.

Key Study Findings

1. Nurses and the nursing profession are essentially invisible in media coverage of health care and, consequently, to the American public.
2. Nurses were cited only 4% of the time in the more than 2000 health-related articles gathered from 16 major news publications.
3. The few references to nurses or nursing that did occur were simply mentioned in passing.
4. In many of the stories, nurses and nursing would have been sources more germane to the story subject matter than the references selected.

5. Health care industry publications were no more likely to take advantage of nursing expertise, focusing more attention on bottom-line issues such as business or policy.

Key Study Recommendations

1. Both media and nursing should take more proactive roles in establishing an ongoing dialogue.
2. The often-repeated advice in media articles and advertisements to "consult your doctor" ignores the role of nurses in health care and needs to be changed to "consult your primary health care provider."
3. Journalists should distinguish researchers with doctoral degrees from medical doctors to add clarity to health care coverage.
4. To provide comprehensive coverage of health care, the media should include information by and about nurses.
5. It is essential to distinguish health care from medicine as subject matter in the media.

Modified from Sigma Theta Tau International: *The Woodhull Study on nursing and the media: health care's invisible partner,* Indianapolis, 1998, Sigma Theta Tau International–Center Nursing Press.

The company's efforts are also focused on increasing the number of individuals choosing nursing careers through recruitment and retention of nursing students. The website www.discovernursing.com is popular among nursing students and prospective students. The site has an easy menu of "who," "what," "why," and "how" with drop-down menus that give thorough information about nursing. This website has three portals: one for persons thinking about nursing as a career, one for nursing students, and one for nurses. Each portal contains information about nursing specific to the needs of the user. This landmark effort by a major American corporation provides a stimulus to the nursing profession to partner with other entities to continue the quest for an accurate image of professional nursing, thereby addressing the nursing shortage.

The Truth about Nursing

The Truth about Nursing is a nonprofit organization with the mission to "increase public understanding of the central, front-line role nurses play in modern health care" (Truth about Nursing, 2018). Currently there are local chapters of The Truth about Nursing in many states and numerous nations around the world. Founded in 2001 by Sandy Summers, RN, and a group of seven graduate students at Johns Hopkins University School of Nursing, The Truth about Nursing uses a variety of social media, including Facebook, Twitter, and LinkedIn, among others, to shape the public's image of nursing. Some of their efforts have included convincing a number of major corporations to change their advertising when they have portrayed nurses in a sexualized or otherwise trivialized manner.

Ultimately all nurses hold the professional responsibility to reinforce positive images of nursing and, equally important, to speak out against negative ones. The nursing profession has the major responsibility for improving its own image. The major avenue for changing the image of nursing occurs one nurse-patient encounter at a time, where nurses demonstrate what nurses do and how to look and behave professionally. In addition, organizations such as the ANA can enhance nursing's image by offering services as consultants to media and setting professional standards.

One way in which nursing can take responsibility for its public image is for nurses to become sensitive to portrayals of nurses and nursing in the media. Box 2.2 contains a checklist for monitoring media images of nurses and nursing on TV and in movies; however, you should keep this checklist in mind as you visit websites, read blogs, books, and other media, and notice commercials and advertisements. Then take action:

- Contact those responsible for negative nursing images on television and in movies.
- Contact the companies that sponsor television programs with negative images of nurses.
- Contact the editors of publications that present nursing in a negative manner.
- Boycott programs, films, and products that promote negative images of nurses and nursing.
- Importantly, contact those responsible for excellent portrayals of nurses and the profession of nursing, letting them know that you have noticed and appreciate their efforts.

National Population Trends

Over the course of American nursing history, nurses have responded as individuals and as a profession to

---

BOX 2.2   Checklist for Monitoring Images of Nurses and Nursing in the Media

Prominence in the Plot

1. Are nurse characters seen in leading or supportive roles?
2. Are nurse characters shown taking an active part in the scene, or are they shown primarily in the background (e.g., handing instruments, carrying trays, pushing wheelchairs)?
3. To what extent are nurse characters shown in professional roles, engaged in nursing practice?
4. Do nurse characters or other characters provide the actual nursing care?
5. In scenes with other health care providers, who does most of the talking?

Demographics

1. Does the portrayal show that men, as well as women, may have careers in nursing?
2. Are nurse characters shown to be of varying ages and ethnicities?

Personality Traits

1. Are nurse characters portrayed as:
   a. Intelligent?
   b. Trustworthy?
   c. Confident?
   d. Problem solvers?
   e. Assertive?
   f. Powerful?
   g. Nurturing?
   h. Compassionate?
   i. Kind?
2. If other health care providers are included in the program, how does their portrayal compare with that of nurse characters?
3. When nurse characters exhibit personality traits listed earlier, are they shown as positive traits?

Primary Values

1. Do nurse characters demonstrate value in:
   a. Service to others?
   b. Scholarship, achievement?
2. How do the values portrayed in nurse characters compare to those portrayed in other health professions?
3. When nurse characters exhibit the primary values of scholarship and achievement, do such portrayals show them to be an aberration in the expected values of nurses?

Sexual Objectification of Nurses

1. Are nurse characters portrayed in a sexualized manner?
2. Are nurse characters referred to in sexually demeaning terms?
3. Are nurse characters presented as appealing because of their physical attractiveness as opposed to their intellectual capacity, professional commitment, or skill?

Role of the Nurse

1. Is the profession of nursing shown to be a fulfilling long-term career?
2. Is the work of the nurse characters shown to be creative and exciting?

Career Orientation

1. How important is the career of nursing to the nurse character portrayed?
2. How does this compare with other professionals depicted in the program?

Professional Competence

1. Do nurse characters exhibit autonomous professional judgment?
2. Does the program send a message that a nurse's role in health care is a supportive rather than central one?

BOX 2.2   Checklist for Monitoring Images of Nurses and Nursing in the Media—cont'd

3. Do nurse characters positively influence patient/family welfare?
4. Are nurse characters shown harming or acting to the detriment of patients?
5. How does the professional competence of nurse characters compare with the professional competence of other health care providers?

Education

1. In programs with nursing students, who actually teaches the nursing students?
2. Who appears to be in charge of nursing education?

3. Is there evidence that the practice of nursing requires special knowledge and skills?
4. What is actually taught to nursing students?

Nursing Administration

1. Are any roles filled by nurse administrators or managers, or are all nurse characters shown as staff nurses or students?
2. Is there evidence of a responsible administrative hierarchy in nursing, or are nurses shown answering to physicians or hospital administrators?
3. Overall, is this a positive or negative portrayal of nursing? Why or why not?

Adapted from Kalisch P, Kalisch B: *The changing image of the nurse,* Menlo Park, CA, 1987, Addison-Wesley, Health Sciences Division.

wars, poverty, epidemics, and various social movements. Contemporary nursing also seeks to respond as a profession to social changes that shape our nation and the world. Two in particular will be examined here: the aging population and increasing diversity.

Aging of America

People in the United States are living longer than they have in the past. The median age of the population in 2015 was 37.8 years (meaning that half the population is older than this); by 2030 the projected median is 40.1 years (U.S. Bureau of the Census, 2015). Between the 2000 and 2010 decennial censuses, the population of persons 62 years of age and older increased 21.1%, with 50 million persons (16.2%) of the population being 62 or older (U.S. Bureau of the Census, 2011). Life expectancy in the United States is currently 78.7 years for people born today—76.2 for males and 81.0 for females (Centers for Disease Control and Prevention [CDC], 2015). This means that the people who have lived to 65 years of age are expected to live into their early to middle 80s. The number of people 75 years or older in 2020—well within the working lives of most of today's nursing students—is projected to reach 21.8 million. The very old (older than 85 years) represent the fastest-growing segment of the total population (Fig. 2.12). In contrast, the number of 35- to 44-year-old Americans is expected to decline from 44.7 million in 2000 to 39.6 million by 2020. This phenomenon is sometimes referred to as the "graying of America." The CDC website (www.cdc.gov) lists a tremendous number of age and health statistics.

Persons older than 75 years are more likely than younger persons to be poor, widowed, female, and living alone and are more likely to have chronic conditions such as arthritis, hypertension, and heart disease. As a consequence of these and other factors, this age group uses a disproportionately higher share of health services than other age groups. The leading causes of death in people 65 years of age and older are heart disease, cancer, and chronic lower respiratory disease (CDC, 2016). The oldest "baby boomers"—those Americans born between 1946 and 1964—are well into their retirement years, and the younger baby boomers are in their 50s. This group of citizens will create an increase in the aging population between 2010 and 2030. As these postwar babies enter their 70s, their large numbers are expected to create an additional strain on the health care system. For the first time in U.S. history, the number of elderly people is increasing as the number of adults in early midlife is decreasing. This new disproportion that is projected to occur in the next 20 years will create stress on the economic and social systems of our nation. The graying of America will have a profound effect on the health care system and the nursing profession, stretching an already challenged capacity to provide adequate medical and nursing care.

The nursing profession has responded to the aging population by increasing courses offered in gerontologic nursing to prepare nurses to care for older patients more effectively. Most nursing programs have integrated basic content on nursing care of the elderly into their curricula, and some baccalaureate programs have separate gerontology courses for their undergraduates. Gerontologic

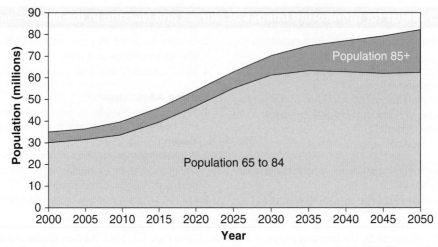

Fig. 2.12 Population projections, ages 65 to 84 years and ages 85 years and older: 2000–2050. (From U.S. Department of Health and Human Services, Health Resources and Services Administration: *Projected Supply, Demand, and Shortages of Registered Nurses: 2000–2020,* Washington, DC, 2002, U.S. Government Printing Office.)

nursing is a specialty in which a nurse can get certification as a generalist, specialist, and NP from the American Nurses Credentialing Center (ANCC). Some schools and colleges of nursing offer master's-level preparation for gerontologic clinical specialists and NPs. In spite of these responses, much remains to be done to prepare nurses for the dramatic increase in the number of aging patients they will encounter in the next few decades.

Diversity

Historically and currently, the United States is widely diverse racially, ethnically, and culturally. The circumstances under which people of varying nationalities have come to the United States range considerably; however, the health care system has always been affected by the change in demographic characteristics of its population. In earlier U.S. history, immigrants were most often from European and Asian countries and often were located in cultural enclaves within major cities. For example, Washington, D.C.; Brooklyn, New York; and San Francisco, California (among many others) are cities with large enclaves of Chinese immigrants in districts known as Chinatown. As described earlier in this chapter, the residents of the tenements of the New York City Lower East Side were often immigrants. Lillian Wald and other nurses responded to their needs by starting what was to become the first visiting nurse association in the United States and had a significant positive effect on the health of residents of the Lower East Side.

Africans were brought to the United States not as immigrants but as slaves. This deeply troubling, shameful, and tragic history continues to affect the lives of African Americans today. Deep distrust of a health care system that exploited African Americans continues. The U.S. Public Health Service Syphilis Study at Tuskegee and the unrestricted use—without permission—of the cell lines of Henrietta Lacks, an African American woman who suffered and died at age 31 of an aggressive adenocarcinoma of the cervix, are examples of exploitation that continue to foment distrust. In a large study of trust in health care institutions across African American, Hispanic, and White populations, Jacobs and colleagues (2011) found that African Americans and Hispanics differed from Whites in that they expected discrimination in the health care system; in particular, African Americans expected to be experimented on, which fostered distrust.

The first decade of the 21st century in the United States was characterized by significant immigration of Latinos from Mexico and other Central and South American countries. People from other nations often have different values, health beliefs, and practices and find that assimilation into the dominant culture is difficult. Instead of blending into American life, individuals from other countries are increasingly appreciated for the uniqueness and flavor they bring to life in the United States. Many prefer to preserve their own cultural heritage rather than becoming "Americanized."

The exact number of persons in the various racial/ethnic groups is difficult to pinpoint. Identifying by race does not necessarily capture all the different cultures that may have migrated from a country. The concept of race as used by the U.S. Census Bureau depends on "self-identification by respondents; that is, the individual's perception of his/her racial identity" (U.S. Bureau of the Census, 2002, p. 5). The U.S. Census Bureau is required to adhere to the Office of Management and Budget's (OMB's) 1997 regulations in classifying race (U.S. Bureau of the Census, 2013). Categories allowable by the OMB are White, Black or African American, American Indian or Alaska Native, Asian, and Native Hawaiian or Other Pacific Islander. People who identify themselves as Hispanic, Latino, or Spanish may be of any race, according to the U.S. Census Bureau (U.S. Bureau of the Census, 2013). People may report being of more than one race. Information on race and ethnicity is critical in policy decision making, including congressional redistricting, civil rights legislation, and promotion of equal employment opportunities. Particularly important to health care is the ability to assess health disparities and environmental risk (CDC, 2013). The next census will occur in 2020 and will likely show significant shifts in race and ethnicity statistics in the United States.

Projections indicate that the White population will become a minority by the middle of the 21st century. This represents a radical change in the historical demographics and attitudes of the nation, with significant implications. Nursing must also change to meet the requirements of persons of varying ethnicities and cultural responses to health and illness. Certain illnesses and health conditions occur disparately across race, ethnicity, and sex. The changing demographics of America represent a significant challenge to nursing.

Diversity in the Profession

To meet the challenge of an increasingly diverse population entering the health care system, nurses need to be educated to be aware and respectful of cultural differences between themselves and their patients and among their patients. The language of cultural education has varied over time, from "cultural competence" to "cultural sensitivity" to a more recent phrase, "cultural humility." This is the view that one understands that he or she cannot be competent in another's culture, but one can take a posture of willingness to learn

and gain experience about other cultures from those who inhabit the culture. Nurses from minority groups are an even smaller minority in nursing, not yet having met the same proportions in the profession as they hold in the population at large. (This is presented in detail in Chapter 1.) Managers, educators, and other nursing leaders will require training so that they can be culturally competent leaders for nurses and students who may have backgrounds different from their own. Attention to the development of nurses who are attuned to culture and cultural differences has become an integral part of progressive nursing education programs. Issues of culture are discussed in detail in Chapter 13.

Technological Developments

The word *technology* seems to be everywhere today and has a place in many domains in health care. For purposes of this basic introduction, four types of technological developments will be discussed: genetic, biomedical, information, and knowledge.

Genetics, genomics, and *epigenetics* are three important words that have shaped and will continue to shape health care for the foreseeable future. Genetics is the science of heredity, and genomics is the study of genomes—DNA sequences. Epigenetics is an important field of study: the examination of the causes of changes in phenotypes or gene expressions not explained by the underlying DNA sequence. The Human Genome Project was a study funded by the National Institutes of Health in which the 20,000 to 25,000 genes on the human genome were mapped out. This took 13 years. The data from the Human Genome Project will continue to have a significant effect on our understanding of health and illness, as well as on predicting who is likely to develop certain conditions, and when.

Pharmacogenetics will have a significant effect on nursing practice eventually, in which the mechanisms and actions of medications can be determined by their genetic structures. This will mean that medications can be prescribed that will be more effective than those that are given generically. For example, advances are being made in chemotherapy for certain cancers, such as leukemias and lymphomas, in which methylation that occurs at the gene level causes the expression of the genes to be aberrant—that is, to go wrong—leading to the development of malignant cell growth. Certain drugs used to treat these cancers are "hypomethylating" agents that reverse the increased, or "hyper," methylation that is occurring in the cells' genetic material.

Biomedical technology involves complex machines or implantable devices used in patient care settings for a variety of reasons—for example, pacemakers, internal automated defibrillators, insulin pumps, artificial organs, and various invasive monitoring systems such as those used to measure intracranial pressure. This form of technology affects nursing practice because nurses assume responsibility for monitoring the data generated from these machines and for assessing the safety and effectiveness of implantable equipment in relation to patient well-being. In many instances, the nurse is called on to react to the data and revise the plan of care. An important consideration in nursing when working in a high-tech environment: do not forget that there is a "human in there" under all of the lines and monitors. The human touch and a word of reassurance are comforting to your patient, and no technology can replace you. Family members usually need help distinguishing monitoring equipment from those technologies that are used to support the patient's basic functions, such as a ventilator. Showing them what you are reading and seeing can be reassuring to them at a time when families are in a great deal of distress.

IT refers to a variety of computer-based applications used to communicate, store, manage, retrieve, and process information. Nurses assumed much of the responsibility for entry and retrieval of data with the development of this technology. Computers are common on nursing units and at the bedside, and with the Centers for Medicare and Medicaid Services' "meaningful use" initiative, most hospitals are moving to electronic health records, as described in Chapter 1. One goal in health care reform includes going "paperless"—that is, that all medical orders, patient records, and other documents will be digitally stored and available for convenient transmittal across various record systems and health care facilities. Any other care provider can access data at any time, as opposed to the single hard copy chart that only one person can view or use at a time.

In some health care organizations, nursing information systems are handheld, allowing nurses to enter and access data about the patient directly from the patient's side, whether in an inpatient, outpatient, or home setting.

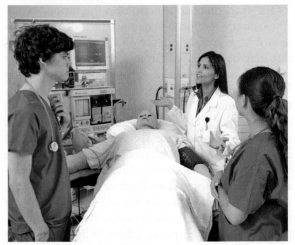

Fig. 2.13 Advanced technology is used to enhance clinical decision making in novices. Here students use a human simulator in a laboratory setting to refine their skills. (Photo courtesy the UNC at Chapel Hill School of Nursing.)

This type of technology allows for more timely documentation of care, and because documentation is done at the time of care, the information is likely to be more accurate. This convenience can come at the expense of patient privacy, and the privacy and confidentiality of patient information are both ethical and legal issues. The Health Insurance Portability and Accountability Act (HIPAA) of 1996 is legislation designed to protect patients' health care information from misuse. A more complete discussion of HIPAA's provisions is found in Chapter 6.

Knowledge technology is described as "technology of the mind." It involves the use of computer systems to transform information into knowledge and to generate new knowledge. Through the creation of "expert systems," this form of technology assists nurses with clinical judgments about patient management problems. An example of knowledge technology includes medication administration systems that prompt the nurse for data before giving a particular medication. Nurse clinicians and nurse leaders should play a role in developing these mechanisms to maximize their effectiveness in improving nursing care and patient outcomes.

In addition, sophisticated human simulation mannequins are gaining popularity in schools of nursing (Fig. 2.13). They make it possible to simulate a clinical event such as cardiac arrest, pneumothorax, or childbirth, allowing the student to practice clinical assessment and intervention skills. One of the benefits of computerized expert systems is that they can provide practice in decision making for novice nurses and nurses who may be working outside their area of expertise without increased risk to a patient. Simulation training is common in other professions such as aviation where the stakes are very high in the event of a mistake. Learning to manage crises in simulated situations allows a person to become confident in his or her skills and accustomed to working under pressure without the risk of harm.

As technology becomes more pervasive, nurses must be very intentional in providing compassionate, personalized care for patients. Technological advances such as telehealth (described in Chapter 1) now allow nurses to monitor their patients' conditions remotely. Without even seeing the patient in person, nurses can gather large amounts of data and make nursing decisions based on that information. As nurses rely more on technology, they may actually spend less time with the patient, with the possibility of creating dissatisfaction for patients and families. Although being able to monitor one's patient on a telemetry unit from the nurses' station is convenient and practical, monitoring of a contraction pattern and fetal heart rate from the nurses' station in a labor and birth suite diminishes the nurse's role to one of labor and fetal surveillance rather than labor support. The use of technology must be applied carefully and never take the place of human-to-human contact and interaction. Successfully combining technology and caring requires sensitivity to patients' physical, emotional, and spiritual needs. This has always been a part of nursing's skill set.

Nursing Shortages

Periodic imbalances are not uncommon between the numbers of nurses working and the number of available nursing positions. Over many decades, there have been rare, brief periods of oversupply of nurses and more frequent and longer-lasting nursing shortages. By far the more common concern is an inadequate supply of RNs to meet the health care needs of the nation.

The term *nursing shortage* can be misleading because actual shortages are usually confined to institutional settings such as hospitals and nursing homes. Causes of shortages may be seen as either external or internal. Internal causes include salary issues, long hours, increased responsibility for unlicensed workers, and significant responsibility with little authority. External causes include changes in demand for nursing services, the increasing age of the American population, greater acuity (degree of illness) of hospitalized individuals, public perceptions of nursing as a profession, and ever-widening career options for women.

A key aspect of recent nursing shortages is the shortage of nursing faculty. Qualified applicants are often denied admission to U.S. schools of nursing because of insufficient numbers of faculty, clinical sites, and classroom space. Faculty shortages are attributed to several factors. First, doctorally prepared and master's degree–prepared faculty are now, on average, more than 50 years of age, foreshadowing a large number of retirements in the next decade. Second, nurses with advanced degrees who are otherwise eligible for faculty appointments are being hired into more lucrative private sector or clinical positions. Third, not enough doctorate- and master's-level graduates are being produced to meet the demands of nursing education. The American Association of Colleges of Nursing (AACN) continues to search for remedies for this situation (AACN, 2012).

In the past, each time a shortage of RNs became serious, two solutions were attempted: (1) increase the supply of nurses, and (2) create a less trained worker to supplement the number of nurses. Practical nursing programs, which produce graduates in only 1 year, were created to meet civilian and military needs of the United States during World War II. The nursing shortage of the 1950s stimulated a desire to shorten basic RN programs, and 2-year associate degree programs were the result. In the 1960s, shortages led to the creation of the position of unit manager; this manager was expected to take over certain tasks to relieve nurses, who could then concentrate on providing patient care. The 1970s produced other new positions, such as emergency medical technicians, physician assistants, respiratory therapists, and others who took on various aspects of patient care formerly performed by nurses. The shortage of nurses in the late 1980s resulted in a proposal by the American Medical Association to create yet another "nurse extender" called the *registered care technician*. However, this initiative was short lived as nurses responded quickly and negatively, with nurse leaders stating that nurses could not be responsible for direct caregivers that nurses had not trained.

Another method of increasing the supply of nurses is to import them from other English-speaking countries. Nurses from the United Kingdom, Australia, New Zealand, certain Caribbean islands, South Africa, and the Philippines are targeted for recruitment. Companies have been established to prepare them to take the National Council Licensure Examination for Registered Nurses (NCLEX-RN®) successfully to practice in this country. The ethics of this solution are addressed in Chapter 7.

Shortages are often limited to certain geographic areas or specialties. In those cases, redistributing RNs who are already licensed can be seen as a solution. Many agencies specialize in providing nurses for short-term assignments, often called *traveling nurses*. Travel nursing can provide individual nurses with opportunities to live in and experience different parts of the country and world, but there is little incentive for traveling nurses to work toward long-term goals on the units where they are, for all practical purposes, filling in until a permanent nurse can be hired.

Explaining why there is a shortage is complex. Like many issues in nursing, there is no simple explanation. What is known is that the shortage exists and is more crucial in traditional settings such as hospitals and long-term care facilities. One reason for the shortage is an increased demand for nurses because of the growth in total population, especially an aging population that has extensive health care needs. The shortage is also compounded by the fact that the nursing workforce is aging, and the number of new entrants to the profession may not keep pace with the numbers who are exiting. Recent data suggests, however, that RNs have been delaying retirement, which resulted in a 5% (136,000) increase in the nursing workforce in 2012 (Auerbach et al., 2014). Auerbach and colleagues (2014) speculated that changes in health care delivery will increase demand for RNs as care coordinators or managers and in ambulatory care, which may be attractive to older RNs who want to move out of hospital settings but continue to work.

Initiatives to Provide a Stable Workforce of Registered Nurses

Recognizing that dramatic swings in the supply of and demand for RNs harm the profession, jeopardize patient care, and are costly to nurses and their employers, organizations inside and outside of nursing have called for mechanisms to ensure more even distribution of the workforce. Here are four major initiatives that made or are making an impact on the nursing workforce:

- The American Recovery and Reinvestment Act of 2009, the goal of which was to stimulate the U.S. economy, had a provision for $500 million to strengthen the U.S. health care workforce. This included the training and education of the next generation of nurses and physicians.
- The Robert Wood Johnson Foundation (RWJF), a private foundation that funds innovative health care initiatives, committed tens of millions of dollars to pursuing programs that help nursing schools, hospitals, and other health care agencies create regional workforce development systems. This initiative was named Colleagues in Caring.
- Johnson & Johnson's Campaign for Nursing's Future was mentioned earlier. Johnson & Johnson is working in partnership with the National Student Nurses Association (NSNA), the NLN, the ANA, the Association of Nurse Executives (AONE), and the STTI Honor Society of Nursing.
- The ANCC Magnet Recognition Program is a model for employers to earn the designation "employer of choice" by implementing a model program designed to attract and retain nurses in acute hospital settings.

Numerous other initiatives by nursing associations, colleges of nursing, and states are also under way.

Nursing faces numerous challenges related to the social context in which it finds itself today. Yet in the history of nursing, nurses have risen to the challenges they face, improving the terrible conditions in war, developing public health initiatives, and becoming proactive in shaping their public image. The challenges to the upcoming generation of nurses may be completely unforeseen, such as the HIV epidemic that challenged nurses in the 1980s. Nurses have confronted the challenges of yesterday and today with ingenuity and intelligence and have set the stage for the next generation to continue this legacy.

CONCEPTS AND CHALLENGES

- *Concept:* In 1860 Florence Nightingale founded a school for nurses at St. Thomas' Hospital, London, which became the model for nursing education in the United States. Formal nursing education programs were established in the United States in 1873.

  Challenge: Nursing must continue to evolve in response to its social context. This means that nursing education must continue to evolve.

- *Concept:* The period between the 1893 World's Fair and 1908 marked a time of organizing for nurses, including the formation of forerunners of the NLN and the ANA.

  Challenge: The evolution of the profession depends on visionary nurses to take leadership roles now and in the future.

- *Concept:* The initiation of state licensure in 1903 meant that nursing education programs would be standardized. Until then, nursing education varied widely.

  Challenge: With the rapid evolution of nursing practice opportunities, consistent, thorough education is particularly important.

- *Concept:* The establishment of the Henry Street Settlement and the rise of community health nursing played a major role in the widespread public acceptance of nurses.

  Challenge: Remembering that nursing has led significant social changes in the past, we can draw inspiration and guidance from the work of nurses such as Lillian Wald, who faced tremendous challenges to care for immigrants and others in poverty, poor living conditions, and poor health.

- *Concept:* Nursing has responded to wars, epidemics, and economic disasters that created a high demand for nursing care. Hospital expansion, technological advances, and social changes have created new and progressively autonomous roles for nurses, especially advanced practice nurses.

  Challenge: The profession of nursing must remain vigilant for new, promising spheres of practice.

- *Concept:* The nursing shortage is projected to increase in the next few years.

  Challenge: Identifying and responding to the cause of shortages, such as the shortage of nursing faculty, will require the attention of nurse leaders.

- *Concept:* New data suggest that men in nursing earn more than $5000 more per year than do women, regardless of setting, specialty, or position.

  Challenge: Nurse leaders and employers must act to correct the injustice of pay inequity.

- *Concept:* Nurses have been stereotyped in the media, which has resulted in misperceptions and lack of clarity by the public about what nurses do and their importance in health care.

  Challenge: Individual nurses must act when nursing is presented in an unfavorable light in the media. Responsibility for the image of the profession belongs to all nurses.

IDEAS FOR FURTHER EXPLORATION

1. Florence Nightingale is often credited with being the first nurse researcher. What were her contributions to the science of nursing?

2. Consider the significance of the events that occurred during the Chicago World's Fair, 1893, to the advancement of the nursing profession. What would nurse leaders address today if they were to hold a leadership summit across all domains of the profession?

3. Think about the role the military had in opening the profession of nursing for African Americans and other minorities, including men. Why did nursing require military conflicts to expand entry into the profession to minorities?

4. How has being a profession in which most practitioners are women influenced the development of nursing?

5. What do you think accounts for the documented pay inequity between women and men in nursing? What challenges do you think nursing leaders and employers should take to correct pay inequity?

6. Describe your idea of the "perfect" nurse. What stereotypes does your description reveal? Does your image of the perfect nurse include a particular gender, race, ethnic group, or generation?

7. Think about social factors that have the potential to stimulate or stifle interest in nursing as a profession. What effects—positive and negative—could these factors have on nursing? What recommendations do you have for the profession to address these factors?

REFERENCES

American Assembly for Men in Nursing (AAMN): *Purpose and objectives*, 2015 (website). Available at: www.aamn.org.

American Association of Colleges of Nursing (AACN): *Media paper on the nursing and nursing faculty shortage*, 2012 (website). Available at: www.aacn.nche.edu/media-relations/fact-sheets/nursing-faculty-shortage.

Auerbach D, Buerhaus P, Staiger D: Registered nurses are delaying retirement, a shift that has contributed to recent growth in the nurse workforce, *Health Aff* 33(8):1474–1480, 2014.

Barton C: *Diary: The papers of Clara Barton (1812–1912)*, Washington, DC, 1862, Library of Congress, Manuscript Division.

Carnegie ME: *The path we tread: blacks in nursing, 1854–1994*, Philadelphia, 1995, JB Lippincott.

Centers for Disease Control and Prevention: *Health, United States*, 2013 (website). Available at: www.cdc.gov/nchs/data/hus/hus13.pdf#016.

Centers for Disease Control and Prevention: *Older persons' health*, 2016 (website). Available at: https://www.cdc.gov/nchs/fastats/older-american-health.htm.

Cherry B, Jacob S: *Contemporary Nursing: Issues, Trends and Management*, St. Louis, 2005, Mosby.

Dock LL, Stewart IM: *A Short History of Nursing*, New York, 1920, Putnam.

Donahue MP: *Nursing: the finest art: an illustrated history*, ed 2, Philadelphia, 1996, Mosby.

Donelan K, Buerhaus PI, Ulrich BT, et al.: Awareness and perceptions of the Johnson & Johnson Campaign for Nursing's Future: Views from nursing students, RNs, and CNOs, *Nurs Econ* 23(4):150–156, 2005.

Gill CJ, Gill GC: Nightingale in Scutari: her legacy reexamined, *Clin Infect Dis* 40(12):1799–1805, 2005.

Gordon S: *Nursing against the odds: health care cost cuts, media stereotypes, and medical hubris undermine nurses and patient care*, Ithaca, NY, 2005, Cornell University Press.

Jacobs EA, Mendenhall E, McAlearney AS, et al.: An exploratory study of how trust in health care institutions varies across African American, Hispanic and white populations, *Commun Med* 8(1):89–98, 2011.

Kalisch PA, Kalisch BJ: *American nursing : a history*, ed 4, Philadelphia, PA, 2004, Lippincott Williams & Wilkins.

Kennedy D: *Birth control in America: the career of Margaret Sanger*, New Haven, CT, 1970, Yale University Press.

Miller HS: *America's first black professional nurse*, Atlanta, 1986, Wright Publishing.

Monsivais DB: Finding the (cultural) clues that make a difference in patient outcomes, *Nurs Clin North Am* 46:xi–xiii, 2011.

Muench U, Sindelar J, Busch SH, Buerhaus PI: Salary differences between male and female registered nurses in the United States, *JAMA* 313(12):1265–1267, 2015.

Nightingale F: *Notes on nursing: what it is and what it is not*, [reprint]. Philadelphia, 1946, JB Lippincott (originally published in 1859).

Oates SB: *A woman of valor*, New York, 1994, The Free Press.

100 Great Black Britons, 2015. Available at: www.100greatblackbritons.com, 2015.

Palmer S: The editor, *Am J Nurs* 1(1):64, 1900.

Pember PY: *A southern woman's story*, Atlanta, 1959, Bill Wiley.

Sigma Theta Tau International (STTI): *The Woodhull study on nursing and the media: health care's invisible partner*, Indianapolis, 1998, Sigma Theta Tau International–Center Nursing Press.

Sleet J: A successful experiment, *Am J Nurs* 2:729, 1901.

Spartacus Educational: Mary Seacole, 2014 (website). Available at: http://spartacus-educational.com/REseacole.htm.

Truth about nursing: mission statement (website). Available at: www.truthaboutnursing.org, 2018.

U.S. Bureau of the Census: *Statistical abstract of the United States: 2002*, Washington, DC, 2002, U.S. Government Printing Office.

U.S. Bureau of the Census: *Age and sex composition, census briefs*, 2011 (website). Available at: www.census.gov/prod/cen2010/briefs/c2010br-03.pdf.

U.S. Bureau of the Census: *Race* (website). Available at: www.census.gov/topics/population/race/about.html, 2013.

U.S. Bureau of the Census: *National summary tables*, 2015 (website). Available at: www.census.gov/population/projections/data/national/2014/summarytables.

Wall BM: Courage to care: the Sisters of the Holy Cross in the Spanish-American War, *Nurs Hist Rev* 3:55–77, 1995.

3

Nursing's Pathway to Professionalism

Beth Perry Black, PhD, RN, FAAN

ⓔ To enhance your understanding of this chapter, try the Student Exercises on the Evolve site at http://evolve.elsevier.com/Black/professional.

LEARNING OUTCOMES

After studying this chapter, students will be able to:

- Identify the characteristics of a profession.
- Distinguish between the characteristics of professions and occupations.
- Describe how professions evolve.
- Identify barriers to nursing's development as a profession.

- Explain the elements of nursing's contract with society.
- Recognize characteristic behaviors that exemplify professional nurses.
- Assess themselves in the development of professional conduct.

The word *professional* shows up in everyday conversation and in the media. A professional athlete is one who is paid and is no longer considered an amateur. A professional stunt actor is one whose dangerous activities should not be "tried at home"—according to warning messages at the bottom of your monitor or TV screen. Job seekers are encouraged to "look professional" when applying for a position. Services such as dry cleaning, lawn care, and plumbing are often referred to as "professional" when they are rendered by someone with specific expertise or tools of their trade.

Historically, physic (medicine), law, and divinity (clergy) were considered "learned professions." Over time, however, the meaning of *profession* has expanded to include other domains of work and career, including nursing. You will learn in this chapter various characteristics of a profession and how nursing fits those characteristics. Furthermore, you will learn what **professionalism** means generally and what professionalism in nursing means specifically.

CHARACTERISTICS OF A PROFESSION

For nearly a century, scholars have grappled with the meaning of **profession**. They have generally agreed that a profession is an occupational group with a set of attitudes or behaviors, or both. In the early 1900s the Carnegie Foundation issued a series of papers about professional schools. In 1910 Abraham Flexner, a sociologist, published what became groundbreaking work for reform in medical education, calling on medical schools to implement high standards for admission and graduation and to follow long-accepted tenets of science in teaching and research (Flexner, 1910). Five years after his initial report, Flexner published a list of criteria that he believed were characteristic of all true professions (Flexner, 1915). These criteria stipulate that a profession:

1. Is basically intellectual (as opposed to physical) and is accompanied by a high degree of individual responsibility

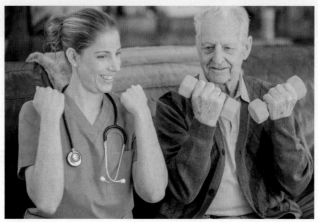

Fig. 3.1 According to experts, professionals are motivated by *altruism,* a desire to help others. (Photo used with permission from iStockphoto.)

2. Is based on a body of knowledge that can be learned and is developed and refined through research
3. Is both practical and theoretical
4. Can be taught through a process of highly specialized professional education
5. Has a strong internal organization of members and a well-developed group consciousness
6. Has practitioners who are motivated by altruism (the desire to help others) and who are responsive to public interests (Fig. 3.1)

Since the 1910 report was published, Flexner's criteria have been widely used as the benchmark for determining the professional status of various occupations and have had a profound influence on professional education in several disciplines, including nursing. In 1968 R. H. Hall, a sociologist, published his work on professionalism. Similar to Flexner's criteria, Hall (1968) described a professional model with five attributes of professions:

1. Use of a professional organization as a primary point of reference
2. Belief in the value of public service
3. Belief in self-regulation
4. Commitment to a profession that goes beyond economic incentives
5. A sense of autonomy in practice

Recognizing the uniqueness of disciplines, Hall recommended each profession develop its own methods of measuring professionalism. In recent years, individuals and groups have continued to identify what professionals believe, think, and do. In the 1990s a pharmacy profession task force spent 5 years studying and promoting pharmacy student professionalism (Task Force on Professionalism, 2000). This task force, in examining the history of professional development in a broad sense, reviewed the work of numerous scholars. From this review they found that members of a profession share the following 10 characteristics:

1. Prolonged specialized training in a body of abstract knowledge
2. A service orientation
3. An ideology based on the original faith professed by members
4. An ethic that is binding on the practitioners
5. A body of knowledge unique to the members
6. A set of skills that forms the technique of the profession
7. A guild of those entitled to practice the profession
8. Authority granted by society in the form of licensure or certification
9. A recognized setting in which the profession is practiced
10. A theory of societal benefits derived from the ideology

Although scholars have not always agreed on the number of criteria and the types of behaviors and characteristics of professions, three criteria consistently appear: service/altruism, specialized knowledge, and autonomy/ethics (Carr-Saunders and Wilson, 1933; Flexner, 1915; Hall, 1968, 1982; Huber, 2000).

FROM OCCUPATION TO PROFESSION

The distinction between an occupation and a profession is not always clear. The term occupation is often used interchangeably with the term *profession,* but their definitions differ. *Collins English Dictionary* (2018) defines *occupation* as "that which chiefly engage one's time; [one's] trade, profession, or business." In this discussion, Huber's (2000) definition of *profession* is used to make the distinction between an occupation and a profession: "a calling, vocation, or form of employment that provides a needed service to society and possesses characteristics of expertise, autonomy, long academic preparation, commitment, and responsibility" (p. 34).

Professions usually evolved from occupations that originally consisted of tasks but developed more specialized educational pathways and publicly legitimized status. The earliest recognized "learned" professions (law, medicine, and divinity) generally followed a sequential development. First, practitioners of these professions performed full-time work in the discipline. They then determined work standards, identified a body of knowledge, and established educational programs in institutions of higher learning. Next, they promoted organization into effective occupational associations and then worked to establish legal protection that limited practice of their unique skills by outsiders. Finally, they established codes of ethics (Carr-Saunders and Wilson, 1933). This is the process known as professionalization.

The evolution from occupation to profession was further analyzed by Houle (1980), who identified a number of characteristics that indicate that an occupational group is moving along the continuum toward professional status. Defining the group's mission and foundations of practice is the first step, followed by the mastery of theoretical knowledge, development of the capacity to solve problems, use of practical knowledge, and self-enhancement (continued learning and development). Finally, Houle described the necessity of the development of a collective identity as an occupation evolves into a profession. Signs of a developing collective identity, and hence a profession, include formal training, credentialing, creation of a subculture, legal right to practice, public acceptance, ethical practice, discipline of incompetent/unethical practitioners, relationship to other practitioners, and formalization of the relationship of practitioners of the profession to users of the practitioners' services.

In an analysis of the concept of professionalism in nursing, Ghadirian and colleagues (2014) determined three attributes of professionalism. First, through nursing education, nurses develop a cognitive framework to understand the profession of nursing, including how and why to conduct oneself in a professional manner, with the goal of learning to prioritize and make decisions correctly in practice. This means that nursing education should be consistent across formal settings for training. Second, nurses acquire professional values (beliefs and ideals) that are consistent across individuals and groups and continue to develop these values through experiences that shape one's professional identity. Third, standards of practice and psychomotor competencies are requirements of professionalism in nursing. Common descriptors of professional behavior were *safety* and *competency.*

Professional Preparation

A profession is different from an occupation in at least two major ways—preparation and commitment (Table 3.1). Professional preparation, typically taking place in a college or university, requires instruction in the specialized body of knowledge and techniques of the profession. In addition to knowledge and skills, professional preparation includes orientation to the beliefs, values, and attitudes expected of the members of the profession, as well as the standards of practice and ethical considerations. These components of professional education are part of the process of socialization into a profession and are discussed in more detail in Chapter 5. This intense preparation enables professional practitioners to act in a logical, rational manner using scientific knowledge and prescribed ways of thinking through problems rather than relying on simple problem solving, custom, intuition, or trial and error. The nursing process, described in detail in Chapter 11, is an example of how the profession of nursing uses scientific knowledge and prescribed ways of thinking through patient problems amenable to nursing care.

Professional Commitment

Professionals are usually highly committed to their work, deriving much of their personal identification from it, and consider it an integral part of their lives; some people even refer to their profession as their "calling" (see Fig. 3.2). Historically, professionals' commitment to their profession has transcended their expectation of

TABLE 3.1	Comparing Occupations and Professions
Occupation	**Profession**
Training may occur on the job.	Education takes place in a college or university.
Length of training varies.	Education is prolonged.
Work is largely manual.	Work involves mental creativity.
Decision making is guided largely by experience or by trial and error.	Decision making is based largely on science or theoretical constructs (evidence-based practice).
Values, beliefs, and ethics are not prominent features of preparation.	Values, beliefs, and ethics are an integral part of preparation.
Commitment and personal identification vary.	Commitment and personal identification are strong.
Workers are supervised.	Workers are autonomous.
People often change jobs.	People are unlikely to change professions.
Material reward is main motivation.	Commitment transcends material reward.
Accountability rests primarily with employer.	Accountability rests with individual.

material reward. The strong identity that professionals develop means that it is common for them to change careers compared with persons involved in occupations, which may not involve such a strong commitment and identity.

Interprofessionality

Educators across health care professions have recognized the importance of the development of core competencies for their students (and future practitioners) in response to initiatives calling for more teamwork across disciplines and team-based care. *Interprofessionality* is a "process by which professionals reflect on and develop ways of practicing that provides an integrated and cohesive answer to the needs of the client/family/population … [involving] continuous interaction and knowledge sharing between professionals" (D'Amour and Oandasan, 2005, p. 9). The World Health Organization (WHO) noted that in the current global climate, "it is no longer enough for health workers to be professional …. [They] also need to be interprofessional" (World Health Organization, 2010, p. 36). The Interprofessional Education Collaborative Expert Panel Report (2011) identified four domains of interprofessional collaborative practice competency:

1. Values/ethics for interprofessional practice
2. Roles/responsibilities
3. Interprofessional communication
4. Teams and teamwork

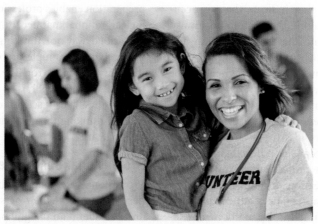

Fig. 3.2 Nurses often put their skills to use as volunteers, as part of their strong commitment to their profession and to helping others. (Photo used with permission from iStockphoto.)

The Institute of Medicine (now the National Academy of Medicine, 2015), in a robust effort to ensure optimal patient outcomes, challenged American health care educators and providers to expand the traditional view of separate professional foci and to consider alternate ways of shaping education and models of care. Interprofessional education (IPE) across disciplines such as nursing, medicine, social work, pharmacy, and others has gained significant momentum. Although IPE is receiving increasing emphasis in health educational settings, there is a current gap in practice that will depend on the development of a workforce for which IPE has provided with skills and knowledge to address the health needs of individuals and communities (Derouin et al., 2018).

NURSING'S PATHWAY TO PROFESSIONALISM

The question of whether nursing is a profession was debated for decades. In the mid-20th century, Roy Bixler and Genevieve Bixler examined nursing's status as a profession. Bixler and Bixler, neither of whom were nurses but both of whom were advocates and supporters of nursing, used seven criteria that are similar to those listed earlier in this chapter. In 1959 they reappraised nursing, noting progress in nursing's professional development (Bixler and Bixler, 1959). More recently, nurse leaders, rather than those outside of nursing, have explored the professionalization of nursing.

Kelly's Criteria

Lucie Kelly, RN, PhD, FAAN, is an outstanding nurse writer, teacher, and influential leader. Now retired from Columbia University, Kelly was editor of the journal *Nursing Outlook* and president of Sigma Theta Tau International Honor Society of Nursing, among many career highlights. Dr. Kelly has spent much of her nursing career exploring the dimensions of professional nursing. Although she compiled the following set of eight characteristics of a profession many years ago, contemporary nursing still embodies these characteristics (Kelly, 1981, p. 157):

1. The services provided are vital to humanity and the welfare of society.
2. There is a special body of knowledge that is continually enlarged through research.

3. The services involve intellectual activities; individual responsibility (**accountability**) is a strong feature.
4. Practitioners are educated in institutions of higher learning.
5. Practitioners are relatively independent and control their own policies and activities (**autonomy**).
6. Practitioners are motivated by service (**altruism**) and consider their work an important component of their lives.
7. There is a code of ethics to guide the decisions and conduct of practitioners.
8. There is an organization (**association**) that encourages and supports high standards of practice.

The Services Provided Are Vital to Humanity and the Welfare of Society

If you ask nursing students why they want to become nurses, the most likely answer would be "to help people." You yourself may have included a statement like this in your application to nursing school. Nursing provides services that are essential to the well-being of people and to society as a whole. The word *services,* however, minimizes the essence of nursing; **caring** is the core of professional nursing, shaping the way that nurses interact with and intervene on behalf of their patients. Nursing interventions in the most general sense are the "services" nurses provide. Nursing is essential in today's world, providing vital care to humanity and the welfare of society.

There Is a Special Body of Knowledge That Is Continually Enlarged Through Research

Nursing has an increasingly well-developed body of knowledge. Nursing has its own doctor of philosophy (PhD), a research degree earned by nurses at the highest levels of education. Through research, the specialized body of knowledge for nursing is developed. In the past, nurse researchers often had PhDs from other academic disciplines, and nursing science was based on principles borrowed from the physical and social sciences. As opposed to practice based in problem-solving earlier in our history, the basis for current nursing practice is theory and research. One of the key principles of **evidence-based practice** is the use of research evidence. You will learn more about theory, research, and evidence-based practice in later chapters.

The Services Involve Intellectual Activities; Individual Responsibility (Accountability) Is a Strong Feature

Nursing is a cognitive (mental) activity that requires both critical and creative thinking and serves as the basis for providing nursing care. Nursing developed and refined its own unique approach to practice, called the *nursing process.* (You will learn more about the nursing process in Chapter 11.)

Individual accountability in nursing has become a hallmark of practice. Accountability, according to the American Nurses Association's (ANA's) *Code of Ethics for Nurses,* is being answerable to someone for something one has done. Provision 4.4 of the Code states, "Nurses are accountable and responsible for the assignment or delegation of nursing activities" (ANA, 2015, p. 17). Furthermore, accountability is firmly rooted in the ethical principles of "fidelity (faithfulness), loyalty, veracity, beneficence, and respect for the dignity, worth, and self-determination of patients" (p. 15).

Practitioners Are Educated in Institutions of Higher Learning

The first university-based nursing program began in 1909 at the University of Minnesota. Three decades later, Esther Lucille Brown (1948) wrote *Nursing for the Future,* calling for nursing education to be based in universities and colleges. In 1965 the ANA published a significant position paper, taking the official position that all nursing education should take place in institutions of higher education (ANA, 1965).

The debate about entry level into practice continues. Despite the ANA's long-held position, associate degree nursing (ADN) programs remain the major source of entry-level registered nurses (RNs) entering the workforce today; however, the number of bachelor of science in nursing (BSN) programs in colleges and universities has increased in the past 30 years, and increasing numbers of RNs with ADN degrees are returning to colleges and universities to earn their BSN degree. In addition, the number of nurses prepared at the master's and doctoral levels continues to increase, although that number is small compared with other health professions.

Practitioners Are Relatively Independent and Control Their Own Policies and Activities (Autonomy)

Licensure by state boards of nursing means that nurses are autonomous practitioners who are responsible for their own practice. *Autonomy* means that one has control over one's practice. Although nursing actions are independent, most RNs are employed in settings in which nurses carry out prescriptions for care or medical regimens by physicians, nurse practitioners, or physician assistants. Recently, nurses who understand that language matters have criticized the use of the phrase "doctor's orders": the word *orders* connotes obedience and thus has outlived its usefulness (Reuter and Fitzsimons, 2013). Although nursing practice acts in many states establish and acknowledge nurses' independent practice, nurses occasionally face constraints on practice in settings in which their scope of practice can be narrowed by their employer or a supervising physician.

Three groups have historically attempted to control nursing practice: organized nursing, organized medicine, and health service administration. *Organized* in this context refers to the collective professional bodies that are the voice speaking for the interests of their respective professions, specifically the ANA and the American Medical Association (AMA), although other organizations have vested interests in these professions too. The interests of these groups are often expressed through lobbying efforts at the state and federal levels to influence legislative decisions that benefit their constituencies. Organizations such as National Nurses United (NNU) and its affiliates use collective bargaining and other strategies to protect the interests of nurses and patients. Although the discussion of nursing unionization is beyond the scope of this chapter, you will find the NNU website (www.nationalnursesunited.org) to be very informative regarding organized nursing's efforts to keep the best interests of nursing, and therefore patients, front and center in the evolution of health care in the United States today.

Both the medical profession and health service administration have attempted to limit the autonomy of nursing to hinder financial competition for patients by nurses in independent practice. Medicine and health service administration are well organized and well funded and have powerful lobbies at state and national levels, posing a major challenge to full autonomy for nurses. Conversely, organized nursing does not yet have available economic resources to compete effectively against these influential forces seeking to minimize nursing autonomy.

The Magnet Recognition Program®, an initiative of the American Nurses Credentialing Center (ANCC), is a credential demonstrating organizational recognition of nursing excellence. By the end of 2016, 445 (9%) hospitals had achieved Magnet designation, most in the United States and a few internationally (ANCC, 2017). The Magnet credential was established to recognize hospitals that attract and retain nurses, acknowledging that this achieves better patient outcomes. Nursing autonomy and control over practice were identified in 1983 as crucial characteristics of these hospitals.

In the 2010 National Survey of Registered Nurses, nurses in Magnet hospitals rated their workplace organization and participation in shared governance higher than did nurses in non-Magnet hospitals; however, there were no differences between Magnet and non-Magnet hospitals with respect to influence on decisions related to patient care, and only 37% of Magnet nurses rated their opportunities to participate in shared governance as very good or excellent (Hess et al., 2011). This implies that nursing still has a significant way to go to become autonomous and to incorporate this value into the culture of nursing.

Practitioners Are Motivated by Service (Altruism) and Consider Their Work an Important Component of Their Lives

As a group, nurses are dedicated to the ideal of service to others, also known as *altruism*. The desire to "help people" is foundational to altruism. Moreover, many, if not most, nurses consider nursing to be a key part of their identity and recognize that their work is important. The ideal of service has sometimes become intertwined with economic issues and historically has been exploited by employers of nurses. Although no one questions the rights of other professionals to charge reasonable fees for the services they render, nurses' altruism is sometimes questioned when they demand higher compensation and better working conditions. Tension exists between organized nursing and those nurses who see collective bargaining as antithetical to the ideal of nursing as altruistic. Nurses must take responsibility for their own financial well-being and for the economic health of the profession. This will, in turn, ensure its continued attractiveness to those considering nursing as a profession.

Commitment to a profession is not a value equally shared by all nurses. Some nurses still regard nursing as simply a job, leaving and returning to practice in response to economic and family needs. This flexible approach, although appealing to many nurses and

---

BOX 3.1 The Florence Nightingale Pledge

I solemnly pledge myself before God and in the presence of this assembly to pass my life in purity and to practice my profession faithfully.

I will abstain from whatever is deleterious and mischievous, and will not take or knowingly administer any harmful drug. I will do all in my power to maintain and elevate the standard of my profession, and will hold in confidence all personal matters committed to my keeping and all family affairs coming to my knowledge in the practice of my calling.

With loyalty will I endeavor to aid the physician in his work and devote myself to the welfare of those committed to my care.

From Dock LL, Stewart IM: *A short history of nursing,* New York, 1920, Putnam.

---

conducive to management of family responsibilities, may inadvertently delay the development of professional attitudes and behaviors for the profession as a whole.

There Is a Code of Ethics to Guide the Decisions and Conduct of Practitioners

A code of ethics provides professional standards and a framework for moral decision making; however, the code does not stipulate how an individual should act in a specific situation. The trust placed in the nursing profession by the public requires that nurses act with integrity. Both the International Council of Nurses and the ANA, among others, have established codes of nursing ethics articulating standards of ethical practice.

In 1893, long before these codes were written, "The Florence Nightingale Pledge" (Box 3.1) was created by a committee headed by Lystra Eggert Gretter and presented to the Farrand Training School for Nurses located at Harper Hospital in Detroit, Michigan (Dock and Stewart, 1920). The Nightingale Pledge functioned as nursing's first code of ethics; it has historical value, and it established the roots for our current code.

There Is an Organization (Association) That Encourages and Supports High Standards of Practice

The ANA is the official voice of nursing and therefore is the primary advocate for nursing interests in general. The ANA is a federation of state nurses associations that all RNs are eligible to join. Membership in a state

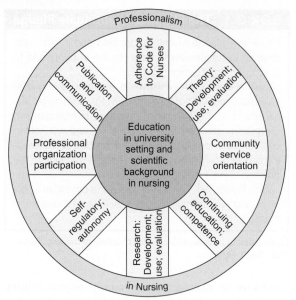

Fig. 3.3 The Wheel of Professionalism in nursing. (Copyright 1984 Barbara Kemp Miller.)

nurses association automatically conveys membership in the ANA. According to the bylaws, the purposes of the ANA are to work for the improvement of health standards and the availability of health care services for all people, to foster high standards of nursing, and to stimulate and promote the professional development of nurses and advance their economic and general welfare (ANA, 2008). The ANA continues to be limited by the relatively low percentage of nurses (fewer than 10%) who belong to the ANA and their constituent state nurses associations. This represents significant political influence that is yet unrealized for the profession.

Miller's Wheel of Professionalism in Nursing

Miller (1985; Adams and Miller, 2001) created a model, the Wheel of Professionalism, based on common themes she identified in the work of sociologists and nursing leaders, as well as statements from *Nursing's Social Policy Statement* and *Code of Ethics for Nurses.* The wheel's center represents the essential foundation of nursing education in an institution of higher learning (Fig. 3.3). According to Adams and associates (1996):

Each of the eight spokes represents other behaviors deemed necessary in maintaining or increasing

nurses' professionalism. They are competence and continuing education; adherence to the code of ethics; participation in the primary and referent professional organization, i.e., ANA and state constituent member association; publication and communication; orientation toward community services; theory and research development and utilization; and self-regulation and autonomy (p. 79).

Standards Established by the Profession Itself

The exploration of the development of nursing as a profession requires discussion of three major documents guiding all nurses in their professional commitments. These are *Nursing's Social Policy Statement: The Essence of the Profession* (ANA, 2010), *Nursing: Scope and Standards of Practice,* 3rd edition (ANA, 2015b), and the *Code of Ethics for Nurses with Interpretive Statements* (ANA, 2015a).

Nursing's Social Policy Statement: The Essence of the Profession
A Contract With Society

Although criteria for professions vary, all professions have one criterion in common: an obligation to the recipients of their services. Nursing therefore has an obligation to those who receive nursing care. The nature of the social contract between the members of the nursing profession and society is summarized in the latest version of *Nursing's Social Policy Statement: The Essence of the Profession,* revised in 2010 (ANA, 2010). This edition was the result of several years of work by many nurses from a variety of settings and holding an assortment of educational degrees and credentials, collectively known as the Congress on Nursing Practice and Economics. The Social Policy Statement serves as a framework for understanding professional nursing's relationship with society and nursing's obligation to those who receive professional nursing care. This statement also includes the ANA's contemporary definition of nursing and pertinent discussions related to the knowledge base of nursing, specialty and advanced practice, and professional regulation. A careful reading of this 45-page document will provide the reader with the essence of nursing's professionalism. It is available online without appendices as a PDF document at https://essentialguidetonursing-practice.files.wordpress.com/2012/07/pages-from-essential-guide-to-nursing-practice-chapter-1.pdf.

Nursing: Scope and Standards of Practice

Nursing: Scope and Standards of Practice, 3rd edition (ANA, 2015b), outlines the expectations of the professional role within which all RNs must practice and delineates the standards of care and associated competencies for professional nursing. The goal of establishing standards is to improve the health and well-being of all recipients of nursing care and to establish the responsibilities for which nurses are accountable. Several editions of *Standards* have been issued by the ANA since the first one was written in 1973. Each edition has been painstakingly revised by large numbers of nurse volunteers under the leadership of the ANA.

The current document (ANA, 2015b) itemizes the Standards of Practice and Standards of Professional Performance. For each standard, there are numerous competencies by which practice for that standard can be assessed. Although all the standards are important to the practice of nursing, the Standards of Professional Performance are particularly germane to this chapter's emphasis on professionalism. The depth and scope of this document are impressive; you should consider adding this book to your professional library.

The Code of Ethics for Nurses

The ANA designated 2015 as the Year of Ethics and published the new revision of the 2001 code. The *Code of Ethics*, like the Social Policy Statement, was revised by a committee of nurses from a variety of roles and settings across the United States. As you recall, most of the early scholars attempting to define *profession* mentioned ethical behavior as a hallmark of a profession. In fact, a code of ethics is generally considered a tool that guides a group toward professional self-definition and provides evidence of professional legitimacy. The health care environment often presents situations that pose ethical problems for nurses. The Code exists to strengthen and guide nurses' decision making as they navigate the ethical dilemmas frequently faced in many practice settings today. The Code empowers nurses to maintain their focus on the patient as the center of health care.

A code of ethics is a written public document that reminds practitioners and the public they serve of the specific responsibilities and obligations accepted by the profession's practitioners. Ever since education was formalized for nurses, the practice of nursing has been guided by ethical standards promoted first by Florence Nightingale and thereafter by nursing groups and organizations. The *Code of Ethics for Nurses* has been modified over the years as nursing and its social context have evolved. It is intended to guide the practice of RNs in all practice settings, with all types of patients, families, groups, and communities receiving care. The *Code of Ethics* serves three distinct purposes: (1) it is a statement of the "ethical values, obligations, duties, and professional ideals of nurses individually and collectively"; (2) it is nursing's "nonnegotiable ethical standard"; and (3) it expresses "nursing's own understanding of its commitment to society" (ANA, 2015a, p. 10).

There are nine provisions in the 2015 Code, each of which is accompanied by interpretive statements intended to clarify the provision. The first three provisions describe "the fundamental values and commitments of the nurse; the next three address boundaries of duty and loyalty; and the last three address aspects of duties beyond individual patient encounters" (p. 16). The entire document, including interpretive statements, can be found here: www.nursingworld.org/MainMenu-Categories/EthicsStandards/CodeofEthicsforNurses/Code-of-Ethics-For-Nurses.html.

COLLEGIALITY IN PROFESSIONAL NURSING

A sometimes overlooked but increasingly important aspect of professionalism in nursing is collegiality. The promotion of a supportive and healthy work environment, cooperation, and recognition of interdependence among members of the nursing profession is the essence of collegiality. Professional nurses demonstrate collegiality by sharing with, supporting, assisting, and counseling other nurses and nursing students. These behaviors can be seen when nurses, for example, share knowledge with colleagues and students, take part in professional organizations, mentor less experienced nurses, willingly serve as role models for nursing students, welcome learners and their instructors in the practice setting, assist researchers with data gathering, publish in professional literature, and support peer-assistance programs for impaired nurses.

As early as 2004, the ANA demonstrated value placed on collegiality as a professional attribute, included collegiality in *Nursing: Scope and Standards of Practice* as one of nine standards of professional performance. The practice of nursing would be enhanced if the commitment to one another, to assistive personnel for whom

BOX 3.2   To Be a Professional

Be respectful. You do not have to like or agree with a person to be civil. Treat him or her as you would want to be treated.

Be ethical. Understand that in professional settings, professional ethics are mandatory.

Be honest. Be trustworthy; do not participate in gossip and rumor.

Be the best. Strive to be better than just good enough.

Be consistent. Behavior should be consistent with professional values and beliefs.

Be a communicator. Invite ideas, opinions, and feedback from patients and colleagues.

Be accountable. Do what you say you will do. Take responsibility for your own actions.

Be collaborative. Collaborations benefit your patients.

Be forgiving. Everyone makes mistakes—including yourself.

Be current. Keep knowledge and skills up-to-date.

Be involved. Be active at local, state, and national levels in professional organizations.

Be a model nurse. What a person says and does reflects on his or her profession.

Be responsible for your own learning. Be assertive in making your learning needs known to teachers and mentors.

Be prepared. Do assignments for classes, and prepare for labs and clinical shifts in advance, making sure that you have a good foundation for your practice.

Modified from Bruhn JG: Being good and doing good: the culture of professionalism in the health professions, *Health Care Manag* 19(4):47–58, 2001; and Cheyne D: Take responsibility for your learning needs, *Nurs Standard* 20(7):88, 2005.

they are legally responsible, and to nurturing the next generation of professional nurses mirrored the commitment nurses have toward their patients.

Box 3.2, To Be a Professional, contains 14 characteristics of professional nurses. Several serve as reminders of the value of collegiality. You may find this list helpful in considering where you are in your development as a professional nurse.

BARRIERS TO PROFESSIONALISM IN NURSING

Nurses own the profession of nursing and thus own the struggle for recognition as a profession. To reduce the barriers to professionalization, the first step is to identify those barriers, several of which are discussed here.

Varying Levels of Education for Entry into Practice

The most obvious barrier to nursing's achievement of professional status is the variability of educational backgrounds for entry into practice. No other profession allows entry into practice at less than the bachelor's level, yet nursing has three entry levels: the BSN, the ADN, and the diploma in nursing. Other health care professions—for example, medicine, dentistry, and physical therapy—require postgraduate preparation for professional practice. Because professional status and power increase with education, a legitimate question is, "How can nursing take its place as a profession, and nurses take their place as professional peers with other health care providers, when most nurses currently in practice do not hold a bachelor's degree?"

David described this "never-ending fracas" (2000, p. 87) over the varying credentials for entry into nursing practice as contributing to the continuing subordination of nursing in the health care arena. Almost two decades later, this "fracas" continues. Nursing's lack of a standardized requirement for a minimum of a BSN, and preferably a master's degree, stands in sharp contrast with other health care professions requiring more education to practice (David, 2000). Nurses prepared in the three different types of basic educational programs have thus far failed to develop a unified identity that would allow the continuing professionalization of nursing. Lack of resolution of these differences threatens to undermine nursing's continued steady development as a profession (Kidder and Cornelius, 2006). This remains a difficult issue for nurses, creating division and defensiveness. A solution would be for nurses to move beyond personal feelings and opinions to look objectively at how nursing compares with other professions with whom we must collaborate and by whom we want to be seen as equals—and adjust our educational and credentialing requirements accordingly.

Gender Issues

Although gender was not identified as a criterion by any of the scholars of professionalism, it continues to play a role in the perceived value of professions dominated by women such as teaching, social work, and nursing. Although the number of men in nursing has increased, a gender balance remains elusive (Fig. 3.4). The persistent devaluing of women's work in our society has created an ongoing struggle for professions such as

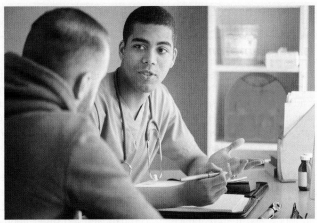

Fig. 3.4 The number of male nurses is increasing.

nursing and teaching to increase their status, increase their compensation, and improve their working conditions. Referenced previously, David (2000) provided an incisive critique of nursing and the detrimental and continuing effects of gender politics on nursing's professional development.

Historical Influences

Nursing's historical connections with religious orders and the military continue to have influence, both positive and negative, today. Aspects that have become liabilities with the passage of time include deference to other professionals, which runs counter to the professional values of autonomy and self-determination, and altruism, which prevents nurses from demanding the fair economic valuation of the work of nursing. Deference to management, physicians, and other stakeholders in the workplace stifles creative and critical thinking required for professional practice. Furthermore, nurses must resist pressure to defend their expectation to be compensated fairly for their complex and demanding work.

Florence Nightingale, the historical figure most strongly associated with the development of modern-day nursing, died in 1910. That same year, Isabelle Hampton Robb died suddenly. As you read in Chapter 2, Robb was a central figure in the women's movement of the late 19th century, and in nursing specifically. Professional Profile Box 3.1 contains a tribute to Robb published in 2011 examining the challenges to nursing Robb faced and the challenges of reenvisioning of the profession today, more than 115 years later.

External Conflicts

As nurses have become more highly educated and advanced practice nurses in particular increasingly assume responsibilities for patient care once considered in the domain of medicine, tensions between nursing and medicine have risen. The influence and resources of organized nursing and professional associations have gone toward lobbying efforts in state legislatures to ensure that the legal scope of nursing practice is protected and appropriately reflects current training and expertise of professional nurses. On the individual level, however, nurses must strive for collaboration, not competition, with physicians and other health care providers with whom they work.

Internal Conflicts

Professional nursing's power and influence are fragmented by subgroups and dissension. Tensions among diploma-educated, associate degree–educated, and bachelor's degree–educated nurses reduce the vitality of the profession. The proliferation of nursing organizations and competition among them for members may diminish rather than increase nursing's influence in the health care arena by diluting concentrations of interested stakeholders across many organizations. Fewer than 10% of the more than 3.1 million RNs in the United States are members of the ANA. The fact that most nurses are not members of any professional organization hampers nursing's ability to govern itself, set standards, and use its collective power to lobby effectively. These are major challenges for nursing if it is to realize its potential collective professional power and autonomy.

PROFESSIONAL PROFILE BOX 3.1
REPAVING THE PATH TO PROFESSIONALISM IN NURSING EDUCATION

In Remembrance of Isabel Hampton Robb

Celebrated as the international year of the nurse, 2010 marked the centennial remembrance of the death of Florence Nightingale in 1910. For nurse educators, it was also a time to remember the contributions of Isabel Hampton Robb, a younger contemporary of Nightingale who died an untimely death the same year. Like many nurses of her day, Robb was an immigrant to the United States who began her second career as a nurse after attending New York Training School for Nurses attached to Bellevue Hospital. After practice abroad, she was recruited into nursing education administration, first in Illinois and then as principal of the Training School and as superintendent at Johns Hopkins Hospital. A politically astute young woman, Robb helped build a path to professionalism for nursing education, drawing on professional and political connections to advance nursing and the quality of patient care. In 1893 she chaired the first major meeting of nursing leaders in Chicago at the Columbian Exhibition and World's Fair, where she presented a paper sent by Nightingale titled "Educational Standards for Nurses." Acknowledging the importance of collaboration in advancing the quality of nursing education and practice, she was a primary founder and first leader of the Association of Nursing Superintendents, the precursor to the National League for Nursing. Her work to unite trained nurses resulted in the Association of Nursing Alumni, which preceded the ANA. Robb set the bar high for nursing education in an era of hospital growth and proliferation of nursing schools. With nursing education highly disorganized, she advocated for admission standards and a formalized curriculum. A scholar of nursing, she took on the task to disseminate teaching materials nationally and wrote reports, articles, and textbooks to provide a sound basis for practice. She addressed the clinical practices of her day, the ethics of nursing, and standards for nursing education. In an era when travel was slow, Robb traveled nationally and internationally and maintained an active correspondence in support of her vision for nursing education. Some 100 years after Robb's death, nursing is again faced with the challenge of reenvisioning standards for the future. The focus now is on the transformation of nursing education to better support the expected changes in a remodeled health care system. Walking along a path initially laid by Robb and her coterie of nursing leaders, a collaboration of nursing and nonnursing leaders set out a call for action in the 2010 Institute of Medicine (IOM) report, *The Future of Nursing: Leading Change, Advancing Health.* This effort to set a national course for nursing education and practice balances optimism for the potential of nurs-

ing and pragmatism grounded in the recognition of barriers to change. In their report, commissioned by the Carnegie Foundation for the Advancement of Teaching, Benner, Sutphen, Leonard, and Day (2010) address the perceived disconnect between the classroom and clinical education. They urge nurse educators to attend to the methods of education and to teach with greater emphasis on clinical reasoning and clinical salience. Noting the challenges that nurses face in practice, from the diversity of patients to the need to manage multiple chronic diseases to the complex and too often fragmented health care system, they underscore the importance of developing in nursing students the ability to readily access and integrate knowledge and skills and transcend discrete classes and clinical experiences. Both the IOM and Carnegie reports reflect the belief, long espoused by nursing leaders, that nurses must be prepared as agents of change. Both reports call for strengthening and empowering nursing leadership. Echoing a call first launched by Robb, the Carnegie report highlights the importance of attending to the socialization, roles, and ethics of nursing graduates as they develop their foundational values, attitudes, and behaviors for leadership. Throughout nursing's history, leaders such as Robb have taken risks to strategically develop, articulate, and promote not simply standards for nursing education but rather a vision of what nursing education and nursing practice offer society. Today, as we reenvision nursing's future and engage in repaving the road of nursing's professionalism, it is fitting to mark the centennial of Isabel Hampton Robb's death and her contributions to nursing education.

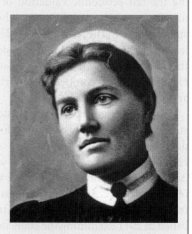

Isabel Hampton Robb

From Wolf KA: End note: Repaving the path to professionalism in nursing education: in remembrance of Isabel Hampton Robb, *Nurs Educ Perspec* 32(2):138, 2011.

⚡ THINKING CRITICALLY BOX 3.1

Rethinking the Professional Image of Nursing: A Content Analysis of Nurse-Authored Blogs

Nursing has suffered from a poor image since the 1800s, which has been perpetuated by the media, physician influence, and societal stereotypes. In much of the literature, image problems have been implicated in contributing to the nursing shortage. The image of nursing has the potential to be influenced by Internet representation. Americans occupying the 18- to 29-year-old age group cite the Internet as their primary source of information because it is convenient and it provides more in-depth and varied viewpoints than does traditional media. The Internet is the number one source of health care information, with more than 12.5 million health-related searches conducted daily, including nurse-authored blogs.

Blogs are increasingly being considered a more credible information source than traditional media. Through blogs, nurses are able to describe their life and experiences—what it means to be a nurse—directly to an audience without many filters or external editing processes. How nurses choose to represent themselves in the media has yet to be described. In this study I systematically reviewed and analyzed blogs written by nurses, examining the authors' portrayal of the profession of nursing with respect to image to yield insight on how nurses represent their profession via Internet blogs and whether these insights support or refute the view that nursing has a poor image.

A sample of 101 blog posts containing information about the professional life of the nurse-author revealed that nurses rarely blogged about the image of nursing (24.85%), with few examples related to actual experience (6.45%). Three themes—"Variety in professional settings," "Nursing as physically/mentally demanding," and "Detailed descriptions of duties/priorities"—accounted for 12.8% of the coding decisions in the analysis. Importantly, 54.5% of coded content fit within the category "Positive or neutral descriptors of nursing," indicating that nurse-authored blogs do not contribute to the poor image of nursing. Furthermore, the experiences nurses blog about do not reinforce the idea that nursing has a poor image.

Beginning with Nightingale's assertion that nursing is a scientific profession with a distinct body of knowledge requiring training, several efforts have transformed the modern landscape of professional nursing: educational requirements have evolved; professional improvement campaigns are progressively being adopted at the institutional level; and image-enhancing advocacy groups work toward correcting misperceptions and stereotypes in the public eye. Considering that the theoretical bases for the poor image argument were formed 20 to 30 years ago when nursing was a very different profession, this study indicates a need to reevaluate the idea that modern nursing has a poor image.

Lindy Beyer, BSN, RN

Janna Dieckmann, PhD, RN

Nursing Image and Professionalism: Are These Related?

In Thinking Critically Box 3.1, you will first read the results of a study completed by a senior honors student of nursing, Lindy Beyer, who has now graduated and is an RN. Ms. Beyer did a systematic review and analysis of nurse-authored blogs, where she found a forum where nurses describe what it means to be a nurse. Once you have read these results, consider these questions:

1. What positive effect does blogging in the public domain have on the profession of nursing?
2. What are possible negative effects that these accounts could have on the profession?
3. Find an example of two nursing blogs, one that promotes a positive view of the nursing profession and another that promotes a negative view of nursing. What are the characteristics of each of these examples?
4. What are your responsibilities as a member of the profession of nursing in responding to the posts on these blogs?
5. What is the relationship of the image of nursing and the professionalization of nursing?

FINAL COMMENTS

Continuing to interrogate the issue of whether nursing is a profession may serve to distract from efforts to improve the professional status of nursing. Debates regarding whether nursing is a profession may actually obscure more pressing issues facing nursing, including improving workplace conditions and compensation, making educational preparation consistent, and implementing evidence-based practice. Nursing has made progress in the past few decades in developing its science and improving its image. Although considerable barriers remain, health care reform in the United States and improvement of health care delivery mean that nurses can establish themselves as primary stakeholders in this debate and move forward.

To summarize this discussion of professionalism in nursing, read Thinking Critically Box 3.2, and identify the professional behaviors exhibited in the case study presented.

 THINKING CRITICALLY BOX 3.2

The Challenge to be a Professional Nurse: Identifying Professional Nursing Behaviors

Instructions: If being a professional nurse is different from practicing the occupation of nursing, there must be certain behaviors that differentiate the two. Read the following case study; then, using various criteria for professions presented in this chapter and the Code of Ethics for Nurses, identify professional behaviors exhibited by Joan. For each behavior you identify, state which source or document, such as the Code or Social Policy Statement, promotes that behavior.

Joan is a 32-year-old married mother of two. She graduated from River City College of Nursing at the age of 26 years and has been practicing since her graduation. Her first position was as a staff nurse at Providence Hospital, a 300-bed private hospital. Nursing administration at Providence encourages nurses to provide individualized nursing care while protecting the dignity and autonomy of each patient and family. She chose Providence because the hospital's philosophy of nursing paralleled her own. Another reason Joan selected this hospital was that she wanted to practice oncology (cancer) nursing, and there is an oncology unit at Providence.

Each day Joan arrives promptly on her nursing unit. Her neat grooming and positive attitude convey pride in herself and her profession. She uses the nursing process in caring for her patients and in dealing with their families. That means she assesses their condition, plans and implements their care, and evaluates the care she has given. Then she documents what she has done in each patient's database in the accepted format. She communicates clearly to the other members of the nursing staff and collaborates with other health care professionals involved in the care of the patients on her unit but is careful not to discuss her patients with others not involved in their direct care.

After 2 years as a staff nurse, Joan accepted a position as a team leader. This means that now she takes responsibility not only for her own practice but also for that of licensed practical/vocational nurses and nursing assistants on her team. To do this effectively, she stays abreast of changes in her state's nurse practice act and Providence

Hospital's policies and procedures. In addition, she updates her knowledge by reading current journals and research periodicals to base her practice on evidence rather than intuition. She makes it a policy to attend at least two nursing conferences each year to stay on top of trends. She belongs to her professional organization and participates as an active member. She finds that this is another source of the latest information on professional issues.

Joan looks forward to working with the nursing students at Providence Hospital. She remembers when she was a student and how a word from a practicing nurse could make or break her day. Of course, students do mean extra work, but she sees this as a part of her role and patiently provides the guidance they need, even when she is busy.

In the course of her daily work, Joan sometimes has questions. She is not embarrassed to seek help from more experienced nurses, from textbooks, or from other health professionals. Sometimes she offers suggestions to the head nurse and the oncology clinical nurse specialist about possible research questions and participates in gathering data when the unit takes on a research study.

Providence Hospital uses a shared governance model, which means nurses serve on committees that develop and interpret nursing policies and procedures. Joan serves on two committees and chairs another. Right now the hospital is preparing a self-study for an upcoming accreditation, so the meetings are frequent. Instead of complaining about the meetings, Joan prepares and organizes her portion of the meeting so that everyone's time is used most effectively. She has to delegate some of her patient care responsibilities to others while she attends meetings. Because she has taken the time to know the other workers' skills and abilities, she does not worry about what happens while she is gone and asks for a full report when she returns to her unit.

At the end of the day when Joan goes home, she occasionally gets a call from a friend with a health-related question or a request to give a neighbor's child an allergy injection. Although she is tired, she recognizes that in

The Challenge to be a Professional Nurse: Identifying Professional Nursing Behaviors

the eyes of others she represents the nursing profession. She is proud to be trusted and respected for her knowledge, skills, and dedication. Helping others through nursing care is something Joan has wanted to do since she was small, and she finds it very fulfilling.

Lately Joan has recognized in herself some troubling signs: She has been irritable and impatient with family and co-workers and generally out of sorts. She has gained weight and is exercising less than usual. She wonders whether working with terminally ill patients and their families is the source of her stress and recognizes that her

work life and personal life are out of balance. Joan's husband has suggested that she take a break from nursing and stay home with the children, but after talking it over with her nurse manager, she has decided to ask for assignment to different nursing responsibilities for a while. She knows that she needs to be her own advocate and take care of herself. Next week she will begin a 3-month stint in outpatient surgery, where she believes the emotional intensity will be somewhat lower. She hopes to return to her first love, oncology nursing, at the end of that time.

CONCEPTS AND CHALLENGES

- *Concept:* Commitment to a profession is different from having a job or an occupation.

  Challenge: The ongoing issue of varying education levels for entry into practice remains a barrier to nursing professionalism.

- *Concept:* A body of knowledge, specialized education, service to society, accountability, autonomy, and ethical standards are a few of the hallmarks of professions.

  Challenge: Nursing is still troubled by lack of autonomy, varying educational preparation, and long-

term commitment to practice that function as barriers to professionalism.

- *Concept:* Nursing has a social contract with society to serve the public safely, competently, and ethically.

  Challenge: Many nurses in practice are not familiar with *Nursing's Social Policy Statement: The Essence of the Profession,* which describes nursing's contract with society, and the *Code of Ethics with Interpretive Statements,* which is the nonnegotiable ethical standard for professional nursing.

IDEAS FOR FURTHER EXPLORATION

1. Determine where nursing currently stands on each of Kelly's criteria for professions.
2. Describe at least five characteristic behaviors of professional nurses.
3. Discuss the Nightingale Pledge (see Box 3.1) as a historical document, as an ethical statement, and as a reflection of Florence Nightingale's social and cultural environment. What value does this document have for today's nurse?
4. Using Miller's Wheel of Professionalism, identify specific activities that fit under each of the "spokes." How might a beginning nurse's behaviors in relation to each spoke differ from those of an experienced nurse? Where does evidence-based practice fit into this model?
5. How might nursing be different today if all nurses viewed it as their profession rather than a job?

REFERENCES

Adams D, Miller BK: Professionalism in nursing behaviors of nurse practitioners, *J Prof Nurs* 17(4):203–210, 2001.

Adams D, Miller BK, Beck L: Professionalism behaviors of hospital nurse executives and middle managers in 10 western states, *West J Nurs Res* 18(1):77–88, 1996.

American Nurses Association (ANA): *Educational preparation for nurse practitioners and assistants to nurses: a position paper*, Kansas City, MO, 1965, The Association.

American Nurses Association (ANA): *Association bylaws*, Silver Spring, MD, 2008, The Association.

American Nurses Association (ANA): *Code of ethics for nurses with interpretive statements*, Washington, DC, 2015a, The Association.

American Nurses Association (ANA): *Nursing: scope and standards of practice*, ed 3, Washington, DC, 2015b, The Association.

American Nurses Association (ANA): *Nursing's social policy statement: the essence of the profession*, ed 2010, Washington, DC, 2010, The Association.

American Nurses Credentialing Center (ANCC): Number of hospitals in the United States with Magnet status (website). Available at: https://campaignforaction.org/number-of-hospitals-united-states-magnet-status/, 2017.

American Nurses Credentialing Center (ANCC): History of the magnet program (website). Available at: www.nursecredentialing.org/Magnet/ProgramOverview/HistoryoftheMagnetProgram, 2015.

Bixler GK, Bixler RW: The professional status of nursing, *Am J Nurs* 59(8):1142–1147, 1959.

Brown EL: *Nursing for the future*, New York, 1948, Russell Sage Foundation.

Carr-Saunders AM, Wilson PA: *The professions*, Oxford, 1933, Clarendon Press.

Collins English Dictionary—Complete and Unabridged (website). Available at: www.collinsdictionary.com/us/dictionary/english, 2018.

D'Amour D, Oandasan I: Interprofessionality as the field of interprofessional practice and interprofessional education: an emerging concept, *J Interprof Care* 19(Suppl 1):8–20, 2005.

David BA: Nursing's gender politics: reformulating the footnotes, *Adv Nurs Sci* 23(1):83–93, 2000.

Derouin A, Holtschneider ME, McDaniel KE, Sanders KA, McNeill DB: Let's work together: interprofessional training of health professionals in North Carolina, *NC Med J* 79(4):223–225, 2018.

Dock LL, Stewart IM: *A short history of nursing*, New York, 1920, Putnam.

Flexner A: *Medical education in the United States and Canada: a report to the Carnegie Foundation for the Advancement of Teaching*, Bethesda, MD, 1910, Science & Health Publications.

Flexner A: Is social work a profession? *School Soc* 1(26):901, 1915.

Ghadirian F, Salsali M, Cheraghi MA: Nursing professionalism: an evolutionary process, *Iran J Nurs Midwifery Res* 19(1):1–10, 2014.

Hall RH: Professionalization and bureaucratization, *Am Sociol Rev* 33:92–104, 1968.

Hall RH: *The professionals, employed professionals, and the professional association. professionalism and the empowerment of nursing*, Kansas City, MO, 1982, American Nurses Association.

Hess R, DesRoches C, Donelan K, Norman L, Buerhaus P: Perceptions of nurses in Magnet® hospitals, non-Magnet hospitals, and hospitals pursuing Magnet status, *J Nurs Admin* 41(7/8):315–323, 2011.

Houle C: *Continuing learning in the professions*, San Francisco, 1980, Jossey-Bass.

Huber D: *Leadership and nursing care management*, Philadelphia, 2000, Saunders.

Institute of Medicine: *Measuring the impact of interprofessional education on collaborative practice and patient outcomes*, Washington, DC, 2015, National Academies Press.

Interprofessional Education Collaborative Expert Panel: *Core competencies for interpersonal collaborative practice: report of an expert panel*, Washington, DC, 2011, Interprofessional Education Collaborative.

Kelly L: *Dimensions of professional nursing*, ed 4, New York, 1981, Macmillan.

Kidder MM, Cornelius PB: Licensure is not synonymous with professionalism: it's time to stop the hypocrisy, *Nurse Educ* 31(1):15–19, 2006.

Miller BK: Just what is a professional? *Nurs Success Today* 2(4):21–27, 1985.

Reuter C, Fitzsimons V: Viewpoint: physician orders, *Am J Nurs* 113(8):8–11, 2013.

Task Force on Professionalism: White paper on pharmacy student professionalism, *J Am Pharm Assoc* 40(1):96–100, 2000.

Wolf KA: End note: Repaving the path to professionalism in nursing education: in remembrance of Isabel Hampton Robb, *Nurs Educ Perspec* 32(2):138, 2011.

World Health Organization (WHO): *Framework for action on interprofessional education and collaborative practice*, Geneva, 2010, World Health Organization (website). Available at: http://whqlibdoc.who.int/HQ/2010/WHO_HRH_HPN_10.3_eng.pdf.

4

Nursing Education in an Evolving Health Care Environment

Maxine Fearrington, MS, RN-BC

ⓔ To enhance your understanding of this chapter, try the Student Exercises on the Evolve site at http://evolve.elsevier.com/Black/professional.

LEARNING OUTCOMES

After studying this chapter, students will be able to:

- Trace the development of basic and graduate education in nursing.
- Discuss the influence of early nursing studies on nursing education.
- Describe traditional and alternative ways of becoming a registered nurse.
- Discuss program options for registered nurses and students with nonnursing bachelor's degrees.
- Differentiate between licensed practical/vocational nurses and registered nurses.
- Differentiate between associate degree and bachelor's degree education.

- Explain the difference between licensure and certification.
- Define *accreditation*, and analyze its influence on the quality and effectiveness of nursing education programs.
- Discuss recommendations of the Institute of Medicine and major nursing organizations regarding transforming nursing education.
- List Quality and Safety Education in Nursing (QSEN) competencies.
- Define *Interprofessional Education* (IPE), and describe its importance in health care today.

Produced almost three decades ago, *Sentimental Women Need Not Apply: A History of the American Nurse* is a classic documentary featuring a comprehensive view of the history of nursing in the United States. In this film, nursing is shown to be both shaping of and shaped by its sociocultural and historical contexts. A century ago, nursing education was often exploitative, with students staffing hospital wards as part of their training, only to be without work at the end of their training. Nursing education was typically hospital based, and students lived together in tightly controlled environments. The film's narrator made the wry observation of mid–20th-century nursing education: "Schools of nursing took women and turned them into girls." Nursing education, although becoming

formalized at the time, did not serve nursing's—or society's—best interests.

Leaders in nursing education today continue to work to evolve nursing education in response to the changing landscape of health care delivery in the United States. Furthermore, nursing education must honor nursing's social contract with the public, recognizing that education of nurses plays a critical role in their ability to achieve optimal outcomes for their patients and to practice safely. In 2009 Patricia Benner, PhD, RN, FAAN, and her team at the Carnegie Foundation for the Advancement of Teaching published a landmark study, *Educating Nurses: A Call for Radical Transformation*. In addition to calling for a bachelor of science in nursing (BSN) as the entry level for registered nurse (RN) practice, this team recommended that all RNs be required to earn a master of science in nursing (MSN) within 10 years of licensure. They found that nurses are undereducated to meet the demands of today's practice. Their recommendations called for a significant shift in basic nursing education, but they made a compelling argument for extending the education of nurses entering the workforce (Benner et al., 2009).

Within a year of the publication of the Carnegie Foundation study, in October 2010 the Institute of Medicine (IOM; now the National Academy of Medicine) published a report, *The Future of Nursing: Leading Change, Advancing Health* (IOM, 2011). This report was compiled as the result of a 2-year initiative by the Robert Wood Johnson Foundation and the IOM to address the need to transform the profession of nursing. Four key messages were at the center of the *Future of Nursing* report:

1. Nurses must practice to the fullest extent of their education and training.
2. Nurses should attain higher education levels through a system of improved education with seamless progression across degrees.
3. As health care in the United States is being transformed, nurses should be full partners with other health care professionals in this effort.
4. Improved data collection and information infrastructure can result in more effective workforce planning and policy development.

In 2012 the results from a survey by the National Council of State Boards of Nursing (NCSBN) indicated that nursing has responded to challenges to increase the sophistication and innovation in nursing education (Spector and Odom, 2012). These innovations included increased use of simulation, integration of Quality and Safety Education for Nurses (QSEN) principles (you will read more about QSEN later in this chapter), development of practice partnerships, and the development of dedicated educational units (DEUs), among others. Also, more attention is being paid to ways to manage a shortage in nursing faculty, which has a direct effect on the number of students that can be educated and added to the nursing workforce.

In addition to the Carnegie and IOM reports, two other important sources called for advancement in nursing education. Linda Aiken, PhD, RN, FAAN, and her colleagues called for increased federal support for the preparation of nurses at the BSN level and higher (Aiken et al., 2009). They suggested policy changes to address the growing need for nursing faculty and in the preparation of advanced practice nurses (APNs) to serve in primary care. In 2010 the Tri-Council for Nursing (an alliance of the American Nurses Association [ANA], American Association of Colleges of Nursing [AACN], American Organization of Nurse Executives, and National League for Nursing [NLN]) released a policy statement that included the following:

Current health care reform initiatives call for a nursing workforce that integrates evidence-based clinical knowledge and research with effective communication and leadership skills. These competencies require increased education at all levels. At this tipping point for the nursing profession, action is needed now to put in place strategies to build a stronger nursing workforce. Without a more educated nursing workforce, the nation's health will be further at risk (Tri-Council for Nursing, 2010).

The ANA continues to support funding for the Title VIII Nursing Workforce Development Programs as contained in the Public Health Service Act, which are administered by the Health Resources and Services Administration (HRSA). Two of the major program areas of HRSA related to nursing are Advanced Education Nursing, grants to schools of nursing to enhance advanced nursing education, including nurse practitioners (NPs), certified nurse-midwives (CNMs), certified registered nurse anesthetists (CRNAs), nurse educators, and others; and Workforce Diversity Grants that increase opportunities for persons from disadvantaged backgrounds and who are underrepresented in the nursing workforce (ANA, 2015; HRSA, 2018).

The contemporaneous release of the IOM report, the Carnegie Foundation report, the Aiken findings, the Tri-Council statement, and the HRSA Title VIII initiatives represent a substantial change in nursing education. Their strong language with regard to the educational basis for nursing required for today's health care environment, combined with the increase in funding for education at a time of serious economic constraints, make it necessary for even the staunchest critic of requirements for higher education for nurses to reconsider.

You are entering nursing at an exciting, challenging time. The remainder of this chapter will focus on nursing education of today and its current structures and requirements. This includes the history behind educational programs, descriptions of the various programs, and trends and future issues.

DEVELOPMENT OF NURSING EDUCATION IN THE UNITED STATES

Florence Nightingale (Fig. 4.1) is credited with founding modern nursing and creating the first educational system for nurses. After hospitals came into existence in Western Europe, and before the influence of Florence Nightingale, nurses had no formal preparation in giving care, because there were no organized programs to educate nurses until the late 1800s. Before this, nursing care was administered by either the patient's relatives, individuals affiliated with religious or military nursing orders, or self-trained persons who were often held in low regard by society.

Nightingale revolutionized and professionalized nursing by arguing that nursing was not a domestic, charitable service but a respected occupation requiring advanced education. In 1860 she opened a school of nursing at St. Thomas' Hospital in London and established the following principles, which were considered highly innovative at the time (Notter and Spalding, 1976):

1. The nurse should be trained in an educational institution supported by public funds and associated with a medical school.
2. The nursing school should be affiliated with a teaching hospital but also should be independent of it.

3. The curriculum should include both theory and practical experience.
4. Professional nurses should be in charge of administration and instruction and should be paid for their instruction.
5. Students should be carefully selected and should reside in "nurses' houses" that form discipline and character. (Nightingale envisioned nursing as a profession only for women.)
6. Students should be required to attend lectures, take quizzes, write papers, and keep diaries. Student records should be maintained.

Nightingale also believed that nursing schools should be financially and administratively separate from the hospitals in which the students trained. This was not the case, however, when nursing schools were first established in the United States.

The first training schools for nurses in the United States were established in 1872. Located at Bellevue Hospital in New York; the New England Hospital for Women and Children in New Haven, Connecticut; and Massachusetts General Hospital in Boston, the programs of study were 1 year long. These schools became known as the "famous trio" of nursing schools. In October 1873, Melinda Anne "Linda" Richards became the first "trained nurse" educated in the United States. By 1879, there were 11 U.S. nursing training schools. Other schools rapidly developed, and by 1900 there were 432 hospital-owned and hospital-operated programs in the United States (Donahue, 1985). These early training programs differed in length from 6 months to 2 years, and each school set its own standards and requirements. On graduation from these programs, students were awarded a diploma. The term *diploma program* was, and still is, used to identify hospital-based nursing education programs. The primary reason for the schools' existence was to staff the hospitals that operated them; therefore high-quality education of student nurses was not always the primary concern of these hospitals.

Early Studies of the Quality of Nursing Education

Nursing leaders of the early 1900s were concerned about the poor quality of many of the recently formed nurse training programs. They initiated studies about nursing and nursing education to prompt changes. October 1899 marked the culmination of approximately 4 years of work by the American Society of Superintendents

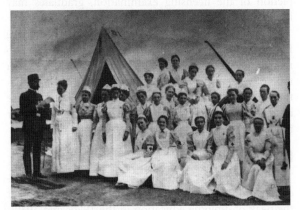

Fig. 4.1 Florence Nightingale's nurses in Scutari, Turkey, during the Crimean War. Nightingale's vision for formalized nursing education transformed nursing.

of Training Schools for Nurses. Isabel Hampton Robb chaired a Society-selected committee to investigate ways to prepare nurses better for leadership in schools of nursing. Teachers College, which had opened in New York 10 years earlier for the training of teachers, seemed the logical location for the leadership training of nurses. A program, originally designed to prepare administrators of nursing service and nursing education, began as an 8-month course in hospital economics (Donahue, 1985).

Mary Adelaide Nutting came to Teachers College in 1907 as the first nursing professor in history and became a pioneer in nursing education. The school at Teachers College became known as the "Mother House" of collegiate education because it fostered the initial movements toward undergraduate and graduate degrees for nurses (Donahue, 1985). In 1912 Nutting conducted a nationwide investigation of nursing education, *The Educational Status of Nursing,* that focused on students' living conditions, nursing education curricula, and teaching methods (Christy, 1969).

Another major and important study of nursing education was published in 1923. Titled *The Study of Nursing and Nursing Education in the United States* and referred to as the **Goldmark Report,** the study focused on the clinical learning experiences of students, hospital control of the schools, the desirability of establishing university schools of nursing, the lack of funds specifically for nursing education, and the lack of prepared teachers (Kalisch and Kalisch, 1995). It is notable that some of the findings of the Goldmark Report in terms of funding and faculty shortages remain applicable to nursing today.

The year 1924 marked another first in nursing education: Yale University opened its School of Nursing, the first nursing school to be established as a separate university department with an independent budget and its own dean, Annie W. Goodrich. The school demonstrated its effectiveness so well that in 1929 the Rockefeller Foundation ensured the permanency of the school by awarding it an endowment of $1 million (Kalisch and Kalisch, 1995). This was an enormous endowment, equivalent to $13.7 million in 2015, and even more astounding given that in 1929 the stock market crash accelerated the collapse of the global economy that spiraled into the Great Depression.

In 1934 a study titled *Nursing Schools Today and Tomorrow* reported the number of schools in existence,

gave detailed descriptions of the schools, described their curricula, and made recommendations for professional collegiate education (National League for Nursing Education, 1934). In 1937 *A Curriculum Guide for Schools of Nursing* was published, outlining a 3-year curriculum and influencing the structure of diploma schools for decades after its publication (National League of Nursing Education, 1937).

Although published over a 30-year period and undertaken by different groups, these early studies consistently made five similar recommendations:

1. Nursing education programs should be established within the system of higher education.
2. Nurses should be highly educated.
3. Students should not be used to staff hospitals.
4. Standards should be established for nursing practice.
5. All students should meet certain minimum qualifications on graduation.

These studies set the stage for the development of the educational programs that exist today.

EDUCATIONAL PATHS TO BECOME A REGISTERED NURSE

Today, preparation for a career as an RN usually begins in one of three ways: in a hospital-based diploma program, a BSN program, or an associate degree in nursing (**ADN**) program. These basic programs vary in the courses offered, length of study, and cost. After the completion of a basic program for RNs, graduates are eligible to take the National Council Licensure Examination for Registered Nurses (NCLEX-RN®). On successful completion of the licensing examination, graduates may legally practice as RNs and use the RN credential.

Having three different educational routes to achieve RN licensure is confusing to the public and even to many nurses themselves. In the following sections, each type of basic program is described, along with its history, unique characteristics, and special issues. These basic programs are discussed in the chronologic order in which they were developed.

Diploma Programs

The hospital-based diploma program was the earliest form of nursing education in the United States. At the peak of diploma education in the 1920s and 1930s, approximately 2000 programs existed, with numerous programs in almost every state. Since their numbers peaked in the first third of the 20th century, the number of diploma programs has decreased, with a dramatic decline since the mid-1960s, when nursing education moved rapidly into collegiate settings. Over the past 50 years, the number of these programs has declined from more than 800 to fewer than 60. This decline in the number of diploma programs is attributable to several factors: the growth of ADN and BSN programs, which moved the education of nurses into the mainstream of higher education; the inability of hospitals to continue to finance nursing education; accreditation standards that have made it difficult for diploma programs to attract qualified faculty; and the increasing complexity of health care, which has required nurses to have greater academic preparation.

Despite the significant decrease in the number of diploma programs, many outstanding nurses practicing today received their basic nursing education in these programs. In the early days of formal nurses' "training" in this country—that is, during the late 1800s and early 1900s—diploma programs provided one of the few avenues for women to obtain formal education and jobs. Most of the early programs followed a modified apprenticeship model. Physicians gave lectures, and students' clinical training was supervised by head nurses and nursing directors. Nursing courses paralleled medical areas and included surgery, obstetrics, pediatrics, operating room experience, and, somewhat later, psychiatry. Students were sometimes sent to affiliated institutions where they could obtain experiences that were not available at the home hospital.

The schedule was demanding, with classes being held after patient care assignments were completed. Critics charged that students were used as inexpensive labor to staff the hospitals and that education was given a lower priority. The truth of those charges varied, depending on which hospital was scrutinized, but there is no question that early nursing students virtually ran the hospitals. Programs lasted 3 years, and, at graduation, students were awarded diplomas in nursing. Today most diploma programs are about 24 months in duration.

A problem that many diploma program graduates faced was that hospitals were not part of the higher education system in the United States. Therefore most colleges and universities did not recognize the nursing diploma as an academic credential and often refused to give college credit for courses taken in diploma programs, regardless of the quality of the courses, students,

and faculty. Most diploma programs today have established agreements with colleges and universities that allow students to earn college credit in courses such as English, psychology, and the sciences, thereby enabling them to attain advanced standing in a bachelor's degree program on completion of the diploma program.

Baccalaureate Programs

Armed with the early studies of nursing education, nursing leaders have continued to push for nursing education to move into the mainstream of higher education—that is, into colleges and universities where other professionals were educated. There is increasing understanding that nurses need a bachelor's degree, the BSN, to qualify nursing as a recognized profession and to provide leadership in administration, teaching, and public health.

By the time the first BSN program was established in 1909 at the University of Minnesota, diploma programs were numerous and firmly entrenched as the system for educating nurses. This first BSN program was part of the university's School of Medicine and followed the 3-year diploma program structure. Despite its many limitations, it was the start of the movement to bring nursing education into the recognized system of higher education.

Seven other BSN programs were established by 1919 (Conley, 1973). Most of the early BSN programs were 5 years in duration. This structure provided for 3 years of nursing education and 2 years of liberal arts. The growth in the numbers of these programs was slow both because of the reluctance of universities to accept nursing as an academic discipline and because of the power of the hospital-based diploma programs. The theoretical, scientific orientation of the BSN program was in sharp contrast to the "hands-on" skill and service orientation that was the hallmark of hospital-based diploma education.

Influences on the Growth of Baccalaureate Education

National studies of nursing and nursing education have reiterated the need for nursing education and practice to be based on knowledge from the sciences and humanities. A forward-looking study was conducted by Esther Lucille Brown, who in 1948 published *Nursing for the Future,* more commonly known as the **Brown Report.** The Brown Report recommended that basic schools of nursing be placed in universities and colleges, with efforts made to recruit men and minorities into nursing education programs (Brown, 1948). This report, sponsored by the Carnegie Foundation, was widely reviewed, discussed, and debated.

In 1965 the ANA published a position paper titled *Educational Preparation for Nurse Practitioners and Assistants to Nurses* (American Nurses Association, 1965). Although not all nursing historians agree, this paper, which subsequently created conflict and division within nursing, had a significant influence on the growth of baccalaureate education in nursing. In preparing the position paper, the ANA studied nursing education, nursing practice, and trends in health care, although the ANA did not refer to a critical, groundbreaking change in American health care that occurred in 1965—the implementation of Medicare and Medicaid. The ANA concluded that baccalaureate education should become the foundation for professional practice. Major recommendations included the following:

1. Education for all those who are licensed to practice nursing should take place in institutions of higher learning.
2. Minimum preparation for entering professional nursing practice should be the baccalaureate degree in nursing.
3. Education for assistants in health service occupations should consist of short, intensive preservice programs in vocational education institutions rather than on-the-job training programs.

Despite tremendous opposition from proponents of diploma and ADN programs, in 1979 the ANA further strengthened its stance by proposing three additional positions (ANA, 1979):

1. By 1985 the minimum preparation for entry into professional nursing practice should be the BSN.
2. Two levels of nursing practice should be identified (professional and technical) and a mechanism to devise competencies for the two categories established by 1980.
3. There should be increased accessibility to high-quality career mobility programs that use flexible approaches for individuals seeking academic degrees in nursing.

The controversy created by the 1965 ANA position paper and the 1979 additions continued for many years. Practicing nurses across the United States, who were mainly diploma program graduates, as well as hospitals supporting diploma programs vehemently protested the recommendations.

In 1970 the National Commission for the Study of Nursing and Nursing Education published a report titled *An Abstract for Action* (Lysaught, 1970). Also known as the Lysaught Report, it made recommendations concerning the supply and demand for nurses, nursing roles and functions, and nursing education. Among the priorities identified by this study were (1) the need for increased research into both the practice and the education of nurses and (2) enhanced educational systems and curricula.

In the mid-1980s, the National Commission on Nursing suggested that the major block to the advancement of nursing was the ongoing conflict within the profession about educational preparation for nurses. The Commission recommended establishing a clear system of nursing education, including pathways for educational mobility and development of additional graduate education programs (De Back, 1991).

The National League for Nursing (NLN) is another major national nursing group supporting the BSN as the entry credential. The organization's membership consists of nurses, faculty, health care agencies, all types of nursing programs, and nonnursing citizens who are supportive of nursing. After much debate, in 1982 the NLN board of directors approved the *Position Statement on Nursing Roles: Scope and Preparation,* which affirmed the BSN as the minimum educational level for professional nursing practice and the ADN or diploma as the preparation for technical nursing practice (NLN, 1982).

In 1996 the AACN board approved a position statement, *The Baccalaureate Degree in Nursing as Minimal Preparation for Professional Practice.* This document supports, among other things, articulated programs, which enable associate degree nurses to attain the BSN (AACN, 1996). This document was last updated in 2000 and still reflects the AACN's current position. It can be found online (www.aacn.nche.edu/Publications/positions/baccmin.htm).

The latest recommendations by influential nursing groups demonstrate a renewed interest in moving toward a BSN as a minimum degree for entry into practice. These recommendations were used to introduce this chapter, which will now focus on the current state of nursing education in the United States.

Today's Baccalaureate Education

Today, baccalaureate programs provide education for students getting their first college degrees in preparation for licensure and RNs holding associate's degrees or diplomas in nursing enrolling in colleges and universities to earn a BSN. This section focuses on the program characteristics of prelicensure baccalaureate education. Baccalaureate programs for RNs are discussed later in this chapter.

Basic BSN programs combine nursing courses with general education courses in a 4-year curriculum in a college or university. Students may be admitted to the nursing program as entering freshmen or after completing certain liberal arts and science courses. Students meet the same admission requirements to the university as other students and often must meet even more stringent requirements to be admitted to the school of nursing with a major in nursing. (Some universities have departments or colleges of nursing rather than schools of nursing.) Courses in the nursing major focus on nursing science, communication, decision making, leadership, and care to persons of all ages in a wide variety of settings (Fig. 4.2).

Faculty qualifications in BSN programs are usually higher than in other basic nursing programs. A minimum of a master's degree for clinical faculty and a doctorate in nursing or a related field is required for permanent, tenure-track faculty. Some colleges and universities now require that all faculty, whether tenure track or clinical track, have an earned doctorate. The requirement of a doctorate ensures that nursing faculty members are able to meet the teaching, research, and service requirements expected of all faculty in universities.

Nursing faculty work leads to many interesting possibilities for collaboration in unexpected places and in distant countries. Professional Profile Box 4.1 describes the experiences of Wendy Woith, PhD, RN, FAAN, in doing her research in Russia with health care workers and tuberculosis, after a lifetime of interest in that country. The editor of this text spent more than 2 memorable weeks in Malawi, a small country in eastern Africa tremendously affected by HIV and malaria, teaching Malawian nurses how to manage two research protocols. Along with Dr. Woith, the editor spent 2 weeks in Russia helping nurses there plan their first nursing research projects and currently has a visiting professorship at a school of nursing in China. Caring for the health of populations takes many different forms across nations. Nursing and the skills you develop provide you with opportunities to experience firsthand how citizens of other countries care for persons across the continuum of ages, development, and health.

BSN graduates are prepared to take the **NCLEX-RN**® and, after licensure, assume beginning practice and ultimately leadership positions in any health care setting,

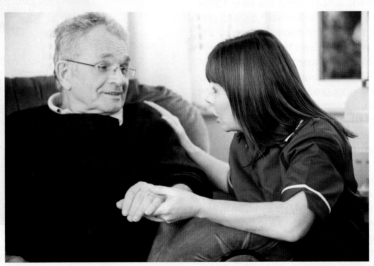

Fig. 4.2 Clinical experience is a vitally important aspect of every basic nursing program. This student is working with her elderly patient in a hospice setting. (Photo used with permission from iStockPhoto.)

PROFESSIONAL PROFILE BOX 4.1
FROM "DUCK AND COVER" TO TUBERCULOSIS PREVENTION

When I was a senior in high school, my mother told me I needed to have a career to "fall back on" (she never mentioned in what case I might need this "fall back" plan). In those days in the Midwest, career choices were pretty much limited to secretary, teacher, or nurse. I could not type, and I was terrified to speak in public, so by default I chose nursing. This was probably the best decision I ever made, because it has afforded me so many opportunities I would never have had otherwise. I started my career as a diploma nurse, and then almost immediately completed a BSN at the first RN-BSN program in my community. I obtained my master's degree in adult health nursing in 1992 and completed work on my PhD in 2006.

I spent 20 years in a hospital setting, moving from critical care to staff development and then to director of clinical practice at a not-for-profit hospital. However, I was one of 60 managers who were downsized at my institution during the reengineering craze of the 1990s. This was a fortuitous event (although I felt far from fortunate at the time!) because I ended up in a university setting where I was asked to provide a presentation of our skills laboratory to nurses visiting from Russia. During our time together, we discussed similarities and differences in nursing education and practice between our countries, and as a result of our conversations I was invited to Vladimir, Russia, to help advance their nursing program. I was asked to return in September 1999 to present at a medical conference, and I was hooked.

I have been intrigued by Russia for as long as I can remember. I attended grade school during the early 1960s where we participated in "duck and cover" drills to prepare us to respond in the event of nuclear attack by the U.S.S.R. I remember watching news reports with Soviet soldiers marching through the iconic Red Square past St. Basil's Cathedral. This had a significant impact on my view of the wider world while growing up. Later, after the fall of the Soviet Empire, I discovered that Russia is truly a beautiful country, and I have been back many times since my initial visit. But it was the desire to help my Russian colleagues expand the professional recognition of nurses that prompted me to seek my doctorate.

Through my work with Russian nurses, I developed an interest in the problem of tuberculosis, and this became the focus for my program of research. My dissertation was a study of treatment delay and poor adherence to tuberculosis medications, and I lived in Russia during the month it took me to conduct my research. This was quite an adventure for a small-town Midwestern girl who does not speak Russian! I remember sitting in my apartment 1 week into the study wondering, "What made me think I could do this?" But it

was affirming when I did complete the study and my dissertation and had my first manuscript accepted for publication.

I have formed close relationships with several nurses and physicians at the Medical College of Vladimir and at some of the area hospitals. These colleagues have served as members of my research team and also as co-investigators. As I build my program of research, I have moved from studying patient-associated issues to the impact nosocomial tuberculosis has on health care workers. My mixed-methods study on barriers and motivators to use of infection control measures, funded by Virginia S. Cleland through the American Nurses Foundation, led to a feasibility study of an intervention using technology to motivate behavior change among Russians working in tuberculosis care; specifically, the intervention was designed to prompt them to wear and fit-check their respirators. Results of the feasibility study are promising, and I plan to expand this into a larger multisite study.

In addition to research, I have been able to assist my Russian colleagues advancing nursing practice and education, including a trip to St. Petersburg with three other American nurses to present a week-long research training course to members of the Russian Nurses Association. Nursing has been an adventure that enabled me to meet people, go places, and do things that changed my life!

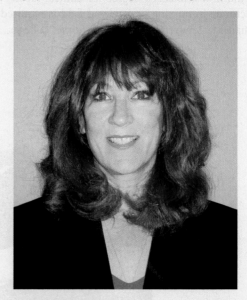

Wendy Woith, PhD, RN, FAAN
Associate Professor of Nursing, Mennonite College of Nursing, Illinois State University

Reference: Courtesy Wendy Woith.

including hospitals, community agencies, schools, clinics, and homes. Graduates with BSN degrees are also prepared to move into graduate programs in nursing and advanced practice certification programs. Programs granting a BSN are the most costly of the basic programs in terms of time and money, but the investment can result in long-term professional advancement. Today, with a great demand for BSN graduates, these nurses have the greatest career mobility among all basic program graduates in nursing.

According to *The Essentials of Baccalaureate Education for Professional Nursing Practice* (AACN, 2008), nurses who graduate from BSN programs are prepared "to practice within complex health care systems and assume the [following] roles: provider of care; designer/manager/coordinator of care; and member of a profession" (p. 3). The AACN document also stressed the concepts of patient-centered care, interprofessional teams, evidence-based practice, quality improvement, patient safety, informatics, clinical reasoning/critical thinking, genetics and genomics, cultural sensitivity, professionalism, and practice across the life span in an increasingly complex health care environment (p. 3).

The challenge to enhance opportunities for students to pursue a career in nursing has been met in an innovative, important way by visionary nurse educators in Rhode Island, who opened the Rhode Island Nurses Institute Middle College Charter High School in Providence. This school is for high school students who are interested in a career in nursing, and they continue at the school through their first year of college. The curriculum focuses on science and math skills that are necessary to be successful in nursing school and then in practice. The mission of the school is "to prepare a diverse group of students to become the highly educated and professional nursing workforce of the future" (Rhode Island Nurses Institute Middle College, 2018).

Associate Degree Programs

ADN (associate degree in nursing) education is the newest form of basic preparation for RN practice, begun in 1952 to address the post–World War II nursing shortage. Based on a model developed by Mildred Montag, EdD, during her doctoral studies, and fueled by interest in community college education after World War II, associate degree programs are now the most common

type of basic nursing education program in the United States and graduate the most RN candidates of all the basic programs.

The popularity of ADN programs can be attributed to several features: accessibility of community colleges, low tuition costs, part-time and evening study opportunities, shorter duration of programs, and graduates' eligibility to take the licensure examination for RNs.

When first envisioned by Dr. Montag, ADN programs were proposed as a solution to a nursing shortage. She suggested a shorter program designed to prepare nurse technicians who would function under the supervision of professional nurses. ADN nurses were to work at the bedside, performing routine nursing skills for patients in acute and long-term care settings. The original ADN program, as outlined by Montag (1951), offered general education courses in the first year and nursing courses in the second year. Montag originally viewed the ADN as a final, end-point degree, not an incremental step to the BSN.

In practice, Montag's original conceptions of ADN programs have been greatly modified. ADN curricula now offer more nursing credits than she suggested. They also include content on leadership and clinical decision making, abilities that Montag did not anticipate as needed in technical nurses. Because of additions to the curriculum, students may need to enroll for more than 2 years to complete the program of study. ADN graduates are employed in a variety of settings and function autonomously with BSN and diploma graduates. In the educational system of nursing today, the ADN can be a step in the progression to the BSN or master's degree.

Since 1990, the NLN Council of Associate Degree Programs has sought to differentiate the competencies of the ADN nurse from those of the BSN nurse. The original document, first written in 1990 (NLN, 1990), was revised in 2000 in response to a changing health care delivery system. Titled *Educational Competencies for Graduates of Associate Degree Nursing Programs,* the revised document identified eight core competencies of ADN education: professional behaviors, communication, assessment, clinical decision making, caring interventions, teaching and learning, collaboration, and managing care (NLN, 2000). The most current version, *Outcomes and Competencies for Graduates of Practice/ Vocational, Diploma, Associate Degree, Baccalaureate, Master's Practice, and Research Doctorate Programs in*

TABLE 4.1	**Landmarks in the History of Nursing Education**
1860	Florence Nightingale founded the first organized program to educate nurses at St. Thomas' Hospital in London.
1872	The "famous trio," the first year-long training schools for nurses, was established in the United States, founded at Bellevue Hospital, the New England Hospital for Women and Children, and Massachusetts General Hospital.
1873	Melinda Anne "Linda" Richards became the first "trained nurse" to graduate in the United States.
1899	Teachers College, Columbia University, offered the first postgraduate course in hospital economics for nurses.
1907	Mary Adelaide Nutting became the first nursing professor at Teachers College, Columbia University.
1909	The first BSN program was established at the University of Minnesota.
1923	The Goldmark Report was published, the first such report focusing on hospital control of schools of nursing and lack of proper teacher preparation.
1924	Yale University established the first nursing school as a separate university department with its own dean, Annie W. Goodrich.
1932	The first EdD in nursing was granted by Teachers College.
1934	The first PhD program in nursing was initiated by New York University.
1948	Esther Lucille Brown's report *Nursing for the Future* was published, recommending that basic nursing programs be situated in colleges and universities rather than in hospitals.
1952	The first ADN program, based on Dr. Mildred Montag's model, was established to prepare nurse technicians.
1954	The University of Pittsburgh started the first PhD program in clinical nursing.
1965	The ANA issued a position paper advocating the BSN degree as the minimum educational preparation for entry into nursing practice.
2004	The AACN passed a resolution to create the DNP degree.

Nursing (2012), addresses four core competencies across all educational levels—human flourishing, nursing judgment, professional identity, and spirit of inquiry (NLN, 2012). Landmarks in the history of nursing education are listed in Table 4.1.

External Degree Programs

External degree programs in nursing are different from traditional basic nursing education in that students attend no classes. Learning is independent and is assessed through highly standardized and validated competency-based outcomes assessments, leading to the description "virtual university." Students are responsible for arranging their own clinical experiences in accordance with established standards.

Excelsior College, formerly known as the New York Regents External Degree Nursing Program, is a well-recognized external degree model. Beginning in 1970 with an ADN program, Excelsior College now offers ADN, BSN, and MSN degrees, all of which are accredited by the National League for Nursing Accreditation Commission (NLNAC). The Excelsior College

School of Nursing was designated by the NLN as a Center of Excellence in Nursing Education, 2011–2016. Excelsior College does not offer clinical experiences to those seeking a basic nursing education and as such they are encouraged to seek basic education that includes clinical instruction.

Since 1981, the California State University Consortium has offered a statewide external BSN program. The California program is for RNs already holding current licenses to practice in the state.

Numerous external degree programs are in existence today, many of which are marketed online and by direct mail. Prospective students must exercise caution to choose only bona fide accredited programs that are affiliated with recognized colleges and universities.

Articulated Programs

In response to the demand for educational mobility, articulation (mobility) among programs has become much more common in today's nursing education system. The purpose of articulation is to facilitate opportunities for nurses to increase their education. An example of a fully articulated system is the licensed practical/vocational nurse/associate degree in nursing/bachelor of science in nursing/master of science in nursing (LPN/LVN/ADN/BSN/MSN) program in which students spend the first year preparing to be an LPN/LVN and the second year completing the ADN. If desired or necessary, students can leave the program at the end of the first year, take the licensure examination for LPN/LVN, and return to the ADN program at a later time. On the other hand, they may continue study in the program after the initial 2 years to earn a BSN degree and even continue for a master's or doctorate.

Multiple-entry, multiple-exit programs are difficult to develop. A tremendous amount of joint institutional planning is needed to create equivalent courses and to keep the programs congruent across institutions. A change in one curriculum dictates changes in all the others. These challenges explain why fully articulated programs have been slow to develop. In increasing numbers, however, articulation agreements between BSN and ADN programs and between ADN and LPN/LVN programs are being established that facilitate student movement among programs and accept transfer credit among institutions. These requirements often result in acceleration or advanced placement within the higher-degree school.

In spite of the difficulties in developing articulated programs, several state legislatures have mandated their public institutions to create these programs to facilitate upward educational mobility for nurses. Other states have statewide voluntary articulation plans, and still others have individual school-to-school agreements in place.

RN-TO-BSN, ACCELERATED BSN, DISTANCE LEARNING: ALTERNATE PATHS IN NURSING EDUCATION

In addition to the basic programs leading to entry-level nursing practice, alternative programs exist.

Baccalaureate Programs for Registered Nurses

After nursing organizations of the 1960s and 1970s publicly advocated for the BSN degree to be the minimum education level for professional practice, the demand for the BSN degree increased. Employers of nurses recognized that broadly educated nurses matched well with the complexities of health care. As a result, many supported the BSN as a requirement for career mobility. Diploma and ADN graduates returned to school in increasing numbers. Today, many students enter ADN programs with plans to earn a BSN ultimately. Baccalaureate programs for RNs allow them, as well as diploma nurses, to accomplish this goal.

Historically, RNs with diplomas and associate degrees did not always find a place in BSN programs. In the early years of baccalaureate education for RNs, many schools required these students to take courses in areas the students had already mastered, constituting barriers for these nurses to complete their BSN degrees. Now, however, BSN programs recognize the importance of RN-to-BSN education and have developed alternative tracks to accommodate the unique learning needs of the RN student.

Baccalaureate programs for RNs are most often offered by universities that also offer basic nursing education in baccalaureate programs. The RN students may be integrated with the traditional BSN students, or they may be enrolled in a separate or partially separate sequence. Some baccalaureate programs for RNs are freestanding; that is, they are offered by colleges that do not have a basic BSN program or in single-purpose institutions. Many of these programs are now offered online.

Most 4-year colleges and universities allow the transfer of general education credits from ADN programs. With increasing frequency, transfer credit is given for nursing courses as well, or there is the option of receiving credit for previous nursing courses through a variety of advanced placement methods such as examinations, demonstrations, and portfolios.

For diploma graduates, transfer credit is usually given for previous college courses, such as English, if they were included as part of the diploma program and taught by college faculty. Options for advanced placement of diploma graduates into BSN programs are extremely variable, and prospective RN students should seek detailed information to select a program that fits individual needs and goals.

The demand for the BSN degree by large numbers of ADN and diploma graduates continues to be strong. More nurses are returning to school to prepare for the wider opportunities offered by the BSN degree. With broad preparation in clinical, scientific, community health, and patient education skills, the baccalaureate nurse is well positioned to move across community-based settings such as home health care, outpatient centers, and neighborhood clinics, where opportunities are fast expanding.

Programs for Second-Degree Students

A noteworthy trend is the significant increase in the number of students with bachelor's degrees in other fields making a career change to nursing. The educational system in nursing has responded to this group of students by offering options to the traditional basic baccalaureate education. Increasingly, baccalaureate programs offer these students an accelerated or fast-track sequence, awarding either a second bachelor's degree or, in some cases, an MSN. Accelerated MSN programs for individuals with bachelor's degrees in another field are known as generic master's degree programs. They usually require about 3 years to complete, depending on the number of prerequisite courses needed. Graduates take the RN licensure examination (NCLEX-RN®) after completing the generic master's program.

Online and Distance Learning Programs

The majority of nursing programs, particularly entry-level programs, are still offered in the traditional way with in-person course work. Technological advances, however, have made it possible for students to take courses online, and a significant percentage of colleges and universities are now offering some or all of their courses online as distance learning (DL). Originally intended to improve educational access for nurses from rural areas, students enrolled in web-based courses today might live in the same town as the educational institution but have significant demands on their time and prefer the flexibility of online offerings.

Master's and doctoral programs in nursing have been at the forefront in the development of online programs, with up to 30% of MSN programs and up to 50% of doctor of nursing practice (DNP) programs now offering half or more of their courses online. According to the AACN, relatively few entry-level BSN programs offer half or more of their courses online, and the majority offer few if any online courses, although this number is increasing. In contrast, RN-to-BSN programs are often offered online.

As more schools of nursing offer coursework and entire degrees through DL, the issue of adequate and properly supervised clinical experience arises. Technology may again provide at least a partial answer to this dilemma through use of virtual environments. DL students validate their clinical competence in a number of traditional ways, including preceptorships, clinical examinations, demonstrations, and clinical portfolios. When the programs are properly structured, well monitored, and offered to carefully selected students, the achievement levels of DL students are comparable with those of traditional students.

Some fraudulent online programs exist in which students are charged very large fees. Other programs may be appealing at the outset, but sometimes enrolled students find serious flaws in how content is delivered online and how their learning is evaluated. Students contemplating enrolling in online programs should be educated consumers and consider several factors when evaluating options, such as the reputation of the college or university offering the courses and access to faculty and student support services such as academic advisement or disability services. Before committing to an online degree program, you should answer these important questions:

1. Do you have the self-discipline needed to keep up with assignments outside a traditional classroom setting?
2. Do you learn best when you can interact with other students and faculty, or do you do well working alone?

ACCREDITATION: ENSURING QUALITY EDUCATION

Accreditation of educational programs in nursing is crucial. Although all nursing programs must be approved by their respective state boards of nursing for graduates to take the licensure examination, nursing programs may also seek accreditation, which goes beyond minimum state approval. Accreditation refers to a voluntary review process of educational programs by a professional organization known as an accrediting agency, which compares the educational quality of the program with established standards and criteria. Accrediting agencies derive their authority from the U.S. Department of Education. Two agencies, the Accreditation Commission for Education in Nursing (ACEN) and the Commission on Collegiate Nursing Education (CCNE), are responsible for accrediting nursing educational programs today.

Accreditation of nursing schools grew out of concerns by leaders of the profession about the lack of quality and standards for nursing education. An accredited program voluntarily adheres to standards that protect the quality of education, safety, and the profession itself—in other words, maintains nursing's social contract with the public. Accreditation provides both a mechanism and a stimulus for programs to initiate periodic self-examination and self-improvement. This process assures students that their educational program is accountable for offering quality education.

Accrediting bodies establish standards by which a program's effectiveness is measured. Programs under review prepare self-study reports that show how the school meets each standard. The self-study report is reviewed by a volunteer team composed of nursing educators from the type of program being reviewed, and an on-site program review is conducted by the same team. After the site visit, the visitors' report and the program's self-study are reviewed by the accrediting organization, and a decision is made about the accreditation status of each nursing program.

Prospective nursing students should inquire about the accreditation status of any nursing program they are considering. Qualifying for certain scholarships, loans, and military service typically requires an accredited program. Acceptance into a graduate program in nursing will likely depend on graduation from an accredited BSN program. Employers of nurses are usually interested in hiring only nurses who are graduates of accredited programs.

Once a program is accredited and in good standing, continuing accreditation reviews take place every 8 to 10 years. Programs that do not meet standards may receive a warning or be placed on probation and given a specific time limit to correct deficiencies. Accreditation can be withdrawn if deficiencies are not corrected within the specified time.

In 1996 the AACN organized the CCNE, which is recognized by the U.S. Department of Education as the national accrediting body for BSN and higher degree nursing programs. CCNE began operation in 1998 and has subsequently established an organizational structure, policies and procedures, and accreditation standards and criteria. In December 1999 CCNE received a recommendation from the National Advisory Committee on Institutional Quality and Integrity, a panel of the U.S. Department of Education, that the Secretary

of Education grant initial recognition of CCNE as a national agency for the accreditation of bachelor's and graduate nursing education programs. This status was renewed in 2002. The establishment of a second national accrediting body for nursing education represented a significant development in the evolution of the nursing profession. Originally commissioned as the National League for Nursing Accrediting Commission (NLNAC), the ACEN is the accreditation agency for LPN/LVN programs, diploma programs, and ADN programs. Bachelor's and higher degree programs may choose which of the two accrediting bodies they wish to use.

TAKING THE NEXT STEPS: ADVANCED DEGREES IN NURSING

A variety of economic, educational, and professional trends are fueling the demand for RNs with **advanced degrees** (master's or doctorate). The evolving health care system requires nurses to possess increasing knowledge, clinical competency, greater independence, and autonomy in clinical judgments. Trends in community-based nursing centers, case management, complexity of home care, sophisticated technologies, and society's orientation to health and self-care are rapidly causing the educational needs of nurses to expand, thereby requiring graduate education. Reforms in health care are expected to increase the demand for nurses with master's and doctoral degrees.

Nurses who have advanced education can become researchers, NPs, clinical specialists, educators, and administrators. Some of the opportunities available to nurses with advanced degrees are described in Chapter 1. Having a workforce of highly educated nurses strengthens the profession.

Master's Education

The purpose of master's education is to prepare people with advanced nursing knowledge and clinical practice skills in a specialized area of practice. Teachers College, Columbia University, is credited with initiating graduate education in nursing. As mentioned, beginning in 1899, the college offered a postgraduate course in hospital economics, which prepared nurses for positions in teaching and hospital administration. From this beginning, there has been consistent growth in the number of master's nursing programs in the United States.

Most nurses in the 1950s and 1960s viewed the master's degree in nursing as the terminal degree—that is, the highest degree in a profession or academic discipline. The master's degree was considered the highest degree nurses would ever need. Early master's programs were longer and more demanding than master's programs in other disciplines. Master's programs in the 1950s and 1960s prepared students for careers in nursing administration and nursing education.

With the rapid development of doctoral programs for nurses during the 1970s, however, the master's degree was no longer considered nursing's terminal degree. Programs were shortened and advanced practice through clinical specialization became the emphasis. Master's programs in nursing are most often found in colleges and universities that have basic BSN programs. These programs may also seek voluntary accreditation from either ANEC or CCNE.

Entrance requirements to master's programs in nursing typically include the following: a BSN degree from an accredited program, licensure as an RN, completion of the Graduate Record Examination or other standard aptitude test, a minimum undergraduate grade point average of 3.0, recent work experience as an RN in an area related to the desired area of specialization, and specific goals for graduate study. These entry requirements vary among colleges and universities, so prospective students need to be aware of specific requirements for the master's programs to which they are applying.

The average traditional program length is 18 to 24 months of full-time study, although part-time study and accelerated curricula are far more common today than in the past. The curriculum includes theory, research, clinical practice, and courses in other disciplines. Master's students generally select both an area of clinical specialization, such as adult health or gerontology, and an area of role preparation, such as informatics, administration, or teaching. Students may be required to write a comprehensive examination and/or to complete a thesis or research project.

Major areas of role preparation include administration, case management, informatics, health policy/health care systems, teacher education, clinical nurse specialist, NP, nurse-midwifery, nurse anesthesia, and other clinical and nonclinical areas of study. With the increasing demand for NPs, master's programs have expanded their practitioner tracks.

The master of science (MS) and the MSN are the two most common graduate degrees offered. Another option in master's education is the RN/MSN track, which allows RNs who are prepared at the associate degree or diploma level and who meet graduate admission requirements to enter a program leading to a master's degree rather than a bachelor's degree. Other recent graduate program options are combined degrees such as the master of science in nursing/master of business administration (MSN/MBA) for nurse administrators or the master of science in nursing/juris doctor (MSN/JD) for nurse attorneys. Clearly diversity in nursing education extends to the graduate as well as the basic level.

Doctoral Education

Doctoral programs in nursing prepare nurses to become faculty members in universities, administrators in schools of nursing or large medical centers, researchers, theorists, and advanced practitioners. Doctoral programs in nursing offer several degree titles. These can be divided into two categories: a research-focused degree—doctor of philosophy (PhD)—and a practice-focused degree—doctor of nursing practice.

History of Doctoral Education in Nursing

Formal doctoral education for nurses began at Columbia University's Teachers College in 1910 with the creation of the Department of Nursing and Health. The first student completed work for the doctor of education (EdD) in nursing education and was awarded the doctorate in 1932. In 2016 the Teachers College of Columbia University began offering an online program leading to an EdD in nursing education.

In 1934 New York University initiated the first PhD program for nurses. The programs at Teachers College and New York University provided many of the profession's early leaders, who worked over the years for improvements in nursing education. From 1934 through 1953, no new nursing doctoral programs were opened. In 1954 the University of Pittsburgh opened the first PhD program in clinical nursing and clinical research in the United States. By the end of the 1950s, only 36 doctoral degrees had been awarded in nursing (Parietti, 1990).

Because of the limited number of nursing doctoral programs, most nurses in the 1950s and 1960s earned doctorates in nonnursing fields, such as education, sociology, and physiology. Doctoral education for nurses moved into a new phase when the federal government initiated nurse scientist programs in 1962, which awarded the doctor of nursing science (DNS, DNSc, DSN) degrees. These programs were created to increase the research skills of nurses and provide faculty for the development of doctoral programs in nursing. The nurse scientist programs were discontinued in 1975 after more universities began offering doctoral programs in nursing. Some universities converted these degrees retroactively to PhD degrees (Ponte and Nicholas, 2015).

Current Status of Doctoral Education in Nursing

The research-focused doctorate for students with prior degrees in nursing is the PhD. The PhD is an academic degree and prepares nurse scholars for research and the development of theory. Nurses with PhDs focus their work on the development of the science of nursing. Some nurses hold the doctor of nursing science degree. It is an academic research degree that has generally been phased out in the United States but is recognized to be the equivalent of a PhD. Other countries award the DNS as the terminal degree (highest academic degree) in nursing. In the United States, the PhD is the terminal degree.

In October 2004 the members of the AACN debated and passed a resolution calling for a new doctorate, the DNP (AACN, 2004). Designed to replace the master's degree, the DNP would be required to be completed by nurses who wish to practice in advanced roles, such as NP or nurse-midwife. Proponents of this change suggested that it would put nursing on an even footing with other health care disciplines that require a clinical doctorate. Detractors argued that the proposed change could increase confusion within and outside the profession about the qualifications of nurses prepared at the doctoral level; it could also discourage nurses from seeking the PhD in nursing and thereby further deepen the shortage of nurse faculty prepared in the manner of other professors on college and university campuses (Dracup and Bryan-Brown, 2005). Despite early concerns, the degree has proven to be popular, and increasing numbers of universities are offering the DNP. The number of programs and graduates has grown rapidly. DNPs may be part of a solution to the shortage of primary care physicians, which will add to the profession's credibility (Croasdale, 2008; Landro, 2008).

Enrollment trends indicate that there is continued demand for all types of doctoral education in nursing. The number of programs, as well as the number of requests for admission to these programs, continues to increase. This trend has partially stemmed from the requirement of a doctorate for academic advancement and tenure for university nursing faculty. A research doctorate is typically required to become a competent researcher who can compete for grants and develop nursing science; PhD-prepared nurses can assist DNP nurses in the development of sound research. DNP-prepared nurses move research into practice. This advances the profession as a whole. Large numbers of nurses with doctorates will continue to be needed in the future as positions requiring this degree expand in universities and throughout the health care system. In Professional Profile Box 4.2 you can read about Tom Bush, DNP, FNP-BC, FAANP, a nurse practitioner who decided to complete his DNP after several years of advanced practice as a family nurse practitioner in an orthopedic clinic in an academic medical center.

BECOMING CERTIFIED: VALIDATING KNOWLEDGE AND PROFICIENCY

Licensure and certification are both forms of credentialing of nurses. **Licensure** refers to state regulation of the practice of nursing. Licensure is required of individuals at the entry point to practice and must be renewed periodically. It is a legal designation that ensures public safety by assessing basic and continuing competence. **Certification** goes beyond licensure by validating a high level of knowledge and proficiency in a particular practice area. Certification has professional but not legal status.

Certification means that a certificate is awarded by a certifying body as validation of specific qualifications demonstrated by an RN in a defined area of practice. A comprehensive examination is required to become certified, as well as documentation of experience, letters of reference, and other documents. You can find a great deal of information about specialty certification at https://www.nursingworld.org/our-certifications.

Certified nurses may have greater earning potential, wider employment opportunities, a broader scope of practice, validation of their skills, knowledge, and abilities, public recognition, a sense of personal satisfaction, and prestige that sets them apart from noncertified

PROFESSIONAL PROFILE BOX 4.2
FNP EARNING HIS DOCTOR OF NURSING PRACTICE DEGREE

Neither of my parents nor extended family attended college so I am the first in my family to earn a college degree. To fund my education, I worked part time while earning an associate's degree in nursing from a local community college in the mountains of eastern Kentucky. I chose nursing because of an interest in biologic and social science and could never have imagined the opportunities gained by choosing a career in nursing.

While working as a registered nurse I soon realized the many rewards and challenges of the nursing profession. I was able to gain valuable on-the-job experience and work toward an advanced degree while earning a living. I quickly enrolled in an innovative bridge program that led to a master's degree in nursing.

My nursing career has included primary care, critical care, and specialty services. For the past 10 years I have split my time between teaching nurse practitioner students at the University of North Carolina at Chapel Hill School of Nursing and clinical practice in the Department of Orthopaedics at the University of North Carolina at Chapel Hill School of Medicine. The dual roles of clinician and educator have positioned me to help others realize the vast opportunities that are the future of nursing.

The landmark report by the Robert Wood Johnson Foundation and the Institute of Medicine, *The Future of Nursing: Leading Change, Advancing Health,* recommends that nurses achieve higher levels of education and training through an education system that promotes seamless academic progression. I have lived this experience, and after two decades of practice I chose to return to school for a doctor of nursing practice degree at East Carolina University in Greenville, North Carolina.

The skills gained from additional education enable me to participate more fully in interprofessional teams to meet the health care needs of individuals and populations in North Carolina and throughout the United States. As our nation moves toward a redesigned health care system, it is imperative that nurses are well positioned to lead the way. Nursing addresses the pathophysiology of disease *and* the human response to illness. This perspec-

tive helps inform my leadership role in interprofessional education among nurse practitioner students and physician residents. Experience as a clinician and educator allows me to share clinical expertise to improve patient outcomes. Demonstrating nursing leadership among multiple health care disciplines has a valuable impact on the next generation of clinicians.

Doctoral nursing education enabled me to apply analytical methodologies for the evaluation of education models for NP transition to practice. Postgraduate NP education (fellowships and residencies) is gaining popularity and is funded primarily by employers interested in recruiting and retaining qualified health care professionals. My DNP project produced the first evidence demonstrating that postgraduate education positively affects NP job satisfaction. Knowledge of factors that influence job satisfaction is valuable to NPs and employers considering formal postgraduate education programs.

It is an excellent time to be a nurse. Together we can improve our nation's health by building on the strengths of all health disciplines, celebrating the differences, and pointing to models of collaboration that serve our citizens well.

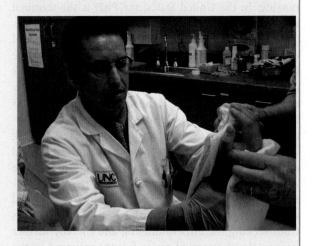

Tom Bush, DNP, FNP-BC, FAANP
East Carolina University, 2015

Reference: Courtesy North Carolina Health News.

nurses. Requirements for admission to certification programs vary, with some requiring only RN licensure and others requiring either a bachelor's or a master's degree. The ANCC, affiliated with the ANA, is

the largest of the certification bodies, providing many certification programs for RNs at the associate degree, bachelor's degree, and advanced practice levels. APNs certified by the ANCC must have master's degrees and demonstrate successful completion of a certification examination based on nationally recognized standards of nursing practice and designed to test their special knowledge and skills. For most specialties, candidates also must show evidence of specified clinical practice experience. Once granted, certification is valid for 3 to 5 years, whereupon the individual must apply for recertification by retesting or by demonstrating continuing education (CE) credits and evidence of ongoing clinical practice.

Nurses holding certification may use the initials RN, C (registered nurse, certified) after their names. Certified bachelor's-prepared nurses are entitled to use RN, BC (registered nurse, board certified). Those certified as clinical specialists use APRN, BC (advanced practice registered nurse, board certified). Box 4.1 lists the areas in which the ANCC offers certification.

Many in the nursing profession believe that nurses should be certified in a standardized manner by nationally recognized certifying boards only and that having multiple standards of certification is confusing and disadvantageous to the profession. The AACN has been particularly vocal in this regard and issued position statements in 1994, 1998, and 2008. The 2008 Consensus Model emphasized standardization goals focusing on APRNs (APRN Consensus Work Group and the National Council of State Boards of Nursing APRN Advisory Committee, 2008). This could become a model for nursing certifications at all levels, thereby unifying certification processes and rendering them more understandable by both employers and the public and thereby benefiting nursing.

MAINTAINING EXPERTISE AND STAYING CURRENT THROUGH CONTINUING EDUCATION

Continuing education (CE), also known as lifelong learning, is a term used to describe ways in which nurses maintain expertise during their professional careers. CE differs from staff development, which refers to how an agency or institution assists its employees in maintaining competence. CE opportunities are those pursued by individual nurses themselves and take place in a variety of settings: colleges, universities, hospitals, community agencies, professional organizations, and professional meetings. CE is available in many formats, such as workshops, institutes, conferences, short courses, evening

---

BOX 4.1 Areas of Certification by the American Nurses Credentialing Center (ANCC) in 2015

Nurse Practitioner (NP) Certification Areas
- Acute care NP
- Adult NP
- Adult—gerontology acute care NP
- Adult—gerontology primary care NP
- Adult psychiatric–mental health NP
- Family NP
- Gerontologic NP
- Pediatric primary care NP
- Psychiatric–mental health NP

Clinical Nurse Specialist (CNS) Certification Areas
- Adult—gerontology CNS
- Adult health CNS
- Adult psychiatric and mental health CNS
- Child/adolescent psychiatric and mental health CNS
- Pediatric CNS

Specialty Certification
- Ambulatory care nursing
- Cardiovascular nursing
- Faith community nursing
- Forensic nursing—advanced
- Genetics nursing—advanced
- Gerontologic nursing
- Hemostasis nursing
- Informatics nursing
- Medical-surgical nursing
- Nurse executive
- Nurse executive—advanced
- Nursing case management
- Nursing professional development
- Pain management nursing
- Pediatric nursing
- Psychiatric–mental health nursing
- Public health nursing—advanced
- Rheumatology nursing

From American Nurses Credentialing Center. Available at www.nursecredentialing.org.

---

courses, DL, and instructional modules offered in professional journals and by professional organizations online.

The ANCC is responsible for standards of CE, accreditation of programs offering CE, transferability of CE credit from state to state, and development of guidelines for recognition systems within states. The **contact hour** is the measure of CE credit. In general, nurses receive 1 contact hour of CE credit for each 50 or 60 minutes they spend in a CE course.

Most states require some evidence of CE for license renewal; the requirements, however, vary from state to state. Once you become licensed, you will need to be aware of the CE requirements for your state to maintain your license. Before renewing their licenses in states and territories with mandatory CE, nurses must provide evidence that they have met contact hour requirements. The requirement for mandatory continuing education is the mechanism through which a regulatory agency (such as a state board of nursing) ensures that nurses remain current in their profession. CE is required in most professions, including medicine, law, pharmacy, and accounting, among others.

CHALLENGES: FACULTY SHORTAGES AND QUALITY AND SAFETY EDUCATION IN TODAY'S COMPLEX HEALTH CARE ENVIRONMENT

A number of challenges face nursing education. Two major challenges are discussed in this section: (1) faculty and other resource shortages resulting in the inability of nursing programs to produce enough nurses to meet society's needs and (2) the need to transform nursing education to meet the need for quality and safety in the complex health care environment.

Faculty and Other Resource Shortages Resulting in Lack of Nurses

Despite the fact that enrollments in ADN and BSN degree programs across the nation have increased in recent years, the number of employed nurses still falls short of current needs and will fall further behind as the population ages. A lack of capacity in nursing schools was explored, and it was found to often be related to insufficient numbers of faculty, clinical sites, or other resources.

As the general population ages, so does the nurse faculty population. The latest available AACN data indicated that the average age of full professors in schools of nursing was 62 years and the average age of associate professors was 58 years (AACN, 2017; http://www.aacn-nursing.org/Portals/42/News/Factsheets/Faculty-Short-age-Factsheet-2017.pdf). This trend will result in increasing numbers of faculty retirements in the next

decade; in 2005 the NLN estimated that as many as 75% of current nursing faculty are expected to retire by 2019 (NLN, 2005). Faculty shortages are severe and seriously affect the nation's supply of RNs. Interest in nursing careers is strong, but access to professional nursing programs is increasingly difficult and is expected to become even more so for the foreseeable future. This represents a formidable challenge for the profession.

Continuing the Evolution of Nursing Education: Quality and Safety Education for Nurses

In response to the challenges of preparing future nurses adequately to "continuously improve the quality and safety of the health care systems," the QSEN project was funded by the Robert Wood Johnson Foundation. In phases 1 and 2 of the QSEN project, Drs. Linda Cronenwett and Gwen Sherwood of the University of North Carolina at Chapel Hill School of Nursing and their team developed and pilot-tested approaches to curricula that would ensure that future nursing graduates had competencies in patient-centered care, teamwork and collaboration, evidence-based practice, quality improvement, and informatics (QSEN, 2012).

In phase 3, which ended in 2012, Dr. Cronenwett and the AACN focused on three goals: (1) promote continuing innovation in the QSEN competencies and dissemination of these innovations; (2) develop faculty expertise required for students to achieve quality and safety competencies; and (3) create mechanisms to sustain the will to change among nursing programs through nursing textbooks, accreditation and certification standards, licensure examinations, and continued competence requirements. In Professional Profile Box 4.3, Linda Cronenwett, PhD, RN, FAAN, describes how the increasing complexity of health care has demanded new ways of thinking about quality and safety in nursing.

Some experts believe that education of all health professions is in need of systemic change. A notable example is the 2003 report of the IOM, *Health Professions Education: A Bridge to Quality*. This report built on the 2001 IOM report, *Crossing the Quality Chasm: A New Health System for the 21st Century*, which recommended a complete restructuring of clinical education across all health professions (IOM, 2001). As a follow-up to the initial report, a multidisciplinary summit of health profession leaders met in 2002; this high-level panel composed of 150 participants recommended the goal of "an

PROFESSIONAL PROFILE BOX 4.3
CHANGING MEANINGS OF QUALITY AND SAFETY IN NURSING EDUCATION

During most of the 20th century, patients were cared for by relatively few people. Even in the hospital, it was often one physician, one nurse per shift (working 5 days a week), and a head nurse who knew everything about each patient's condition. A nurse could know every medication she gave, and disruptions during medication rounds were few.

The sole purpose of nursing education was to prepare nurses to care for individual patients. Quality and safety were considered dependent on the knowledge and skills of individual professionals. A nurse could say, "I'm the best nurse on this unit. If your mother were sick, you'd want me caring for her. But don't bother me with committees or performance improvement teams or being a better team player. That's not the work I care to do." No one challenged that nurse's definition of what it meant to be a good nurse.

Today, health care is a complex enterprise. Multiple physicians and other health care professionals are involved in a hospitalized patient's care. Patients and families rarely have the same nurse 2 days in a row, and much nursing care is delivered by various types of assistants and technicians. There are thousands of pieces of medical equipment, multiple procedures and medications, and complex systems for documenting care. If you had to identify which professionals were responsible for the quality and safety of a patient's care, it would be hard to know who to hold accountable. In fact, quality and safety are more likely to be related to the way a health care microsystem (unit, clinic, or community-based setting) is designed to work than to the traits and skills of individual professionals. The reliability of the system is what meets or fails to meet patient needs, and although system reliability includes, it is not limited to, the quality of care any one professional gives any one patient.

With the 2003 IOM Report, *Health Professions Education: A Bridge to Quality,* all educators were challenged to alter the process of professional development so that health professionals, including nurses, would graduate understanding and accepting that their jobs consisted of both caring for individual patients and continuously improving the quality, safety, and reliability of the health care systems within which they worked. The development of specific competencies related to patient-centered care, interprofessional teamwork and collaboration,

evidence-based practice, safety sciences, quality improvement methods, and informatics was considered an essential element of future curricula. QSEN was an initiative funded by the Robert Wood Johnson Foundation to support faculty development to accomplish this paradigm shift in nursing education.

To be a good health professional into the future will mean knowing what constitutes good care (as it has in the past), but it will also mean knowing something about how the actual care delivered in one's unit or clinic compares to expected or best practices in the world at large. Furthermore, if there is a gap between good care and the results of care in one's own system, being a good health professional will mean knowing what one can do to close that gap.

Gradually, nursing curricula are changing to meet these new expectations. We want you to be good nurses in this new world—ones who know what quality of care is all about.

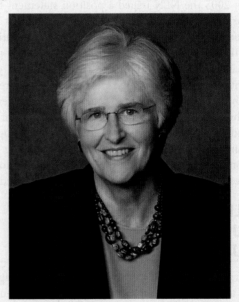

Linda R. Cronenwett, PhD, RN, FAAN
*Principal Investigator, Quality and Safety Education for Nurses
(QSEN), Distinguished Professor and Former Dean, School of Nursing,
University of North Carolina at Chapel Hill*

Reference: Courtesy Linda R. Cronenwett.

outcome-based education system that better prepares clinicians to meet both the needs of patients and the requirements of a changing health system" (IOM, 2003). Five major problems were identified in professional health education across disciplines (IOM, 2003):

1. Students are not being educated to care for the increasingly diverse, elderly, and chronically ill patient populations.
2. Students are not being prepared to work in teams, but once in practice, they are usually expected to work in interdisciplinary teams.
3. Students are not consistently educated in how to find, evaluate, and use the rapidly expanding scientific evidence on which practice should be based.
4. There is little opportunity to learn how to identify, analyze, and eliminate the root causes of errors and other quality problems in health care delivery systems.
5. Students often are not provided basic informatics training to enable them to access information and use computerized order entry systems.

In 2005 the NLN issued a position statement titled *Transforming Nursing Education.* This statement promoted evidence-based education—that is, educational practices based on research into best educational practices rather than "tradition, past practices, and good intentions" (NLN, 2005, p. 1). There is an increased emphasis on evidence-based practice in today's evolving health care environment. The NLN statement of a decade ago shaped the view of the faculties of schools of nursing in terms of designing and implementing educational practices in which the focus is on developing professional nursing practice that is evidence based.

COLLABORATION IN HEALTH CARE EDUCATION: INTERPROFESSIONAL EDUCATION

Interprofessional education (IPE) is a highly significant and recent development in the training of nurses, physicians, social workers, pharmacists, and other health care professionals, in which students in these disciplines take courses and have clinical experiences together. IPE involves structural changes in health care education to think beyond the traditional model in which health care professionals are educated separately, often without understanding the focus and expertise of practitioners in other disciplines. IPE enhances the development of respect across disciplines, increased understanding of the roles of other disciplines, and better communication among practitioners. Health care is more effective when delivered collaboratively using teamwork among health care professionals. Interprofessional teamwork and collaboration has the potential to increase patient satisfaction, decrease errors and improve safety, and be more cost effective (Derouin et al., 2018). In 2011 the IOM encouraged the health care professions to think differently about education, given the increasingly obvious need for collaboration among the professions to provide optimal health care and improve outcomes (IOM, 2015). Early adopters of IPE have begun to publish their experiences, with one noting that "IPE and practice are crucial to the development of future health care professionals" (Derouin et al., 2018, p. 225).

The important thing for students of nursing to recognize is that nursing organizations and leaders are constantly analyzing the changes in the health care system and working to set standards by which high-quality education nursing programs can be designed, implemented, and evaluated. The complexity of health care delivery systems, the various populations served, the shortage of faculty, and the lack of human and financial resources make this a challenging task. However, there is no question that nursing education—including movement toward interprofessional education—will continue to evolve and to be responsive to the significant changes in today's health care environment.

■ CONCEPTS AND CHALLENGES

- *Concept:* First provided in hospitals, entry-level nursing education has evolved into three major types of basic programs, diploma, ADN, and BSN, each of which has a range of features.
  Challenge: The differing levels of education for entry into practice pose a problem for nursing that has yet to be resolved, although an increasing number of employers are requiring at least a BSN.
- *Concept:* Alternatives such as bachelor's degree programs for RNs, external degree programs, accelerated options for postbaccalaureate students, and online programs contribute to a rich yet complex educational picture for RNs.

Challenge: Standardization of nursing education across the various programs becomes a challenge across these various educational offerings.

- *Concept:* Voluntary accreditation is designed to ensure the quality of nursing education programs.

  Challenge: Students are often not aware of their program's accreditation status. Graduate programs require that applicants be graduates of accredited schools of nursing.

- *Concept:* Schools have found it necessary to restrict enrollments because of faculty shortages, lack of clinical sites, and budget constraints.

  Challenge: Nursing leaders must work to make nurse faculty positions attractive in terms of compensation and work environment. At a time of economic volatility, this is a particularly difficult challenge for nursing.

- *Concept:* Lifelong learning through CE is considered essential for all professionals, particularly in practice-based disciplines such as nursing.

  Challenge: States vary on their requirements for CE for license renewal. Even if your state does not require CE, your professional responsibility is to stay current in practice through CE opportunities.

- *Concept:* The problem of reduced resources in nursing education may soon reach crisis proportions and poses a threat to smaller schools and universities.

Challenge: The underfunding of higher education in general and, in particular, diminishing sources of federal and state funding for schools of nursing require the attention of nurse leaders to ensure an adequate workforce of well-educated nurses to manage today's complex health care problems.

- *Concept:* QSEN was developed to meet the challenge of ensuring competencies of nursing graduates in patient-centered care, teamwork and collaboration, evidence-based practice, quality improvement, and informatics.

  Challenge: QSEN and other initiatives required a change in thinking about nursing education and the way nurses practice to ensure the best possible patient outcomes in a health care environment where resources are strained.

- *Concept:* IPE is a new and developing model of education for health care providers across disciplines in response to the increasing need for professional collaboration to optimize patients' health outcomes.

  Challenge: IPE is not yet widespread; however, nursing stands to benefit from IPE through its potential to elevate communication, create shared goals, and increase respect across health care disciplines.

IDEAS FOR FURTHER EXPLORATION

1. Watch *Sentimental Women Need Not Apply* (available on DVD). How does your experience of nursing school compare with that of students a century ago? What challenges to nursing have not changed over time?

2. How did you determine which type of basic nursing program you entered? Knowing what you know now, what changes, if any, would you make in your choice? How would you advise a high school student interested in nursing to select a program?

3. Consider the challenge that states face in determining whether a BSN should be the educational degree for entry into practice. Discuss the pros and cons of requiring a BSN to take the NCLEX-RN®. In what ways would the unification of nursing education strengthen the profession? What are the drawbacks to this approach?

4. If you could create a curriculum for nursing school, what would you include? What courses have surprised you by being included in your nursing education?

5. Discuss the merits and drawbacks of mandatory CE from viewpoints of both nurses and consumers of nursing care.

6. What unique contributions to nursing are possible by nurses with master's-degree–level education? With doctorates?

7. Find out if your school has implemented QSEN competencies. How prepared are you in each of the competencies?

8. Find out if your school offers any interprofessional courses or experiences with other health care disciplines. If so, consider enrolling in one or more to enhance your education and understanding of the focus and values of other health professionals.

REFERENCES

Aiken LH, Cheung RB, Olds DM: *Education policy initiatives to address the nurse shortage in the United States, Health Affairs Web Exclusive*, 2009 (website). Available at: http://content.healthaffairs.org/content/28/4/w646.full.

American Association of Colleges of Nursing (AACN): *Position statement: certification and regulation of advanced practice nurses*, Washington, DC, 1994, The Association (revised 1998).

American Association of Colleges of Nursing (AACN): *Position statement: the baccalaureate degree in nursing as minimal preparation for professional practice*, Washington, DC, 1996, The Association.

American Association of Colleges of Nursing (AACN): *Position statement: the practice doctorate in nursing*, Washington, DC, 2004, The Association.

American Association of Colleges of Nursing (AACN): *The Essentials of baccalaureate education for professional nursing practice*, Washington, DC, 2008, The Association. http://www.aacnnursing.org/Portals/42/News/Factsheets/Faculty-Shortage-Factsheet-2017.pdf.

American Nurses Association (ANA): *Position paper: educational preparation for nurse practitioners and assistants to nurses*, Kansas City, MO, 1965, The Association.

American Nurses Association (ANA): *A case for baccalaureate preparation in nursing*, Kansas City, MO, 1979, The Association.

American Nurses Association (ANA): *Funding for nursing workforce development*, 2015 (website). Available at: http://nursingworld.org/DocumentVault/GOVA/Federal/Federal-Issues/NursingWorkforceDevelopment.html.

APRN Consensus Work Group, National Council of State Boards of Nursing APRN Advisory Committee: *Consensus model for APRN regulation: licensure, accreditation, certification and education*, American Association of Colleges of Nursing, 2008 (website). Available at: www.aacn.nche.edu/education/pdf/APRNReport.pdf.

Benner P, Sutphen M, Leonard V, et al.: *Educating nurses: a call for radical transformation*, San Francisco, 2009, Jossey-Bass.

Brown EL: *Nursing for the future*, New York, 1948, Russell Sage Foundation.

Christy T: Portrait of a leader: M. Adelaide nutting, *Nurs Outlook* 17(1):20–24, 1969.

Conley V: *Curriculum and instruction in nursing*, Boston, 1973, Little, Brown.

Croasdale M: *Medical testing board to introduce doctor of nursing certification*, American Medical Association, 2008 (website). Available at: www.ama-assn.org/amednews/2008/06/16/prl10616.htm.

De Back V: The National commission on nursing implementation project, *Nurs Outlook* 39(3):124–127, 1991.

Derouin A, Holtschneider ME, McDaniel KE, Sanders KA, McNeill DB: Let's work together: interprofessional training of health professionals in North Carolina, *NC Med J* 79(4):223–225, 2018.

Donahue MP: *Nursing: the finest art: an illustrated history*, St. Louis, 1985, Mosby.

Dracup K, Bryan-Brown CW: Doctor of nursing practice: MRI or total body scan, *Am J Crit Care* 14(4):278–281, 2005.

Health Resources and Services Administration (HRSA): HRSA health workforce: nursing. (website). Available at: https://bhw.hrsa.gov/grants/nursing.

Institute of Medicine (IOM): *Crossing the quality chasm: a new health system for the 21st century*, Washington, DC, 2001, National Academies Press.

Institute of Medicine (IOM): *Health professions education: a bridge to quality*, Washington, DC, 2003, National Academies Press.

Institute of Medicine (IOM): *The future of nursing: leading change, advancing health*, Washington, DC, 2011, National Academies Press.

Institute of Medicine (IOM): *Measuring the impact of interprofessional education on collaborative practice and patient outcomes*, Washington, DC, 2015, National Academies Press.

Kalisch P, Kalisch B: *The advance of American nursing*, ed 3, Boston, 1995, Little, Brown.

Landro L: Making room for "Dr. Nurse," *Wall Street Journal*, April 2, 2008, p D-1.

Lysaught J: *An abstract for action*, New York, 1970, McGraw-Hill.

Montag M: *The education of nursing technicians*, New York, 1951, Putnam.

National League for Nursing Education: *Nursing schools today and tomorrow*, New York, 1934, The League.

National League of Nursing Education: *A curriculum guide for schools of nursing*, New York, 1937, The League.

National League for Nursing (NLN): *Position statement on nursing roles: scope and preparation*, New York, 1982, The League.

National League for Nursing (NLN): *Council of associate degree programs: educational outcomes of associate degree nursing programs: roles and competencies*, New York, 1990, The League.

National League for Nursing (NLN): *Educational competencies for graduates of associate degree nursing programs*, New York, 2000, The League.

National League for Nursing (NLN): *Transforming nursing education* (website). Available at www.nln.org/aboutnln/PositionStatements/index.htm, 2005.

National League for Nursing (NLN): Preparing the next generation of nurses to practice in a technology-rich environment: an informatics agenda, 2008 (website). Available at: www.nln.org/aboutnln/PositionStatements/index.htm.

Notter L, Spalding E: *Professional nursing: foundations, perspectives and relationships*, ed 9, Philadelphia, 1976, JB Lippincott.

Parietti E: The development of doctoral education in nursing: a historical overview. In Allen J, editor: *Consumer's guide to doctoral degree programs in nursing*, New York, 1990, National League for Nursing, p 1532.

Ponte RP, Nicholas PK: Addressing the confusion related to DNS, DNSc, and DSN degrees, with lessons for the nursing profession, *J Nurs Scholarsh* 42(4):347–353, 2015.

QSEN: *Quality and safety education for nurses*, 2012 (website). Available at: www.qsen.org.

Rhode Island Nurses Institute Middle College: Mission and vision, 2018 (website). Available at: www.rinimc.org.

Spector N, Odom S: The initiative to advance innovations in nursing education: three years later, *J Nurs Regul* 3(2):40–44, 2012.

Tri-Council for Nursing: Tri-Council for Nursing issues new consensus policy statement on educational advancement of registered nurses, 2010 (website). Available at: www.nln.org/newsroom/news-releases/news-release/2010/05/14/tri-council-for-nursing-issues-new-consensus-policy-statement-on-the-educational-advancement-of-registered-nurses.

5

Becoming a Professional Nurse: Defining Nursing and Socialization Into Practice

Maureen J. Baker, BSN, MSN, PhD

Ⓔ To enhance your understanding of this chapter, try the Student Exercises on the Evolve site at http://evolve.elsevier.com/Black/professional.

LEARNING OUTCOMES

After studying this chapter, students will be able to:

- Describe the benefits of defining nursing and how this is related to professional socialization.
- Compare early definitions of nursing with contemporary ones.
- Recognize the impact of historical, social, economic, and political events on evolving definitions of nursing.
- Identify commonalities in existing definitions of nursing.

- Understand how students' initial images of nursing are transformed through professional education and experiences.
- Differentiate between formal and informal socialization.
- Identify factors that influence an individual's professional socialization.
- Describe two developmental models of professional socialization, and explain how they are used.
- Describe strategies to ease the transition from student to professional nurse.

Suppose you were to ask someone, "What do nurses do?" Then think about how you as a nursing student would answer the same question. You might be tempted to respond with a list of psychomotor skills such as injections, medication administration, and physical assessments you have been practicing in your clinical setting. You might use some of your communication skills to turn the question back on the person: "You are wondering about nurses. What is it that *you* think nurses do?" This might be your best means of buying some time until you come up with an answer—describing the work of nursing is not always easy.

This chapter will help you answer this question. Definitions of nursing and nursing's scope of practice delineate who nurses are and what they do. Definitions provide answers to these questions: "What is nursing?" "What is the role of the nurse?" "What is unique about nursing?" and "What are the boundaries of nursing practice?" Although the answers to these questions

seem simple, agreement on a single definition of nursing has been elusive; however, the careful crafting of definitions of nursing by noteworthy nursing organizations has resulted in definitions that are increasingly similar and specific about what nursing is.

In this chapter, definitions of nursing are explored to determine how they have evolved over time. Once you have a clear understanding of definitions of nursing, you will learn how to make the move from student to nursing student and then from nursing student to professional nurse. This developmental trajectory from student to professional nurse involves a process known as *socialization*, which occurs over time but ultimately guides you in developing a safe and informed professional nursing practice. Defining nursing is an important first step in socialization. Having a clearer understanding of what nursing is (and, as Nightingale said, "What it is not") helps you move closer to incorporating the values of professional practice.

DEFINING NURSING: HARDER THAN IT SEEMS

You may be surprised to learn that finding a universally acceptable definition of nursing has been difficult historically. Common responses to your question, "What do nurses do?" might be "They take care of people in the hospital" and "They help doctors." Few people outside of the health care setting understand who nurses are and what they do.

Even nurses themselves have been unable to agree on one definition. For more than 150 years, individuals and organizations around the world such as the International Council of Nurses (ICN), the United Kingdom's Royal College of Nursing (RCN), and the American Nurses Association (ANA) have attempted to achieve a consensus on a definition of nursing. In 1859 Florence Nightingale wrote a famous text, *Notes on Nursing: What It Is and What It Is Not,* an early attempt to define who and what nurses are and do. Some efforts have been more successful than others.

The definitions reviewed in this chapter have become increasingly aligned over time. Considering the variations in knowledge and technology during the different points in history when these definitions were written, the similarities are remarkable. All the definitions are rooted in history and were affected by significant political, economic, and social events that shaped nursing.

Why Define Nursing?

Having an accepted definition of nursing provides a framework for nursing practice. A definition establishes the parameters (or boundaries) of the profession and delineates the purposes and functions of the work of nursing. In addition, a definition guides the educational preparation of aspiring practitioners and guides nursing research and theory development. Importantly, a clear definition makes the work of nursing visible and valuable to the public and to policymakers who determine when, where, and how nurses can practice. Norma Lang, Professor and Dean Emerita at the University of Pennsylvania, described the need for definition succinctly: "If we cannot name it, we cannot control it, finance it, research it, teach it, or put it into public policy. It's just that blunt!" (Styles, 1991).

Definitions Clarify Purposes and Functions

Nursing is a complex enterprise that is often confusing to its own practitioners as well as to the public. Defining nursing assists people to grasp its nuances, many of which are not readily observable. The profession of nursing benefits when the public, other health care providers, policy makers, insurers, and journalists, among others, understand who nurses are and what they do.

Definitions Differentiate Nursing from Other Health Occupations

Five million allied health care providers in more than 80 different occupations represent approximately 60% of all health care providers (Explore Health Careers, 2018). Advances in technology require providers who need to be educated, hired, and oriented to their specific work setting and who are paid with limited health care dollars. These resulting costs figured greatly into the redesign of the health care system over the past decade and required the redefining of roles within the system. Defining nursing amid these new providers became even more important to avoid losing the core identity of nursing. Nurses have had to name and claim for their own what it is that nurses do.

Furthermore, with the implementation of health care reforms, nursing must be clearly defined and its importance within the health care system unmistakable. Nurses understand that they have the skills and expertise to address a wide variety of health issues; keeping nurses in key positions of influence as the health care system continues to take shape in the next few years is crucial to fulfilling nursing's social contract with the public, which you read about in previous chapters. The ANA's *Nursing's Social Policy Statement: The Essence of the Profession* explicates this contract.

Definitions Influence Health Policy at Local, State, and National Levels

Policymakers, such as legislators and regulators, need a clear understanding of the role and scope of nursing. Without that understanding, they cannot institute good health care policy that maximizes use of nurses' particular skills to protect and improve the health of the public.

A key reason to define nursing is that nursing practice is regulated at the state level. Nursing practice acts of each state need to reflect the widening expertise and autonomy of nurses. When the roles of professional registered nurses (RNs), advanced practice nurses, licensed practical/vocational nurses, and nursing assistants are well defined, legislators can pass progressive laws regulating and expanding nursing practice. Otherwise, nursing practice acts that are legislated by state governing bodies may restrict nursing practice and inhibit professional growth.

Definitions Focus Educational Curricula and Research Agendas

When nursing faculty plan the curriculum of a school of nursing, one of the major determinants of the design is their definition of nursing. A definition of nursing provides a good starting point for curriculum development. Without the foundation of a clear definition, deciding what to include in a nursing curriculum and how to prioritize educational needs would be very difficult and unwieldy. In much the same way, nurse researchers cannot easily determine phenomena of interest for nursing unless they are clear about the boundaries and purposes of nursing actions that a definition of nursing sets in place.

Evolution of Definitions of Nursing

While nursing was progressing as a more formal academic discipline and practice profession over the past 150 years, a number of attempts were made to define nursing that reflect the profession's evolution over the years.

Nightingale Defines Nursing

Florence Nightingale was the first person to recognize the complexities of nursing that led to difficulty in defining it. Considering how relatively undeveloped nursing was during her time, Nightingale's definitions contain what today we recognize as contemporary concepts. Remember that during Nightingale's day, formal education in nursing was just beginning. In *Notes on Nursing: What It Is and What It Is Not* (originally published in 1859), she became the first person to attempt a written definition of nursing, stating, "And what nursing has to do … is put the patient in the best condition for nature to act upon him" (Nightingale, 1946, p. 75). She also wrote:

> I use the word nursing for want of a better. It has been limited to signify little more than the administration of medicines and the application of poultices. It ought to signify the proper use of fresh air, light, warmth, cleanliness, quiet, and the proper selection and administration of diet—all at the least expense of vital power to the patient. (Nightingale, 1946, p. 6)

Although Nightingale lived in a time when little was known about disease processes and effective treatments were extremely limited, these definitions foreshadowed contemporary nursing's focus on the therapeutic environment as well as the modern emphasis on health promotion and health maintenance. She accurately observed that, although simply possessing observational skills does not make someone a good nurse, without these skills a nurse is ineffective. Indeed, informed observation has always been an integral part of the processes of nursing. Nightingale was also the first person to differentiate between nursing provided by a professional nurse using a unique body of knowledge and physical care provided by a layperson such as a mother caring for a sick child.

Early 20th-Century Definitions

Fifty years after Nightingale wrote *Notes on Nursing*, the search for a definition began in earnest. Following the English model, many schools of nursing had been established in the United States, and many nurses with formal education were practicing. These nurses sought to develop a professional identity for their rapidly expanding discipline. Shaw's *Textbook of Nursing* (1907) defined nursing as an art: "It properly includes, as well as the execution of specific orders, the administration of food and medicine, the personal care of the patient" (pp. 1–2). Harmer's *Textbook of the Principles and Practice of Nursing* (1922) elaborated on Shaw's bare-bones definition: "The object of nursing is not only to cure the sick … but to bring health and ease, rest and comfort to mind and body. Its object is to prevent disease and to preserve health" (p. 3). The fourth edition of the Harmer text, which showed the influence of coauthor and visionary Virginia Henderson, redefined nursing: "Nursing may be defined as that service to an individual that helps him to attain or maintain a healthy state of mind or body" (Harmer and Henderson, 1939, p. 2). Henderson's perceptions represented the emergence of contemporary nursing and were so inclusive that they remained useful over a long time. We will encounter her influence again in the next section.

Post–World War II Definitions

World War II helped advance the technologies available to treat people, which, in turn, influenced nursing. The war also made nurses aware of the influential role emotions play in health, illness, and nursing care. Hildegard Peplau (1952), widely regarded as a pioneer among contemporary nursing theorists and herself a psychiatric nurse, defined nursing in interpersonal terms: "Nursing is a significant, therapeutic, interpersonal process. Nursing is an educative instrument that aims to promote forward movement of personality in the direction of creative, constructive, productive, personal, and community living" (p. 16). Peplau reinforced the idea of the patient as an active collaborator in his or her own care. Recently, Peplau's notion of patient participation and collaboration in their health and health care has reemerged and is referred to as active patient engagement. Patient engagement, or when patients take purposeful action in improving their health, is a crucial factor in helping transform the current health care paradigm. During the late 1950s and early 1960s, the number of master's programs in nursing rapidly increased. As more nurses were educated at the graduate level and learned about the research process, they were eager to test new ideas about nursing. Nursing theory was born. (See Chapter 9 for an in-depth discussion of nursing theory.)

Dorothea Orem was one of the important theorists who began work during this early period of theory development. Her 1959 definition captures the flavor of her later, more completely elaborated self-care theory of nursing: "Nursing is perhaps best described as the giving of direct assistance to a person, as required, because of the person's specific inabilities in self-care resulting from a situation of personal health" (Orem, 1959, p. 5). Orem's belief that nurses should do for a person only those things the person cannot do without assistance emphasized the patient's active role.

By 1960, Henderson's earlier definition had evolved into a statement with such universal appeal it was adopted by the ICN:

The unique function of the nurse is to assist the individual, sick or well, in the performance of those activities contributing to health or its recovery (or to a peaceful death) that he would perform unaided if he had the necessary strength, will or knowledge. And to do this in such a way as to help him gain independence as rapidly as possible. (Henderson, 1960, p. 3)

This definition of nursing was widely accepted both in the United States and across the world. Many believe it is still the most comprehensive and appropriate definition of nursing in existence.

Another pioneer nursing theorist, Martha Rogers, included the concept of the nursing process in her definition: "Nursing aims to assist people in achieving their maximum health potential. Maintenance and promotion of health, prevention of disease, nursing diagnosis, intervention, and rehabilitation encompass the scope of nursing's goals" (Rogers, 1961, p. 86).

Professional Association Definitions

Nursing organizations worldwide have worked to define nursing, developing and revising them over time. Definitions reviewed here include those of the ANA, the RCN, and the ICN. As you study these definitions, notice that some new concepts and terms are introduced in the more recent American definitions. In the United States nursing has defined itself as the health discipline that "cares," although recent discussion suggests that limiting nursing to "caring" only overlooks the significant role that nurses have in the curative processes of health care (Gordon, 2005).

American Nurses Association. The ANA has published several definitions of nursing over the years. As of 2015, the ANA continued to define nursing as "the protection, promotion and optimization of health and ability, prevention of illness and injury, alleviation of suffering through the diagnosis and treatment of human response, and advocacy in the care of individuals, families, communities and populations" (ANA, 2015b). This is the definition published in both the 2003 and 2010 editions of *Nursing's Social Policy Statement: The Essence of the Profession.* This definition includes six essential features of contemporary nursing practice (ANA, 2003, p. 5) that the ANA still recognizes:

- Provision of a caring relationship that facilitates health and healing
- Attention to the range of human experiences and responses to health and illness within the physical and social environments
- Integration of objective data with knowledge gained from an appreciation of the patient or group's subjective experience
- Application of scientific knowledge to the processes of diagnosis and treatment through the use of judgment and critical thinking
- Advancement of professional nursing knowledge through scholarly inquiry
- Influence on social and public policy to promote social justice

The wide focus of the practice of nursing is described in the preface to the *Code of Ethics for Nurses* (ANA, 2015a): "Nursing encompasses the prevention of illness, the alleviation of suffering, and the protection, promotion, and restoration of health in the care of individuals, families, groups, and communities" (p. 10). The definition of nursing and the ethics to which nurses are bound are intertwined.

Royal College of Nursing. The RCN is the United Kingdom's voice of nursing and is the largest professional union of nurses in the world. This organization embarked on an 18-month-long initiative to define nursing, culminating in the April 2003 publication of the document titled *Defining Nursing* (RCN, 2003). In 2014 the RCN's Nursing Policy and Practice Committee upheld and affirmed the continuing appropriateness of the 2003 definition because it described nursing to persons who do not understand nursing; it clarified the role of nurses in multidisciplinary teams and identified areas of research that nursing needs to strengthen its science (RCN, 2015).

The RCN definition of nursing has a core statement supported by six defining characteristics:

> *Nursing is the use of clinical judgment in the provision of care to enable people to improve, maintain, or recover health, to cope with health problems, and to achieve the best possible quality of life, whatever their disease or disability, until death.*
> **Royal College of Nursing. (2003). Defining Nursing.**
> **RCN, London**

The six defining characteristics are delineated by statements of the "particulars of nursing": purpose, mode of intervention, domain, focus, value base, and commitment to partnership. A full description of the particulars is available at www.rcn.org.uk.

International Council of Nurses. The ICN is a federation of national nurses associations representing more than 13 million nurses worldwide in more than 130 countries. Although ICN's membership is diverse, its definition of nursing is similar to that of single-nation organizations such as the ANA and RCN. According to the ICN:

> *Nursing encompasses autonomous and collaborative care of individuals of all ages, families, groups and communities, sick or well and in all settings. Nursing includes the promotion of health, prevention of illness, and the care of ill, disabled and dying people. Advocacy, promotion of a safe environment, research, participation in shaping health policy and in patient and health systems management, and education are also key nursing roles. (ICN, 2015)*

You can learn much more about the ICN online at www.icn.ch.

Definitions Developed by State Legislatures

One of the most significant definitions of nursing is contained in the nursing practice act of the state in which a nurse practices. Regardless of how restrictive or permissive it may be, the definition contained in a nursing practice act constitutes the legal definition of nursing in a particular state. Professional nurses must maintain familiarity with the latest version of the act. North Carolina's Nursing Practice Act, most recently revised in 2009, contains particularly specific language defining nursing (North Carolina Board of Nursing, 2009):

> *"Nursing" is a dynamic discipline which includes the assessing, caring, counseling, teaching, referring and implementing of prescribed treatment in the maintenance of health, prevention and management of illness, injury, disability or the achievement of a dignified death. It is ministering to, assisting, and sustained, vigilant, and continuous care of those acutely or chronically ill; supervising patients during convalescence and rehabilitation; the supportive and restorative care given to maintain the optimum health level of individuals, groups, and communities; the supervision, teaching, and evaluation of those who perform or are preparing to perform these functions; and the administration of nursing programs and nursing services.*

Furthermore, the North Carolina Board of Nursing describes nursing as a dynamic discipline, described as both a science and an art:

> *The practice of nursing is a scientific process founded on a professional body of knowledge. It is a learned profession based on an understanding of the human condition across the life span and the relationship of a client with others and within the environment. The practice of nursing is an art dedicated to caring and to assisting clients by providing sustained, vigilant, and continuous care to those acutely or chronically ill. Nurses assist clients to attain or maintain optimal health, implementing a strategy of care to accomplish defined goals within the context of a client centered health care plan. Nursing is a dynamic discipline that increasingly involves more sophisticated knowledge, technologies and client care activities. (North Carolina Board of Nursing, 2017)*

? THINKING CRITICALLY BOX 5.1

What Would You Do?

Imagine you are dining out and are seated next to a table where an 18-year-old woman tells her parents she wants to be a nurse. The parents' reaction is one of disdain. They reply, "Are you serious? You want to be a nurse? You want to clean backsides and sling around bedpans for the rest of your life? Why don't you think about medical school—that is much better and much more respectable." The daughter, visibly upset, leaves the table. The parents turn to you and say, "Why would anyone want to be a nurse?"

What would you do and what would you say to these parents? Using your thoughts and experience, as well as elements of definitions from this chapter, how would you explain and define nursing to them? You may want to save your response and refer to it after you graduate from nursing school. As you become more socialized into nursing, your definition will likely evolve.

The language in this nursing practice act sounds like familiar nursing language. State nurses associations and boards of nursing actively assist legislators in drafting laws that accurately reflect the nature and scope of nursing. The current nursing practice act in each state can be obtained online or by calling or writing the state board of nursing. The website www.cybernurse.com/state-boards.html lists the contact person and contact information for all 50 states and the U.S. territories of Guam, the Virgin Islands, and the Northern Mariana Islands.

Before moving on to the next discussion on socialization, take time to look at the question posed in Thinking Critically Box 5.1. What would you do?

BECOMING A NURSE: SHAPING YOUR PROFESSIONAL IDENTITY

Defining nursing means that you have determined the essential elements of being a nurse: what a nurse is and what a nurse does. When you first decided to become a nurse, you had certain preconceived notions about what nursing was and how you saw yourself as a nurse. Your desire to be a nurse may have been shaped by an illness experience of your own or a family member. Becoming a nurse may simply be something that you have always wanted to do without a specific event that spurred this desire. Or you may be pragmatic in your career choice by selecting a profession in which demand is high, the risk of unemployment is low, and the compensation is adequate. Whatever the reason you decided pursue a career in nursing, your view of nursing and what it entails is almost certainly going to be challenged while in nursing school. Your thinking about nursing should evolve and mature over the course of your education and career.

Although many students enter the profession of nursing with the goal of "taking care of people," how this goal is translated into practice remains something of a mystery until you begin your education as a nursing student. Being a student of nursing is the first of many steps in socializing you into professional practice: the goal of socialization is the development of professionalism. The goal of your nursing education is not simply teaching you the tasks of nursing, although they are important elements of your practice. The overriding goal of your education is to teach you to think like a nurse, to see the world of health care through the lens of nursing, and to respond to your educational and clinical experiences with the development of professionalism.

This process requires that students internalize, or take in, new knowledge, skills, attitudes, behaviors, values, and ethical standards and make these a part of their own professional identity. For the RN returning to school for a bachelor of science in nursing (BSN) degree, a modification of an already formed professional identity occurs. This process of internalization and development or modification of an occupational identity are known as *professional socialization*; it begins during the period when students are in formal nursing programs and continues as they practice in the "real world."

Lai and Lim (2012) described two conditions—structural and cultural—that are part of professional socialization in nursing. Structural conditions are those in which one's professional role is shaped by rules (e.g., job descriptions, workplace policies, carrying out prescriptions for care by physicians and other providers). Cultural conditions are those in which traditions, symbols, language, and other idea systems in a society are at work in shaping how one becomes a fully socialized professional nurse. The goal, then, of socialization as a professional nurse is the development of a professional identity such that the attributes of nursing become "part of a nurse's personal and professional self-image and behavior" (p. 32).

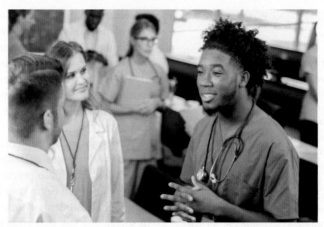

Fig. 5.1 During formal socialization, students internalize the knowledge, skills, and beliefs of nursing in planned educational experiences and interactions with faculty and other nurses. (Photo used with permission from iStockphoto.)

FROM STUDENT TO NURSE: FACILITATING THE TRANSITION

Nursing faculty are concerned with creating educational experiences that encourage and facilitate the transition from student to professional nurse. You may wonder how this transition occurs, especially when you are faced with the challenges of simply figuring out what is going on in your classes, labs, and clinical sites.

Learning any new role is derived from a mixture of formal and informal socialization. We have all been socialized into a variety of roles over the course of our lives. One that is so familiar to you now is the role of student in a generic sense. You learned in kindergarten that there are particular ways to behave in class, times to sit quietly and times to play, ways to get the teacher's attention, and ways that you did not want to get the teacher's attention. You learned the unwritten rules of being a student, and, unless you were particularly incorrigible, you learned your role as a student early and well.

In nursing, formal socialization includes lectures, online activities, assignments, and clinical experiences, such as planning nursing care, writing a paper on professional ethics, learning steps of a physical examination of a healthy child, starting an intravenous line, practicing communication skills with a psychiatric patient, or spending time with a mentor (Fig. 5.1). A faculty member may serve as your first nursing mentor. Formal socialization proceeds in an orderly, building-block fashion, such that new information is based on previous information. For that reason, more advanced nursing students are often encouraged to manage a larger number of patients than they did as novice students, when their skills were fewer and less tested.

Informal socialization includes lessons that occur incidentally, such as the unplanned observation of a nurse teaching a young mother how to care for her premature infant, participating in a student nurse association, or hearing nurses discuss patient care in the nurses' lounge. Part of professional socialization is simply absorbing the culture of nursing—that is, the rites, rituals, and valued behaviors of the profession. This requires that students spend enough time with nurses in work settings for adequate exposure to the nursing culture to occur. Most nurses agree that informal socialization experiences were often more powerful and memorable than formal socialization in their own development.

Learning a new vocabulary is also part of professional socialization. Each profession has its own jargon that is generally not well understood by outsiders. Professional students in any field usually enjoy acquiring the new vocabulary and practicing it among themselves. Although the vocabulary of any profession can be confusing and complex, students quickly become fluent as a function of both formal and informal socialization. Students should be aware, however, that certain informal vocabulary overheard on nursing units is not always appropriate in professional settings and may actually be denigrating to patients or their families. Deciding early to forgo these sorts of negative characterizations is a step toward maturity in your professional socialization.

Learning any new role creates some degree of anxiety. You likely remember your nervousness and anxiety as you started college or a new job. New students may find themselves particularly anxious as clinical experiences begin—the uncertainty of the situation, the unfamiliar language, the presence of patients with serious medical diagnoses, and a keen sense of the importance of the work of nursing can all contribute to this anxiety. Once the initial anxiety and excitement of entering nursing school have worn off, students may find themselves dealing with disappointment and frustration when their learning expectations come into conflict with educational realities. Students' ideas of what they need to learn, when they need to learn it, and what might be the best way to learn it may differ from how their education actually unfolds. Students sometimes become disillusioned when they observe nurses behaving in ways that conflict with their ideas and ideals about how nurses should behave. Knowing in advance that these things may happen can help students accurately assess the sources of their anxiety and manage it more effectively.

Factors Influencing Socialization

As students progress through nursing programs, a variety of factors challenge their customary ways of thinking. These include personal feelings and beliefs, some of which may conflict with professional values. For example, if students have strong religious beliefs, they may be uncomfortable working with patients who have no such belief or whose beliefs are different from their own. Yet the very first statement in the *Code of Ethics for Nurses* (ANA, 2001) requires that nurses work with all patients regardless of their beliefs. However, if you have a strong moral objection to a particular belief system of a patient or a negative reaction to a patient based on some characteristic of the patient, you should seek out your clinical faculty or other professional mentor to discuss your reaction and determine how to handle your conflicted feelings in an appropriate and professional way. This is not an uncommon response in nursing students as their sphere of contact with others different from themselves grows.

When children are growing up, they are first influenced by the values, beliefs, and behaviors of the significant adults around them. Later, peers become a significant influence. These influences also shape ideas about health, health care, and nursing. A common issue in nursing practice revolves around negative health behaviors of patients. If a nurse's family valued fitness,

for example, that nurse may have difficulty empathizing with an obese patient with heart disease who refuses to exercise despite the clear health benefits. In this example, a personal value (fitness) comes into conflict with a professional value (nonjudgmental acceptance of patients). Other patient issues that sometimes challenge students' personal values are substance abuse, self-destructive behaviors, abortion, issues related to sexuality, sexual orientation, expression of gender identity, fertility treatments, and care at the end of life.

All people have biases; however, unexamined biases are more likely to influence behavior than examined ones. Nurses need to be aware of their biases and discuss them with peers, faculty, and professional role models or mentors. Failure to address one's biases may adversely affect the nursing care provided to certain patients. Professional nurses make every effort to avoid imposing their personal beliefs on others. (See Chapter 12 for further discussion of self-awareness and nonjudgmental acceptance as necessary attributes of professional nurses.) Becoming a professional nurse requires learning how to deal with conflicts in values such as these while respecting patients' differing viewpoints. This cannot be taught but is the responsibility of each aspiring professional. Having a systematic way to examine and think about your actions and responses to patient situations is a tenet of reflective practice (Sherwood and Horton-Deutsch, 2012). Reflective practice can help nurses cope with their role in a complex, emotionally charged health care system and concurrently help them develop their knowledge and nursing practice (Sherwood and Zomorodi, 2014). The key point is that you should begin to identify and reflect on those "hot button" issues that seem to affect you negatively so that you can understand your own responses and how to set them aside while still providing excellent care of your patients.

As seen from this brief overview, socialization is much more than the transmission of knowledge and skills. Socialization serves to develop a common nursing consciousness and is the key to keeping the profession vital and dynamic while preserving its fundamental focus on human responses in health and illness.

A New Factor Influencing Socialization: Distance Learning

Distance learning in nursing has become common. Increasing numbers of nursing schools are using technology to deliver education to students who do not have access to traditional on-campus programs. Initially, single courses or continuing education short courses were offered by distance education. Today, entire nursing curricula are offered via video teleconferencing and online courses, with limited time spent on campus. This trend is expected to continue as demand increases. Even in traditional nursing curricula, some content is taught online combined with occasional classroom sessions (also known as "hybrid" courses).

Students have found distance education to be useful; "millennials" born in the late 1990s and early 2000s now at college age use technology easily and would like to see faculty develop courses that appeal to their comfort with technology and distance learning (Fichten et al., 2015; McHaney, 2012). Questions then arise about whether professional attitudes and values—in other words, professional socialization—can be effectively achieved through distance education. In a compelling large-sample study from Canada related to distance learning and socialization published by Loisier in 2014 (tonybates.ca, 2015), researchers found that despite the support of the idea of collaborative learning and socialization via distance education, socialization does not occur automatically online in collaborative work and in fact it may conflict with distance students' desire for flexible and individual learning. This finding is somewhat at odds with Peddle, Bearman, and Nestel's integrative review (2016) suggesting that at least with regard to undergraduate health professional education, distance learning, including the use of virtual patients and environments, may be used successfully and with adequate socialization.

"JUST GOING THROUGH A STAGE": MODELS OF SOCIALIZATION

The transition from student to nurse is a topic of importance to nurse researchers interested in creating effective means of professional socialization. During the 1970s and 1980s, a number of models of professional socialization of basic and RN students were developed. Cohen (1981) and Hinshaw (1976) described developmental models appropriate for beginning nursing students. Bandura (1977) described a type of socialization he called *modeling*, which is useful when learning any new behavior. Benner (1984) identified five stages nurses pass through in the transition from novice to expert. Cohen's and Benner's models are explained in

more detail subsequently. Although these models were developed in the early 1980s, they serve to describe processes of transition and socialization that many faculty have come to recognize as almost universal among nursing students.

Cohen's Model of Basic Student Socialization

Cohen (1981) proposed a model of professional socialization consisting of four stages. Basing her work on developmental theories and studies of beginning students' attitudes toward nursing, she asserted, "Students must experience each stage in sequence to feel comfortable in the professional role" (p. 16). She believed that a positive outcome in all four stages is necessary for satisfactory socialization to occur. You may find yourself determining where you and your classmates stand amid these four stages. A reminder, however: although it is interesting and potentially useful, this model has not been subjected to rigorous testing or scientific validation. However, this model does appear to fit the behaviors that experienced faculty note in the development of students' socialization into professional practice.

Cohen identified the first stage in her model, stage I, as unilateral dependence. Because they are inexperienced and lack knowledge, students at this stage rely on external limits and controls established by authority figures such as teachers. During stage I, students are unlikely to question or analyze critically the concepts teachers present, because they lack the necessary background to do so. An example of a student operating in a unilateral dependent stage would be the student who agrees to a clinical assignment without questioning the clinical faculty's thinking about the appropriateness of the assignment or what the student may gain from the assignment. The student absorbs the faculty's direction and discussion about the patient without yet making linkages of his or her own in thinking about the patient's condition. Fundamentally, students at this stage do as they are told because they lack the experience and knowledge to question.

In stage II (negativity/independence), students' critical thinking abilities and knowledge bases expand. They begin to question authority figures. Cohen called this occurrence cognitive rebellion. Students at this level begin to free themselves from external controls and to rely more on their own judgment. They think critically about what they are being taught. This is a stage when students begin to question, "Why do I have to learn about this? This isn't nursing!" or complain, "I will never learn to give an injection to a patient if I have to sit here reading about the nursing process!" This can be a stage where a student's fledgling independence may cause some lack of judgment in the clinical setting; at this stage, students might not consult with their clinical faculty before attempting a new procedure because they do not appreciate the safety net the clinical faculty brings to the situation. In addition, students at this stage may begin to demand to care for additional or more complex patients, resisting their faculty's (more informed) judgment that the student is not yet ready.

Stage III (dependence/mutuality) is characterized by what Cohen described as students' more reasoned evaluation of others' ideas. They develop an increasingly realistic appraisal process and learn to test concepts, facts, ideas, and models objectively. Students at this stage are more impartial; they accept some ideas and reject others. This is a time when students begin to appreciate the usefulness of the nursing process in organizing care and begin to use more sophisticated critical thinking skills.

In stage IV (interdependence), students' needs for both independence and mutuality (sharing jointly with others) come together. Students develop the capacity to make decisions in collaboration with others. The successfully socialized student completes stage IV with a self-concept that includes a professional role identity that is personally and professionally acceptable and compatible with other life roles. Faculty appreciate the maturity and trustworthiness that students exhibit when they reach this stage in their professional development. These students are often highly self-directed, seeking out learning experiences to maximize their knowledge before the completion of their formal education. Table 5.1 summarizes the key behaviors associated with each of Cohen's stages.

Benner's Stages of Nursing Proficiency (Basic Student Socialization)

Patricia Benner, a nurse, was curious about how nurses made the transition from inexpert beginners to highly expert practitioners. She described a process consisting of five stages of nursing practice, on which she based her 1984 book, *From Novice to Expert.* The stages Benner described are "novice," "advanced beginner," "competent practitioner," "proficient practitioner," and "expert practitioner." Advancing from stage to stage occurs gradually as nurses gain more experience in patient care. Clinical

TABLE 5.1   Cohen's Model of Basic Student Socialization

Stage	Key Behaviors
I: Unilateral dependence	Reliant on external authority; limited questioning or critical analysis
II: Negativity/ independence	Cognitive rebellion; diminished reliance on external authority
III: Dependence/ mutuality	Reasoned appraisal; begins integration of facts and opinions following objective testing
IV: Interdependence	Collaborative decision making; commitment to professional role; self-concept now includes professional role identity

Data from Cohen HA: *The nurse's quest for professional identity,* Menlo Park, CA, 1981, Addison-Wesley.

judgment is stimulated when the nurse's "preconceived notions and expectations" (p. 3) collide with, or are confirmed by, the realities of everyday practice.

Since its generation and publication in 1984, Benner's model has received and continues to receive significant attention from researchers testing how learning theories apply to adult skill acquisition (e.g., reflective thinking, clinical decision-making skills). Researchers have tested and confirmed that Benner's model is valid and suggested that her stages and theory can be used for all adult learning situations associated with nursing care (Oshvandi et al., 2016).

Benner's novice stage, or stage I, begins when students first enroll in nursing school. Because they generally have little background on which to base their clinical behavior, they must depend rather rigidly on rules and expectations established for them. Their practical skills are limited. For example, a novice nurse is faced with the request of a man who is terminally ill and wants to see and pet his beloved dog and faithful companion just one more time. The novice is very uncomfortable with the request because it is against the rules. The novice denies the request, citing the hospital rules.

By the time learners enter the advanced beginner period, or stage II, they have discerned that a particular order exists in clinical settings (Benner et al., 1996). Their performance is marginally competent. They can base their actions on both theory and principles but tend to experience difficulty in establishing priorities, viewing many nursing actions as equally important. When faced with the same situation as the novice nurse and the man approaching death who wants to cuddle and pet his dog just one last time, the advanced beginner nurse also has an understanding of the needs of the man to continue his familiar ritual, bringing him the comfort and companionship he had at home with his dog. The advanced beginner suggests that the family bring a picture of the dog so the man can see his dog and reflect and reminisce about the good times and friendship they had together.

Competent practitioners, or stage III learners, usually have 2 to 3 years' experience in a setting. As a result, they feel competent, organized, and efficient most of the time. These feelings of mastery are a result of planning and goal-setting skills and the ability to think abstractly and analytically. These learners can coordinate several complex demands simultaneously. For example, the competent nurse spends a few moments at the start of his or her shift examining the needs of each patient and planning fundamental care. At this stage, the competent nurse understands that situations change quickly and that planning is the best way to ensure that care gets implemented even when emergencies or unexpected events arise. This nurse may or may not allow the beloved dog in the patient's room; however, the nurse will examine the needs of everyone carefully and many of the exigencies involved before making a final decision.

Proficient practitioners (stage IV) have typically been in practice 3 to 5 years. These nurses are able to see patient situations holistically rather than in parts, to recognize and interpret subtleties of meaning, and to easily recognize priorities for care. They can focus on long-term goals and desired outcomes. These experienced nurses are likely to be leaders on their units, having a wealth of experience and commitment to nursing. Concerned with patient outcomes rather than institutional rules, the proficient nurse would likely understand in a holistic way the needs of the man whose life is nearing its end and his desire to continue a cherished ritual of petting and cuddling with his dog. This nurse is likely to allow the "rules" to be broken in deference to the needs of the man.

Expert practitioner, or stage V, status is reached only after extensive practice experience. These nurses perform intuitively, without conscious thought, automatically grasping the significance of the patient's complete

TABLE 5.2	**Benner's Stages of Nursing Proficiency (Basic Student Socialization)**
Stage	**Nurse Behaviors**
I: Novice	Has little background and limited practical skills; relies on rules and expectations of others for direction
II: Advanced beginner	Has marginally competent skills; uses theory and principles much of the time; experiences difficulty establishing priorities
III: Competent practitioner	Feels competent, organized; plans and sets goals; thinks abstractly and analytically; coordinates several tasks simultaneously
IV: Proficient practitioner	Views patients holistically; recognizes subtle changes; sets priorities with ease; focuses on long-term goals
V: Expert practitioner	Performs fluidly; grasps patient needs automatically; responses are integrated; expertise comes naturally

Data from Benner P: *From novice to expert: excellence and power in clinical nursing practice.,* Menlo Park, CA, 1984, Addison-Wesley.

experience. They move fluidly through nursing interventions, acting on the basis of their feeling of rightness of nursing action. They may find it difficult to express verbally why they selected certain actions, so integrated are their responses. To observers, their expertise seems to come naturally. Expert nurses on occasion have difficulty deconstructing their work—that is, being able to describe what they experience clinically, because it comes so naturally to them. The expert nurse might even initiate a suggestion to the family that they bring the dog to the man's bedside, because the expert recognizes and understands that this ritual that brings comfort and peace is even more important to honor as death approaches.

Table 5.2 summarizes Benner's stages from novice to expert. Professional Profile Box 5.1 contains a description of an experience very early in the nursing education of this text's author that demonstrated the clear difference between novice and expert nursing; Professional Profile Box 5.2 contains the description of a memorable night shift early in the career of Maureen Baker, PhD, CNL, RN, who as an advanced beginner faced an onslaught of patient complications on a postoperative step-down unit.

PROFESSIONAL PROFILE BOX 5.1
FROM NOVICE TO EXPERT

"How did she know that?"

The difference between a novice and an expert nurse was demonstrated to me in a very stark way when I was in my first semester of nursing school. I was assigned to a surgical unit with other junior students. Our clinical instructor, Janie, had 8 years of surgical intensive care unit experience as an RN and had been a faculty member for several years. The fact that she was 7 months pregnant never slowed her down in any way. Janie just always seemed to know when we needed her, even when we did not know we needed her.

I had finished morning care for my patient, a kind elderly man who was going to be transferred to a long-term care facility later that morning. Because I was not busy, I asked one of the other students on the unit if she needed any help. Her patient's situation was complex, having been transferred from the surgical intensive care unit (ICU) the night before. He had a deep sacral decubitus ulcer that needed to be assessed, in addition to gangrene in his lower extremities. She asked me to help turn him so she could assess his sacral area. Using our best communication skills, we told the patient exactly what we were going to do, that we were going to turn him on his side, and assured him that we were not going to hurt him.

Being the two novices that we were, we were fascinated by the size and depth of the ulcer and spent what seemed like several minutes staring at it. The patient never complained about the position we were holding him in. We continued to try to figure out what to do with regard to his pressure sore. I finally took a look at his face and began to reassure him that we were almost done. Then I realized that he was not responding. My novice assessment: "He looks funny" ("funny" in an odd way, not in a humorous way).

Thank goodness Janie, the expert nurse and clinical faculty member, was walking past the patient's door. She heard my novice assessment and immediately understood the severity of "looking funny" to a new student. In my memory she became airborne as she dashed into the room; in reality she simply walked in, made an immediate and correct assessment of the patient, and called a code. He was in a full cardiac arrest. My novice classmate and I stood cowering in the corner as the room quickly filled with persons responding to the emergency. I wondered aloud, *"How did she know that?"*—with so little effort, on intuition, and with incredible calm, Janie took in the disastrous situation. I found myself envying her expertise in the resuscitation effort, the placement of a pacemaker in the patient, and coordination of his transfer back to the ICU.

My novice assessment: "He looks funny." Her expert assessment: "New students, can't describe patient. Complex patient. Risk for variety of complications due to prolonged bed rest and postop infection, unresponsive, cyanotic, eyes open, not breathing, no heart rate. Call code, lower head of bed, start CPR, make sure IV is patent, make sure oxygen is available, etc."

Thankfully, Janie took my classmate and me to lunch that day, encouraging us to discuss what had happened and reassuring us that nothing we did caused him to have an arrest. She allowed us to work through our own considerable distress (reflective practice). And I knew that I wanted to be "just like her" when I first became an RN and later when I became a nursing faculty member. I will always be grateful for her example of expert nursing and compassionate mentoring.

Beth Perry Black, PhD, RN, FAAN
School of Nursing, University of North Carolina at Chapel Hill

PROFESSIONAL PROFILE BOX 5.2
FROM ADVANCED BEGINNER TO EXPERT

"Why didn't I think of that?"

I was only 6 months out of new nurse orientation and received report on the four patients I would be caring for that evening in the postoperative unit. The unit, often referred to as "the pit," had a history of accommodating "heavy"—labor-intensive—and complex patients. As I listened to the day nurse give me report, my to-do list for each patient was growing by the second.

- A nurse for 6 months and four complex postop patients. Four patients.
- In bed 1, a large man who'd had coronary artery bypass surgery the day before had two chest tubes, a Foley, and an external pacemaker. In bed 2, an elderly man who had an active gastrointestinal (GI) bleed needed to be prepped for tomorrow's bowel surgery. The GoLYTELY regimen was to begin at 6 p.m. (GoLYTELY ... anything but!) In bed 3, a fragile woman with a history of pulmonary disease was recovering from abdominal surgery. And one empty bed—I was awaiting an admission from the postanesthesia care unit (PACU).

"I got this!" I thought as I gazed over my to-do list, set my priorities, and got to work. But as the sun began to set

PROFESSIONAL PROFILE BOX 5.2 —cont'd
FROM ADVANCED BEGINNER TO EXPERT

on New York City that evening, the atmosphere in "the pit" began to change.

The man in bed 1, still calm and cooperative, asked if we were underwater. The bubbling of the chest tubes confused him. I quickly reassured him that we weren't underwater and adjusted the suction strength on the chest tube units.

I began to focus my efforts on the woman, who was now having difficulty breathing (dyspnea). I sat her up in bed, listened to her lungs, adjusted her oxygen, assessed urine output, and gave her a scheduled dose of Lasix. At that time, Barbara, a gruff woman and my nursing leadership for the evening, strode into the room with the pace and manner of a drill sergeant and asked me for the unit's "bullet"—a quick rundown of what is happening on the unit.

I implemented SBAR (*S*ituation *B*ackground *A*ssessment *R*ecommendation) on each patient and expressed concern for my dyspneic patient. Barbara listened as I methodically went through my nursing interventions as she looked over the unit, then she abruptly handed me her clipboard. Barbara immediately walked over to bed 3 and, with a calm, confident, yet tender voice, introduced herself. She gently assisted the woman, who was breathing rapidly, to a sitting position with her legs dangling at the side of the bed. In a reassuring tone, Barbara told the patient that gravity works on the excess fluid in her lungs when she sits up and dangles, making it easier to breathe. I sensed such relief from the woman while her breathing improved and anxiety dissipated. And I thought to myself … *"Why didn't I think of that?"*

Just then, the man with the GI bleed and GI prep began to have explosive bloody diarrhea, over and over again, and was moaning in discomfort. His daughter at the bedside was distraught. The lovely man in bed 1—the man who was calling me "sweetheart" earlier in my shift—became more confused. Imagine a 250-pound man with multiple tubes and wires calling for the cops. He said he was leaving and would not be held prisoner. He was going to have me arrested and began to spit at me as he attempted to pull at his chest tubes and hurdle the bed rails. The phone was ringing because the PACU was getting "slammed" with postop patients, and the nurse wanted to give me the report for the patient who was on his way up to the empty bed in my unit.

I became paralyzed with fear and doubt, not knowing what to do first. I was not in control of this unit, but rather the unit was in control of me. Karen, a resource nurse, floated in with calmness amid the chaos. Karen enlisted a nursing assistant to help her with the man with the GI bleed while I tried to calm down and attend to the confused patient in bed 1.

Somehow that night, we restored order. I looked at my "to-do" list, which barely had a dent in it because all of my time and energy was spent on gaining control in a frenzied evening. Karen saw I was overwhelmed and exhausted at that point. She quietly reassured me and reminded me that nursing is a 24-hour/7-day-a-week profession, and if I could not get to every last thing, the next nurse would. What was important that night was that we took care of our patients, not our "to-do" lists. Again I thought to myself, *"Why didn't I think of that?"*

This is the difference between an expert and advanced beginner nurse. The advanced beginner—me—defaulted to task-oriented behavior in an attempt to gain some semblance of control. The expert nurses—Barbara and Karen—used prior experience, knowledge, and intuition amid what I thought was chaos to deliver effective, professional care.

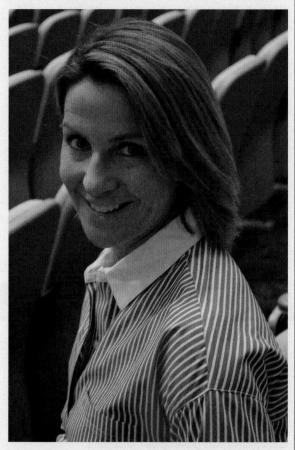

Maureen J. Baker, PhD, CNL, RN
Molloy College 1995, Rockville Centre, New York

Courtesy Maureen J. Baker.

Actively Participating in One's Own Professional Socialization

Many schools of nursing have programs for RNs with associate degrees or diplomas to return for completion of their BSN degree. These students have special socialization needs as they return to the classroom, sometimes after many years of practice. Comfortable with their identities as nurses, becoming a student again can challenge adults returning to school. These are a few strategies for RN to BSN students to decrease stress associated with transition back to school; many of these strategies will be useful for students in their basic nursing education:

- Do not lose sight of your reason for returning to school. Your stress is temporary, but your efforts will get you where you want to go professionally (e.g., certification, promotion, personal growth, or graduate school).
- Be actively involved in your studies, including being proactive on your own behalf in approaching your faculty for assistance and clarification.
- You may be troubled by others' opinions of your return to school; however, set aside their ideas for your own. Remember that those who criticize you for going back to school may be at least a little envious of your drive to reach your important career goal.
- Advanced education requires that you think conceptually. Not all content that you encounter is immediately applicable to the clinical setting; it is important nonetheless.
- Become an excellent time manager, and be disciplined about how you spend your study time.
- A mentor—another nurse, a more advanced student, or a faculty member—is an invaluable source of support.
- Trust your faculty to help you, but remember that despite all appearances, they cannot read your mind. Ask for their help and guidance.

For other ideas about how to become an active participant in your own socialization process, use the checklist in Box 5.1.

FROM STUDENT TO EMPLOYED NURSE: SOCIALIZATION SPECIFIC TO THE WORK SETTING

When nurses graduate, professional socialization is not over. In fact, the intensity of their socialization is likely

---

BOX 5.1 A Do-It-Yourself Guide to Professional Socialization

The following are 20 possible behaviors demonstrated by students who take responsibility for their own professional socialization. Place a check next to the behaviors you regularly exhibit. Be honest with yourself.

1. I interact with other students in and out of class.
2. I participate in class by asking intelligent questions and initiating discussion occasionally.
3. I have formed or joined a study group.
4. I use the library, labs, and teachers as resources.
5. I organize my work so that I can meet deadlines.
6. If I have a conflict with another student or a teacher, I take the initiative to resolve it.
7. I do not let minor personality problems distract me from my goals.
8. I seek out new learning experiences and sometimes volunteer to demonstrate new skills to others.
9. I have chosen professional role models.
10. I am realistic about my performance.
11. I try to accept constructive criticism without becoming defensive.
12. I recognize that trying to do good work is not the same as doing good work.
13. I recognize that each teacher has different expectations, and it is my responsibility to learn what is expected by each.
14. I demonstrate respect for my teachers' time by making appointments whenever possible.
15. I demonstrate respect for my classmates, patients, and teachers by never coming to class or clinical unprepared.
16. I recognize my responsibility to help create an interactive learning environment and am not satisfied to be merely an academic spectator.
17. I participate in the student nurse association and encourage others to do the same.
18. I represent my school with pride.
19. I project a professional appearance.
20. One of my goals is to become a self-directed, lifelong learner.

Scoring

1–10 checks: You need to examine your behavior and think about taking more responsibility for your own socialization.

11–15 checks: You are active on your own behalf; try to begin using some of the remaining behaviors on the list, or come up with your own.

More than 15 checks: You are a role model of positive action in your own professional socialization process.

to increase as their exposure to nursing and the culture of nursing increases. Most experts believe that socialization, similar to learning, is a lifelong activity. The transition from student to professional nurse is another of life's challenges, and, similar to most challenges, it is one that helps people grow.

Just about the time that students become well socialized to the culture of the educational setting, they graduate and face socialization to a work setting. Most new nursing graduates feel somewhat unprepared and overwhelmed with the responsibilities of their first positions. Although agencies that employ new graduates realize that the orientation period will take time, graduates may have unrealistic expectations of themselves and others.

During the early days of practice, most graduate nurses quickly realize that the ideals taught in school are difficult to achieve in everyday practice. This is largely a result of time constraints and can result in feelings of conflict and even guilt. In school, students are taught to spend time with patients and to consider their emotional as well as physical needs, and nursing students are likely to have a lighter patient assignment than they will have once they are licensed RNs in practice. Once in practice, new nurses may find that much emphasis seems to be placed on finishing tasks and on documentation. Talking with patients, engaging in patient teaching, or counseling family members may not be considered central to care on a busy nursing unit. Early in professional practice, having time to do comprehensive, individualized nursing care planning, a staple of life for nursing students, may seem like an unrealistic luxury.

Optimal transitions for graduate nurses to professional practice often occur within the context of a positive and supportive working environment (Rush et al., 2013). Supportive relationships between nurses, demonstrating both recognition and acknowledgment of the learning and support needs of new nurses, can have a long-lasting impact on effectiveness in the work setting (Laschinger et al., 2016, p. 83). One way to strengthen supportive professional relationships and enhance professional development is through the use of social media (George et al., 2013). Social media is defined as forms of electronic communication (such as websites for social networking and microblogging) through which users create online communities to share information, ideas, personal messages, and other content (such as videos) (Merriam-Webster online dictionary, 2018). Social media can provide a professional space for nurses to build supportive professional relationships, help develop nursing expertise and knowledge, and serve as an outlet for reflective practice in the forms of blogging or journaling. However, when using social media, nurses need to be extremely mindful of their employers' policies and their ethical and legal responsibilities in keeping specific patient information private and confidential (National Council of State Boards of Nursing, 2011).

An interesting suggestion offered by Kopp (2008) is to "listen to gossip." This can help you determine who is integral to the culture of the unit and give you insight into the idiosyncratic behaviors or responses of co-workers. Participating in malicious gossip is unprofessional and hurtful to others, but being aware of comments that give you insight into your new colleagues can help you understand the culture of the unit more quickly. For instance, you may overhear two co-workers discussing a third: "Alan is in the middle of everything. He manages to get appointed to every task force in the hospital, it seems." Now you know that Alan is a key person on the unit; however, if your co-workers had been speculating about the cause of Alan's recent breakup with his partner, you need to remove yourself from the conversation because that is unprofessional and no one's business except Alan's.

Speed of functioning is another area in which new nurses vary widely. By the end of a well-planned orientation, new graduates should be able to manage an average patient load without too much difficulty. Time management is a skill that is closely related to speed of functioning. Managing your time well means managing yourself well and requires self-discipline. The ability to organize and prioritize nursing care for a group of patients is the key to good time management. Box 5.2 and Fig. 5.2 provide guidance on how to keep poor time management from becoming a problem while you are a student. Once you have established good time management skills, they will carry over to your practice setting both as a student in clinical and in professional practice.

New nurses also must adapt to working with other care personnel, such as unlicensed assistive personnel (UAP; e.g., nursing assistants, patient care technicians) and other unlicensed persons whose help is important in caring for patients. Some nurses may find working with UAPs uncomfortable when they are unaccustomed to delegating, are unsure of the abilities of others, or believe only they can provide quality care.

BOX 5.2   Time Management Self-Assessment

Effective time management is a skill that can be developed. Listed are principles reflecting good time management. For each of the statements A through J, circle the answer that most closely characterizes how you manage your time.

A. I spend some time each day planning how to accomplish school and other responsibilities.
   0. Rarely
   1. Sometimes
   2. Frequently

B. I set specific goals and dates for accomplishing tasks.
   0. Rarely
   1. Sometimes
   2. Frequently

C. Each day I make a "to-do" list and prioritize it. I complete the most important tasks first.
   0. Rarely
   1. Sometimes
   2. Frequently

D. I plan time in my schedule for unexpected problems and unanticipated delays.
   0. Rarely
   1. Sometimes
   2. Frequently

E. I ask others for help when possible.
   0. Rarely
   1. Sometimes
   2. Frequently

F. I take advantage of short but regular breaks to refresh myself and stay alert.
   0. Rarely
   1. Sometimes
   2. Frequently

G. When I really need to concentrate, I work in a specific area that is free from distractions and interruptions.
   0. Rarely
   1. Sometimes
   2. Frequently

H. When working, I turn down other people's requests that interfere with completing my priority tasks.
   0. Rarely
   1. Sometimes
   2. Frequently

I. I avoid unproductive and prolonged socializing with fellow students or employees during my workday.
   0. Rarely
   1. Sometimes
   2. Frequently

J. I keep a calendar of important meetings, dates, and deadlines and carry it with me.
   0. Rarely
   1. Sometimes
   2. Frequently

Scoring

Give yourself 2 points for each "Frequently," 1 point for each "Sometimes," and 0 points for each "Rarely."

0–10 points: You need to improve your time management skills.

11–15 points: You are doing fine but can still improve.

16–18 points: You have very good time management skills.

19–20 points: Your time management skills are superior.

An overlooked aspect of stress in new graduates is the sheer physical fatigue caused by 8- to 12-hour shifts accompanied by the standing, walking, lifting, bending, and stooping that patient care requires. Some new graduates will have never spent an entire shift on a unit while in school. When physical fatigue is combined with the mental and emotional stress of decision making, efforts to become integrated into a peer group, uncertainty about policies or procedures, and lack of role clarity, sensory overload is almost certain to occur.

With all of this content about fatigue, gossip, demands of the job, and mental and emotional stress of decision making, it may have become evident to you that sometimes nursing units are difficult places to maintain one's good humor, much less create a culture

of civility (Regan et al., 2017). Ariza-Montes and colleagues (2013) described the issues facing nurses in terms of incivility, which includes bullying, and noted that organizational structures that are hierarchical, are downsizing, or whose employees do not feel empowered contribute to incivility. This conduct is a form of workplace violence that most often occurs with new nurses, particularly inexperienced nurses.

A culture of civility involves respecting one another, honoring differences, listening and seeking common ground, and engaging in social discourse (Clark and Carnosso, 2008). Although the culture in many hospital units may be characterized by some degree of incivility, there are ways to turn the culture into one of civility. This starts with recognizing that incivility needs to be

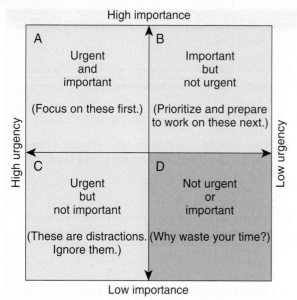

High importance

A	B
Urgent and important	Important but not urgent
(Focus on these first.)	(Prioritize and prepare to work on these next.)
C	D
Urgent but not important	Not urgent or important
(These are distractions. Ignore them.)	(Why waste your time?)

High urgency — Low urgency

Low importance

Fig. 5.2 Setting priorities is an important aspect of time management. Use this grid to determine whether a task should go to the top, middle, or bottom of your daily "to-do" list—or if it belongs on the list at all.

addressed, developing a framework at the institutional level setting and operationalizing behavioral standards, and being patient but persistent in creating a civil culture from one that is toxic. Nurses have the responsibility to intervene on behalf of their colleagues who are being harassed or bullied; silence from the other nurses is a form of acquiescence to bullying (Houck and Colbert, 2017). Similarly, not enforcing mandates for civility in the workplace implies that bullies in fact have permission to harass (Hébert, 2017). Bullying or allowing others to bully is antithetical to caring, the core value of nursing.

"Reality Shock": When Ideals and Reality Collide

A reality of nursing today is that nurses are expected to provide care in a complex health care system with an aging population and more persons living with chronic illness. Working conditions are sometimes very difficult, especially when acuity (severity of illness) of the patients is high and staffing is low. Despite the rewards of a career spent in nursing, nursing can be difficult at times. A current challenge in nursing is retention: keeping nurses in nursing. Replacing nurses who leave is extremely expensive for hospitals and other health care facilities. Many

of the difficulties faced by nurses now are not very different from other times of shortage when the needs of the health care system were greater than the profession of nursing could address. This section is intended to leave you in a more powerful position to understand some of the negative feelings you may experience as you make the transition into professional nursing. Because "forewarned is forearmed," discussion is included of not only how to recognize these feelings but also how to manage them so that you will remain an involved, well-prepared, and productive professional nurse.

"Reality shock" (Kramer, 1974) was a term used to describe the feelings of powerlessness and ineffectiveness experienced by new graduates, a term that is still relevant more than four decades later. Psychological stresses generated by reality shock decrease the ability of individuals to cope effectively with the demands of the new role. Causes of reality shock include the following:

- Absence of positive reinforcement (such as one gets from clinical faculty) and lack of frequent communication
- Lack of support, such as the availability of faculty that students have
- The gap between the ideals taught in school and the actual work setting
- The inability to provide nursing care effectively because of circumstances such as a heavy case load or time constraints

Unfortunately, some new nurses "drop out" at this point, rather than taking steps to resolve reality shock. Kramer identified several ways nurses may drop out:

- Disengaging mentally and emotionally
- Driving oneself and others to the breaking point by trying to do it all
- "Job hopping"—looking for the perfect, nonstressful job that is completely compatible with professional values
- Prematurely returning to school (seeking the routine and known expectations of a student)
- Burning out—a condition of unresolved reality shock with subsequent emotional exhaustion
- Leaving the nursing profession entirely, which neither nursing nor society can afford

Much can be done to reduce reality shock in the transition from student to professional. Students must recognize that schools cannot provide enough clinical experience to make graduates comfortable on their first day as new nurses. They can take responsibility for obtaining as much practical experience as possible outside of school. Working in a health care setting during summers, on school breaks, and on weekends may be helpful. The current difficult economy requires some students to work in addition to going to school. To the extent possible, they should avoid work during the school week or keep it to a minimum because academic responsibilities take priority during that time, and exhausted students make poor learners. Also, exhausted students are at risk for making clinical errors. If you are a student who must work in addition to going to school, consider letting your faculty know. They may be helpful to you in helping you balance your study and work time.

Some schools offer programs in which students are paired with practicing nurses (preceptors) and work closely with them to experience life as an RN. These are sometimes called *shadowing* programs. If your school offers such a program, take advantage of it. If not, seek out information about similar programs at area hospitals. Many agencies, including hospitals and the military, are now providing excellent opportunities for students nearing graduation to function in expanded roles.

Nursing residency programs are 1-year programs that offer the new nurse graduate clinical and educational activities to facilitate the transition to professional practice and enhance competence, confidence, and professional development. Nursing residency programs can help to bridge the gap between academic preparation and competency development in the clinical setting (Letourneau and Fater, 2015). In the 2010 report *The Future of Nursing: Leading Change, Advancing Health*, the Institute of Medicine (IOM) (now the National Academy of Medicine) recommended nurses should have the benefit of a residency program at the start of their careers and during career transitions. Nursing residency programs, increasing in both popularity and availability, are structured programs and focus on specific institutional policies, procedures, and standards of care to help new nurses assimilate, develop, and transition into their professional nursing role and practice. Nurses receive education and training in technical skills, critical thinking, organizational skills, prioritization skills, professionalism, and interprofessional communication, helping to ease the "reality shock" and transition from the role of nursing student to professional nurse.

Existing nursing residency programs are listed by state and can be found at the following American Association of Colleges of Nursing link: http://www.aacnnursing-.org/Portals/42/AcademicNursing/NRP/NRP-Partici-pants-by-State.pdf?ver=2017-07-17-151637-730.

Talking with other new graduates about your feelings is one of the best ways to combat reality shock. Take the initiative to form a group for mutual support—others need it too. Another interpersonal strategy is to seek a professional mentor. A mentor is an experienced nurse who is committed to nursing and to sharing knowledge with less experienced nurses to help advance their careers. A mentor can be a great source of all types of knowledge, as well as another source of support. Having a mentor is different from having a preceptor. Mentoring involves the formation of a long-term relationship through which ideas, experiences, and successful behavior patterns are shared.

Ask a nurse whose work you wish to emulate to be your mentor, and identify what he or she can offer. Some inexperienced nurses are fearful of approaching potential mentors with this request. They should remember that this process is not a one-way street; it has benefits to both parties because it complements and validates the mentor's knowledge and self-esteem, as well as provides important information and support to the nurse being mentored. To get the most from a mentoring relationship, first understand your professional and personal needs, and select a mentor who seems to share your values and beliefs. Set up specific times to meet, and be willing to communicate openly with your mentor. A mentoring relationship is a powerful tool by which a new nurse can benefit from the experience, wisdom, and feedback from someone who has "been there"— who understands your experience because he or she has experienced the same thing.

The Internet provides opportunities for nursing students to learn more about the profession of nursing and to assist with socialization into practice. As noted in Chapter 3, nurses often blog about work and work issues. You may find that these serve as a good outlet for you, both to read and to contribute to. Writing serves as a means of organizing one's thoughts and helps you make sense of them; writing can also help you manage uncomfortable feelings and distress.

Care of self is an important activity as you begin your career in the care of others. Recall that when you are traveling by plane, the flight attendants instruct you to put on your oxygen mask first in the case of an emergency. You are then prepared to help those around you. The same principle applies here. You will provide better care to others if you care for yourself first, such as eating nutritiously, exercising regularly, avoiding tobacco and

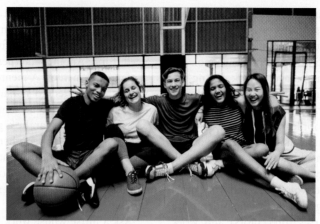

Fig. 5.3 Self-care, including time with friends, is an important aspect of managing the stress of a new career. (Photo used with permission from iStockphoto.)

excessive alcohol use, seeking spiritual support if that is important to you, and having friends outside of work—all of those things that you know are good for you. The stronger and healthier you are physically, psychologically, and spiritually, the better prepared you are to face the demands of your transition into the important work of nursing (Fig. 5.3).

In the final analysis, you—and only you—are responsible for your own lifelong professional socialization. Those nurses who maintain a good balance between their work and personal lives and who have reasonable expectations of the work of nursing without sacrificing their own values and ideals have great potential to be effective nurses over a long career.

CONCEPTS AND CHALLENGES

- *Concept:* Nursing has been difficult to define, although definitions distinguish nursing from other health care professions.

  Challenge: Although the definitions of nursing in this chapter have more in common than they have differences, the fluid nature and complexity of nursing, society, and health care may prevent the development of one standard definition of nursing.

- *Concept:* Nurses move across a trajectory from novice to expert, progressing from an orientation toward rules and procedures to a patient-centered approach to care that is intuitive.

  Challenge: Novices and advanced beginners should be alert to situations in which they need help from more experienced nurses in setting priorities and addressing patient needs.

- *Concept:* A critical process through which novices become well-functioning professional nurses, socialization occurs in both educational settings and in the workplace.

- *Challenge:* Individuals have the responsibility to participate actively in their own professional socialization by seeking out experiences that enhance socialization.

- *Concept:* Reality shock occurs during a stressful period new nurses may encounter when entering nursing practice.

  Challenge: Identifying and understanding the stages of reality shock and how to resolve them can assist new graduates through the transition from nursing student to practicing nurse.

- *Concept:* Mentors can be valuable resources in enhancing and enriching the professional socialization experience.

  Challenge: Identify an experienced nurse, colleague, or faculty member to help you through the transition to practice. Then be available to mentor new nurses as you gain experience and move along the trajectory from novice to expert.

IDEAS FOR FURTHER EXPLORATION

1. Examine your state's nursing practice act for its definition of nursing. How is it similar to or different from definitions in this chapter?
2. From among the definitions of nursing in this chapter, determine the one you think fits most closely with your understanding of nursing, and explain your choice.
3. How might new technologies, economic factors, social trends, and evolving practice options for nurses affect future definitions of nursing? How might these factors affect the scope of nursing?
4. If you are already a practicing nurse, how has your personal definition of nursing changed over time? How have you seen the scope of nursing change since you entered practice?
5. Describe how both formal and informal socialization experiences in school are affecting your understanding and image of nursing.
6. Examine one of the two models of socialization discussed in this chapter, and determine at which stage you are in your development as a student and nurse. Give your rationale for that placement. If none of the models or stages fits your experience, create your own model (or stage).
7. Talk to an experienced nurse about his or her experience with reality shock. How is this individual handling the transition from student to practicing nurse? What can you learn from his or her experience?
8. Identify several personal and professional areas in which you think you could use mentoring and support. Select a potential mentor, and ask if you can have an honest conversation about how he or she can be helpful to you in your personal and professional development.

REFERENCES

American Nurses Association (ANA): *Code of ethics for nurses*, Washington, DC, 2001, American Nurses Publishing.

American Nurses Association (ANA): *Nursing's social policy statement*, ed 2, 2003, Washington, DC.

American Nurses Association (ANA): *Code of ethics for nurses* (website), 2015. Available at: www.nursingworld.org/MainMenuCategories/EthicsStandards/CodeofEthicsforNurses/Code-of-Ethics-For-Nurses.html.

American Nurses Association (ANA): What is nursing? 2015 (website). Available at: www.nursingworld.org/Especially-ForYou/What-is-Nursing.

Ariza-Montes A, Muniz NM, Montero-Simó MMJ, Araque-Padilla RA: Workplace bullying among healthcare workers, *Intern J Environ Res and Pub Health* 10(8):3121–3139, 2013. http://doi.org/10.3390/ijerph10083121.

Bandura A: *Social learning theory*, Englewood Cliffs, NJ, 1977, Prentice-Hall.

Benner P: *From novice to expert: excellence and power in clinical nursing practice*, Menlo Park, CA, 1984, Addison-Wesley.

Benner P, Tanner CA, Chesla CA: *Expertise in nursing practice: caring, clinical judgment, and ethics*, New York, 1996, Springer.

Clark CM, Carnosso J: Civility: a concept analysis, *J Theory Constr & Testing* 12(1):11, 2008.

Cohen HA: *The nurse's quest for professional identity*, Menlo Park, CA, 1981, Addison-Wesley.

Explore Health Careers: Allied health professions overview, 2018 (website). Available at: https://explorehealthcareers.org/field/allied-health-professions/.

Fichten CCS, King L, Jorgensen M, et al.: What do college students really want when it comes to their instructors' use of information and communication technologies (ICTs) in their teaching? *Online Submission* 14(2):173–191, 2015.

George DR, Rovniak LS, Kraschnewski JL: Dangers and opportunities for social media in medicine, *Clin Obstet Gynecol* 56(3), 2013. http://doi.org/10.1097/GRF.0b013e318297dc38.

Gordon S: *Nursing against the odds: how health care cost cuts, media stereotypes, and medical hubris undermine nurses and patient care*, Ithaca, NY, 2005, Cornell University Press.

Harmer B: *Textbook of the principles and practice of nursing*, New York, 1922, Macmillan.

Harmer B, Henderson V: *Textbook of the principles and practice of nursing*, ed 4, New York, 1939, Macmillan.

Henderson V: *Basic principles of nursing care*, London, 1960, International Council of Nurses (ICN).

Hébert LLC: Protections from workplace bullying and psychological harassment in the united states: a problem in search of a cause of action. In *Psychosocial risks in labour and social security law*, Cham, 2017, Springer Press, pp 269–287.

Hinshaw AS: *Socialization and resocialization of nurses for professional nursing practice*, New York, 1976, National League for Nursing.

Houck NM, Colbert AM: Patient safety and workplace bullying: an integrative review, *J Nurs Care Qual* 32(2):164–171, 2017.

Institute of Medicine (US), Committee on the Robert Wood Johnson Foundation initiative on the future of nursing: *The future of nursing: Leading change, advancing health*, Washington, DC, 2011, National Academies Press.

International Council of Nurses (ICN): *The ICN definition of nursing*, 2015 (website). Available at: www.icn.ch/definition.htm.

Kopp G: How to fit in fast at your new job, *Am Nurse Today* 3(1):40–41, 2008.

Kramer M: *Reality shock: why nurses leave nursing*, St. Louis, 1974, Mosby.

Lai PK, Lim PH: Concept of professional socialization in nursing, *Int e-J Sci Med Educ* 6(1):31–35, 2012.

Laschinger HKS, Cummings G, Leiter M, et al.: Starting out: a time-lagged study of new graduate nurses' transition to practice, *Internat J Nursing Studies* 57:82–95, 2016.

Letourneau RM, Fater KH: Nurse residency programs: an integrative review of the literature, *Nurs Educ Perspect* 36(2):96–101, 2015.

McHaney R: *The new digital shoreline: how Web 2.0 and millennials are revolutionizing higher education*, Stylus Publishing, 2012.

Merriam-Webster.com: Social media, 2018 (website). Available at: https://www.merriam-webster.com/dictionary/social%20media.

National Council of State Boards of Nursing, 2011 (website). Available at: https://www.ncsbn.org/NCSBN_SocialMedia.pdf.

Nightingale F: *Notes on nursing: what it is and what it is not*, Philadelphia, 1946, JB Lippincott. Reprint (originally published in 1859).

North Carolina Board of Nursing: *Nurse practice act*, 20, 2009 (website). Available at: www.ncbon.com.

North Carolina Board of Nursing: *Practice/Overview*, 2017 (website). Available at: https://www.ncbon.com/practice-overview.

Orem D: *Guidelines for developing curricula for the education of practical nurses*, Washington, DC, 1959, U.S. Government Printing Office.

Oshvandi K, Sadeghi Moghadam A, Khatiban M, Cheraghi F, Borzu R, Moradi Y: On the application of novice to expert theory in nursing: a systematic review, *J Chem Pharm Sciences* 9(4):3014–3020, 2016.

Peddle M, Bearman M, Nestel D: Virtual patients and nontechnical skills in undergraduate health professional education: an integrative review, *Clin Simul Nurs* 12(9):400–410, 2016.

Peplau H: *Interpersonal relations in nursing: a conceptual frame of reference for psychodynamic nursing*, New York, 1952, GP Putnam's Sons.

Regan S, Wong C, Laschinger HK, et al.: Starting out: qualitative perspectives of new graduate nurses and nurse leaders on transition to practice, *J Nurs Manag* 25(4):246–255, 2017.

Rogers M: *Educational revolution in nursing*, New York, 1961, Macmillan.

Royal College of Nursing (RCN): *Defining nursing*, 2003 (website). Available at: www.rcn.org.uk.

Royal College of Nursing (RCN): *Defining nursing*, 2015 (website). Available at: www.rcn.org.uk/__data/assets/pdf_file/0003/604038/Defining_Nursing_Web.pdf.

Rush KL, Adamack M, Gordon J, Lilly M, Janke R: Best practices of formal new graduate nurse transition programs: an integrative review, *International J Nurs Stud* 50(3):345–356, 2013.

Shaw CW: *Textbook of nursing*, ed 3, New York, 1907, Appleton.

Sherwood G, Horton-Deutsch S: *Turning vision into action: reflection to build a spirit of inquiry. Reflective practice: transforming education and improving outcomes*, Sigma Theta Tau International, 2012, pp. 3–19.

Sherwood G, Zomorodi M: A new mindset for quality and safety: the QSEN competencies redefine nurses' roles in practice, *Nephrology Nurs J* 41(1):15, 2014.

Styles MM: Bridging the gap between competence and excellence, *ANNA J* 18(4):353–366, 1991.

tonybates.ca: *Does distance education socialize students? A study from Québec*, 2015 (website). Available at: www.tonybates.ca/2014/04/04/does-distance-education-socialize-students-a-study-from-quebec/.

6

Nursing as a Regulated Practice: Legal Issues

Beverly Brown Foster, MN, MPH, PhD, RN

ⓔ To enhance your understanding of this chapter, try the Student Exercises on the Evolve site at http://evolve.elsevier.com/Black/professional.

LEARNING OUTCOMES

After studying this chapter, students will be able to:
- Describe the components of a model nursing practice act.
- Discuss the authority of state boards of nursing.
- Explain the conditions that must be present for malpractice to occur.
- Identify nursing responsibilities related to delegation, informed consent, and confidentiality.

- Explain the legal responsibilities of nurses to enforce professional boundaries, including the use of social media.
- Describe strategies nurses can use to protect their patients, thereby protecting themselves from legal actions.

Few aspects of professional nursing practice seem more daunting than those related to laws, rules, and regulations. Laws, rules, and regulations that shape any professional practice serve to protect the public from practitioners who are unsafe or otherwise unqualified. Sometimes you may feel like the "nursing police" are looking over your shoulder and a malpractice attorney is waiting around every corner. In this chapter the goal is to clarify some of the basic legal issues related to nursing practice so you can understand their importance while not feeling overwhelmed. In fact, understanding nursing as a regulated profession can give you confidence by understanding the purpose of boards of nursing responsible for setting limits on practice, knowing the scope of your practice, and knowing how to protect your career by practicing within accepted standards of care.

Maintaining basic knowledge of the law as it relates to professional nursing practice is especially important now in this time of change in health care with expansion of nursing roles and practice settings. This chapter will give you a foundation of knowledge about the various ways that nursing practice is shaped and regulated by legislation and regulations. Nurses, especially early in their careers, are sometimes concerned about "breaking the law" regarding nursing practice or misinterpret the meaning and purposes of laws. Laws and regulations serve to protect both nurses and the patients for whom they are providing care.

AMERICAN LEGAL SYSTEM

The U.S. Constitution is the framework on which governance in this country is built. The purpose of the law in the United States is found in the Preamble to the U.S. Constitution: to ensure order, protect the individual person, resolve disputes, and promote the general welfare.

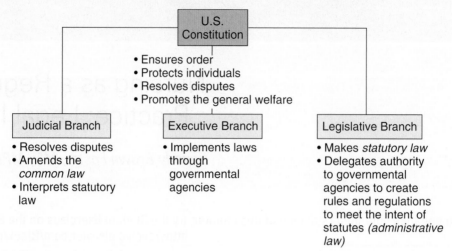

Fig. 6.1 Branches of the U.S. federal government were established by the Constitution to provide for a balance of power.

To achieve these broad objectives, the law concerns itself with the legal relationships between persons and the government. All law in the United States flows from the U.S. Constitution and must conform to its principles. This means that, although states themselves have the power to set laws for their citizens, no state or municipality can make laws that are not in accordance with the intentions of the framers of the Constitution. These intentions are subject to interpretation; hence the constitutionality of a particular law or ruling is argued in the court system.

The Constitution established a government in which the balance of power was divided among three separate but equal branches: (1) the executive branch, charged to implement law and which includes the office of the president at its highest level; (2) the legislative branch, charged to create law and which includes the U.S. Congress and other regulatory agencies that set law; and (3) the judicial branch, charged to interpret law and which includes the Supreme Court and federal court system (Fig. 6.1). The separate but equal branches constitute a form of government with a built-in system of checks and balances to keep one body from claiming authority not recognized in the Constitution.

Laws are rules of conduct that are authored and enforced by formal authorities and hold people accountable for compliance. Three major types of laws govern American society: common law, statutory law, and administrative law. Common law is decisional, meaning that judges' rulings become law. U.S. law has its

foundation in centuries-old English common law. Every time a judge makes a legal decision, the body of common law expands.

Statutory laws (statutes) are those established through formal legislative processes. Every time the U.S. Congress or a state legislature or assembly passes legislation, the body of statutory law expands.

Administrative laws are created when the legislative branch of a government delegates authority to governmental agencies to create laws that meet the intent of a statute. Both federal and state administrative laws have the force and effect of statutory law.

Laws are further categorized as either civil or criminal. Civil law recognizes and enforces the rights of individuals in disputes over legal rights or duties of individuals in relation to one another. In civil cases the party judged responsible for the harm may be required to pay compensation to the injured party. In contrast, criminal law involves public concerns regarding an individual's unlawful behavior that threatens society, such as murder, robbery, kidnapping, or domestic violence. The criminal court system both defines what constitutes a crime and also may mandate specific punishments, within limits set by legislative bodies and the Constitution. Individuals convicted of criminal charges are punished, usually through the loss of some degree of their freedom, ranging from probation to imprisonment. They may also be required to pay fines.

Administrative cases result when a person violates the regulations and rules established by administrative law. In nursing, examples of administrative cases would be when a nurse practices without a valid license or beyond the scope of nursing practice. These cases are reviewed by state boards of nursing, which administer laws related to nursing practice and determine the appropriate sanctions for the infraction. This is discussed in more detail later in this chapter.

STATE BOARDS OF NURSING, NURSING PRACTICE ACTS, AND LICENSURE

The boundaries of the practice of nursing, medicine, dentistry, law, and many others are established and regulated at the state level. This means that the legislative body in each state sets practice law and then assigns authority to implement the law to appropriate regulatory agencies and boards. These laws are in the form of professional practice acts, which set the licensing standards for various professions.

The purpose of licensing certain professions is to protect the public health, safety, and welfare. The statute that defines and controls nursing is called a *nursing practice act*. All 50 states, the District of Columbia, and several U.S. territories have nursing practice acts passed by their legislatures. State boards of nursing (SBNs) are the regulatory bodies by which nursing practice acts are administered and enforced. Ultimately, SBNs regulate nursing to protect the public from harm by unprepared or incompetent practitioners (Russell, 2017).

Statutory Authority of State Nursing Practice Acts

Nurses, as health care providers, have certain rights, responsibilities, and recognitions through various state laws, or statutes. The nursing practice act in each state accomplishes the following objectives (Russell, 2017):

1. Defines the standards and scope of professional nursing
2. Describes the authority, power, and composition of the board of nursing
3. Defines educational program standards
4. Sets the minimum educational qualifications and other requirements for licensure
5. Determines and protects the legal titles and abbreviations nurses may use
6. Provides for disciplinary action of licensees for certain causes

In many states, nursing practice acts also define the responsibilities and authorities of the SBN; thus the nursing practice act of the state in which nurses practice is statutory law affecting nursing practice within the bounds of that state. For example, a registered nurse (RN) who works in Virginia practices under the nursing practice act of Virginia, although the nurse's home address may be in Maryland. Maryland's state board of nursing has no jurisdiction over the nurse's practice as long as the nurse is working in Virginia.

Once the law regarding nursing practice is established or amended by the legislature, the legislative branch delegates authority to enforce the law to an executive agency, usually the SBN. SBNs are responsible for enforcing the nursing practice acts in the various states. The SBN publicizes rules and regulations that expand the law. The statutory law plus the rules and regulations propagated by the SBN give full meaning to the nursing practice act in each state. The board of nursing in each state has a comprehensive website containing crucial information for nurses practicing in that state. You should familiarize yourself with your SBN's website, which will include details of how you apply for and maintain your nursing license once you have passed the licensing examination. In addition, the nursing practice act for your state will be featured on the website so that you can be informed as to the specific rules and regulations under which you will practice and the "scope of practice," which defines your care (Ballard et al., 2016; National Council of State Boards of Nursing [NCSBN], 2016). Nursing practice acts are revised periodically to keep up with new developments in health care and changes in nursing practice. State nurses associations are usually instrumental in lobbying their state legislators for appropriate updating of nursing practice acts.

Because of the importance of practice acts to professional nurses, the American Nurses Association (ANA) and the NCSBN have collaborated to develop suggested language for the content of state nursing practice acts. Discussions over the past two decades at the national level, facilitated by both the NCSBN and ANA, have brought a national perspective on nursing regulation to the state level, fostered dialogue and the development of more consistent standards across state lines, and provided increased protection for the public. The current NCSBN's Model Nursing Practice Act (2014) is a comprehensive document developed to guide individual states' development and revisions of their nursing practice acts. The NCSBN describes the current model as both a standard toward which states may strive and a reflection of the current and changing regulatory and health care system environments.

Executive Authority of State Boards of Nursing

At both the federal and state government levels, the executive branch administers and implements law. The governor, who holds the state's highest executive office, generally delegates the responsibility for administering the nursing practice act to the SBN, the agency charged with executing (carrying out) laws. In most states, the SBN consists of RNs representing different areas of practice and education, licensed practical/vocational nurses (LPNs/LVNs), and consumers (members of the general public). In a few states, nurses elect members of the SBN; otherwise, they are appointed by the governor. The governor typically appoints consumers to the board.

The SBN's authority is limited. It can adopt rules that clarify general provisions of the nursing practice act, but it does not have the authority to enlarge the law. The law is set by the state governing body (legislature or assembly), and legislation is usually proposed by the SBNs, often in collaboration with state professional organizations. Within these confines, SBNs have three functions similar to those of the federal and state governments:

1. Executive, with the authority to administer the nursing practice act
2. Legislative, with authority to adopt rules necessary to implement the act (note that rules are different from laws, which are made by the state's legislative body)
3. Judicial, with authority to deny, suspend, or revoke a license or to otherwise discipline a licensee or to deny an application for licensure

Each of these functions is as broad or as limited as the state legislature specifies in the nursing practice act and related laws.

SBNs can be independent agencies in the executive branch of state government or part of a department or bureau such as a department of licensure and regulation. Some state boards have authority to carry out the nursing practice act without review of their actions by other state officials. Others must recommend action to another department or bureau and receive approval of the recommendation before the decision is finalized.

Licensing Powers

Because nursing is a regulated practice, nurses must hold a valid license to practice. Being granted a license to practice nursing takes several years of hard work, and keeping one's license active and in good standing is a professional priority. Each state determines who is qualified to receive a license to practice nursing, as well as the limits on the license. Licensure laws may be either mandatory or permissive. A mandatory law requires any person who practices the profession or occupation to be licensed. A permissive law on the other hand protects and limits the use of the title granted in the law but does not prohibit persons from practicing the profession or occupation if they do not use the title. In other words, persons could practice nursing if they did not refer to themselves as a nurse. All states now have a mandatory licensure law for the practice of nursing to safeguard the public. This means that only licensed nurses—RNs or LPN/LVNs—can practice nursing and call themselves nurses. Unlicensed assistive personnel (UAP) such as certified nursing assistants (CNAs) may not refer to themselves as nurses. Patients often mistake the roles of various practitioners who are providing care; however, the CNAs and other UAP need to clarify with patients that they are not nurses when patients refer to them as such.

In most states, SBNs have the authority to set and enforce minimum criteria for nursing education programs. The practice act usually stipulates that an applicant for licensure must graduate from a state-approved nursing education program as a prerequisite to being admitted to the licensure examination. This means that schools of nursing must have state approval to operate. State approval requirements are generally less stringent than are national accreditation standards. Schools may voluntarily seek national accreditation to demonstrate that they meet higher than minimum standards. Although many other professions and occupations require graduation from a nationally accredited educational program as a prerequisite of licensure, only state approval is currently required in nursing. Some states are currently undertaking rule changes to require that nursing programs have national accreditation to achieve state approval.

Not only does the state, through the SBN, grant licenses, but it also has the power to sanction a nurse for performing professional functions in a manner that is dangerous to patients or the general public.

Sanctions range from probation, a predetermined period during which the nurse may not have any further complaints made against him or her; suspension of the nursing license for a specific period, after which the nurse may resume practice; or revocation of the license if the infraction is especially egregious or the nurse shows a pattern of unsafe practice. The most common reason nurses are disciplined by SBNs is for practicing while under the influence of alcohol or other substance, often a narcotic taken ("diverted") from the workplace.

Historically the nursing profession has demonstrated a commitment to the rehabilitation of nurses whose practice is impaired by mental health issues or substance abuse. The ANA first published a recommendation that a Nursing Disciplinary Diversion Act be implemented by states through their boards of nursing (ANA, 1990). Later the NCSBN published *Substance Use Disorder in Nursing*, a comprehensive resource to assist with the evaluation, treatment, and management of nurses with a substance problem (NCSBN, 2015). Nurses are estimated to misuse drugs and alcohol at approximately the same rate—10% to 15%—as the general population; however, only a small percentage of nurses are disciplined each year for substance abuse. The goal of SBNs is to return to safe practice those nurses who have been identified as having a problem with drugs and/or alcohol use. This is accomplished through the use of interventions that have evidence of effectiveness.

Licensure Examinations

Individuals who have successfully completed their basic nursing education from a state-approved school of nursing are eligible to sit for the licensing examination. The nurse licensure examination for RNs is the National Council Licensure Examination for Registered Nurses (NCLEX-RN®). The NCLEX-RN®, which is updated regularly, tests critical thinking and nursing competence in all phases of the nursing process. The current test plan can be found at the NCSBN website (www.ncbsn.org), where you can download a comprehensive document available as a PDF file. Search for "test plan" on the website to find a list of the most recent and up-to-date test plans; they are updated every 3 years. Through the NCSBN, each state participates in the licensing process through test plan and item development, periodic validation of the examination content with current practice, and adoption of a minimum passing score.

The NCLEX-RN® is administered by computerized adaptive testing (CAT) at various testing centers across each state at a time scheduled by the test taker. CAT means that the computer will determine the level of difficulty of the next question based on whether you answered the previous question correctly. This form of testing is believed to be as objective as possible. The minimum number of questions is 75; the maximum is 265. Each person taking the examination has 6 hours to complete it, including breaks. You will likely hear much speculation about the NCLEX-RN® from classmates. The test stopping at 75 questions is not an indication that you passed or failed. What it does indicate is that you either clearly passed with the minimum number of questions or clearly failed. Because around 88% of first-time test takers educated in the United States pass the examination, the significance of "75 questions" is not clear or predictable.

Test takers who are not successful in passing the NCLEX-RN® may take the examination again after paying the examination fees. A waiting period of 45 days is required before a retake is permitted. Passing rates for graduates of different nursing schools are published online on SBNs' websites. Passing rates for first-time test takers reflect the quality of the education that specific programs are providing. Schools with consistently high scores among their first-time test takers are providing excellent education and preparation of their graduates for professional nursing practice. Most if not all states include the first-time pass rate for each nursing school in their respective states. You can likely find your own school's first-time pass rate on your SBN's website.

Mobility of Nurses: Licensure by Endorsement

Since 1944, most SBNs have participated in a cooperative effort to assist in the interstate mobility of nurses. The NCLEX-RN® is a national examination; therefore, all states recognize the licensure awarded in other states because the nurses have passed the NCLEX-RN®. This is called *licensure by endorsement*. Endorsement means that RNs may practice in different states without having to take another licensing examination. To receive a license in a different state, nurses submit proof of licensure in another state, pay a licensure fee and meet any other requirements imposed by the state, and they receive a license in the new state by endorsement. Licensure by endorsement is not available in all practice disciplines. Nursing's plan serves as a national model for other licensed professions and occupations.

Nurse Licensure Compact

Because the United States has a mobile society, a regulatory approach known as a Nurse Licensure Compact (NLC)—a mutual recognition model of licensure—was developed by the NCSBN in 2000. In 2015 an extensive revision of the NLC was undertaken, and the enhanced NLC (eNLC) was implemented in 2018 (Puente, 2017). The NLC and the eNLC were developed to improve mobility of nurses while still protecting the public health, safety, and welfare. Mobility occurs in travel nursing, in crossing state lines from one's home to one's workplace, in the telehealth practices (being physically present in one state while providing nursing care to a patient in another state through digital technology), and simply moving to another state for personal or career purposes. Having a mobile nursing workforce able to respond to regional and national disasters is an advantage for states in the compact.

The eNLC allows an RN to have one license (in the state of residency) yet practice in other compact member states without an additional license in the state of employment. Importantly, the nurse is subject to the nursing practice act in the state where she or he is practicing, not to that of the state of licensure. A single license for each nurse and the concomitant reduction of state barriers provide better protection for the public through improved tracking of nurses for disciplinary purposes and information sharing.

Each state that wishes to participate in the compact must pass legislation enabling the board of nursing to enter into the interstate NLC. Utah, Texas, and Wisconsin were the first states to implement the compact on January 1, 2000. Nurses licensed in any state that has implemented the compact can practice in their own states, as well as in any other compact state without applying for licensure by endorsement before beginning work. A nurse who has changed permanent residence from one compact state to another may practice under the license from his or her former state of residence for up to 90 days, which starts on the nurse's first day of work. The license in the new state of residence will be granted under endorsement rules if the nurse is in good standing with the SBN of the state from which the nurse is moving. This means that a nurse moving between compact states does not have to delay working as a nurse until a new license is granted. Updated information about states participating in or seeking legislation to participate can be found on the NCSBN website. Based on a demand from nurses educated abroad, the NCSBN began administering the NCLEX-RN® internationally to otherwise qualified nurses applying for U.S. licensure in January 2005. Testing sites are available abroad and are published at https://www.ncsbn.org/testing-locations.htm. Performance scores on the NCLEX™ for United States and abroad are published annually by the NCSBN at https://www.ncsbn.org/12171.htm. Chapter 7 contains a fuller discussion of the significant issues surrounding recruiting nurses from other countries to practice in the United States.

LEGAL RISKS IN PROFESSIONAL NURSING PRACTICE

Nurses make decisions daily affecting the well-being of their patients. Because they have access to personal information about patients and interact with them during stressful times, they are in positions of responsibility and trust. Several areas of nursing practice—delegation, informed consent, and confidentiality—are particularly important in terms of risk. Furthermore, nurses may also be charged with malpractice or assault and battery. Being fully informed, however, will help you minimize risks related to these areas.

Malpractice

Malpractice is the primary legal concern of health care professionals. Nurses are accountable for their own practice and can be named in a malpractice suit, just as any practitioner can be named. Malpractice suits are very complex. This discussion will give you basic information about malpractice and, importantly, how to protect yourself from practices that make you susceptible to claims of malpractice.

Negligence is the central issue in malpractice. Negligence is the failure to act as a reasonably prudent person would have acted in the same circumstances. For example, a person parks his car on a steep hill and does not engage the parking brake. The car then rolls down the hill and into the porch of a nearby house. The homeowner may seek damages in a civil suit on charges of negligence. Because a reasonably prudent person would

BOX 6.1   Malpractice: Professional Negligence

Malpractice is not limited to what a nurse *does* (commission); it also refers to what a nurse *fails to do* (omission) in a nursing care situation. The following is an example in which an RN is negligent in both ways.

A patient had surgery one morning for an abdominal mass. He was given morphine 8 mg intravenously (IV) at 5 p.m. At 5:20 p.m., he was very drowsy, but when the nurse woke him and asked about his pain, he complained that his "stomach still hurts some." She gave him a second dose of morphine 8 mg IV. When the nurse went back to check on him an hour later, he was in respiratory arrest. After aggressive resuscitation, the patient was placed on a ventilator and admitted to the intensive care unit, where he stayed for 4 days after showing signs of new-onset neurologic impairments.

The nurse was negligent by commission when she gave the patient a second dose of morphine because (1) the nurse had to awaken the patient to ask him about his pain, and (2) the patient's complaint of "some pain" likely did not warrant a second dose of intravenous morphine so soon after the first dose. A reasonably prudent nurse in the same situation would not have given a relatively large dose of morphine so soon after the first, especially given that the patient was drowsy and had to be awakened to assess his pain.

The nurse was negligent by omission because she failed to check on her patient for an hour after giving a second substantial dose of morphine. The first dose made him very drowsy after 20 minutes; this would indicate that he had a significant response to the first dose. The nurse also failed to assess the patient for causes of his continuing pain, such as examining his abdomen and checking his vital signs for evidence of a surgical complication.

---

have set the parking brake, the result—the damage to the porch—can be shown to be a direct result of the failure to act reasonably.

Malpractice is negligence applied to the acts of a professional. In other words, malpractice occurs when a professional—for example, a nurse or a physician—fails to act as a reasonably prudent professional would have acted under the same circumstances. Malpractice does not have to be intentional; that is, the professional did not mean to act in a negligent manner. Malpractice may occur in two ways: (1) by commission (doing something that that should not have been done) and (2) by omission (failing to do things that should have been done) (Box 6.1).

A patient or someone acting on behalf of the patient who brings a claim of malpractice against a nurse (or other professional) is known in the legal system as the plaintiff. Malpractice suits are civil, not criminal, cases. The nurse becomes the defendant. Getting a malpractice case to be argued in front of a judge and jury is a long process and is actually unlikely to get this far. Often, malpractice cases are settled out of court, meaning that the outcome is negotiated between attorneys for the plaintiffs and defendant(s) (Thinking Critically Box 6.1).

The central question in any charge of malpractice is, "Was the prevailing standard of care met?" The nursing standard of care is what a reasonably prudent

 THINKING CRITICALLY BOX 6.1

What or Who Needs the Most Attention—the EHR or Your Patients?

You hear nursing colleagues discussing prevention of malpractice, and you notice that some nurses are spending more time attending to patients' medical records than they are in providing care to patients. Think about how this emphasis on "defensive practice"—that is, making sure that your patient's medical record is perfect—may actually impede the delivery of safe care. As you think about this issue, consider what the purpose of documentation is. How can you use the medical record to enhance the care of your patients? How might excessive documentation harm you in a malpractice suit?

EHR, Electronic health record.

nurse, under similar circumstances, would have done. Standard of care reflects a basic minimum level of prudent care based on the ethical principle of nonmaleficence ("do no harm"). Nurses, not practitioners from other disciplines, determine whether standard of care is met. For instance, a physician cannot testify what the standards of care are for nurses. Nurse expert witnesses are hired by both the plaintiff and the defendant and will testify as to whether the nurse met the prevailing standard of care.

"Prevailing" is an important qualifier. As practice changes and develops, standards of care change accordingly. The issue in malpractice cases is the standard of care that prevailed—or was in effect—at the time the negligent act occurred. What may be considered negligent now may not have been considered negligent at the time. The standard of care prevailing at the time is key and is ascertained through expert witness testimony; documents, including national standards of nursing practice; the patient record; and other pertinent evidence, such as the direct testimony of the patient, the nurse, and others. Box 6.2 illustrates the presumed failure of an RN to meet the prevailing standard of care.

There are two requirements of a malpractice action. First, the defendant (nurse) has specialized knowledge and skills, and, second, through the practice of that specialized knowledge the defendant causes the plaintiff's (patient's) injury. All four elements of a cause of action for negligence must be proved (Reising, 2012). These elements are the same for any professional accused of malpractice:

1. The professional (nurse) has assumed the duty of care (responsibility for the patient's care).
2. The professional (nurse) breached the duty of care by failing to meet the standard of care.
3. The failure of the professional (nurse) to meet the standard of care was the proximate cause of the injury.
4. The injury is proved.

A high degree of proof is needed in each of these four elements. Monetary damages are awarded when a plaintiff prevails. These awards are based on proved economic losses, such as time missed from work or out-of-pocket health care costs, and on remuneration for pain and suffering caused by the injury. In the case of a death, the next of kin can become the plaintiff on behalf of the deceased patient. In a clinical setting, you may occasionally hear a nurse or other provider complain about a patient's care as being "malpractice." This term is often misused and applied to what may be bad practice, but remember that to be sued for malpractice, an injury must have occurred that is directly and demonstrably caused by the act.

In the past, only some malpractice lawsuits involved nurses, but the physician or hospital defendants were typically sued for damages even when nurses provided the substandard care. In these instances, physicians were implicated through the "captain of the ship" doctrine. This archaic doctrine implied that the physician is ultimately in charge of all patient care and thus should be responsible financially. Hospitals were implicated through the legal theory of *respondeat superior* (from Latin, meaning "let the master answer"), which attributes the acts of employees to their employer. However, as nurses have obtained more credentials and their expertise, autonomy, and authority for nursing practice have increased, direct liability for nursing care has risen correspondingly.

BOX 6.2 Standards of Care: A Case Example

An 8-month-old infant was brought by his parents to the emergency department (ED) with significant fever and dehydration. The family with the infant was Spanish speaking and included a family member trained in nursing in her country of origin.

Intravenous (IV) fluids were ordered for rehydration. Because of the need for the infant to be able to move from bed to the arms of his caregivers, the IV line was set up before IV catheter insertion with both regular- and extension-length tubing. The ED RN, in her second year in the ED, failed to flush the line to clear air from the extension tubing and then inserted the catheter and began the infusion. This was noted by the family, and an unsuccessful attempt was made to alert the nursing and medical staff. The infant subsequently died of a significant air embolus. The family engaged an attorney, who eventually filed a malpractice suit against the hospital and the nurse. The following standards of care were considered in this case.

1. Hospital policy indicated that an interpreter should have been called for communication with family.
2. Hospital policies and orientation competency guidelines, completed by this nurse, indicated that flushing of an IV line was a required step in the process.
3. Local schools of nursing indicated that flushing of an IV line was part of basic skills training, and current textbooks about fundamentals of nursing confirmed this content.
4. Other nurses in local EDs were interviewed, and all reported that flushing of an IV line before infusion was standard practice.
5. The company manufacturing the IV tubing had visual and written instructions on the box indicating proper use of the product, including flushing of the line.

BOX 6.3   Six Major Categories of Negligence That Result in Malpractice Lawsuits

1. Failure to follow standards of care, including failure to
   - Perform a complete admission assessment or design a plan of care
   - Adhere to standardized protocols or institutional policies and procedures (for example, using an improper injection site)
   - Follow a physician's verbal or written orders
2. Failure to use equipment in a responsible manner, including failure to
   - Follow the manufacturer's recommendations for operating equipment
   - Check equipment for safety before use
   - Place equipment properly during treatment
   - Learn how equipment functions
3. Failure to communicate, including failure to
   - Notify a physician in a timely manner when conditions warrant it
   - Listen to a patient's complaints and act on them
   - Communicate effectively with a patient (for example, inadequate or ineffective communication of discharge instructions)

- Seek higher medical authorization for a treatment
4. Failure to document, including failure to note in the patient's medical record
   - A patient's progress and response to treatment
   - A patient's injuries
     - Pertinent nursing assessment information (for example, drug allergies)
     - A physician's medical orders
     - Information about telephone conversations with physicians, including time, content of communication between nurse and physician, and actions taken
5. Failure to assess and monitor, including failure to
   - Complete a shift assessment
   - Implement a plan of care
   - Observe a patient's ongoing progress
   - Interpret a patient's signs and symptoms
6. Failure to act as a patient advocate, including failure to
   - Question discharge orders when a patient's condition warrants it
   - Question incomplete or illegible medical orders
   - Provide a safe environment

Reprinted with permission from Croke EM: Nurses, negligence, and malpractice: An analysis based on more than 250 cases against nurses, *Am J Nurs* 103(9):54–63, 2003.

In a paper that is still widely cited, Croke (2003) conducted a review of more than 350 trial, appellate, and supreme court case summaries from a variety of legal research sources and analyzed 253 cases that met the following criteria: a nurse was engaged in the practice of nursing as defined by his or her state's nursing practice act; a nurse was a defendant in a civil lawsuit as the result of an unintentional action (no criminal cases were considered); and a trial was held between 1995 and 2001. Sixty percent of the cases occurred in acute care hospitals. Six major categories of negligence resulted in malpractice lawsuits against nurses: failure to follow standards of care, failure to use equipment in a responsible manner, failure to communicate, failure to document, failure to assess and monitor, and failure to act as a patient advocate. More details of Croke's analysis are presented in Box 6.3. The findings from this review paper remain relevant today.

The key point is that professional nurses must consider carefully the legal implications of practice and be willing to and capable of conforming to prevailing professional standards and all legal expectations. Among factors leading to the increase in the number of malpractice cases against nurses is delegation.

Delegation

Delegation—giving someone authority to act for another—is an issue that carries great legal and safety implications in nursing practice. The ability to delegate has generally been reserved for professionals because they hold licenses that sanction the entire scope of practice for a particular profession. Professional nurses, for example, may delegate independent nursing activities (as well as medical functions that have been delegated to them) to other nursing personnel. State nursing practice acts do not give LPNs or LVNs the authority to delegate.

Professional RNs retain accountability for acts delegated to another person. This means that the RN is responsible for determining that the delegated person (delegatee) is competent to perform the delegated act. Likewise, the delegatee is responsible for carrying out the delegated act safely. The professional nurse remains legally liable, however, for the nursing acts delegated to others unless the delegatee is also a licensed professional whose scope includes the assigned act. For example, an RN can assign an unlicensed CNA who has been properly trained to take vital signs of all the patients under the RN's care. The nursing assistant cannot, however, reassign this responsibility to another person. The RN remains accountable for the data that the CNA collects, because it is not the CNA's responsibility, nor is it within his or her training, to interpret those data. However, if the RN asks another RN to take the vital signs of a patient, and the second RN agrees, the second RN then becomes responsible for carrying this out, interpreting the data, and acting on them accordingly.

Delegation must also be considered in terms of ethical implications. The ANA's Code of Ethics for Nurses, Provision 4.4, Delegation of Nurse Activities (2015), states,

The nurse must make reasonable efforts to assess individual competence when assigning selected components of nursing care to other healthcare workers. This assessment involves evaluating the knowledge, skills, and experience of the individual to whom the care is assigned, the complexity of the assigned tasks, and the health status of the patient.... Nurses may not delegate responsibilities such as assessment and evaluation; they may delegate tasks.... Employer policies or directives do not relieve the nurse of responsibility for making judgments about the delegation and assignment of nursing care tasks. (p. 2)

Importantly, the Code of Ethics is clear that workplace policies or directives do not supersede the ethical standards described in the Code.

Delegation is an important liability and one not fully appreciated by many practicing nurses. The professional nurse's primary legal and ethical consideration must be the patient's right to safe, effective nursing care. Box 6.4 contains a list of "five rights" to ensure safe delegation of tasks to nursing assistants and other UAP. With the present nursing shortage, the use of UAP has expanded, further increasing the RN's liability related to delegation. Additional information on delegation can be found on the NCSBN website at www.ncsbn.org.

In an attempt to further clarify issues of delegation, the ANA (2005) also defined the responsibilities of the nurse when delegating to nursing assistive personnel. They reinforce the stance that the RN may delegate elements of care but cannot delegate the nursing process

---

BOX 6.4   Five Rights to Ensure Safe Delegation

The following are standards that delineate responsibility for the RN who is delegating responsibility to unlicensed personnel such as nursing assistants.

1. *Right task:* Is the task appropriate for delegation in a specific care situation?
2. *Right circumstances:* Is delegation appropriate in this case? Consider the patient's health status, care delivery setting, complexity of the activity and delegate's competency, and available resources, and determine any other relevant factors.
3. *Right person:* Can the nurse verify that the person delegated to do the task is competent to complete this task?
4. *Right direction/communication:* Has the RN given clear, specific instructions? These include identifying the patient clearly, the objective of the task, time frames, and expected results.
5. *Right supervision/evaluation:* Can the RN or other licensed nurse provide supervision and evaluation of the patient and the performance of the task?

Data from National Council of State Boards of Nursing: *The Five Rights of Delegation,* approved August 1997 by the Delegate Assembly. Retrieved from www.ncsbn.org.

itself. Furthermore, they reaffirm that the judgment of the nurse is primary in determining the patients, environments, and care situations for safe delegation and that the nurse remains responsible for evaluating the outcomes of nursing care.

Significantly, the ANA and the NCSBN published a joint statement on delegation (NCSBN, 2015), noting that there is more to do for patients than there are nurses to do the work, and the increasingly complex therapies have created a demand for nursing care. Therefore, delegating, assigning, and supervising assistive personnel are "critical competencies for the 21st century nurse" (p. 1, introduction).

Informed Consent

All patients or their guardians (e.g., parents of minor children) must be given an opportunity to grant informed consent before treatment unless there is a life-threatening emergency. The following are the three major conditions of informed consent:

1. Consent must be given voluntarily.
2. Consent must be given by an individual with the capacity and competence to understand.

3. The patient must be given enough information so that the locus of the decisions lies with the patient and not the provider; in other words, the provider cannot influence the patient unduly by giving incomplete information or obscuring data that the patient should have to make a truly informed decision.

Informed consent, then, is a full, knowing authorization by the patient for care, treatment, and procedures and must include information about the risks, benefits, side effects, costs, and alternatives. Consumers of health care need a great deal of information and should be told everything they would consider significant in making a treatment decision. This is a long-standing element of health care law (*Canterbury v. Spence,* 464 F2 772, 1972).

For informed consent to be legally valid, elements of completeness, competency, and voluntariness are evaluated. *Completeness* refers to the quality of the information provided. *Competency* takes into account the capability of a particular patient to understand the information given and make a choice. *Voluntariness* refers to the freedom the patient has to accept or reject alternatives. *Autonomy* is the key ethical principle that supports voluntariness as foundational to informed consent. When patients are minors, are under the effects of drugs or alcohol (including preoperative medications), or otherwise have cognitive deficits or impairments, competency to consent is in question. In these situations, consent needs to be granted by the patient's spouse, next of kin, or court-ordered guardian or health care proxy.

The role of nurses in informed consent, unless they are themselves primary providers, is to collaborate with the primary provider, most often a physician. A nurse may witness a patient's signing of informed consent documents but is not responsible for explaining the proposed treatment (Fig. 6.2). The nurse is not responsible for evaluating whether the physician has truly explained the significant risks, benefits, and alternative treatments. However, professional nurses are responsible for determining that the elements for valid consent are in place, providing feedback if the patient wishes to withdraw consent or grant consent previously withheld, and communicating the patient's need for further information to the primary provider. Advocacy is a key nursing responsibility when the nurse is not certain that a patient is fully informed or understands what he or she has signed.

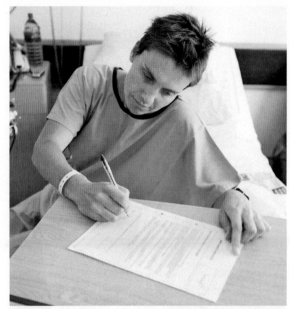

Fig. 6.2 Professional nurses may be called on to witness a patient's signing of informed consent documents. The primary provider, however, is responsible for providing necessary information to the patient or legal guardian. (Photo used with permission from iStockPhoto.)

CONFIDENTIALITY: THE CHALLENGE TO PROTECT PRIVACY

Confidentiality is both a legal and an ethical concern in nursing practice. Confidentiality is the protection of private information gathered about a patient during the provision of health care services. The Code of Ethics for Nurses Provision 3.1 states that "the nurse has a duty to maintain confidentiality of all patient information, both personal and clinical in the work setting and off duty in all venues, including social media and any other means of communication.... Nurses are responsible for providing accurate, relevant data to members of the health care team and others who have a need to know" (ANA, 2015).

The Code acknowledges exceptions to the obligation of confidentiality. These include discussing the care of patients with others involved in their direct care, quality assurance activities, legally mandated disclosure to public health authorities, and information required by third-party payers (ANA, 2015). The Code also recognizes the need to disclose information without the patient's consent when the safety of

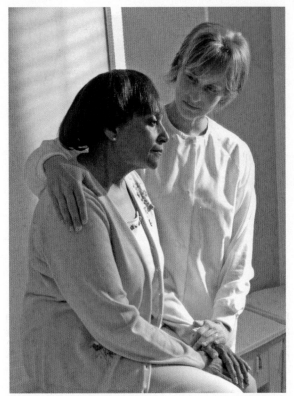

Fig. 6.3 Nurses have an obligation for confidentiality but are not protected by privileged communication statutes. In some cases, nurses are required to report what a patient has told them. (Photo used with permission from Photos.com.)

innocent parties is in question (*Tarasoff v. Board of Regents of the University of California*, 551 P2 334, 1976).

The principle of confidentiality is protected by state and federal statutes, but there are exceptions and limitations. Although some professions have statutorily protected privileged communication, such as attorneys and priests, nurses are usually not included in such statutes (Fig. 6.3). Nurses then may be ordered by a court to share information without the patient's consent. The professional nurse must understand these legal limitations to confidentiality.

Based on common, state, or municipal law, nurses have the duty to report or disclose certain information such as suspected abuse or neglect of a child (or elder, in some states), gunshot wounds, certain communicable diseases, and threats toward third parties. These laws vary by state and may be the responsibility of institutions providing health care services and not of an

individual practitioner. Nurses should be aware of these requirements, however, and make sure their appropriate supervisor is informed.

The Health Insurance Portability and Accountability Act of 1996

The Health Insurance Portability and Accountability Act (HIPAA) of 1996 is the first federal privacy standard governing protection of patients' medical records. The privacy provisions in the act began as a 337-word guideline, but as the final regulations were written, the provisions expanded to 101,000 words. HIPAA was designed, in part, to reinforce the protection of patient information as it is transmitted electronically, but the final act goes far beyond that goal. The regulations protect medical records and other individually identifiable health information, whether on paper, electronically, or communicated orally.

HIPAA requires all health care providers, including physicians, hospitals, health plans, pharmacies, public health authorities, insurance companies, billing agencies, information systems sales and service providers, and others, to ensure the privacy and confidentiality of patients. Although passed in 1996, the confidentiality regulations were not implemented until April 2003 to give providers time to prepare the necessary safeguards and documents and to train workers in their use.

HIPAA regulations require several major patient protections:

- Patients are able to see and obtain copies of their medical records, generally within 30 days of their request, and to request corrections if they detect errors. Providers may charge patients for the cost of copying and mailing the records.
- Providers must give patients written notice describing the provider's information practices and explaining patients' rights. Patients must be asked to agree to these practices by signing or initialing the notice.
- Limitations are placed on the length of time records can be retrieved, what information can be shared, where it can be shared, and who can be present when it is shared.

A number of other protections are provided in this comprehensive federal legislation. A current guide to the complicated HIPAA regulations can be found online at the Department of Health and Human Services (2018). The increasingly widespread use of electronic health records and digital transmission of health information has necessitated the development of comprehensive guidelines ("Guide to Privacy and Security of Electronic Health Information") to help with the implementation of the Meaningful Use programs while still protecting the privacy and security of patient information (U.S. Department of Health and Human Services, 2015). The integration of HIPAA into clinical practice was not easy because it necessitated changing many aspects of day-to-day care on nursing units, such as having patients' names on whiteboards at nursing stations with detailed information about their diagnoses, care teams, and plans. HIPAA regulations, however, served to remind nurses and other practitioners of the importance of determining what and how much information on patients to share, and who actually needed to know information. For many nurses, then, HIPAA affirmed nursing's long-standing responsibility to our patients.

Social Media: Maintaining Confidentiality and HIPAA Standards

In 2011 the NCSBN published a white paper, "A Nurse's Guide to the Use of Social Media," in response to the burgeoning social media outlets, such as social networking sites (e.g., Facebook, LinkedIn), blogs and microblogs (e.g., Twitter), photo and video sites (e.g., YouTube, Instagram, Snapchat), and other online forums, including sites specifically for nurses and nursing students (NCSBN, 2011). Health care settings now generally have policies in place to govern the use of social media from workplace settings, as do many non–health-related employers. However, the use of social media outside of nursing school or the workplace can cause tremendous consequences if used in ways that interfere with the privacy of patients, even if the nurse's or student's intentions are not malicious. *The ethical principle of confidentiality and HIPAA regulations place significant limitations on the content of nurses' social media activities and comments.* In a 2010 survey, NCSBN found that 33 boards of nursing had received complaints of nurses who have violated patient privacy by posting photos or identifiable information on social networking sites (NCSBN, 2011). Violating HIPAA regulations means that the nurse has broken federal law and may have also broken state laws in the process.

NCSBN identified six common myths and misunderstandings regarding social media. You should be aware of these and structure your online communication accordingly. It is a professional obligation with important ethical

and legal ramifications. The following is a list of these pervasive myths and misunderstandings (you can find the full white paper at the NCSBN website for details):

- *Myth 1:* Posts and photos are private and accessible only to the intended recipient.
  - *Fact:* They can be reposted, "retweeted," and otherwise disseminated in ways completely beyond your control.
- *Myth 2:* Once content has been deleted, it is no longer accessible.
  - *Fact:* There is no "erasing" digital content. Cached versions and screenshots of posts and photos are available. Even sites such as Snapchat in which content quickly "disappears" retain digital evidence of the content.
- *Myth 3:* No harm is done if patient information is disclosed only to the intended recipient.
  - *Fact:* This is still a breach of confidentiality, just as if you used spoken words to share private information about patients. As soon as you write or tell something, you have lost control of the message. You cannot control what happens to the information you have passed along.
- *Myth 4:* It is acceptable to refer to a patient by a nickname, room number, or diagnosis/condition.
  - *Fact:* This still remains a breach of confidentiality and is disrespectful to the patient.
- *Myth 5:* If your patient is posting about his or her health condition, you may also post about it.
  - *Fact:* The patient can say or write anything about himself or herself; however, this does not in any way release you from the obligations of confidentiality and HIPAA regulations.
- *Myth 6:* Social media blurs the distinction between one's professional and personal lives.
  - *Fact:* This is an illusion. Professional boundaries are still firmly in place, although social media may cause you to believe that they are not.

The use of social media makes it tempting to respond to online social contact with patients and former patients. For instance, you may get a "friend" request on Facebook from a former patient that you liked very much. As difficult as this is to do, you should ignore that request or decline it for the sake of your professional boundaries. Establishing an online relationship will interfere with your ability to provide care for that patient if and when you encounter that person in the health care setting in the future.

Furthermore, the quick availability of mobile phone cameras makes it easy to take photos of patients of whom you are fond, or of their new baby, or of milestones in the patient's recovery. Your employer or school of nursing is likely to have a policy in place prohibiting the use of cameras in the clinical setting. Although there are certain times in which photography in the clinical setting is appropriate, it is in very circumscribed situations and will involve the use of the institution's camera, not your personal smartphone. Box 6.5 contains an example of a situation in which a mobile phone photo taken by a nursing student in a clinical setting led to unforeseen problems.

Assault and Battery

Assault and battery is occasionally the basis for legal action against a nurse defendant. Assault is a threat or an attempt to make bodily contact with another person without the person's consent. Assault precedes battery; it causes the person to fear that battery is about to occur. Battery is the assault carried out: the impermissible, unprivileged touching of one person by another. Actual harm may or may not occur as a result of assault and battery.

If, for example, a nurse threatens a patient with a vitamin injection if the patient does not eat his or her meals, the patient may charge assault. Actually giving the patient a vitamin injection against his or her will leaves the nurse open to charges of battery, even if there is a physician's prescription for this treatment. Patients have the right to refuse treatment, even if the treatment would be in their best interest. This is both a legal and an ethical principle (autonomy). Both by common law and by statute, informed consent is required in the health care context as a defense to battery (42 U.S.C. 1395 cc., 1990).

EVOLVING LEGAL ISSUES AFFECTING NURSING

As the health care system and the profession of nursing evolve, legal issues affecting nursing practice are also evolving. Specific legal issues illustrating the changing nature of nursing practice are related to role changes, supervision of UAP, payment mechanisms, and issues associated with the implementation of the Patient Self-Determination Act (PSDA). Each of these issues is discussed briefly in the following sections.

> ### BOX 6.5   A Cautionary Tale: The Far-Reaching Effect of Digital Technology
>
> During her rotation in the maternity unit, a nursing student really enjoyed taking care of the infants in the newborn nursery. One evening, a baby with a rare and distinctive facial defect was admitted to the nursery. The baby's parents had come from another state so the mother could give birth at this institution because of its known expertise in the management of craniofacial defects. The defect was severe, and the student was curious about it. She took a photo of the baby in his bassinet with her cell phone, wanting to use the photo in a presentation she was preparing on genetic defects for another class.
>
> She consequently downloaded the photo onto her computer and included it in her PowerPoint presentation, which was posted online for her classmates. A few weeks later, she was called to the office of the director of her nursing program. A complaint had been filed against her and her school by the infant's parents, who had neither known about nor consented to having their baby photographed. They found the photo while using a search engine's "image" function as they were seeking more information about their infant's genetic condition. The photo was embedded in the student's PowerPoint presentation, which was available online, with the student's name, school, and course number on the title slide. It was not difficult for them to figure out where and when the photo was made. Tracing their identity would not be difficult, and their privacy was compromised.
>
> The student was dismissed from her nursing program because there was a policy in place at both the school and the clinical institution forbidding use of cell phone photography. Although she tried to defend herself that the baby's name band was obscured, the presence of the rare facial defect served as enough of an identifier to compromise the family's privacy. She was reminded that even without the clear policy forbidding photography, she had committed an egregious ethical violation by not protecting the family's privacy. One seemingly simple photograph created a career-threatening situation for this student who failed to understand the far-reaching effects of digital technologies.

Role Changes in Health Care

Just as a nurse's knowledge base and the nurse's accountability for nursing practice have increased over time, so too has the need to expand the legal authority for nursing practice. Professional nurses realize the importance of states' nursing practice acts to reflect nursing practice accurately and to keep up with changes in health care delivery as they occur. In other words, states' nursing practice acts must be responsive to changes in practice. Advanced practice nurses set the pace for evolving nursing practice, and the nursing practice act must support their ability to offer nursing services to consumers in various settings. Otherwise, the legal basis for nursing practice is unclear and nurses are vulnerable to litigation.

Nurses face legal exposure and are vulnerable when their state's nursing practice act is not updated periodically to support explicitly an expanded scope of practice. Working collaboratively within the constituent member (state nurses) association and the SBN to expand the evolving scope of nursing practice appropriately ensures the growth of the profession and increases the number of primary care providers needed by the public. Professional nurses should support their professional associations and SBN, which guide the development of legislation that accurately reflects current nursing practice at all levels. Your practice is directly affected by the work of professional organizations at the legislative levels.

An interesting role for nurses has been developed over the past 25 years—legal nurse consulting. The American Association of Legal Nurse Consultants was founded in 1989. It is a nonprofit organization that is dedicated to the professional enhancement of RNs who practice as consultants in the legal field. Box 6.6 contains more information about legal nurse consulting and the interesting work legal nurse consultants do.

Prescriptive Authority

An important role expansion for advanced practice nurses is prescriptive authority. *Prescriptive authority* is defined as the legal acknowledgment of prescription writing as an appropriate act of nursing practice. The ANA, the American Academy of Nurse Practitioners, and others support prescriptive authority for advanced practice nurses, as distinguished from generalist RNs.

By 2006, advanced practice nurses had some type of prescriptive authority in all 50 states. This authority ranged from completely independent authority with no collaborative requirements to a limited authority in which nurse practitioners can prescribe (excluding controlled substances) with some degree of physician involvement or delegation of prescription writing. In other states, nurse practitioners can prescribe (including controlled substances) with some degree of physician

---

BOX 6.6 What Is a Legal Nurse Consultant?

A legal nurse consultant (LNC) is an experienced nurse who brings expertise from his or her professional nursing education and clinical experience to the evaluation of standard of care, causation, damages, and other medically related issues in medicolegal cases or claims. For instance, if a nurse is named in a malpractice suit, the attorneys for both the plaintiffs (the person/persons who filed the suit) and the defendants (the persons being sued) will seek the expertise of nurses who can evaluate if the nurse met the standard of care and other important aspects of the case. LNCs have additional education and experience regarding applicable legal standards and/or strategy to the evaluation of medicolegal cases or claims. LNCs know how to analyze health care records and medical literature critically, as well as other relevant legal documents and other information to the case or claim on which they are consulting.

LNCs practice in a variety of settings, such as law firms, governmental agencies, health care facilities, forensic environments, and LNC consulting firms, among others. Some LNCs are self-employed in their own practices. In addition to medical malpractice, LNCs practice in a variety of areas such as personal injury, long-term care litigation/elder law, product liability, workers' compensation, life care planning, and forensic/criminal settings. Among their many activities, LNCs serve as expert witnesses; they interview clients, evaluate the strengths and weaknesses of cases, and locate or prepare evidence for trial.

LNCs can become board certified through the Legal Nurse Consultant Certified program, which allows them to use the LNCC credential. This certification demonstrates that the nurse has met the experience and education requirements and has passed the certification examination. For more information about this very interesting and challenging career, you can contact the American Association of Legal Nurse Consultants (AALNC) at info@aalnc.org or visit their website at www.aalnc.org. You can also find them on Facebook and LinkedIn (AALNC, 2013).

---

involvement or delegation of prescription writing). This is an evolving area of practice, and advanced practice nurses must be aware of the boundaries on prescriptive authority given to them in the state where they are practicing. Your state's board of nursing website will give you the most up-to-date information regarding prescriptive authority for advanced practice nurses in your state. The ultimate goal is a uniform consensus practice model across all states. Progress toward this goal may be viewed online at https://www.ncsbn.org/5397.htm.

Both generalist and advanced practice nurses must understand prescriptive authority of advanced practice in their states. Generalist nurses must know from whom they can accept medication prescriptions, and advanced practice nurses must stay within their legal scope of practice.

Supervision of Unlicensed Assistive Personnel

Another evolving legal issue is the continued role expansion of UAP or limited licensed (LPN/LVN) personnel within health care institutions. Nursing assistants (i.e., UAP) are increasingly being substituted for nurses, thus creating greater risks to patients and increasing the liability of nurses, who supervise their work. The important findings from a landmark research study described in the Evidence-Based Practice Box 6.1 indicate that lack of professional nurse supervision and the educational level of nurses themselves significantly affect patients, institutions, and nurses alike (Aiken et al., 2003; Buerhaus et al., 2002; Institute of Medicine, 1996). Convening expert panels of educators, researchers, and practitioners to develop standards for delegation, the NCSBN published a comprehensive National Guidelines for Nursing Delegation NCSBN, (2016) to provide guidance for the complex process of delegation and patient care assignment across both licensed and unlicensed personnel.

The substitution of unlicensed personnel for RNs is a strategy used by health care facilities to hold down costs. Such substitution jeopardizes quality of care and places the RN at increased risk for patient injury liability because of acts performed or omitted by UAP. Over the long term, professional nursing care may actually be less expensive than care provided by unlicensed personnel, who are less likely to provide patient teaching and recognize complications.

The licensure or state approval of unlicensed personnel is a complex issue that has relevance for RNs because professional nurses are legally responsible for the tasks delegated to unlicensed persons. Nationally standardized education and training for these workers would assure nurses that their co-workers have a minimum level of competence. The NCSBN has developed the National Nurse Aide Assessment Program (NNAAP) examination, a test of both cognitive and skill performance to certify nurse aide competency. The Medication

EVIDENCE-BASED PRACTICE BOX 6.1

A Landmark Study on Nurse Staffing and Patient Safety

This study changed the way that health care providers and administrators understood the importance of professional RNs in safeguarding the well-being of hospitalized patients. Linda Aiken, PhD, FAAN, RN, and her many colleagues have continued to address issues of staffing and safety throughout her distinguished career in nursing. An interdisciplinary group of researchers, led by Dr. Aiken at the University of Pennsylvania, was concerned about nurse understaffing and the resulting threats to patient safety in hospitals. The group members decided to study the educational composition of RNs in relation to patient outcomes. Their objective was "to examine whether the proportion of hospital RNs educated at the baccalaureate level or higher is associated with risk-adjusted mortality and failure to rescue (deaths in surgical patients with serious complications)" (p. 1617).

The researchers analyzed outcome data for 232,342 general, orthopedic, and vascular surgery patients discharged from 168 nonfederal adult general Pennsylvania hospitals between April 1, 1998, and November 30, 1999. These figures were linked to data on educational composition, staffing, and other characteristics.

The percentage of RNs with a bachelor's or higher degree ranged from 0% to 77% in the various hospitals in the study.

After adjusting for patient characteristics and hospital structural characteristics (size, teaching status, level of technology), as well as for nurse staffing, nurse experience, and whether the patient's surgeon was board certified, a 10% increase in the proportion of bedside nurses holding a bachelor's degree was associated with a 5% decrease in both the likelihood of patients dying within 30 days of admission and the odds of failure to rescue (p. 1617).

These researchers concluded that significantly lower mortality and failure to rescue rates were found in hospitals with higher proportions of bachelor of science in nursing (BSN)-prepared nurses. They recommended that investments in public funds be made to increase the number of BSN-prepared nurses to substantially improve the quality of care in the nation.

Aiken LH, Clarke SP, Cheung RB, et al.: Educational levels of hospital nurses and surgical patient mortality, *JAMA* 290(12):1617–1623, 2003.

Aide Certification Examination (MACE) also administered by the NCSBN, certifies competency in administration of simple medications by UAP. Regardless of certifications by UAP, it remains the responsibility of professional nurses to know the limitations of the particular assistive personnel under their supervision.

Payment Mechanisms for Nurses

Nurses may practice in nontraditional roles and settings. Many professional nurses are both capable of and interested in offering nursing services as private practitioners, but payment mechanisms may limit such activities. Nurses are concerned about offering services for which consumers are unable to obtain reimbursement from their insurance carriers, and third-party reimbursement has traditionally been limited to care provided by physicians.

Over time, nurses and nursing professional associations have supported state and federal legislation to provide direct and indirect payments to nurses for nursing services rendered. Advanced practice nurses and their advocates scored a major legislative victory with the passage of the 1997 Balanced Budget Act after an 8-year fight to obtain direct reimbursement. The resistance to advanced practice nurse reimbursement was significant and protracted. This legislation authorized nurse practitioners and clinical specialists, beginning in January 1998, to bill the Medicare program directly for nursing services furnished in any setting. Even now, it remains a regulatory challenge to devise a fair and equitable payment system for advanced practice nurses, whose scopes of practice vary from state to state. Nurses are concerned that these changes are often not implemented or that advanced practice nurses are paid less for services similar to those provided by other health care professionals who are paid at a higher rate.

Laws are passed that are sometimes not implemented. This occurs when the group affected by the law (for example, the insurance industry) is unwilling to implement the changes and no "watchdog" agency is created to ensure that changes occur. For example, federal legislation was enacted requiring state Medicaid agencies to pay certain nurses (nurse practitioners, nurse-midwives, and nurse anesthetists) directly for services provided to Medicaid recipients. As with the laws affecting private insurers, these requirements were not implemented in every state. Nurses may need to seek legal remedies to require implementation of policies mandated by federal law (*Nurse Midwifery Associates v. Hibbett,* 918 Fed 2 605, 1990).

The Patient Protection and Affordable Care Act (ACA) was passed in 2010 and enacted with a number of initiatives implemented incrementally. This law reformed health care and health insurance industries in the United States, with the goal of increasing quality, availability, and affordability of health insurance. In 2008 President Barack Obama campaigned on a platform of health insurance for all Americans. The debate about health care in general over the course of the debate over the ACA in particular brought health care inequities, high costs, and poor access to preventive care into the spotlight. As a result of the new spotlight on these issues of great concern to the profession of nursing, the ANA and constituent member (state) associations are working to ensure that nurses are included in discussions and roundtables addressing the management of health care reform in the United States. The ACA faced two significant challenges before the U.S. Supreme Court (*National Federation of Independent Business v. Sebelius,* 2011-2012; *King et al. v. Burwell,* 2014-2-15). In each case the court ruled to uphold key provisions of the ACA. Further challenges to the ACA are expected, and currently many provisions of the ACA remain vulnerable to repeal, including coverage for persons with preexisting medical conditions, among others.

Patient Self-Determination Act

Although the PSDA became effective in 1991, many problems in its implementation remain. Nurses are in a position to help patients and families understand this law and how it can assist them to have the end-of-life care they prefer. The PSDA applies to acute care and long-term care facilities receiving Medicare and Medicaid funds. It encourages patients to consider which life-prolonging treatment options they desire and to document their preferences in the event they become incapable of participating in the decision-making process. Written instructions recognized by state law describing an individual's preferences in regard to medical intervention should the individual become incapacitated are called an *advance directive.* Additional details about the PSDA are included in Chapter 7.

This Act was passed partly in response to the U.S. Supreme Court's decision in *Cruzan v. Director Missouri Department of Health* (110 Supreme Court 2841, 1990), which was viewed as limiting an individual's ability to direct health care when unable to do so. The Cruzan case is explained in more detail in Chapter 2. The PSDA requires the health care facility to document whether the patient has completed an advance directive.

The PSDA's basic assumption is that each person has legal and moral rights to informed consent about medical treatments with a focus on the person's right to choose (the ethical principle of autonomy). The Act does not create any new rights, and no patient is required to execute an advance directive.

According to the PSDA, acute care (hospitals) and long-term care facilities must do the following:

1. Provide written information to all adult patients about their rights under state law
2. Ensure institutional compliance with state laws on advance directives
3. Provide for education of staff and the community on advance directives
4. Document in the medical record whether the patient has an advance directive

The Agency for Health Care Policy and Research (now called the Agency for Healthcare Research and Quality) reported that even when patients had advance directives in place, the directives were not guiding end-of-life care as legislators and advocates had anticipated. This was attributable to several factors: patients were not considered ill enough to implement their advance directives; family members were not available, were too overwhelmed to implement the patient's wishes, or disagreed with the patient's wishes; and the advance directive itself was not specific enough or did not cover pertinent clinical issues. A model for advanced directives developed by the American Association of Retired Persons, the American Bar Association, and the American Medical Association seeks to address these issues and can be accessed at the American Bar Association website (American Bar Association, 2018). Documentation of the existence of advance directives and use of them in planning care is an important patient advocacy role for nurses and is a legal requirement that needs careful implementation in clinical settings.

PROTECTING YOURSELF FROM LEGAL PROBLEMS

Although the discussion about legal issues related to nursing practice has covered many topics, it is important that new nurses realize that the vast majority of nurses never encounter a legal problem during their professional careers. This is because there are a number of effective strategies that professional nurses can use to limit the possibility of legal action (Butler and Lostritto, 2015).

Practice in a Safe Setting

To be truly safe, facilities in which nurses work must be committed to safe patient care. The safest situation is one in which the agency does the following:

1. Employs an appropriate number personnel with a variety of skills to care adequately for the number of agency patients at all levels of acuity
2. Has policies, procedures, and personnel practices promoting quality and safety (Smith, 2018)
3. Keeps equipment in good working order
4. Provides comprehensive orientation to new employees, supervises all levels of employees, and provides opportunities for employees to learn new procedures consistent with the level of health care services provided by the agency (note that a comprehensive orientation is not "on-the-job training") (Paradiso, 2018)

Risk management is a key part of an active quality and safety program. Risk management seeks to identify and eliminate potential safety hazards, thereby reducing patient and staff injuries. Common areas of risk include a wide range generally and specifically involving failure to ensure patient safety: medication errors, failure to monitor or respond to a patient, patient falls, failure to follow workplace procedures, and failure to supervise when delegating, among others.

In a desire to promote improvements in patient safety, The Joint Commission on Accreditation of Healthcare Organizations (i.e., The Joint Commission) adopted patient safety goals in 2005 that were revisited in 2012 and again in 2015. A summary of these goals is online (The Joint Commission, 2018). These goals identify significant ways in which patient safety can be enhanced through environmental, educational, practice, and policy changes. They are far-reaching and affect patients at almost every level and setting of care, from hospitals to office-based surgery to laboratory services.

Communicate With Other Health Professionals, Patients, and Families

The professional nurse must have open and clear communication with nurses, physicians, and other health care professionals. Safe nurses trust their own assessments, inform physicians and others of changes in patients' conditions, and question unclear or inaccurate physicians' prescriptions or treatment plans. A key aspect of communication essential in preventing legal problems is keeping good patient records. This written form of communication is called *documentation*.

The medical record (often referred to as the electronic health record [EHR]), particularly the nurse's notes, provides the core of evidence about each patient's nursing care. No matter how good the nursing care, if the nurse fails to document it in the medical record, from the perspective of the law the care did not take place. (You may hear nurses remind each other, "Not documented—not done.") Be sure to document accurately, in a timely manner, and concisely. Know the documentation policies of your agency and your unit, particularly the acceptable abbreviations.

Current and descriptive documentation of patient care is essential, not only to provide quality care but also to protect the nurse. Assessments, plans, interventions, and evaluation of the patient's progress must be reflected in the patient's medical record in case malpractice is alleged. Nurses must also document phone conversations with patients, family members, physicians, and other health care providers.

If a patient is angry, not adhering to his or her treatment plan, or complaining, nurses should be even more careful to document thoroughly. Professional nurses recognize that establishing and maintaining good communication and rapport with patients and their families not only is an aspect of best practice but also is a means of protection from lawsuits. If you encounter a negative patient or family situation that you sense is escalating, seek the advice and guidance of a nurse manager or other person in a position of authority in your organization. You do not have to settle problems with patients and families by yourself, and in fact it is wise to involve those in leadership situations to help deescalate difficult situations.

Accountability for accurate documentation has increased in recent years because of the advent of electronic documentation and multiple uses of recorded data, such as reimbursement, research, and quality assurance audits. The importance of the patient record as the basis for safe practice remains. You will learn how to document correctly as you advance through nursing school. Common problems in documentation include gaps in data or entries, subjectivity or bias, and deviating from policies and procedures established by your place of employment.

Meet the Standard of Care

The most important protective strategy for the nurse is to be a knowledgeable and safe practitioner and to meet the standard of care with all patients (Strong, 2016). Meeting the standard of care involves being technically competent, keeping up-to-date with health care innovations, being aware of peer expectations, and participating as an equal on the health care team.

Nurses must familiarize themselves with the policies and procedures of the agency in which they work, and if policies deviate from the current standard of care, they must take steps through organizational processes to bring institutional practices in line with standards and law. They must know how to use equipment properly and know when that equipment is malfunctioning. Safe nurses keep up with the current evidence to guide their practice by reading the professional literature and attending continuing education conferences and workshops. Professional nurses must use national standards of practice, care planning, and care evaluation. The ANA has developed generic and specialty standards of nursing practice and published these in the document *Nursing: Scope and Standards of Practice,* described in more detail elsewhere in this text. These national standards can be used by quality improvement programs in individual hospitals in establishing their own specific standards of nursing care appropriate for the setting.

Continued competence is an issue the nursing profession has not uniformly addressed (Strong, 2016). At this time, different states have differing requirements for continuing education as a prerequisite for license renewal. Professional nurses recognize that continuing education and maintaining competence are essential to safe practice, regardless of state requirements.

In the final analysis, the best protection a nurse can have is to know the limits of his or her own education and expertise and the provisions of the state's nursing practice act. Staying within those limits may sometimes require nurses to enlist assistance from more experienced nurses to be able to meet the standard of care. This should be viewed as a learning opportunity and an indication of maturity rather than as a failure or evidence of incompetence. Box 6.7 contains information about documents that all professional nurses should own, read, and understand to ensure that they meet the standard of care.

Carry and Understand Professional Liability Insurance

Despite the efforts of dedicated professionals, sometimes they make mistakes and patients are injured. It is

BOX 6.7   Four Documents You Should Own

Professional nurses are accountable for practicing within their scope of practice. To stay current with changes that may affect the scope of nursing practice, you should always have the latest revision of the following four documents. You must read and understand them and be mindful of their provisions as you practice.

1. A copy of the nursing practice act of the state in which you practice. These are generally available for downloading from states' board of nursing websites. Familiarity with the law in your state is a key safeguard against inadvertently overstepping your limits of practice while understanding the full set of responsibilities that your state requires you to fulfill as a professional RN.

2. *Nursing's Social Policy Statement: The Essence of the Profession.* Available from the ANA (www.nursingworld.org), this short but important document lays out in concise language the most current definition of nursing; the knowledge base for nursing, including specialization and advanced practice roles; and the regulation of practice. It represents "an expression of the social contract between society and professional nursing" (p. v) in the United States. The ANA has taken the position that the scope of nursing practice should flow from the definition of nursing that is contained in this document. It therefore has considerable impact on the national scope of practice.

3. *Nursing: Scope and Standards of Practice.* Also published by the ANA, this document expands on the *Social Policy Statement.* It focuses on defining and delimiting clinical practice and its safe implementation. *Scope and Standards'* statements, in conjunction with other documents, are widely used in legal cases to determine whether a nurse has met the "standard of care" in a particular case. In addition to this general document, the ANA has published standards for numerous specialized areas of practice, such as hospice and palliative care and gerontologic, pediatric, neuroscience, vascular, and psychiatric–mental health nursing, among others.

4. ANA's *Code of Ethics for Nurses with Interpretive Statements.* This document is available for viewing only (http://www.nursingworld.org/MainMenuCategories/EthicsStandards/CodeofEthicsforNurses) and may be purchased even if you are not yet a member of the ANA. It describes the ethical provisions that cover all aspects of nursing practice. In addition, it adds a number of clarifying ("interpretive") statements for each of the provisions. Knowledge of your professional organization's code of ethics is an important protection for you as you begin or continue your nursing practice.

The three ANA documents are available on the ANA website, www.nursingworld.org.

---

essential for nurses to carry professional liability insurance to protect their assets and income in case they are required to pay monetary compensation to an injured patient (Pohlman, 2015). Nursing students should also carry insurance, and most nursing education programs require that they do so. In addition to carrying the insurance, nurses must read and understand the provisions of their malpractice coverage.

Professional liability insurance policies vary. Typically they provide up to $2 million of coverage for a single incident and up to $4 million total, but this varies by insurance carrier, so you must become familiar with your policy and coverage. The amount of coverage depends on the nurse's specialty. Certified nurse-midwives, for example, pay higher liability insurance premiums than do psychiatric nurses because a nurse-midwife's potential for being sued is greater. Look for a policy that has portable coverage, and make sure that it covers court judgments, out-of-court settlements, legal fees, and court costs (Watson, 2014). Furthermore, a good policy covers incidents occurring any

time, as long as the incident took place while the policy was in force, even if you no longer carry the insurance (occurrence policy).

Professional liability insurance is available through most state nurses associations, nursing students associations, and private insurers. Group policies, such as those available through professional associations, are usually less expensive than individual policies and are an important benefit of association membership. Box 6.8 provides information about the two main types of professional liability policies.

Promote Positive Interpersonal Relationships

Even in the face of untoward outcomes from a health care provider, it is usually only the disgruntled patient who sues. Therefore the best strategy for the professional nurse is prevention of legal actions through positive interpersonal relationships.

Prevention includes giving personalized, concerned care; including the patient and the family in planning and implementing care; and promoting positive, open

---

BOX 6.8 Basic Types of Professional Liability Insurance Policies

Occurrence Policies

Cover injuries that occur during the period covered by the policy, whether or not the policy is still in effect at the time the suit is brought.

Claims-Made Policies

Cover injuries only if the injury occurs within the policy period and the claim is reported to the insurance company during the policy period or during the "tail." A tail is an uninterrupted extension of the policy period and is also known as the extending reporting endorsement.

BOX 6.9 Guidelines for Preventing Legal Problems in Nursing Practice

- Practice safely in a safe setting.
- Communicate with other health professionals, patients, and—with the patient's permission—family members. Document fully, carefully, and in a timely manner.
- Delegate wisely, remembering the "five rights" of delegation.
- Meet or exceed the standard of care by staying on top of new developments and skills.
- Carry professional liability insurance, and know the specifics of the policy.
- Promote positive interpersonal relationships and a nondefensive manner while practicing caring, compassionate, holistic nursing care.

---

interpersonal relationships that communicate caring and compassion. When confronted with angry patients or family members, you must avoid criticizing or blaming other health care providers and maintain a concerned and nondefensive manner.

The professional nurse who is clinically competent and caring, communicates openly with patients, and acknowledges the holism of the patient is likely to prevent most legal problems. Box 6.9 summarizes the important steps nurses can take to avoid legal problems in professional practice. When or if you commit an error, follow your agency's reporting requirements, learn from the experience, and then begin the process of self-compassion, "being warm and understanding toward yourself when you make a mistake, rather than punishing yourself with self-criticism" (Curtin, 2017, p. 64).

CONCEPTS AND CHALLENGES

- *Concept:* Law is a system of rules that governs conduct and attaches consequences to certain behavior. These consequences include civil or criminal action or both.

   Challenge: Nursing is subject to and limited by the definition of practice in the state nursing practice act and the qualifications for licensure to practice nursing in that state. Become familiar with your state's nursing practice act.

- *Concept:* The law is dynamic and must be responsive to society's needs.

   Challenge: Being responsive has broadened the scope of nursing practice and increased the possibility for legal actions involving nurses.

- *Concept:* Technological advances have increased concern about informed consent and patients' rights to direct the care they choose to receive or refuse.

   Challenge: The use of social media may blur the lines between personal and professional boundaries; however, the nurse needs to maintain firm professional boundaries with current and former patients when using social media.

IDEAS FOR FURTHER EXPLORATION

1. Using your state's nursing practice act, describe the scope of practice of the RN. When was the last time the law was modified? Does it accurately reflect current nursing practice?

2. Read the section of the nursing practice act relating to advanced practice. What differences are identified between the scope of practice of the general RN and that of the advanced practice nurse?

3. If a physician writes a prescription for an unusually high dose of a medication, what steps should the nurse take to ensure patient safety?

4. What are the liability issues for a nurse who fails to raise the side rails on a postoperative patient's bed if the patient is injured in a fall?

5. Do you have an advance directive in place? Think about what you would want if you become

incapacitated. Write your wishes down, and then consider taking whatever steps your state requires to create an official advance directives document. Be willing to have that "hard conversation" about end-of-life wishes with your family or close friends.

6. It will not be long before you will be interviewing for your first nursing position. What questions should you ask to determine whether it is a legally safe setting in which to practice?

7. Discuss ways that social media have complicated how you determine where your professional and personal boundaries are.

REFERENCES

Aiken LH, Clarke SP, Cheung RB, et al.: Educational levels of hospital nurses and surgical patient mortality, *JAMA* 290(12):1617–1623, 2003.

American Association of Legal Nurse Consultants: *What Is a Legal Nurse Consultant?* Information Brochure, 2013 (website). Available at: nlcnc.org.

American Bar Association: *Health Care for Advance Directives*, 2018. Available at: https://www.american-bar.org/groups/public_education/resources/law_issues_for_consumers/directive_whatis.html.

American Nurses Association (ANA): *Code of Ethics for Nurses, Provision 4.4 Delegation of Nurse Activities*, 2015 (website). Available at: www.nursingworld.org.

Ballard K, Haagenson D, Christiansen L, et al.: Scope of nursing practice decision-making framework, *J Nurs Adm* 7(3):19–21, 2016.

Buerhaus PI, Needleman J, Mattke S, Stewart M: Strengthening hospital nursing, *Health Aff* 21(5):123–132, 2002.

Butler KA, Lostritto MD: Malpractice 101:strategies for defending your practice, *J Radiol Nurs* 34(1):13–24, 2015.

Croke EM: Nurses, negligence and malpractice: an analysis based on more than 250 cases against nurses, *Am J Nurs* 103(9):54–63, 2003.

Curtin L: Self-compassion, mistakes and moral behavior, *Am Nurse Today* 12(3):64, 2017.

Heyland DK, Barwich D, Pichhora D, et al.: Failure to engage hospitalized elderly patients and their families in advance care planning, *JAMA Intern Med* 173:778–787, 2013.

Institute of Medicine (IOM): *Nursing Staff in Hospitals and Nursing Homes: Is It adequate?* Washington, DC, 1996, National Academies Press.

The Joint Commission: *National Patient Safety Goals* (website), 2018. Available at: https://www.jointcommission.org/assets/1/6/2018_HAP_NPSG_goals_final.pdf.

National Council of State Boards of Nursing: *Scope of Nursing Practice Decision-Making Framework*, 2016. Available at: https://www.ncsbn.org/decision-making-framework.htm.

National Council of State Boards of Nursing (NCSBN): *White Paper: A Nurse's Guide to the Use of Social Media*, 2011 (website). Available at: https://www.ncsbn.org/3739.htm.

National Council of State Boards of Nursing (NCSBN): *Model Nursing Practice Acts*, 2014. Available at: https://www.ncsbn.org/legislative-initiatives-and-resources.htm.

National Council of State Boards of Nursing (NCSBN): *Substance Use Disorder in Nursing*, (website), 2015. Available at: https:www.ncsbn.org/10369.htm.

National Council of State Boards of Nursing (NCSBN): National guidelines for nursing delegation, *J Nurs Regul* 7(1):5–14.

Paradiso L: Everyone is responsible for a culture of safety, *Am Nurse Today* 13(3):33–34, 2018.

Puente J: The enhanced nurse licensure compact, *Am Nurse Today* 12(10):50–53, 2017.

Pohlman KJ: Why you need your own malpractice insurance, *Am Nurse Today* 10(11):28–30, 2015.

Reising DL: Make your nursing care malpractice-proof, *Am Nurse Today* 7(1):24–29, 2012.

Russell KA: Nurse practice acts guide and govern, *J Nurs Regulation* 8(3):18–25, 2017.

Smith CA: Promoting high reliability on the front-line, *Am Nurse Today* 13(3):30–34, 2018.

Strong M: Maintaining clinical competency is your responsibility, *Am Nurse Today* 11(7):46–47, 2016.

U.S. Department of Health and Human Services: *Privacy and Security Guide*, 2015. Available at: https://www.healthit.gov/sites/default/files/pdf/privacy/privacy-and-security-guide.pdf.

Watson E: Nursing malpractice: costs, trends, and issues, *J Leg Nurse Consulting* 25(1):26–31, 2014.

Ethics: Basic Concepts for Professional Nursing Practice

Josie K. Christian, DNP, MSN, BSN, RN, PHN

To enhance your understanding of this chapter, try the Student Exercises on the Evolve site at http://evolve.elsevier.com/Black/professional.

LEARNING OUTCOMES

After studying this chapter, students will be able to:

- Differentiate between values, morals, ethics, and bioethics.
- Explain the difference between Kohlberg's and Gilligan's approaches to moral reasoning.
- Compare and contrast the three normative ethical theories.
- Identify and define basic ethical principles.
- Discuss the concept of justice as an ethical principle in health care delivery.
- Discuss the relevance of a code of ethics for the profession of nursing.
- Understand how professional ethics override personal ethics in professional settings.

- Describe ethical dilemmas resulting from conflicts between patients, health care professionals, family members, and institutions.
- Identify a model for ethical decision making, and discuss the steps of the model.
- Recognize sociocultural challenges to professional ethical behavior, including social media and substance abuse.
- Understand the important ethical issues related to immigration, migration, and health care.
- Recognize moral distress, and describe the individual and organizational issues resulting from unaddressed moral distress.
- Describe the process of using moral courage with the CODE Moral Courage Model.

In our everyday, nonwork lives, the "rightness" or "wrongness" of a situation or how to act can seem very clear. We sometimes refer to these sharply, clearly delineated acts or decisions as being "black or white." Often in health care, nurses face an uncertain space known as the "gray area" where what are right or wrong acts is not clear or sharply delineated. You have learned that nursing focuses on human responses, so as with all endeavors that deal with humans and responses, nurses face the messiness—the gray area—that is inherent in individuals' lives and actions. Understanding ethical principles, frameworks, nursing's code of ethics, and your values and beliefs can help you face the complex ethical issues that confront nurses. You will learn to act in accord with nursing's code of ethics, which will give you a firm foundation on which to practice nursing ethically.

Scholars have devoted their entire careers to the study of *ethics,* the examination of questions of right and wrong, how values are determined, and how ethics are applied in specific situations. Ethics are also known as moral philosophy. There are three general types of ethics: (1) *metaethics,* which focus on universal truths, and where and how ethical principles are developed; (2) *normative ethics,* which focus on the moral standards that regulate behaviors; and (3) *applied ethics,* which focus on specific difficult issues such as euthanasia, capital punishment, abortion, and health disparities. In a practice profession such as nursing, ethical issues often arise, created by the very nature of the work of nursing. The purpose of this chapter is to give you a basic introduction to the very complex issues of ethics so that you will be better prepared to recognize and work through situations with ethical implications.

Common situations with ethical implications for nurses include making decisions about the allocation of time and resources, what and how much information to share with patients and their families, how to manage and deal with colleagues professionally, and how to resolve problems when the desires and needs of patients and families conflict with institutional policies or the values of those providing the care. More dramatic ethical issues for nurses include assisting families making end-of-life decisions, allocating care in emergency situations (triage), managing pain near the end of life with large doses of narcotics, and advocating for a patient even when the nurse does not agree with the patient.

To manage the complex ethical issues they face, nurses need an understanding of the theoretical basis for ethical decision making.

Throughout their education and practice, nurses must exercise judgment when making clinical decisions. However, when nurses encounter ethical dilemmas, they need an ethical decision-making model to apply to the situation and one that works for individual nurses in the context of his or her value system. Box 7.1, "To Be Guardians of the Ethical Treatment of Patients," describes the importance of the role of nurses and nursing faculty in achieving high standards of integrity to provide ethical care for our vulnerable patients.

DEFINITIONS OF BASIC CONCEPTS IN ETHICS

Defining *values, morals, ethics,* and *bioethics* is useful as a first step in understanding ethics and their relationship to health care. **Values** are attitudes, ideals, or

---

BOX 7.1   To Be Guardians of the Ethical Treatment of Patients

Anne Bavier (2009), PhD, RN, FAAN, Dean of the University of Texas at Arlington College of Nursing and President-elect of the National League for Nursing, wrote to nursing students and their faculty in an editorial about the high standards of integrity for themselves and for all who serve patients:

To become the guardians of patients' well-being and of the nursing profession, nurses must learn more than technical skills, even more than just critical thinking or ethical criteria.... The topic is timely: If recent headlines are any indication, professional ethics are in critical condition. We are all familiar with reports of financial dishonesty that have contributed to a contracted global economy, and we have seen recent surveys about student cheating and plagiarism. It seems that a chronic ailment, human frailty, is the underlying disorder.

For nurses and nurse faculty, the outcomes of dishonesty are, without hyperbole, a matter of life and death. When a math student or an English student cheats without learning, society is impaired, to be sure. However, if a nursing student cheats without learning, patients may sicken or die.... When the (National League for Nursing [NLN]) adopted its core values, it included integrity, "evident when organizational principles of communication, ethical decision making, and humility are encouraged, expected, and demonstrated consistently." The NLN

states that "not only is doing the right thing simply how we do business, but our actions reveal our commitment to truth-telling and to how we always see ourselves from the perspective of others in a larger community" (http://www.nln.org/about/core-values). *Most schools and universities have similar codes of conduct that stress the greater good of individual actions and the pursuit of truth.*

Nurses and nurse faculty must be the guardians of the ethical treatment of patients. Aristotle's deceptively simple rationale for living well and doing good seems exquisitely suited to nursing education: "Every art and every inquiry, and similarly every action and choice, is thought to aim at some good; and for this reason the good has rightly been declared to be that at which all things aim." Nursing, as both art and inquiry, action and choice, must always reflect on its aims. That is what Aristotle called phronesis, practical wisdom, change for good by planning an effective route to a desirable goal. Thus, a nurse educator (whether in classroom or clinic) is not just a master of skills conveyed to the student but also a teacher of practical wisdom: ethical action.

Deeply mentored by nurse faculty, they must become confident, autonomous health care professionals who have high standards of integrity for themselves and for all who serve patients.

From *Nursing Education Perspectives* by Anne Bavier. Copyright 2009 by National League for Nursing. Reproduced with permission of National League for Nursing in the format Textbook via Copyright Clearance Center.

beliefs that an individual or a group holds and uses to guide behavior. Values are usually expressed in terms of right and wrong, hierarchies of importance, or how one should behave. Values are freely chosen and indicate what the individual considers important, such as honesty and hard work. Values are assimilated from and influenced by personal and professional experiences and are deeply rooted in an individual's culture. Attitudes are integrated with values and can shape nurses' judgments and actions. Attitudes may, however, result in nurse bias if the nurse is not cognizant of how the beliefs may affect the nurse's judgment. The terms *morals* and *ethics* are often used interchangeably, but for the purposes of this book, a distinction is made. Philosophers and scholars have conflicting views on how to define these terms. **Morals** provide standards of behavior that guide the actions of an individual or social group and are established rules of conduct to be used in situations where a decision about right and wrong must be made. Morals typically focus on behaviors and actions of what to do (good) and what to avoid (harm). An example of a moral standard is "One should not lie." Morals are learned over time and are influenced by life experiences and culture.

Ethics is a term used to reflect what actions an individual should take and maybe "codified," as in the ethical code of a profession. "Ethics" is derived from the Greek word "ethos," which means habits or customs. Ethics are process oriented and involve a critical analysis of actions. If ethicists (persons who study ethics) reflected on the moral statement "One should not lie," they would clarify definitions of lying and explore whether there are circumstances under which lying might be acceptable.

Bioethics are the application of ethical theories and principles to moral issues or problems in health care. Bioethics (also referred to as *biomedical ethics*) as an area of ethical inquiry came into existence around 1970, when health care providers began to embrace a holistic view of the patient and the rights of patients, in addition to treating and curing disease. Bioethics are concerned with determining what should be done in a specific situation by applying ethical principles. For instance, discussions about genetic testing often have a strong bioethical component surrounding use of knowledge from this type of testing. The website www.bioethics.net is a source of comprehensive and up-to-date information about issues related to bioethics that you may find interesting.

Advances in science and medical technologies have allowed health care providers to sustain lives under circumstances that once would have caused a patient's death. On the one hand, these technologies are excellent tools in the management of some problems—for example, in assisting with ventilation until a patient can breathe without assistance, as sometimes happens in the case of a life-threatening but reversible condition (e.g., severe pneumonia, moderately severe head injury). Conversely, these advances sometimes create ethical dilemmas for health care providers. For example, a patient may be "kept alive" even when there is no discernible brain activity or hope for the return of spontaneous respiration. Nurses struggle with situations such as these, asking whether a patient should be sustained ("kept alive") under these circumstances. These situations sometimes raise serious questions for nurses about the meaning of life and what constitutes being "alive."

A critical attribute of providing care in a professional setting is that professional ethics override personal morals and values. The American Nurses Association (ANA) published a position statement in 1983 that remains in effect today and that contains this statement: "The ANA believes the Code [of Ethics] for Nurses is nonnegotiable and that each nurse has an obligation to uphold and adhere to the code of ethics" (ANA, 1994). Holding all nurses accountable to the same ethical code is a means of protecting patients by establishing a clear standard by which nurses make ethical decisions and carry out their duties. Provision 2 of the Code of Ethics describes the nurse's primary commitment to the patient; provision 5 describes the responsibility of nurses to maintain their own integrity. These two provisions are not in conflict, but they do underscore the importance of understanding nursing's primary ethical obligations to the care of patients.

Nurses, then, must think carefully about personal values and morals. Being clear on where one stands personally on a situation will help the nurse make careful choices about their work environment and the types of patients with whom he or she would like to work. For instance, if a nurse's personal moral belief is that abortion is wrong under any circumstances, he or she would find untenable the requirements of a work setting in which pregnancy terminations are performed for genetic disorders. Similarly, if a nurse believes that drug addiction represents a moral shortcoming, seeking employment on an infectious disease unit where many patients have addiction problems would be a poor choice. By understanding their personal values, nurses can anticipate situations in which their personal morals and professional ethics may be in conflict. A thoughtful nurse who is aware of deep personal values and moral standards will make decisions regarding practice setting so that the nurse's own personal integrity remains intact, while putting patients and their needs first.

Moral reflection—critical analysis of one's morals, beliefs, and actions—is a process through which a person develops and maintains moral integrity. Moral integrity in a professional setting is a goal in which one's professional beliefs and actions are assessed and analyzed (reflected on) so that professional ethics continue to mature and respond to changes in practice (Hardingham, 2001). In any complex ethical situation, nurses should analyze their own actions so that they can reduce inner conflicts between their personal values and morals and their professional ethics. A model of nurses' ethical reasoning developed by Roseanne Fairchild, PhD, RN, CNE, NE-BC, is featured in Professional Profile Box 7.1.

Moral distress is a phenomenon of spiritual, emotional, and behavioral anguish (Burston and Tuckett, 2013). Moral distress may arise when one knows the

---

PROFESSIONAL PROFILE BOX 7.1
NURSES' ETHICAL REASONING SKILLS MODEL

A dynamic, ethically based reasoning process became apparent to me over a period of years as I worked with patients and families as a registered nurse (RN) in the emergency department and in hospice/palliative care. This dynamic is proposed to involve the interplay of several important internal cognitive processes, as depicted in the nurses' ethical reasoning skills (NERS) model (Fairchild, 2010). With this theory, I propose that when faced with an ethical dilemma, the professional nurse's cognitive processes include reflection, reasoning, and a review of competing values, ultimately leading to purposeful *action* on behalf of patients and families in the nurse's care.

I developed this model during my doctoral studies at Indiana University, based on my work experiences as an RN, and also based on current evidence in ethical decision making, and in nursing and health systems theory and research (Fairchild, 2010). During my studies, a diverse mix of coursework in ethics and theory seemed to coalesce, allowing me to visualize the complexity of patient care decision-making processes as a unique and ongoing cycle for nurses, akin to a phenomenon called *systems thinking* (Pesut and Herman, 1999). In systems thinking, we continually take experiences in and reflect on them from a holistic, values-based, knowledge-driven stance. Thus what nurses and other health care providers strive to accomplish every day in emergent and/or crisis situations needs to be represented and supported by a fluid, interactive thought dynamic that promotes sound ethical decision making at the "sharp end" (Cook and Woods, 1994) of care.

As challenges in patient care are managed on a daily basis in practice, I believe that practical ethical decision-making skills need to be pushed to the forefront of health care

delivery, based on ever-changing characteristics of today's complex health care systems. In addition, as nurses, our experiences teach us that *context* is of utmost importance as we strive to follow basic tenets of our profession; that is, to do good, and above all, to do no harm (Gilligan, 1987) on behalf of patients and families. Nurses' unique commitment and calling to apply both higher level knowledge and humanistic, holistic caring are what set us apart from the medically based disease model of care. Knowing and cooperatively manifesting our uniqueness allow us to act wholeheartedly and in good faith with other members of the health care team, because we are consciously realizing the complexity, as well as the fragility, of the human caring work we engage in each day.

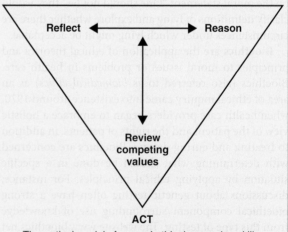

Theoretical model of nurses' ethical reasoning skills.

Roseanne M. Fairchild, PhD, RN, CNE, NE-BC
Indiana State University, Clayton, IN

morally correct action to take but is unable to act as a result of internal constraints (such as lack of moral courage) or external constraints, including power differentials (Saureland et al., 2014). Moral distress may also occur when a nurse's moral action is ineffective in ensuring the moral outcome, often because of constraints beyond the nurse's control (Rushton et al., 2016).

Repercussions of moral distress affect not only the nurse but also the broader health care context, including risk to health care quality and patient outcomes, job satisfaction, and retention, as well as the physical, spiritual, and emotional wellness of the nurse (Burston and Tuckett, 2013). Unaddressed moral distress can lead to nurse behaviors that exacerbate an integrity-compromising situation, including nurse apathy, indifference, avoidance, disengagement in patient care situations, feelings of powerlessness, and loss of moral sensitivity (McCarthy and Gastmans, 2015).

The following scenario and the one later in this chapter have several important ethical implications that cause a moral dilemma for the health care team and the family. Examine the scenarios for various ethical issues, and think about what parts of this situation might pose a moral dilemma or moral distress for you.

Scenario 1: What are the implications of "doing everything"? A newborn infant was admitted to the neonatal intensive care unit (NICU). She was born very prematurely and weighs only 520 grams (about 1 pound). The parents want "everything done" for the infant to ensure her survival; the infant, however, has multiple setbacks including serious infections; feeding problems; and then a grade IV intraventricular hemorrhage, which is severe bleeding into the ventricles of the brain. The neonatologists are convinced that the infant will have profound physical, cognitive, and developmental problems if she even survives and ask for a meeting with the parents to discuss discontinuing the infant's life support. The parents want life support to be continued and for the infant to be a "full code," meaning that all efforts will be made to resuscitate her in case her heart stops. The infant's primary care nurse understands the parents' deep desire to give their child every chance to live; however, he also understands the severe physical and neurologic complications of extreme prematurity. He is concerned about pain and suffering the infant may be experiencing because of her numerous treatments and extensive supportive technology. He thinks about the resources in terms of time and money that continuing support of this infant requires, and although he does not like thinking about patient care in those terms, he recognizes

the tension he feels about the effort the infant is requiring. The nurse realizes that he dreads going in to work every day to take care of this infant and finds himself dwelling on the situation when he is not at work. After a long shift one night, he goes home and blurts out to his wife, "This just isn't right, and I don't know what to do about it."

This example demonstrates numerous aspects of moral dilemmas and resulting moral distress. The nurse experienced moral distress, a sense of being unable to act in a way that he believes is moral in this situation. The nurse recognized the parents' desire for their child to live; the possibility of pain and suffering of the infant; the real possibility of severe, long-term problems if she lives; the expense in terms of time and money; the emotional toll of care of the infant; and his own discomfort and sense of helplessness. This nurse also demonstrated that he was reflecting on his own practice and beliefs, which will help maintain his moral integrity. He will also use the lessons from this patient situation as he matures as a nurse, so that similar situations in the future may not be so distressful for him. Thinking Critically Box 7.1 refers to this patient situation; once you have studied the remainder of this chapter, you will have additional

---

❓ THINKING CRITICALLY BOX 7.1
Addressing Distressful Ethical Situations

Reflect on the clinical example of the nurse's moral distress related to the prematurely born infant in the NICU. Now that you have some basic knowledge about ethics, consider these questions:

1. What would a deontologist's position be with regard to the sustaining of the infant's life?
2. What would a utilitarian's position be in this case?
3. What virtues of the nurse do you see at work in this case?
4. What basic ethical principles do you think the nurse may be using in analyzing this moral dilemma?
5. What are your own personal beliefs and values regarding the sustaining of a very premature infant on extensive life support?
6. What are alternative ethical viewpoints that someone else may hold regarding this situation?
7. Who holds the primary responsibility for determining what should happen in this case—the parents or the health care providers? Defend your response from an ethical perspective.
8. What is the state's (government's) role in intervening in this type of situation?

knowledge, tools, and perspective with which to consider the complexities of this scenario.

To function effectively in today's complex health care arena, nurses need to understand approaches to moral reasoning, theories of ethics, basic ethical principles, and ethical decision-making models. A significant advance in the professionalization of a traditional occupation such as nursing is the adoption of a formal code of ethics (Baker, 2009). Professional ethical codes such as that of the ANA provide substantial guidance in determining how to respond and act in practice settings when faced with an ethical dilemma. The remainder of this chapter will provide a basic orientation to these complex topics.

APPROACHES TO MORAL REASONING

Similar to other forms of human development, moral reasoning is a process in which maturation occurs over time as persons become more abstract in their thinking and understanding of the world. Moral development describes how a person learns to handle moral dilemmas from childhood through adulthood. Two important theorists in moral development and reasoning are Lawrence Kohlberg and Carol Gilligan.

Kohlberg's Stages of Moral Reasoning

Kohlberg (1976, 1986) proposed three levels of moral reasoning as a function of cognitive development: (1) preconventional, (2) conventional, and (3) postconventional. Each of these three levels is then considered in terms of stages. In the preconventional level, the individual is inattentive to the norms of society when responding to moral problems. Instead, the individual's perspective is self-centered. At this level, what the individual wants or needs takes precedence over right or wrong. A person in stage 1 of the preconventional level responds to punishment. In stage 2, the person responds to the prospect of personal reward. Kohlberg observed the preconventional level of moral development in children younger than 9 years of age, as well as in some adolescents and adult criminal offenders. A more typical example, however, is that of a toddler for whom the word *no* has yet to have meaning as he or she persists in reaching for a breakable object on a table.

The conventional level is characterized by moral decisions that conform to the expectations of one's family, group, or society. The person making moral choices based on what is pleasing to others characterizes stage

3 within this level. An individual in stage 4 of the conventional level makes moral choices based on a larger notion of what is desired by society. When confronted with a moral choice, people functioning at the conventional level follow family or cultural group norms. According to Kohlberg, most adolescents and adults generally function at this level. "Because it's the law" is a common explanation of persons operating at a conventional level of moral reasoning.

The postconventional level consists of stage 5 and stage 6 and involves more independent modes of thinking than previous stages. The individual has developed the ability to define his or her own moral values. Individuals who apply moral reasoning at the postconventional level may ignore both self-interest and group norms in making moral choices. For example, they may sacrifice themselves on behalf of the group. Part of their moral reasoning and behavior is based on a socially agreed-on standard of human rights (Haynes et al., 2004). In this highest level of moral development, people create their own morality, which may differ from society's norms. Kohlberg believed that only a minority of adults achieves this level.

Progression through Kohlberg's levels and their corresponding stages occur over varying lengths of time for different individuals. The stages are sequential, they build on each other, and each stage is characterized by a higher capacity for moral reasoning than the preceding stage. Kohlberg (1976) suggested that certain conditions might stimulate higher levels of moral development. Intellectual development is one necessary characteristic. Individuals at higher levels intellectually generally operate at a higher stage of moral reasoning than those with lower levels of intellect. An environment that offers people opportunities for group participation, shared decision-making processes, and responsibility for the consequences of their actions also promotes higher levels of moral reasoning. Moral development is stimulated by the creation of conflict in settings in which the individual recognizes the limitations of present modes of thinking. For example, students have been stimulated to higher levels of moral reasoning through participating in courses on moral discussion and ethics (Kohlberg, 1973).

Gilligan's Stages of Moral Reasoning

Gilligan (1982) was concerned that Kohlberg did not adequately recognize women's experiences in the development of moral reasoning. She noted that Kohlberg's theories had largely been generated from research with men and boys, and when women were tested by using Kohlberg's stages of moral reasoning, they scored lower than men. Gilligan believed that women's and girls' relational orientation to the world shaped their moral reasoning differently from that of men and boys. Women do not have inadequate moral development but different development because of their gender. Kohlberg's inattention to gender differences meant that his theory was inadequate in explaining women's moral development.

Gilligan described a moral development perspective focused on care. In Gilligan's view, the moral person is one who responds to need and demonstrates consideration of care and responsibility in relationships. This perspective differed from the orientation toward justice described by Kohlberg (1973, 1976). In Gilligan's research on moral reasoning, women most often exhibited a focus on care, whereas men more often exhibited a focus on justice. Gilligan described the differences between women's and men's moral reasoning not as a matter of better or worse, or mature or immature, but simply as a matter of having "a different voice" in moral reasoning.

Gilligan (1982) suggested that women view moral dilemmas in terms of conflicting responsibilities. She described women's development of moral reasoning as a sequence of three levels and two transitions, with each level representing a more complex understanding of the relationship between self and others. Each transition resulted in a critical reevaluation of the conflict between selfishness and responsibility. Gilligan's levels of moral development are (1) orientation to individual survival; (2) a focus on goodness with recognition of self-sacrifice; and (3) the morality of caring and being responsible for others, as well as self. The focus of nursing on care as a moral attribute is congruent with Gilligan's assertion that the dynamics of human relationships are "central to moral understanding, joining the heart and the eye in an ethic that ties the activity of thought to the activity of care" (p. 149). Critical thinking within a caring professional relationship is a sound basis for nursing practice.

Nurses at times combine the care/justice perspective when forced to make ethical decisions. Nurses have shifted from the moral perspective of care to a justice orientation where universal rules and principles are used in moral decision making (Zickmund, 2004).

Furthermore, as economics and scarcity of resources shape the delivery of health care, nurses may find themselves less able to use critical thinking, reflection, and higher stages of moral reasoning in their practice setting.

The nature of the practice of nursing has deeply ethical implications. Some implications are clear, such as those described in the case of the NICU earlier in this chapter. The ethical implications of day-to-day practice and decisions are often obscured by more dramatic scenarios. In scenario 2, a nurse organizes her day and addresses her patients' needs by a strategy she calls "time management."

Scenario 2: At the beginning of her shift on an orthopedic trauma unit, Michelle, a registered nurse with 3 years' experience, identified and prioritized several tasks that she needed to complete during her shift, listing times for scheduled medications, three complex dressing changes, helping a patient on postoperative day 1 to get out of bed, and discharge teaching for her patient Mr. Thomas, who was going home after a long hospitalization for the treatment of a severe compound fracture of his lower leg. Michelle knew that there was another patient in the emergency department (ED) waiting for admission to the unit, but there were no empty beds; the only bed that was going to be available was the one Mr. Thomas now occupied. Michelle anticipated a busy shift.

Also, Michelle's patient Mr. Dillard complained of pain in his abdomen and asked for medication frequently. After assessing each of her six patients, Michelle collected the discharge papers for Mr. Thomas and started her teaching with him and his wife, who was going to continue care of the large wound in Mr. Thomas' leg at home. Mrs. Thomas had numerous questions and what seemed to be a routine discharge became more complicated when she asked Michelle for a home health referral so a nurse could help them manage Mr. Thomas' wound at home. Soon, Mr. Dillard rang his call light and asked for pain medication; a nurse colleague stepped into the room to tell Michelle, "Your frequent flyer in Room 312 rang again." Several minutes later, the ED charge nurse called to ask when a bed was going to be ready. The patient in the ED had been there since 10 p.m. the previous evening. Michelle began to feel a bit of stress but decided to reprioritize her day.

As she stood at the med cart and reviewed Mr. Dillard's pain med use, she noted to her colleague, "He has got to be drug seeking. That is the only explanation."

She decided that she could forgo for the time being getting a home health referral for Mr. Thomas; she understood that until he went home, she would not have to do the long admission process for the new patient coming from the ED. When Mr. Dillard asked for pain medication a second time, Michelle rolled her eyes and continued to check the morning laboratory reports; when Mrs. Thomas came to the nurses' station to ask about the home health referral, Michelle told her, "I called the social worker to come up to see you, but she is busy and can't get here until midafternoon." Mrs. Thomas thanked Michelle and walked away, at which point Michelle turned to a new nurse in orientation and told her, "And that's the time management skill they don't teach you in nursing school" and high-fived another colleague.

In Thinking Critically Box 7.2, you will be considering this scenario and how day-to-day nursing acts have ethical implications.

 THINKING CRITICALLY BOX 7.2

Day-to-Day Ethical Considerations

Reread scenario 2 carefully, and then consider the perspectives from various persons described in it.

1. You are the new nurse in orientation. Describe the scenario from your perspective, and identify what you understand as elements of the scenario with ethical implications.

2. You are Michelle. Describe the scenario from your perspective as a competent nurse with a busy day ahead.

3. You are Mr. Dillard. Your pain in your abdomen was not part of your original admission diagnosis. You are hospitalized for treatment for injuries after an automobile accident in which the air bag deployed. You ask Michelle to call your doctor because you are not getting pain relief. Michelle tells you that you are to get pain medication every 4 to 6 hours, and it has only been 3.5 hours. Consider the ethical implications of pain management. What did Michelle mean in referring to Mr. Dillard as "drug seeking"? What does "being ethical" mean for a nurse in this situation? Was Michelle being ethical?

4. You are Mrs. Thomas, and as you walk away you hear Michelle's "time management" comment. You return to the desk to ask Michelle if she had even called a social worker yet. From an ethical perspective, how should Michelle respond?

The article described in this chapter's Evidence-Based Practice Box 7.1 demonstrates that nurses often fall short of established ethical standards to complete their daily work. This problem is not exclusive to American nurses: the problem exists across nursing internationally.

THEORIES OF ETHICS

Theories of ethics, like all theories, are conceptual descriptions of phenomena. In ethics, the phenomena described are understandings of behaviors in terms of their moral implications. Theories are broad descriptions, and no single ethical theory can be applied universally in health care situations. As previously introduced, there are three general types of ethics: (1) *metaethics,* which focuses on universal truths, and where and how ethical principles are developed; (2) *normative ethics,* which focuses on the moral standards that regulate behaviors; and (3) *applied ethics,* which focuses on specific difficult issues such as euthanasia, capital punishment, abortion, and health disparities. In this section, selected ethical theories useful to nurses are introduced with emphasis on the normative ethical theories (virtue ethics, deontological ethics, and utilitarian ethics), and principalism ethics. Table 7.1 provides the highlights and contrasts among the three normative ethical theories, and Table 7.2 summarizes principalism ethics.

Deontology

The term *deontology* has its origins from the Greek word *deon,* which means "obligation" or "duty." German philosopher Immanuel Kant (1724–1804) was a preeminent deontologist. He believed that an act was moral if its motives or intentions were good, regardless of the outcome. An ethical action consists of doing one's duty or honoring one's obligations to human beings: to do one's duty was right; to not do one's duty was wrong. The deontological perspective does not look primarily at the consequences of actions or outcomes; rather, it focuses on the intent of the act. For example, a nursing student was providing care to a senior man who was dying and who had been estranged from his son for many years. From his wallet, he pulled out a tattered piece of paper with a phone number on it. Handing it to the nursing student, he asked her to promise him that she would call his son and ask him to come for a final visit. She promised.

Although she was filled with dread, the nursing student recognized her obligation to her patient to honor her promise to him. With trembling hands, she called the number. The man who answered listened to her for a few moments; then he said, "I wouldn't go to see him if you paid me. Tell him I am glad he's dying." And then he hung up on her. The student was horrified and was very upset about what to tell her dying patient. From a deontological perspective, the nursing student acted ethically, because she had a duty to respond to her patient's request and to keep her promise, despite the outcome.

Deontology can be further divided into act deontology and rule deontology. Act deontologists determine the right thing to do by gathering all the facts and then making a decision. Much time and energy are needed to judge each situation carefully. Once a decision is made, there is a commitment to universalizing it. In other words, if one makes a moral judgment in one situation, the same judgment will be made in any similar situation. Rule deontologists, on the other hand, emphasize that principles guide our actions. Examples of rules might be "Always keep a promise" or "Never tell a lie."

EVIDENCE-BASED PRACTICE BOX 7.1

Nurses' Ethical Decision Making: Conformist Practice

A growing concern exists regarding nurses' ethical competence. Barriers to ethical practice compromise nurses' ability to care for patients in a manner that they consider to be moral. De Casterlé and colleagues (2009), an international team of nurse researchers, conducted a meta-analysis using data from nine different studies in four countries to determine how nurses became involved in ethical decision making and action in their daily practice. A meta-analysis is a means of using similar data from different studies that address similar hypotheses and research questions to get results from a larger sample. By combining data, these researchers were able to pool the responses of 1592 RNs who completed the Ethical Behavior Test, which is based on an adaptation of Kohlberg's theory of moral development.

De Casterlé and colleagues first reviewed the existing literature about nurses' ethical decision making in practice. They found in their review that nurses typically were often poorly prepared to address ethical dilemmas and that nurses do not use critical thinking in making ethical decisions. Nurses were also found to experience conflicts between their personal values and professional ethics, and few nurses were able to express ethical problems to the health care team. In addition, nurses found that their work environment hindered their ability to practice nursing in a manner that they believed was ethical. Heavy workloads, time and financial constraints, and staffing problems all interfered with nurses' ability to make ethical decision making a priority.

Among the 1592 RNs included in the sample of this meta-analysis, 58 nurses were recruited specifically because they were known to demonstrate high-level ethical reasoning and practice. These nurses constituted the "expert group." This strategy is known as "purposeful sampling," to include in a study a very specific group of participants as a comparison group.

The expert group exhibited a significantly higher likelihood to make ethical decisions from a postconventional level of moral reasoning, usually at Kohlberg's sixth stage. The nonexpert group (the other 1534 nurses) generally preferred moral decisions that corresponded to Kohlberg's fourth stage, the conventional level of moral reasoning. The nonexpert nurses were significantly more likely than expert nurses to prefer moral decisions from the preconventional level, at Kohlberg's second stage.

The findings suggested that nurses typically make ethical decisions at a conventional level and that this is an international phenomenon among nurses. The researchers referred to this as "conformist practice" that "excludes a critical and creative search for the best caring answer" (p. 547) to ethical dilemmas. The conventions of practice—medical prescriptions, rules of the nursing unit, and policies and procedures—serve as a framework for practice but should not preclude individualized patient care. The findings of this study confirmed much of what the researchers had seen from their review of the literature: that nurses often face ethical challenges, that workplace conditions hinder nurses from ethical practice, and that there is a growing concern about nurses' ability to practice ethically. In addition, de Casterlé and colleagues found that nurses tend to conform to workplace rules and norms rather than using creativity and reflecting critically on their practice. The researchers suggest that, to provide the best care possible for patients, nurses must develop maturity in their moral reasoning, especially at a time when economic values tend to predominate in shaping workplace decisions.

Data from de Casterlé BD, Izumi S, Godfrey NS, et al.: Nurses' responses to ethical dilemmas in nursing practice: meta-analysis, *J Adv Nurs* 63(6):540–549, 2009.

TABLE 7.1   Highlights and Contrasts Among the Three Normative Ethical Theories

Framework	Virtue	Consequentialist	Duty
Deliberative Process	What kind of person should I be (or try to be), and what will my actions show about my character?	What kinds of outcomes should I produce (or try to produce)?	What are my obligations in this situation, and what are the things I should never do?
Focus	Person: Attempts to discern character traits (virtues and vices) that are, or could be, motivating the people involved in the situation.	Outcome: Directs attention to the future effects of an action, for all people who will be directly or indirectly affected by the action.	Duty: Directs attention to the duties that exist prior to the situation and determines obligations.
Definition of Ethical Conduct	Ethical conduct is whatever a fully virtuous person would do in the circumstances.	Ethical conduct is the action that will achieve the best consequences.	Ethical conduct involves always doing the right thing: never failing to do one's duty.
Motivation	Aim is to develop one's character.	Aim is to produce the most good.	Aim is to perform the right action.
Limitations	Assumes everyone has moral motives and strives to develop virtues. Requires a case-by-case approach without a defined decision-making process.	In interest of benefiting the majority, the interests of the minority are overlooked. Impossible to calculate all consequences.	Assumes humans make moral judgments. Life situations vary, and rules for all circumstances are unrealistic. Disregard for consequences of actions.

Adapted by Brown University, 2017.
Acknowledgement: This framework for thinking ethically is the product of dialogue and debate in the seminar Making Choices: Ethical Decisions at the Frontier of Global Science held at Brown University in the spring semester 2011. It relies on the Ethical Framework developed at the Markkula Center for Applied Ethics at Santa Clara University (http://www.scu.edu/ethics/practicing/decision/) and the Ethical Framework developed by the Center for Ethical Deliberation at the University of Northern Colorado as well as the Ethical Frameworks for Academic Decision-Making on the Faculty Focus website (https://www.facultyfocus.com/articles/faculty-development/ethical-frameworks-for-academic-decision-making/), which in turn relies on Understanding Ethical Frameworks for E-Learning Decision-Making, December 1, 2008, Distance Education Report. Primary contributors include Sheila Bonde and Paul Firenze, with critical input from James Green, Margot Grinberg, Josephine Korijn, Emily Levoy, Alysha Naik, Laura Ucik, and Liza Weisberg. It was last revised in May 2013.

In all situations, the rule is to be followed. Deontologists are not concerned with the consequences of adhering to certain rules or actions. If one's guiding principle is "Always keep a promise," a deontologist will keep promises, even if circumstances have changed. For the nursing student in the previous example, by judging that making a call under these circumstances was ethical, she set for herself a precedent—that she would act the same way in each circumstance like this one. Similarly, if she acted on the principle to never tell a lie, she would find a caring way to tell her patient not to expect his son to visit when he asked.

One of the limitations of this duty-based theory is there is an assumption that humans will all make moral judgments. Additionally, life situations vary, and a guide (rules of duty) for all circumstances is unrealistic. Last, a significant theory limitation of deontology is the disregard of consequences of actions.

Utilitarianism

Utilitarianism is based on a fundamental belief that the moral rightness of an action is determined solely by its consequence. Utilitarianism was first described by David Hume (1711–1776) and was developed further by many notable philosophers, including Jeremy Bentham (1748–1832) and John Stuart Mill (1806–1873). Mill had a significant influence on utilitarian ethics as it is known today.

Those who subscribe to utilitarian ethics believe that "what makes an action right or wrong is its utility, with

TABLE 7.2	Summary of Principalism Theory		
Ethical Principle	**Moral Basis**	**Overemphasis/ Downside**	**Challenges in Health Care**
Autonomy (includes confidentiality)	Respect for individuals	Lack of caring, not interfering with decision making	Some patients defer autonomy to their provider. Who is granted the autonomy with incompetent or unconscious patients, minors, and those with cultural power differentials? Autonomy as a principle is typically weighted highest in health care.
Beneficence (includes patient advocacy)	Do good	Paternalism—inflicting own values	Context of patient's life and situation must be considered. Beneficence may conflict with informed refusal.
Nonmaleficence	Do no harm	Lack of action, questionable treatments not offered	Therapeutic interventions may cause harm. Often conflicts with autonomy. Rule of double effect used to justify actions that may cause harm.
Justice	Be fair; provide care appropriate to needs	With lack of resources impossible to be fair or individualize	Is health care a right or a privilege? Should nonadherent patients continue to receive health care resources? Health disparities highlight the lack of health care justice.
Fidelity (includes confidentiality and synergistic with veracity)	Loyalty and truthfulness	Confidentiality may impede efficiency and quality of care	No absolute duty to keep promises; in each situation, the harmful consequences of the promised action must be weighed against the benefits of promise keeping.
Veracity	Truth telling or not lying	Truth may cause harm	Cultural variances existing regarding truth telling with health care information. Sometimes a desire to justify why deceit is best in situations occurs.

useful actions bringing about the greatest good for the greatest number of people" (Guido, 2006, p. 4). In other words, maximizing the greatest good for the benefit, happiness, or pleasure of the greatest number of people is moral. Utilitarianism assumes that it is possible to balance good and evil with a goal that most people experience good rather than evil. Professional health care providers use utilitarian theory in many situations. Consider, for example, the concept of *triage,* in which the sick or injured are classified by the severity of their condition to determine the priority of treatment. Imagine that there is a plane crash in a remote area in which many of the survivors are severely burned. The local health care facility cannot manage all of the patients, and although air transport is available from a large medical facility 3 hours away, only those with the possibility of surviving can be transported. Those with less serious burns can be managed at a smaller hospital. This means that someone must decide who will and will not be treated. The most gravely injured will not be treated until those with a reasonable chance of survival

are taken care of, although this means that some of the more severely injured will die awaiting care. As a function of utilitarianism, triage is accepted worldwide as an ethical basis for determining treatment.

Often, utilitarianism is the basis for deciding how health care dollars should be spent. For example, money is more likely to be spent on research for diseases that affect large numbers of people than for research on diseases that affect relatively few. Some health care systems, such as the National Health Service in the United Kingdom, depend on utilitarian ethics as one determinant of who receives treatment. For example, inexpensive procedures that benefit large numbers of people, such as cataract surgeries, are easier to access than expensive ones, such as organ transplantations, that benefit a few. A difficulty inherent in utilitarianism is that in the interests of benefiting the majority, the interests of the individual or minority, who also deserve help, may be overlooked. Another limitation of utilitarianism is that it is impossible to calculate all consequences of an action.

Virtue Ethics

Virtue ethics was first noted in the works of Plato, Aristotle, and early Christians. According to Aristotle, virtues are tendencies to act, feel, and judge that develop through appropriate training but come from natural tendencies. This suggests that individuals' actions are built from a degree of inborn moral virtue (Burkhardt and Nathaniel, 2002).

More recently, bioethics literature has emphasized the character of the decision maker. *Virtues* are specific character traits, including truth telling, honesty, courage, kindness, respectfulness, compassion, fairness, and integrity, among others. These virtues become obvious through one's actions and are expressions of specific ethical principles. Truthfulness, for example, embodies the principle of veracity, which will be discussed in the next section of this chapter. When virtuous people are faced with ethical dilemmas, they will instinctively choose to do the right thing because they have developed character through life experiences (Butts and Rich, 2005).

Descriptions of character in terms of virtues portray an individual's way of being, rather than the process of decision making. One's actions in both personal and professional domains extend from this way of being. This does not guarantee right behavior, but it may predispose an individual to right behavior. Similarly, the development of a profession's code of ethics provides a framework of virtues and qualities of character that shape the behaviors of persons engaged in that profession; however, there is no guarantee that members of the profession will act ethically. In other words, a limitation of virtue ethics is the assumption everyone has moral motives and strives to develop their virtues.

The ability to respond to ethical dilemmas or situations in the health care arena is dependent on the nurse's own integrity, honesty, courage, or other personal attributes. Practicing ethically requires a decision to act within the ethical code of the profession, demanding commitment, personal investment, and the intention and motivation to become a good nurse. Nurses' ways of being and acting are essential to the integrity of nursing practice and patient care. Nurses often practice in challenging circumstances in which they must rely on their own integrity to ensure that care is given conscientiously and consistently. Virtues may be what separate the competent nurse from the exemplary nurse. Another limitation of virtue ethics is that it requires a case-by-case approach without a defined decision-making process.

Principalism

In 1976 the Belmont Report formalized principalism as a moral decision-making approach to assess the ethics of research with human subjects in response to the horrific history of biomedical research, including the thalidomide case and the Tuskegee syphilis study (Bulger, 2007). Ethical principles, rather than theories, are emphasized in the Belmont Report. Application of ethical principles is a practical approach to ethical decision making that brings together the best elements of each ethical theory while aligning with most societal and religious belief systems.

Principalism uses key ethical principles of beneficence (do good), nonmaleficence (do no harm), autonomy (respect for the person's ability to act in his or her own best interests), and justice in the resolution of ethical conflicts or dilemmas. Fidelity (faithfulness) and veracity (truth telling) are also important ethical principles that may be at work in managing ethical dilemmas. Nurses are often more knowledgeable about ethical principles than theories and are more likely to use a combination of these principles when critically analyzing ethical dilemmas. Although judging ethical dilemmas with ethical principles is useful, principalism does have limitations when applied to health care ethical dilemmas. Principalism provides no guidance on which ethical principle is prioritized when two or more ethical principles are in conflict. In other words, principalism does not provide a clear process for arriving at a decision; rather, it allows the principles to guide a decision.

SIX ETHICAL PRINCIPLES BASED ON HUMAN DIGNITY AND RESPECT

Respect for humans as a function of human dignity is the primary ethical responsibility for nurses in practice. The *Code of Ethics for Nurses* states that "the nurse practices with compassion and respect for the inherent dignity, worth, and uniqueness of every individual, unrestricted by considerations of social or economic status, personal attributes, or the nature of health problems" (ANA, 2015a). Respect for persons requires that each person be valued as a unique individual equal to all others and that every aspect of a person's life is valued. This can be difficult, because it is sometimes hard to value those parts of human lives that differ from our own. Human dignity and respect for persons are the foundation of the six ethical principles discussed in this section: autonomy, beneficence, nonmaleficence, justice, fidelity, and veracity. Table 7.2 summarizes the moral basis for each principle, the downside of overemphasis of each principle, and the potential challenges with each ethical principle within the health care context.

Autonomy

The principle of *autonomy* asserts that individuals have the right to determine their own actions and the freedom to make their own decisions. Respect for the individual is the cornerstone of this principle. Autonomous decisions are based on (1) individuals' values, (2) adequate information, (3) freedom from coercion, and (4) reason and deliberation. Autonomous decisions lead to independent, autonomous actions. Autonomous actions by a patient include deciding to refuse treatment; giving consent for treatment or procedures; and obtaining information regarding results of diagnostic tests, diagnosis, and treatment options.

Regard for autonomy, however, is often missing in the health care system. Health care professionals often take actions that affect patients' lives profoundly without adequate consultation with the patients themselves. Some health care providers, including physicians and nurses, may operate unknowingly in a paternalistic way that assumes that health care providers are better equipped than patients to make health care decisions for patients. Some patients, however, prefer to have decisions made for them, possibly because of a lack of information, fear of making a poor choice, or trusting that a care provider will make the right decision for them.

Incorporating the principle of autonomy in all health care situations can be difficult. Autonomy poses a problem for health care workers when the patient is incompetent to make decisions because of physical condition, psychological or mental status, or developmental age. Examples of those unable to participate in decisions include infants or small children, mentally incompetent patients, and unconscious patients. Other patients may be unable to participate in decision making because of external constraints, such as the lack of necessary information, or the norms of their culture. Nevertheless, the principle of autonomy is an increasingly important principle in health care and nursing. In fact when two or more principles are in conflict, often autonomy is weighted higher in health care.

Beneficence

Beneficence is commonly defined as "the doing of good" and is one of the critical ethical principles in health care. In determining what is "good," nurses should always consider one's actions in the context of the patient's life and situation. Although this sounds simple, health care providers are challenged daily when what is good for the patient may also cause harm to the patient or is in conflict with what the patient wants. Suppose, for example, that an elderly patient has become confused, especially at night, and is at high risk for falls. She has fallen at home twice. Now that she is confused, she is at even more risk for a fall, especially because confusion can become worse at night in the elderly. The health care team decides that the patient needs a sitter to stay with her in her room all night. The patient objects stridently, because she is very dignified and proud and enjoys her privacy. She complains that she "doesn't need a babysitter" and cries for a long time. The patient is prevented from falling but is psychologically distressed because of limitations on her independence, freedom, privacy, and dignity.

Virtually everyone would agree that promoting good and avoiding harm are important to all human beings—and certainly to health care professionals. It may seem surprising, therefore, how often conflicts occur surrounding the principle of beneficence. A beneficent act may conflict with other ethical principles, most often autonomy. Even though a nurse or physician may understand that a particular treatment has a benefit for the patient, the patient may decide to forgo that treatment (autonomy) for a variety of reasons. In this instance, the health care provider should avoid acting paternalistically and recognize that the patient remains in a position of self-determination.

Nonmaleficence

Nonmaleficence is defined as the duty to do no harm. This principle is the foundation of the medical profession's Hippocratic Oath; it is likewise critical to the nursing profession. Inherent in the *Code of Ethics for Nurses* (ANA, 2015a), the nurse must not act in a manner that would intentionally harm the patient. Although this point appears straightforward, the nature of health care dictates that some therapeutic interventions carry risks of harm for the patient, but the treatment will eventually produce great good for the patient. Classic examples of this are chemotherapy and bone marrow or stem cell transplantation procedures. Both interventions can make patients sicker for a time, posing a risk for complications such as opportunistic infections, but the possibility of achieving a cure or remission of disease may justify the temporary harm. The concept that justifies risking harm is referred to as the rule of "double effect."

Double effect considers the intended foreseen effects of actions by the professional nurse. The doctrine states that as moral agents we may not intentionally produce harm. It is ethically permissible, however, to do what may produce a distressful or undesirable result if the intent is to produce an overall good effect (Beauchamp and Childress, 2001).

The rule of double effect justifies that an individual may rightfully perform an act that produces a good and bad effect provided the following four conditions are met at one and the same time (Buckley et al., 2012):

1. The action must be good or at least morally indifferent (neutral).
2. The health care provider must intend only the good effect, and the bad effect is unintended.
3. The good effect is not achieved by means of the bad effect.
4. There is a favorable balance between the desirable and undesirable effects (the good outweighs the bad).

Justice

The principle of *justice* is that equals should be treated the same and that unequals should be treated differently. In other words, patients with the same diagnosis and health care needs should receive the same care, and those with greater or lesser needs should receive care that is appropriate to their needs.

Basic to the principle of justice are questions of who receives health care and whether health is a right or a privilege. These questions have been central to discussions surrounding health care reform in the United States in the past several years. Such questions involve the allocation of resources: how much of our national resources should be appropriated to health care; what health care problems should receive the most financial resources; what persons should have access to health care services?

Numerous models have been developed for distributing health care resources. These models include the following (Jameton, 1984):

- To each equally
- To each according to merit (this may include past or future contributions to society)

- To each according to what can be acquired in the marketplace
- To each according to need

You may disagree with each or all of these models of resource distribution; certainly, no single one is adequate in ensuring a just model for the distribution of health care resources. In an ideal world, all people would receive all available treatment and resources for their health needs, including disease prevention and health promotion. Unfortunately, this is not possible because of costs and limited resources. When people with wealth have advantageous access to the best quality health care available, which may include lifesaving medical devices or innovations, how does one apply the concept of justice? Conversely, how does the issue of justice apply when access to care that is known to be cost effective and simple, such as prenatal care, is difficult or impossible for working-class women who are on the job during clinic hours?

Health disparities among ethnic minorities with regard to types of treatments and services that are available represent a difficult problem in terms of an ethic of justice. Research has demonstrated that allocation of resources in the health care system is not equitable among racial groups and that "racial disparity exists in health care access, treatment options and outcomes" (Harrison and Falco, 2005, p. 252). Thinking Critically Box 7.3 describes lessons learned by nursing students who participate in international learning experiences and how to continue one's growth of social consciousness and sense of justice.

Furthermore, how does one decide what is just when a natural disaster strikes, crippling health care facilities, and providers are left with critically ill patients in dire circumstances? The situation of Memorial Medical Center (now Oschner Baptist Medical Center) in New Orleans, Louisiana, in the aftermath of the devastating Hurricane Katrina in 2005 brought these questions of justice and ethical decision making in a disaster to the general public in a way that was unprecedented in modern American history. Desperate health care providers were in a dire situation with no electricity, rising water, unbearable heat, and no reasonable hope of rescue for their many patients, many of whom were critically ill even before the hurricane struck. An investigation later found that nurses and physicians had administered lethal doses of morphine and midazolam to more than 20 patients whom the providers determined were unlikely to survive the disaster. A physician and two

THINKING CRITICALLY BOX 7.3

To Keep the Vision of Social Justice

Nursing students often have a great deal of interest in and energy for international learning experiences. These experiences expose students to the huge gap in health care practices and availability between developed and undeveloped nations. In an article by Kirkham and colleagues (2009), they describe the challenge of "keeping the vision" for nursing students and their faculty as they return home—sustaining the social consciousness that is raised during these international experiences.

Kirkham and colleagues (2009) defined social consciousness in terms of "personal awareness of social injustice," borrowed from Giddings (2005, p. 224). Specifically, they described social injustice as unfairness in the burdens and rewards of a society in which there is inequitable access to health care services. Social injustice is the foundation of health disparities, a serious ethical issue that challenges the human right to health and health care.

In their study of student learning that took place in international settings and the long-term benefits and effects of these experiences, Kirkham and colleagues sought to describe students' experiences but also to find ways to integrate and maintain the students' learning once they returned home (in this case, Canada).

Students had many experiences that opened their eyes to the health care practices and accessibility of care in an underdeveloped country (Guatemala). Students related the realization that "statistics … became faces of people I know" (p. 6) and that "people are the same everywhere" (p. 6). They also recognized the significant prosperity and power gradients that exist between North and Central America. From these realizations, the students began to have a deep sense of social injustice and the consequences of short-term international efforts that are not sustained. These insights challenged the students' worldview.

Despite the immense learning and intense reflection that resulted from these experiences, "keeping the vision" became hard as students returned home. Kirkham and colleagues (p. 9) suggested four strategies that may help students in translating their learning and sustaining their new vision for social justice. Individually, students can write journals of their reflections and insights, read journals, and maintain contact with their host families. In formal groups, students can mentor new students who will go through the same experiences, participate in forums and focus groups, and become involved in other humanitarian projects. In informal groups, students can reflect on and share their experiences with other students and faculty who participated in the international experience. And last, nursing school curricula can be shaped to integrate themes of social justice.

Data from Kirkham SR, Van Hofwegen L, Pankratz D: Keeping the vision: sustaining social consciousness with nursing students following international learning experiences, *Int J Nurs Educ Scholarsh* (online) *6*(1):article 3, 2009.

nurses were eventually charged with second-degree murder. The charges were dropped against the nurses, and a grand jury did not indict the physician. Other questions were raised related to whom nurses had primary ethical responsibilities during the storm: their patients or their own families?

In 2015 the ANA sponsored an ethics symposium that featured an interactive address with Sheri Fink, MD, PhD, who won the Pulitzer Prize for her book *Five Days at Memorial,* an investigation of the patients' deaths after Katrina. Dr. Fink noted that thinking about situations in disasters in advance is a way to prepare for the troublesome ethical situations that arise under conditions that are barely imaginable under normal circumstances (ANA, 2015b).

Justice as a principle often leaves us with more questions than answers. It raises our consciousness in identifying unjust situations and in shaping resolutions to

those situations, but applying the principle of justice does not determine what the answer should be. A single ethical principle cannot typically be used to resolve complex ethical dilemmas such as those encountered in health care settings.

Fidelity

The principle of *fidelity* refers to faithfulness or honoring one's commitments or promises. For nurses, this specifically refers to fidelity to patients. Through the process of licensure, nurses are granted the privilege to practice. The licensure process is intended to ensure that only a qualified nurse, appropriately trained and educated, can practice nursing. When nurses are licensed and become a part of the profession, they accept certain responsibilities as part of the contract with society. Nurses must be faithful in keeping their promises of respecting all individuals, upholding the *Code of Ethics for Nurses* (ANA, 2015a), practicing within the scope of nursing practice, keeping nursing skills current, abiding by an employer's policies, and keeping promises to patients. Fidelity entails meeting reasonable expectations in all these areas. Fidelity is a key foundation for the nurse-patient relationship. When nurses receive patient assignments and accept hand-off reports on those patients, they are committed to providing care to those assigned to them. Failure to carry out the prescribed care is unethical (provided that the prescribed care is safe and consistent with good practice) and may constitute patient abandonment or neglect. This is a serious charge that would likely require the state board of nursing review of the specific details of the case to determine whether the nurse failed to carry out this responsibility ethically.

Fidelity suggests that one is faithful to the promises, agreements, and commitments made. This faithfulness creates the trust that is essential to any relationship. Most ethicists believe there is no absolute duty to keep promises, however. In every situation the harmful consequences of the promised action must be weighed against the benefits of promise keeping (Burkhardt and Nathaniel, 2002). This is an ethical posture that may explain decisions by some nurses during Hurricane Katrina, described earlier, to stay at home with their families rather than going to the hospitals for their shifts.

Veracity

Veracity is defined as telling the truth, or not lying. Truth-telling is fundamental to the development and continuance of trust among human beings. Telling the truth is expected. It is necessary to basic communication, and societal relationships are built on the individual's right to know the truth, or not to be deceived. Inherent in nurse-patient relationships is the understanding that nurses will be honest with their patients. However, in some (rare) instances nurses are constrained in some health care systems that place limits on what a nurse can tell a patient. These situations, however, can pose an ethical dilemma for nurses who believe that it is unethical to withhold information from patients, especially when patients ask for information about their condition or diagnosis. A nurse can still remain truthful by telling the patient, "Dr. Roberts always prefers to discuss her findings with her patients directly. I will page her and ask when you can expect her to make rounds tonight to talk to you." Intentional deception, however, is considered morally wrong. (Consider the situation again of Michelle, the nurse who was challenged by Mrs. Thomas, her patient's wife, about whether she had even

called a social worker yet: caught in a lie, what was the best thing Michelle could do?)

Some health care providers attempt to justify deceiving their patients. For the most part, these justifications are related to the idea that patients would be better off not knowing certain information or that they are not capable of understanding the information. This reflects a posture toward patients known as "paternalism," in which someone believes that he or she knows what is best for another person who is competent to make his or her own autonomous judgments about a course of action. Some justify not being truthful with a patient if they perceive that the patient might refuse medical treatment if he or she knew the "complete" truth. However, if both patient and health care provider are respectful of each other as individuals, it is difficult to accept that deception is ever justified. Two exceptions exist, however. If a patient asks not to be told the truth, the nurse can, under the ethical principles of beneficence and nonmaleficence, withhold the truth. This does not mean that the nurse must lie but that the nurse is released from the obligation to report to the patient what he or she may know. Furthermore, if a patient is mentally incompetent, autonomy and the capacity for self-determination are diminished, thereby justifying the withholding of health care information.

Hines (2008) made an interesting observation that true cultural humility (a posture that requires that clinicians make every effort to understand their patients' beliefs and how their patients want themselves and their illness to be treated) is tied to respecting patient preferences for information and treatment. Although Hines was writing about care in an oncology setting, her observation that "goals of care can be established, refined, or refocused at any point in the trajectory of care, whether truth-telling or not telling is occurring" (p. 415) holds true for any practice setting for nurses.

CODES OF ETHICS FOR NURSING

A code of ethics is a hallmark of mature professions and a social contract through which the profession informs society of the principles and rules by which it functions. Ethical codes shape professional self-regulation, serving as guidelines to the members of the profession, who then meet their responsibility as trustworthy, qualified, and accountable caregivers. Codes of ethics, however, are useful only to the extent that they are known and upheld by the members of the profession in practice.

American Nurses Association's Code of Ethics for Nurses

Ethical practice has been a priority for nurses in America since the late 19th century. In 1893 the Nightingale Pledge (Box 7.2) became the first public evidence of an ethical code in nursing. In 1896 the Nurses' Associated Alumnae of the United States and Canada, which later became the ANA, was organized with the purpose to establish and maintain a code of ethics. A suggested code was developed in 1926 and published in the *American Journal of Nursing (AJN)* but was never formally adopted. Similarly, a "tentative" code was published in the *AJN* in 1940, but this version also was never formally adopted. Finally, in 1950, with the addition of 17 provisions, the 1940 version was formally adopted as the Code of Ethics for Nurses. Between 1950 and 1985, the Code was revised and refined six times; the ANA's House of Delegates adopted a complete revision of the Code in 2001.

The *Code of Ethics for Nurses with Interpretive Statements* is the nursing profession's expression of its ethical values and duties to the public (ANA, 2015a). The Code has undergone no fewer than eight revisions, each clarifying meanings, defining terms, and making the Code more relevant to nursing practice at the time. Codes through the years have also reflected trends in social awareness issues, such as women's and patients' rights. The consequences of breaking the Code have become more specific with later versions.

In 2015 the ANA published the latest version of the *Code of Ethics for Nurses with Interpretive Statements*. A view-only version is available at http://www.nursing-world.org/code-of-ethics for both ANA members and nonmembers. The ANA is responsible for the periodic review of the code to ensure that it reflects the contemporary issues of this dynamic profession and is consistent with the ethical standards of the society in which we live.

The ANA's *Nursing: Scope and Standards of Practice* (3rd edition) is another very important document for professional nurses. It defines standards of practice and standards of professional performance. The standards describe the minimal expectations and duties a registered nurse should perform competently regardless of role or population served. The current version of the *Nursing: Scope and Standards of Practice* was published in 2015. Standard 7: Ethics emphasizes that an ethical practice spans across all roles and settings and is integral to nursing professionalism (ANA, 2015c). Standard 7 also incorporates the ANA *Code of Ethics for Nurses* recognizing its moral foundation for nursing practice. Chapter 6 contains more detailed information on the Scope and Standards of Practice.

International Council of Nurses Code of Ethics for Nurses

The International Council of Nurses (ICN) also has published a code of ethics for the profession (ICN, 2012). This document discusses the rights and responsibilities of nurses related to people, practice, society, co-workers, and the profession. The ICN first adopted a code of ethics in 1953. Its last revision, adopted in 2012, represents an agreement by more than 80 national nursing associations that participate in the international association. The preamble of *The ICN Code of Ethics for Nurses* (Box 7.3) is unchanged from the previous version and details the four fundamental responsibilities for nurses and describes the ethical foundations of nursing practice. The *ICN Code of Ethics for Nurses* can be viewed online (http://www.icn.ch/who-we-are/code-of-ethics-for-nurses/).

BOX 7.2   The Florence Nightingale Pledge

The Florence Nightingale Pledge was written in 1893 by Lystra Gretter at the Farrand Training School in Detroit, Michigan. It was modeled after the Hippocratic Oath taken by physicians as they begin their medical careers. The pledge is dated in its wording and gender references; however, key ethical principles discussed in this chapter and elsewhere in this text are present in this early statement intended to hold nurses to a high standard of professional ethical behavior. These principles are noted parenthetically in **bold italics**.

I solemnly pledge myself before God and presence of this assembly; to pass my life in purity and to practice my profession faithfully **(fidelity)**.

I will abstain from whatever is deleterious and mischievous and will not take or knowingly administer any harmful drug **(nonmaleficence)**.

I will do all in my power to maintain and elevate the standard of my profession **(beneficence)** and will hold in confidence all personal matters committed to my keeping and family affairs coming to my knowledge in the practice of my calling **(confidentiality)**.

With loyalty will I endeavor to aid the physician in his work **(fidelity)**, and devote myself to the welfare of those committed to my care **(justice)**.

NAVIGATING THE GRAY AREAS: ETHICAL DECISION MAKING

The gray area of ethical decision making in nursing practice entails addressing ethical dilemmas. An ethical dilemma is a moral conflict in which the decision maker experiences indecision because the available choices or alternatives result in conflicting values or ethical principles. With an ethical dilemma, there is no one good decision; however, two or more decisions may be deemed as right (also known as a right versus right dilemma). Table 7.3 illustrates the complexity of an ethical dilemma and the black and white clarity resulting when an issue is not a dilemma.

Nurses encounter situations daily that require them to make professional judgments and act on those judgments. The judgments or decisions are usually made in collaboration with other persons involved in the situation: patients, families, and other health care professionals. Ethical decision making requires that the nurse make judgments or decisions when two or more of their values are incongruent. When an ethical decision is made, respect and valuing of the perspectives held by others, even when all do not agree on the resolution, is important professional behavior. Through respectful collaboration, the best decision can be reached in even the most difficult dilemma. Note that the "best decision" will be made in response to an ethical dilemma. There is no clear-cut right or wrong decision to address an ethical dilemma because there would not be a dilemma if it were clear what action to take.

Ethical Decision-Making Model

Whether involved in a collective or individual decision, nurses need to be knowledgeable about suggested steps in ethical decision making. Table 7.4 demonstrates the

---

BOX 7.3 International Council of Nurses Code of Ethics for Nurses: Preamble

Nurses have four fundamental responsibilities: to promote health, to prevent illness, to restore health, and to alleviate suffering. The need for nursing is universal.

Inherent in nursing is respect for human rights, including cultural rights, the right to life and choice, to dignity, and to be treated with respect. Nursing care is respectful of and unrestricted by considerations of age, color, creed, culture, disability or illness, gender, sexual orientation, nationality, politics, race, or social status.

Nurses render health services to the individual, the family, and the community and coordinate their services with those of related groups.

From *ICN Code of Ethics for Nurses*, International Council of Nurses, Geneva, Switzerland, Copyright 2012.

TABLE 7.3 The Gray Area of an Ethical Dilemma

No Ethical Dilemma = Wrong versus Right	Ethical Dilemma = Gray Area with Right versus Right	No Ethical Dilemma = Right versus Wrong
	• Includes a conflict of two or more ethical principles and possible conflict of values/beliefs. • Two or more equally unfavorable choices to resolve the dilemma.	
It is clear after morally and ethically analyzing the situation there is clearly one or more wrong choices that should not be pursued and one right choice.	Ethical Decision Making Requires a Contextual Factor Analysis: • Ethical principles at stake/in conflict • Beliefs and values of the stakeholders • Legal mandates, organizational policy • Professional Codes of Ethics Note—most professional codes of ethics allow for conscientious objection to participate in care against individual values/beliefs as long as the patient has competent professionals to care for him or her.	It is clear after morally and ethically analyzing the situation there is only one or more clear "right" action(s) to take, and the other action(s) are wrong and should not be pursued.

TABLE 7.4   Comparison of the Nursing Process, Ethical Decision-Making Model, and CODE Moral Courage Model

Nursing Process	Ethical Decision-Making Model	CODE Moral Courage Model (Lachman, 2010)
Assess	Clarify the dilemma, gather additional data	Courage: Critically evaluate does action need to be taken to address the situation?
Analyze/ diagnose	Identify options	Obligation to honor: Analyze/reflect—what is the right thing to do? Consider what is at risk with the ANA Code of Ethics for Nurses, stakeholder beliefs and values, and ethical principles.
Plan	Make a decision	Danger management: What do I need to do to handle my fear?
Evaluate	Evaluate	(Should reflect on situation and outcome.)

similarity in the processes required in ethical decision making and the nursing process, both of which are based on sound critical thinking. A variety of ethical decision-making models are available in published literature across many disciplines and share more similarities than differences. The steps are not always necessarily sequential, nor are they intended to be rigid processes. Instead, ethical decision making is a process that guides exploration of the dilemma and examination of options to determine the best solution to a difficult situation.

The following steps can be used in ethical decision making:

1. Clarify the ethical dilemma.
2. Gather additional data.
3. Identify options.
4. Make a decision.

- What is the specific issue in question? Who should actually make the decision? Who is affected by the dilemma? Determine the ethical principle or theory related to the dilemma. Are there value conflicts? What is the timeframe for the decision?
- After the ethical dilemma is clarified, in most instances more information needs to be collected. Clarity is enhanced when you have as many facts as possible about the situation. Make sure you are up-to-date on any legal cases or precedents related to the situation, because ethical and legal issues often overlap.
- Most ethical dilemmas have multiple solutions, some of which are more feasible than others. The more options that are identified, the more likely it is that an acceptable solution can be identified. Brainstorm with others, and consider every possible alternative.
- To make a decision, think through the options that are identified, and determine the impact of each option. Ethical principles and theories, as well as universal basic human values, may help determine

the significance of each option. When a nurse is confronted with an ethical dilemma, an active decision should be made, as opposed to refusing to make a decision (being nonactive), which is irresponsible professional behavior.

- Once a course of action has been determined, the decision must be carried out. Implementing the decision usually involves working collaboratively with others.
- Unexpected outcomes are common in crisis situations that result in ethical dilemmas. Decision makers should consider the effect an immediate decision may have on future ones. Reflecting on a decision and action can help determine whether a different course of action might have resulted in a better outcome. If the action accomplished its purpose, the ethical dilemma should be resolved. If the dilemma has not been resolved, engage in additional deliberation, and reexamine alternative options. Consider the six suggested ethical decision-making steps in the context of Case Study 7.1 of Daniel, a terminally ill man who wants you—his nurse—to help him end his life.

5. Act.
6. Evaluate.
    (1) *Clarify the ethical dilemma.* The specific issue is the patient's right to autonomy versus the nurse's professional ethics and personal morals.
    (2) *Gather additional data.* Is Daniel responding to something that happened before you even got to his home today, such as an argument or a confrontation? Is he becoming depressed?
    (3) *Identify options.* Options may include the following:
        (a) Simply tell Daniel you will not help him die.
        (b) Respond to his dire request with compassion, and try to determine what is behind his sudden sense that he wants to die.

CASE STUDY 7.1

Your Hospice Patient Wants to Die ... and He Wants You to Help Him

Daniel is a 55-year-old gay man with advanced lung cancer and is positive for human immunodeficiency virus (HIV). He has a longtime partner, Liam, with whom he has lived for more than 20 years. Daniel is miserable, with profuse secretions from his lungs; every breath is a struggle. Yet despite his weakened physical condition, he is still very alert. He is getting oxygen via nasal cannula. He is very image conscious, and part of each of your visits is spent helping him groom himself and put on fresh designer pajamas. His mother is staying with him and Liam, and she has never been told that Daniel is gay or that he has HIV. He confides to you that trying to maintain the secret that he has kept from his mother is exhausting and is becoming burdensome. In the middle of your visit, he asks for a mirror to see what he looks like. You hand him a small mirror, and he is shocked at what he sees—a gray, shrunken, emaciated image looking back at him. He sets the mirror down carefully on the bedside table, looks at you evenly, and with great seriousness says, "I am ready to die, and I want you to help me."

As a new nurse, you are not ready for this. You know that in his bedside drawer there is enough oral morphine to stop his breathing. You know that his death is still probably days away, and you are very sad for him in his misery. When you say, "I can't do that, Daniel," he starts crying and says, "I trusted you to help me...."

What should you do in response to this situation? What does the ANA say about assisted suicide and euthanasia? What is your personal moral code in this situation?

(c) Determine whether there is better symptom management that you can implement to make him more comfortable.

(d) Consider what would happen if Daniel told his mother the truth about his sexual orientation and HIV status.

(e) With Daniel and his partner's support, enlist the assistance of other hospice services such as pastoral care to help him ease his spiritual distress. (*Note:* There are many choices available here. These are just some suggestions.)

(4) *Make a decision.* Make sure that everyone, especially Daniel, agrees with the plan.

(5) *Act.* This may include a number of interventions, both physical and psychoemotional.

(6) *Evaluate.* Does Daniel continue to express his desire to die now? Is he more comfortable? Is his distress less troublesome? Is he at some level of peace with his partner, his mother, and his life? Did your actions enhance the nurse-patient relationship with mutual trust and caring?

EXPLORING ETHICAL DILEMMAS IN NURSING

Ethical dilemmas are a common occurrence in nursing practice. Many ethical dilemmas arise in nursing because of conflicts among patients, their families, health care professionals, and institutions. The following section will explore the major issues involved in these conflicts: (1) personal value systems, (2) peers' and other professionals' behaviors, (3) patients' rights, (4) institutional and societal issues, and (5) patient data access issues.

Dilemmas Resulting From Personal Value Systems

Values are important preferences that influence the behavior of individuals. Values are learned beliefs that help people choose among difficult alternatives, even when there may not be a good choice.

Each person has a set of values that was shaped by the beliefs, purposes, attitudes, qualities, and objects of a child's early caregivers. In time, individuals develop their own value systems that are grounded in their culture and life experiences. Variations in value systems become highly significant when dealing with critical issues such as health and illness or life and death. Value systems enable people to resolve conflicts and decide on a course of action based on a priority of importance.

Professions have a "built-in" value system known as a code of ethics, discussed earlier in this chapter. A very difficult issue for nursing students to come to terms with on occasion is when their personal values conflict with their professional values, or, more specifically, when they are faced with a professional situation that has some elements that are not in keeping with the nurse's personal moral code or values. The overriding concern in this situation is that professional ethics outweigh personal ethics in a professional setting. It is incumbent on the nurse to find a work situation in which his or her personal ethics are not routinely challenged by situations that occur with patients.

BOX 7.4   Childhood Value Messages

By the time we are about 10 years old, most of our values have already been "programmed." Values are taught to us by family members and friends, through the media, in churches and schools, and by watching other people. What are the value messages you learned as a child?

Recall as many values as you can remember hearing as a child, and write them in the blanks provided below. Here are a few examples to get you thinking:

"Be nice."

"You can do anything you want to if you try hard enough."

"Clean your plate; there are starving children in _____!"

"Making money is the number one goal in life."

"You always have to tell the truth, no matter what."

"Crying is a sign of weakness. You have to be strong."

Now it is your turn to write some of your childhood values. How many of these values still influence the way you think and act today? Which ones influence you professionally? If you want to further explore your values, you may do the following:

1. Next to each value on your list, write the person's name who taught or modeled that value.
2. Put a star next to those messages that are still your values today.
3. Put a check mark next to those messages that you need to alter.
4. How are some of these values still influencing you today? Is this a positive or negative influence?

- _____
- _____
- _____
- _____
- _____
- _____
- _____

Reprinted with permission of Uustal DB: *Clinical ethics and values: issues and insights in a changing healthcare environment*, East Greenwich, RI, 1993, Educational Resources in Healthcare.

Nurses must have a good sense of their own values and be able to identify clearly what they believe to be good or right. We each develop our own value systems based on a variety of messages that we received in our formative years from our parents, siblings, friends, teachers, and religious training. The "childhood value messages" exercise (Box 7.4) can help you identify values learned as a child that may still influence you today.

To understand how personal and professional values can conflict in nursing practice, consider the following situation: Marta had been a nurse on a postpartum unit for a number of years. Over time, an increasing number of pregnant women (antepartum) with serious problems related to the pregnancy were admitted to the unit where Marta worked. Although Marta preferred to work with new mothers and their infants, she occasionally took care of antepartum patients. One day in report, she learned that there was a newly admitted patient, Mrs. Anderson, who was 11 weeks pregnant with triplets. Mrs. Anderson had a history of serious heart disease, but her condition was thought to be stable. Marta agreed to take care of her, having very little information about her.

Shortly after receiving her hand-off report, Marta went into Mrs. Anderson's room to do her usual assessment, only to find that Mrs. Anderson was crying, being comforted by her husband, who was also crying. Mrs. Anderson related to Marta that the maternal-fetal medicine specialist and her cardiologist had recommended that they do what is known as a selective reduction (also known as multifetal pregnancy reduction [MFPR]), a form of pregnancy termination in which a multiple pregnancy (meaning more than one embryo or fetus) is reduced to one or two remaining embryos. Mrs. Anderson was already having signs of cardiac decompensation early in pregnancy, evidenced by her increasing difficulty breathing, especially while lying down, so remaining pregnant at all put her health at great risk. Already it was clear that Mrs. Anderson was not going to be able to tolerate the demands on her heart of a multiple pregnancy. She and her husband, although sad, understood that the selective reduction was their only chance of having a child at all and that without it her own life was in serious danger.

Marta was very upset with this news. As a practicing Catholic, she had a very strong moral stance against abortion, and as a nurse, she had worked specifically with mothers and their new infants to avoid issues related to pregnancy termination. The procedure was going to be performed in Mrs. Anderson's room under ultrasound guidance within the next few minutes. Marta faced a serious moral dilemma in determining what to do. She sought the advice and counsel of a colleague whose wisdom she admired and trusted. In a few moments, Marta decided that her responsibility was to her patient and that, although she was present during the termination, she was not participating in performing it in any way. She understood her patient's deep distress and sadness. Before reentering the room, Marta took a moment to calm herself to be in a better state of mind to provide care for her patient. After taking a deep breath, she went into Mrs. Anderson's room and encouraged Mr. Anderson to sit near his wife where they could see each other; then she took Mrs. Anderson's hand, saying "I will be with you through this." Mrs. Anderson whispered, "Thank you."

Marta had set aside her personal values to take excellent care of her patient as a trained and caring professional nurse.

Dilemmas Involving Peers' and Other Professionals' Behavior

All practicing nurses participate as members of the health care team. This involves cooperation and collaboration with other professionals. As is true in all situations involving human beings, conflicts can easily develop, particularly in stressful circumstances. These conflicts may be between two nurses, the nurse and physician, the nurse and agency policies, or the nurse and any other health care professional (Professional Profile Box 7.2).

As discussed previously, conflicts can evolve because of differing value systems, cultures, education levels, or a variety of other factors. Like Marta in the previous example, a nurse may believe that abortions are wrong under any circumstances, whereas the institution in which he or she is employed routinely performs them. This creates a conflict between the nurse's value system and the institution's practices, which can be the source of distress. Conflicts relevant to human rights often center around one of the ethical principles discussed earlier: autonomy, beneficence, nonmaleficence, veracity, or justice.

A disturbing reality in health care is the presence of providers in all disciplines who fail to meet standards of care routinely, who may simply be incompetent, or who participate in actions that are considered unethical by other professionals. An incompetent worker may suffer from a physical or mental impairment or may be indifferent to standards of care. Unethical actions result when health care workers break basic norms of conduct toward others, especially the patient, whatever the reason.

Sociocultural Influences Posing Ethical Challenges: Social Media and Substance Abuse

Nurses face two serious ethical challenges in today's sociocultural context: (1) the use of social media and (2) substance use/abuse. Substance use/abuse by health care providers is not new but still poses a tremendous dilemma for nurses who may suspect that a colleague is impaired at work or has developed a substance abuse problem. More recently, social media has changed the landscape of communication; ethical problems have arisen in nursing related to the use of social media.

The widespread use of social media, such as Facebook, Twitter, and blogs, has created two distinct problems: (1) the transmission of potentially identifiable patient information and (2) the blurring of professional and personal boundaries (remember, however, that—as you read in Chapter 6 on legal issues—this blurring is a myth, and in fact distinct boundaries still exist). Moreover, nurses who are posting on sites such as these may fail to realize that their posts are widely available to professional and personal contacts, including their employers and colleagues. In response to the ethical challenges posed by social networking, the ANA and the National Council of State Boards of Nursing (NCSBN) have both issued guidelines for maintaining professional boundaries within social networking.

The ANA has developed a Social Networking Principles Toolkit available on its website (www.nursingworld.org) to help nurses understand their responsibilities when using social media (ANA, 2012). In August 2011 the NCSBN published a white paper, *A Nurse's Guide to the Use of Social Media* (www.ncsbn.org), a guideline that details the challenges related to ethical use of social media (NCSBN, 2012). The ANA and NCSBN have mutually endorsed their positions regarding nurses' professional use of social media (ANA, 2012) and their endorsement still stands. It is important to realize that the principles undergirding the protection of patients regarding social media do not change, even as digital media continue to grow and thrive. In other words, what is not appropriate for posting on Facebook is also not appropriate for Instagram, Snapchat, or any other forms of digital communication yet to be developed. Box 7.5 contains five basic principles related to the ethical use of social media.

Consider the following situation, and think about the ethical considerations related to the use of social media: You and your colleague who works on the same nursing unit enjoy sports and share a passion for the local university's football program. You are both members

PROFESSIONAL PROFILE BOX 7.2
DISTRESS IN AN EXPERT LABOR AND DELIVERY NURSE

This is a true account of a moral dilemma and moral distress in a labor and delivery nurse, Mary Tilghman, RN, who had been in practice for 6 years at the time of this event. She asked to use a pseudonym in recounting this story, because she does not want anyone to identify her situation or the location where this event happened. But the story itself is true and illustrates the very difficult ethical situations that nurses find themselves in and the lingering distress that these situations can cause. Here is her story:

I was working on a slow evening in a labor and delivery unit. We got a call from our dispatcher that emergency medical services (EMS) was bringing in a patient who was 25 weeks, pregnant and having some vaginal bleeding. This is not really unusual, but it can be serious. I notified the resident doctor and another nurse, and I set about getting a labor room ready. In about 10 minutes, EMS arrived with a young woman who was very pale and crying loudly. Her young husband was with her.

When we moved her to the labor bed, it was obvious that "some bleeding" was an understatement. She was bleeding from everywhere—even her gums, nose, and a small crack in her lip were bleeding. I listened for fetal heart tones, and when I could not hear them, I asked her when the last time was that she had felt the baby move. I suspected that she had DIC—disseminated intravascular coagulopathy—a severe problem that sometimes occurs when a fetus is dead but labor does not begin. She said it had been "2, maybe 3 weeks." Her husband was shocked, because she had not told him that she had not been feeling the baby move. I called for the doctor right away, and then I paged the anesthesiologist to come to labor and delivery STAT. This was a severe emergency. I started a large-gauge intravenous (IV) line so that we could give her blood and fluids, and sent some blood samples for laboratory testing, including a type and cross-match.

The doctor confirmed the fetal death by doing a quick ultrasound examination. The doctor explained to the woman that this was an emergency and had her sign a consent form. We hurried the patient to the operating room (OR) for an emergency dilation and evacuation (D&E). At the time, I had seen a lot as an obstetric nurse in a high-risk unit, but I was horrified at her huge and rapid blood loss. The anesthesiologist ordered as many units of O-negative blood (universal donor) as we could get until donor blood could be matched to hers in the blood bank. Weakly but as firmly as she could, the woman declared, "No blood. No blood. I am a Jehovah's Witness. Please no blood. If I die, I will be all right. No blood. Please." Everyone in the room heard her. The anesthesiologist patted her shoulder and told her that she would "be okay."

Everybody in the room could tell that this woman was bleeding to death. The anesthesiologist prepared to give her medications to increase her blood pressure and perfusion. By then the senior resident doctor and the attending physician were working quickly to perform the D&E. The junior obstetric resident was very concerned by the situation. He left the room in a hurry and found the woman's husband, who was pacing outside in the hallway. The resident asked him, "Were you planning to be with your wife when she gave birth to your baby?" The husband said yes. The resident then told him, "Your wife is going to die. I think that you might want to be with her as she dies."

He gave the husband some scrubs to put on over his clothes and started toward the OR. By then, the woman's blood had begun to run out from under the OR door and into the hallway. When the husband saw it, he threw up his hands, saying, "Just give her the blood. Give her the blood…." The resident patted him on the back and told him it was a good decision. The husband left the OR, and the anesthesiologist began infusing unit after unit of blood and blood products into the woman. I reminded them of her plea not to give her blood, but the physicians agreed that her husband's verbal consent was enough for them. The junior resident said, "I just don't think they understand what it means to bleed to death. I thought he'd change his mind if I showed him."

The patient went to intensive care for many days but recovered. I never saw her again. But I was very distressed over what I thought—and still think—was coercion on the part of the resident physician, showing the husband his wife's blood, and overriding the woman's clear and unmistakable pleas for no blood products. She was willing to die rather than break her deep religious conviction. No matter what I believed about her religious views, my role was to advocate on her behalf—to be her voice. This situation is still distressful to me many years after it happened. I was so relieved that she lived, but I also felt like I was part of something that she had made clear she didn't want. Sometimes ethical dilemmas in nursing are unforgettable. For me, this is the one that stands out most clearly, the one that still haunts me.

BOX 7.5   Ethical Use of Social Media

The use of social media has created professional and personal opportunities, yet it can pose significant ethical challenges. Keep these principles in mind when you engage in blogging, including microblogs, or communicating via social networking sites.

1. You must not post anything about your patients that may violate their rights to privacy and confidentiality. Their privacy is not ensured by your use of "privacy settings." This is both an ethical and a legal obligation.
2. Never post images of patients. You are likely to be restricted by your school or employer in your use of personal devices for taking photos of patients. Even though it is tempting to take a photo of a favorite patient, a cute baby, or some curiosity you encounter in the clinical setting, you must not.
3. Online contact with patients blurs professional and personal boundaries. Although it is difficult to turn down a patient's (or former patient's) request that you "friend" them, you are obligated to enforce the professional boundary that separates you.
4. You are ethically obligated to report any breach in confidentiality or privacy that you encounter online.
5. Remember that posting anything leaves a digital footprint forever. Even deleting a post or photo leaves evidence behind. If you have the slightest question as to the appropriateness of a blog entry or update, err on the side of extreme caution. Your patients and your career will thank you.

From National Council of State Boards of Nursing (NCSBN): *White paper: a nurse's guide to the use of social media*, 2012. Retrieved from www.ncsbn.org/2930.htm; American Nurses Association (ANA): *Social networking principles toolkit*, 2012. Retrieved from www.nursingworld.org/FunctionalMenuCategories/AboutANA/Social-Media/Social-Networking-Principles-Toolkit.aspx.

of a sports website that features a message board, and you know each other's screen names under which you post anonymous comments. One of the team's star athletes sustained a serious neck injury during a game and was admitted to the trauma center where you work, although not on your unit. The following day, you see a comment posted by your colleague under his screen name that details the injured player's condition. You realize that your colleague has obtained information about the player from the hospital's electronic health record (EHR) system and has posted it on the website.

What is your responsibility in this situation? What do you do next?

The second sociocultural problem is the number of nurses and other health care professionals impaired by drug dependence, alcohol abuse, or other addictions. Deciding how and when to confront a colleague who is impaired may constitute an ethical dilemma. When a colleague appears to be under the influence of some type of substance (e.g., exhibiting slurred speech, unsteady gait, combativeness, the smell of alcohol on his or her breath), the decision to report is usually easy, even if personally painful. Be aware, however, that certain acute medical conditions may be responsible for changes in behavior or gait; your colleague may be experiencing a medical emergency. It is crucial that you engage the assistance of a nurse manager or supervisor before confronting your colleague if you suspect your colleague is impaired in some way.

When a colleague is showing a pattern of behavior that may indicate a substance abuse problem (e.g., frequent tardiness, excuse making, excessive absences, leaving the work setting frequently, increasingly poor clinical judgment), the dilemma can be overwhelming. Nurses agonize over whether to report suspected instances of unethical conduct or incompetent care, including an impairment caused by alcohol or drugs. Fortunately, some employers and state nurses associations have developed plans to assist impaired nurses in getting the help they need and make provisions for them to return to the profession once they are far enough along in their recovery process. The board of nursing in each state, as well as each state nurses association, can provide information on specific programs for impaired nurses in the state. However, the process must begin with a co-worker who follows the ANA ethical standard that obligates professional nurses to report colleagues who "pose a threat or danger to patients, self or others" (ANA, 2015a, p. 13).

To understand how the suspicion of substance abuse can be triggered, consider the following situation: Gloria is a registered nurse (RN) who works on a surgical floor. She has just assisted in the transfer of Mr. Hudson to his room from the postanesthesia care unit (PACU) after surgery and heard the PACU nurse report that Mr. Hudson had received 6 mg of morphine intravenously before transfer, and he is resting comfortably. Gloria sees another nurse drawing up morphine, a narcotic, in a syringe and then leaving the medications room. Ten minutes later, she returns with an empty syringe. Gloria asks, "Who needed pain medication?" The other nurse replies, "Mr. Hudson. He was in pain after surgery." Confused, Gloria checks Mr. Hudson's room and learns from his wife that he has neither asked for nor received pain medication since arriving on the surgical floor.

What should Gloria do now? What are her options, and how should she best manage this situation?

Dilemmas Regarding Patients' Rights

As health care has changed over the years, so too has the nature of relationships between providers and patients. Years ago, health professionals, particularly physicians, were considered to have the final word on care decisions and treatment options. Now consumers of health care are increasingly demanding to have a voice in their health care decisions. A number of special interest groups have developed and published lists of patient rights. In 1971 the United Nations passed a resolution known as the Declaration of the Rights of Mentally Retarded Persons, an early model that recognized the interests of a particular group of persons with disabilities. In 1990 the Congress of the United States passed the Americans with Disabilities Act, which was amended in 2008. This extensive act has provided a significant improvement in the lives of persons with a variety of mental and physical disabilities, recognizing their rights to participate fully in all aspects of society.

Other less formal interest groups have written guidelines such as the Dying Person's Bill of Rights, Pregnant Patient's Bill of Rights, and Rights of Senior Citizens. The health care system has responded to consumers' awareness of their rights. Many of the rights demanded by patients as consumers of health care are legal rights that have been upheld by the judicial system. The American Hospital Association (AHA) has an extensive website that addresses the wide range of rights of patients in the hospital setting. Replacing the former Patient Bill of Rights, the document "The Patient Care Partnership" was published in 2003 and is still currently used. The document describes what patients can and should expect while hospitalized, including a safe, clean environment; quality care; involvement in one's own care that includes a discussion regarding the treatment plan; help with understanding the bill and filing insurance claims; and preparation to leave the hospital (AHA, 2003). Some of the rights described in these documents are the right to privacy, the right to informed consent, the right to die, the right to confidentiality and respectful care, the right to care without discrimination, and the right to information concerning medical condition and treatment (AHA, 2003).

Patient Self-Determination Act

Congress passed the Patient Self-Determination Act (PSDA) in 1990; it was enacted in December 1991. The PSDA is a safeguard for patients' rights, giving patients the legal right to determine how vigorously they wish to be treated in life-or-death situations, and calls for hospitals to abide by patients' advance directives. The PSDA specifies that any organization receiving Medicare or Medicaid funds must inform patients of state laws regarding directives, document the existence of directives in the patient's medical record, educate staff regarding directives, and educate the community about directives. This Act encourages individuals to think about the type of medical and nursing treatment they would want if they were to become critically injured or ill. At the time questions arise, the patient is often unconscious or too sick to make decisions or communicate personal wishes.

Advance directives are designed to ensure individuals the rights of autonomy, refusal of medical intervention, and death with dignity. Advance directives are legal documents that indicate the wishes of individuals in regard to end-of-life issues. Critically ill individuals can remain in charge of their own end-of-life decisions if their advance directives are carried out. Each time they enter a health care institution, patients should have in their possession their advance directives. In addition, copies should be given to significant others, primary care providers, and any legal counsel that may be involved with the patient. The best directive is one that has been notarized or developed in conjunction with a legal expert, and the contents of which have been discussed with family or the person with designated health care power of attorney who will carry out one's directives in the event of a sudden catastrophic or terminal illness.

Families should talk about how each member wants critical situations to be handled. Individual preferences can then be understood. Ideally, family members, caregivers, and courts (in very extreme cases) will not need to make decisions for the patient. Too often the first time a patient learns about advance directives is on admission to a health care facility. The question then arises as to who is responsible for discussing this sensitive issue with the patient. The ideal time for patients to make difficult end-of-life decisions is well in advance of the need.

Advance directives have not been without controversy. One problem is that states have passed different legislation so there is no guarantee that one state will honor another's advance directives. A trusted person may be appointed to make decisions on behalf of the patient when the patient cannot make them on his or her own. This is known as the assignment of the health care power of attorney, as mentioned. Rarely, persons have been designated by a family member to hold health care power of attorney without their prior knowledge. Ideally, the person making this designation and the trusted person being assigned this important responsibility should have a detailed discussion and prior understanding about what he or she is to do on behalf of the person. Holding health care power of attorney and making decisions based on the unambiguous wishes of the patient is a serious moral obligation, requiring that this designee act as the moral agent for the patient. Prior assignment of one's health care power of attorney can minimize, but in some cases not altogether avoid, disagreements among family members. When family members are left to make difficult treatment and end-of-life decisions, conflicts can occur at a time when families are already in distress and are vulnerable. Health care providers sometimes convene family meetings to work out these types of difficult situations.

Ethical Issues Related to Immigration and Migration

The movement of people among nations—population migration—has become a topic of great interest across the world. The United States is no exception and faces a number of ethical issues that affect health care. Two distinct issues are addressed here that affect nursing and have ethical implications: (1) communication/language problems between patients and heath care providers and (2) the migration of nurses.

Communication is fundamental to safe, effective health care, the moral commitment to patients. Patients who do not speak English, and who hold a variety of health care beliefs and practices to which American health care workers may not be accustomed, pose a challenge. Many health care institutions, especially larger medical centers, have addressed the issue of language by hiring professional medical interpreters. Interpretation involves the spoken word, and translation refers to the written word.

Medical interpretation is a specialty that requires extensive knowledge of medical terminology, in addition to cultural humility and sensitivity to the needs of the patient. Many American nursing students have some working knowledge of another language, often Spanish. The level of fluency needed for safe interpretation, however, is not typically achieved in language coursework. Nurses who are not bilingual or fluent in medical terminology should defer to a professional medical interpreter for explanations of procedures, diagnoses, obtaining informed consent, and other complex health care–related issues. Furthermore, although it is tempting to enlist the assistance of a patient's family member to interpret, this is not a safe practice. Children of patients should never be asked to interpret under any circumstances. The International Medical Interpreters Association (IMIA) works to define educational requirements and qualifications for medical interpreters and to establish norms of practice. IMIA's website (http://imiaweb.org) addresses many issues of interest to nurses.

The second issue with significant ethical implications for health care delivery is international nurse migration—that is, the influx of nurses from other countries coming to the United States seeking better pay and working conditions. This poses two distinct ethical problems. First, this exacerbates nursing shortages in other countries. Countries particularly hard hit by this phenomenon include the Philippines, which already loses several thousand nurses a year to this country; India; South Africa; and, possibly, China. The ANA is on record as opposing measures to "uncap" limits on nurses immigrating to the United States, expressing support instead to increase appropriations to expand nursing programs in this country. This comes at a time when a majority of qualified applicants to American schools of nursing are not admitted because of inadequate numbers of faculty and facilities.

In a statement in 2008 before the Congressional Committee on the Judiciary Subcommittee on Immigration, Citizenship, Refugees, Border Security, and International Law, Cheryl Peterson, MSN, RN, representing the ANA, laid out the ANA's position in opposition of the use of immigration to solve the nursing workforce shortage. Peterson cited these three reasons: (1) Congress had failed to provide adequate funding for domestic schools of nursing; (2) the health care industry had failed to establish a workplace environment conducive to the retention of experienced U.S. nurses in patient care; and (3) the United States had failed to engage in active workforce planning to sustain nursing's and other health care professions' workforces into the future (ANA, 2008). The ANA was joined by Physicians for Human Rights in opposing any legislation that would increase the United States' reliance on foreign nurses to mediate a shortage of nurses. In a scathing critique of this practice, one physician member of the Physicians for Human Rights described an open-immigration policy as having the potential to "undermine our multibillion-dollar effort to combat AIDS and malaria by potentially worsening the shortage of health workers in developing countries. We're pouring water in a bucket with a hole in it, and we drilled the hole" (Dugger, 2006).

The second ethical issue this raises is the documentation of competency to provide safe nursing care, which occurs in the passing of the National Council Licensure Examination (NCLEX®) by graduates of approved American nursing schools. Nurses who may come to the United States expecting to find well-paying jobs as professional registered nurses (RNs) may find that their education and skills may not be sufficient to practice as a registered nurse. English as a second language for nurses who migrate to the United States poses similar communication difficulties, as described previously, and cultural acclimation to the United States may pose particular challenges for these nurses. Moreover, there has been an increase in exploitative and highly unethical recruitment practices by companies that, after collecting huge fees for their services, mislead foreign nurses and/or misrepresent work opportunities in the United States available to these nurses (Stubenrauch, 2008).

Dilemmas Created by Institutional and Social Issues

Health care institutions must comply with many governmental regulations that affect both workers and patients. In turn, hospitals and other health care institutions implement their own policies and procedures. Nurses may experience moral dilemmas when they disagree with the policies of their institutions. Health care organizations are subject to public scrutiny and accountability, and those that receive public funds through the Centers for Medicare and Medicaid Services (CMS) are under particular scrutiny. Ethical dilemmas between nurses and the organizations that employ them may develop over policies dictated by the organizations or mandated by governmental agencies. Nurses experience moral distress when the correct course of action is known, but they are unable to act because of internal or external

constraints. If moral distress results for the nurse, it may negatively affect not only patients but the nurse as well (McCarthy and Gastmans, 2015). Thoughtful and conscious action is required to address moral distress, which may lead to greater self-awareness and resilience (McCarthy and Gastmans, 2015).

Ethics committees were created to assist with ethical dilemmas in institutional settings. These committees are multidisciplinary groups charged with the responsibility of providing consultation and emotional support in situations in which difficult ethical choices are necessary. The recommendation from an ethics committee poses no obligation for action; however, they should receive serious consideration by the decision makers. Those desiring help, usually clinical caregivers such as physicians and nurses, refer cases to the committee for additional direction.

Dilemmas Created by Patient Data Access Issues

Digital technologies and EHRs are powerful sources for the storage and transmission of information about patients across health care specialties and disciplines. However, these technologies have created a digital portal into patients' confidential medical information (as in the example given earlier about the injured athlete). Those in positions to access health care information share a great responsibility to protect this information from unauthorized use.

Informational technology, particularly the EHR, places great responsibilities in the hands of health care providers. Computer ethics have been in existence since the 1970s, but in recent years there has been renewed interest in scholarly inquiry in nursing informatics as the use of technology has become standard in health care institutions. The following example illustrates the type of ethical dilemma that can result from the inappropriate access of a patient's EHR.

Tom, a third-year nursing student, observed Susan, a first-year nursing student, sitting at the nurses' station reading patient information about a faculty member's child who was hospitalized with a serious illness in the same hospital. Neither Susan nor Tom was directly involved in the patient's care.

Considering Susan's inexperience, what steps should Tom take? Does Susan's inexperience factor into your thinking about this situation?

TABLE 7.5 **The Situational Briefing Model (SBAR)**	
Situation	Concise statement on the problem/issue.
	• What is going on?
Background	Provide background detail that is pertinent to the situation/issue.
	• What is the context?
Assessment	Present subjective and objective data pertinent to the issue.
	• What do you think is going on?
	• Analyze options and risks
	• What are you ruling out (if indicated)?
Recommendation	State the action needed to correct the problem identified in the situation.
	• What do you want to happen, by when and by whom?
	• Will the situation need to be reevaluated? Describe.

THE PRACTICE OF MORAL COURAGE

Registered nurses may face a variety of barriers that limit the provision of optimal health care, leading to moral and ethical challenges (McLeod-Sordjan, 2014). Nurses must speak up to address these barriers. Nevertheless, nurses in some situations fail to speak up and are unable to maintain integrity because of fear, resulting from hierarchical organization relationships, or because of uncertainty regarding the best action to take (Goethals et al., 2010; Woods, 2005). Nurses have a professional obligation, as emphasized in the ANA (2015a) *Nursing Code of Ethics,* to speak up, maintaining personal integrity and the integrity of the profession, as well as to advocate for social justice and human rights. There is an ethical mandate for nurses to be prepared to address situations that compromise personal and professional integrity through the use of moral courage (McLeod-Sordjan, 2014).

Moral courage is an individual's capacity to overcome fear and stand up for his or her core values with awareness, despite the potential risk (Lachman, 2010). In other words, moral courage is necessary when moral integrity is in jeopardy, and action to maintain integrity entails risk. Lachman (2010) coined a moral courage model using the acronym *CODE* to signify the necessity to respond to an integrity-compromising situation: *C*ourage, *O*bligation to honor, *D*anger management, and *E*xpression and action. Lachman's (2010) model illustrates the essential elements of being a moral agent.

• **Courage:** The nurse in this step recognizes courage may be necessary to maintain integrity. The nurse

analyzes the situation to determine whether an action is required to address the situation.

• **Obligations to honor:** The nurse considers his or her values and beliefs, the ethical principles at stake with the situation, and the ANA (2015a) *Code of Ethics for Nurses* provisions to determine what obligations require honoring.

• **Danger management:** The nurse identifies strategies to manage the fear of repercussions when maintaining integrity. Managing danger may include sharing the situation with a trusted nurse or mentor and seeking feedback on how to address the situation. Nurses may also rehearse and practice how they will address the situation and speak up to manage fear. Communicating concerns in an organized manner in an SBAR format guides communication also addressing fear. See Table 7.5, The Situational Briefing Model (SBAR), for additional detail. Another useful tool for managing danger is the CUS Method, coined by the Agency for Healthcare Quality and Research (2014) with Teamstepps. The CUS Method includes first stating the **c**oncern ("I am concerned about…"), next sharing why the situation is **u**ncomfortable ("I am uncomfortable with…"), and last if the conflict is unresolved and is a potential **s**afety issue, stating the specific concerns ("this is a safety issue…").

• **Expression and Action:** In the final step, the nurse determines what action is required to maintain integrity considering personal values and beliefs and the obligations to honor. The action may direct (addressing the concern directly with the

PROFESSIONAL PROFILE BOX 7.3
MODERN-DAY MORALLY COURAGEOUS NURSE ALEX WUBBELS

Many nurses in the profession of nursing history (such as Florence Nightingale, Mary Eliza Mahoney, and Mary Seacole) faced oppression, barriers, and risk when advocating for what is right, demonstrating moral courage. Alex Wubbels is a modern-day nurse who demonstrated moral courage and integrity to advocate for a patient's rights (ANA Enterprise, 2017). On July 26, 2017, Wubbels was ordered by a police officer to allow him to draw blood on an unconscious patient who was a motor vehicle crash victim. The patient's car was struck by a car being chased by police. The patient was not under arrest. Wubbels refused to allow the blood to be drawn, upholding a hospital policy requiring a warrant or the patient's consent. Wubbels protected the patient's privacy and rights and was aggressively arrested as a result. Although no charges were filed, the incident resulted in a national outrage as it was captured on police body cameras. One officer involved in the incident was fired and the other demoted. The hospital also updated its policy regarding obtaining evidence related to a crime scene so that nurses are no longer directly involved with the officers. Wubbels was courageous as she advocated for the patient's rights, and her courage made a national impact. Considering your own practice, what actions would you take to preserve a patient's rights?

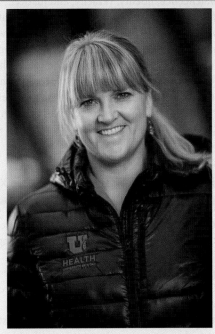

Alex Wubbels, RN
University Hospital, Salt Lake City, Utah

American Nurses Association Enterprise: *American Nurses Association calls for action in wake of police abuse of registered nurse*, 2017. Retrieved from http://www.nursingworld.org/FunctionalMenuCategories/MediaResources/PressReleases/American-Nurses-Association-Calls-for-Action-in-Wake-of-Police-Abuse-of-Registered-Nurse.html

source) or indirect (addressing the concern with a secondary source such as a manager or supervisor). See Professional Profile Box 7.3 to learn more about a morally courageous modern-day nurse, Alex Wubbels.

The safe practice of nursing is inextricable from ethical challenges. You as students of nursing are encouraged to be aware of your own values, morals, and ethics and to become sensitive to the values, morals, and ethics at work in every nursing situation.

CONCEPTS AND CHALLENGES

- *Concept:* Professional ethics override personal ethics in a professional setting.
  Challenge: Patient situations that conflict with a nurse's personal ethics can be very troublesome; however, the ANA's *Code of Ethics for Nurses* is nonnegotiable for nurses regarding ethical behavior.
- *Concept:* The terms *morals* and *ethics* are often used interchangeably. Technically, however, morals reflect what is done in a situation, whereas ethics are concerned with what should be done. Values are beliefs, ideals, and attitudes that one uses to guide behavior.

Challenge: Being familiar with ethical theories and principles, moral development, and decision-making models prepares nurses to participate actively in resolving ethical dilemmas that commonly occur in health care settings.
- *Concept:* Ethical dilemmas occur in all areas of nursing practice, and in fact, each nursing situation has ethical implications.
  Challenge: Nurses need to understand that even simple decisions such as prioritizing care have an ethical basis.

- *Concept:* Respect for humans is the foundation for the six ethical principles of autonomy, beneficence, nonmaleficence, fidelity, veracity, and justice.

  Challenge: These principles are more than a matter of opinion about what constitutes right and wrong. Understanding basic ethical principles involved in a situation can clarify, rather than complicate, how to act ethically and are helpful in determining the best action to take when faced with an ethical dilemma.

- *Concept:* Nurses must protect patients' privacy and confidentiality at all times when using social media.

  Challenge: Social media has blurred professional and personal boundaries, making it particularly important for nurses to be vigilant to protect their patients when using social media.

- *Concept:* Use of technology such as electronic health records has compounded common ethical dilemmas and created new ones for health care workers.

  Challenge: Access to health records are increasingly monitored in health care institutions; however, nurses can ensure that they manage digital information correctly by simply asking themselves, "Do I need to know this?"

IDEAS FOR FURTHER EXPLORATION

1. Explain the differences among morals, values, and ethics, using the definitions from this chapter. Describe a patient situation in which you would feel challenged in terms of your own morals, values, and ethics.

2. Compare the ANA's Code of Ethics for Nurses with the ICN's Code of Ethics for Nurses. How are they similar, and how are they different?

3. Select an ethical theory or principle that is most congruent with your approach to ethical dilemmas. Use it as a basis for considering the ethical dilemmas in this chapter. How helpful to you is this particular theory or principle in determining how you would act?

4. Discuss your reactions to the following scenarios and questions in a small group:

   a. Mrs. Otto has recently undergone extensive surgery for gynecologic cancer. The day after surgery, she asks for more pain medication than the physician has prescribed. You call for an order to increase the pain medication dosage, but she still complains every 2 hours that she cannot tolerate the pain. What should be done?

   b. Mrs. Loriz suffers from severe chronic pain, the cause of which has not been definitely diagnosed. Her husband has brought her into the emergency department for the fifth time this month asking for narcotic relief from the pain. In tears she states, "A shot of a narcotic is the only thing that takes the edge off." She threatens suicide if she is sent home without some help. The physician has ordered a placebo. What is the nurse's responsibility?

   c. Mr. Nelson, age 87 years, suffered a serious stroke. His wife of 65 years keeps a constant vigil at his bedside. After 4 weeks, he remains unresponsive and develops pneumonia. He is being fed through a feeding tube and ventilated through a tracheotomy. Mrs. Nelson feels that agreeing to a do-not-resuscitate (DNR) order is letting her husband down but recognizes he has no quality of life. How should the nurse counsel Mrs. Nelson?

   d. Emily and Michael are parents of a young child dying of Tay-Sachs disease. Emily recently found out she is pregnant again and wants to know whether their second child is affected with the same disease. She undergoes genetic testing and learns that the fetus also has Tay-Sachs disease. Emily and Michael are considering whether to terminate the pregnancy, knowing that their expected baby will have a fatal condition. How can the nurse assist these parents in making their decision?

5. Answer the following questions, basing your answers on identified ethical principles:

   a. When is it acceptable to refuse an assignment?

   b. What is the nurse's duty when a patient confides the desire to self-harm?

   c. Is health care a right?

   d. What should the nurse do when his or her personal values are in conflict with those of the patient?

REFERENCES

Agency for Healthcare Research and Quality: *Pocket guide: Teamstepps*, 2014. Retrieved from: http://www.ahrq.gov/professionals/education/curriculum-tools/teamstepps/instructor/essentials/pocketguide.html.

American Hospital Association (AHA): *The patient care partnership: understanding expectations, rights and responsibilities, (website)*, 2003. Available at: http://www.aha.org/advocacy-issues/communicatingpts/pt-care-partnership.shtml.

American Nurses Association (ANA): *Position statement: the nonnegotiable nature of the ANA code for nurses with interpretive statements (website)*, 1994. Available at: http://gm6.nursingworld.org/MainMenuCategories/Policy-Advocacy/Positions-and-Resolutions/ANAPositionStatements/Position-Statements-Alphabetically/prtetcode14446.html.

American Nurses Association (ANA): *Immigration, citizenship, refugees, border security, and international law (website)*, 2008. Available at: www.nursingworld.org/DocumentVault/GOVA/Federal/Testimonies/Testimony061208.pdf.

American Nurses Association (ANA): *Social networking principles toolkit (website)*, 2012. Available at: www.nursingworld.org/FunctionalMenuCategories/AboutANA/Social-Media/Social-Networking-Principles-Toolkit.aspx.

American Nurses Association (ANA): *Code of ethics for nurses with interpretive statements*, Washington, DC, 2015a, American Nurses Publishing.

American Nurses Association (ANA): *Courage: acting on your convictions, (website)*, 2015b. Available at: www.theamericannurse.org/index.php/2015/06/05/courage-acting-on-your-convictions/.

America Nurses Association (ANA): *Nursing: scope and standards of practice*, Silver Spring, MD, 2015c, American Nurses Association.

American Nurses Association Enterprise: *Learn how to cultivate moral courage*, 2017. Retrieved from: https://engage.healthy-nursehealthynation.org/blogs/8/685.

Baker R: In defense of bioethics, *J Law Med Ethics* 37(1):83–92, 2009.

Bavier A: Holding students accountable when integrity is challenged, *Nurs Educ Perspect* 30(1):5, 2009.

Beauchamp TL, Childress JF: *Principles of biomedical ethics*, ed 4, New York, 2001, Oxford University Press.

Brown University: *A framework for making ethical decisions*, 2017. Retrieved from: https://www.brown.edu/academics/science-and-technology-studies/framework-making-ethical-decisions.

Buckley WJ, Sulmasy DP, Mackler A, Sachedina A: Ethics of palliative sedation and medical disasters: four traditions advance public consensus on three issues, *Ethics Med* 28(10):35–63, 2012.

Bulger JW: *Principalism*, 2007. Retrieved from: https://www.uvu.edu/ethics/seac/Bulger-Principlism.pdf.

Burkhardt MA, Nathaniel AK: *Ethics and issues in contemporary nursing*, ed 2, Albany, NY, 2002, Delmar.

Burston A, Tuckett A: Moral distress in nursing: contributing factors, outcomes and interventions, *Nursing Ethics* 20(3):312–324, 2013.

Butts J, Rich K: *Nursing ethics: across the curriculum and into practice*, Sudbury, MA, 2005, Jones & Bartlett.

Cook RI, Woods DD: Operating at the sharp end: the complexity of human error. In Bogner ME, editor: *Human error in medicine*, Hillsdale, NJ, 1994, Lawrence Erlbaum Associates, pp 255–310.

de Casterlé BD, Izumi S, Godfrey NS, et al.: Nurses' responses to ethical dilemmas in nursing practice: meta-analysis, *J Adv Nurs* 63(6):540–549, 2009.

Dugger CW: U.S. plan to lure nurses may hurt poor nations, *New York Times*, May 24, 2006. Available at: www.nytimes.com/2006/05/24/world/americas/24nurses.html?pagewanted=all&_r=0.

Fairchild RM: Practical ethical theory for nurses responding to complexity in care, *Nurs Ethics* 17(3):353–362, 2010.

Giddings L: A theoretical model of social consciousness, *Adv Nurs Sci* 28:224–239, 2005.

Gilligan C: *In a different voice: psychological theory and women's development*, Cambridge, MA, 1982, Harvard University Press.

Gilligan C: Moral orientation and moral development. In Kittay EF, Meyers DT, editors: *Women and moral theory*, Savage, MD, 1987, Rowman.

Goethals S, Gastmans C, Dierckx de Casterle B: Nurses' ethical reasoning and behavior: a literature review, *Int J Nurs Stud* 47(5):635–650, 2010.

Guido GW: *Legal and ethical issues in nursing*, ed 4, Upper Saddle River, NJ, 2006, Pearson Education.

Hardingham LB: Ethics in the workplace: reflective practice, *Alberta RN* 57(3):28–29, 2001.

Harrison E, Falco SM: Health disparity and the nurse advocate: reaching out to alleviate suffering, *Adv Nurs Sci* 28(3):252–264, 2005.

Haynes L, Boese T, Butcher H: *Nursing in contemporary society: issues, trends, and transition to practice*, Upper Saddle River, NJ, 2004, Pearson Prentice-Hall.

Hines PS: Truth-telling, not telling, and listening, *Cancer Nurs* 31(6):415–416, 2008.

International Council of Nurses (ICN): *The International Council of Nurses code for nurses*, Geneva, Switzerland, 2012, International Council of Nurses.

Jameton A: *Nursing practice: the ethical issues*, Englewood Cliffs, NJ, 1984, Prentice-Hall.

Kirkham SR, Van Hofwegen L, Pankratz D: Keeping the vision: sustaining social consciousness with nursing students following international learning experiences, *Int J Nurs Educ Scholarsh* (online) 6(1), 2009, Article 3.

Kohlberg L: Continuities and discontinuities in childhood and adult moral development revisited. In Kohlberg L, editor: *Collected papers on moral development and moral education*, Cambridge, MA, 1973, Moral Education Research Foundation.

Kohlberg L: Moral stages and moralization: the cognitive developmental approach. In Lickona T, editor: *Moral development and behavior*, New York, 1976, Holt, Rinehart and Winston, pp 31–53.

Kohlberg L: A current statement on some theoretical issues. In Modgil S, Modgil C, editors: *Lawrence Kohlberg: consensus and controversy*, Philadelphia, 1986, Falmer, pp 485–546.

Lachman V: Strategies necessary for MC, *Online J Issues Nurs* 15(3), 2010. Manuscript 3, Retrieved from: http://www.nursingworld.org/MainMenuCategories/EthicsStandards/Courage-and-Distress/Strategies-and-Moral-Courage.html.

McCarthy J, Gastmans C: Moral distress: a review of the argument-based nursing ethics literature, *Nurs Ethics* 23(1):131–152, 2015.

McLeod-Sordjan R: Evaluating moral reasoning in nursing education, *Nursing Ethics* 21(4):473–483, 2014.

Pesut DJ, Herman J: *Clinical reasoning: the art and science of creative and critical thinking*, Albany, NY, 1999, Dell.

Rushton CH, Caldwell M, Kurtz M: CE: Moral distress: a catalyst for building moral resilience, *Am J Nurs* 116(7):40–49, 2016.

Saureland J, Marotta K, Peinemann A, Berndt A, Robichaux C: Assessing and addressing moral distress and ethical climate, part I, *Dimens Crit Care Nurs* 33(40):234–245, 2014.

Stubenrauch JM: The ethics of recruiting foreign-educated nurses, *Am J Nurs* 108(12):25–26, 2008.

Uustal DB: *Clinical ethics and values: issues and insights in a changing healthcare environment*, East Greenwich, RI, 1993, Educational Resources in HealthCare.

Woods M: Nursing ethics education: are we really delivering the good(s)? *Nursing Ethics* 12(1):5–18, 2005.

Zickmund SL: Care and justice: the impact of gender and profession on ethical decision making in the healthcare arena, *J Clin Ethics* 15(2):176–187, 2004.

8

Conceptual and Philosophical Foundations of Professional Nursing Practice

Anita Tesh, BSN, MSN, PhD, CNE, ANEF, RN

To enhance your understanding of this chapter, try the Student Exercises on the Evolve site at http://evolve.elsevier.com/Black/professional.

LEARNING OUTCOMES

After studying this chapter, students will be able to:

- Describe the components and processes of systems.
- Explain Maslow's hierarchy of human needs and its relationship to motivation.
- Recognize how environmental factors such as family, culture, social support, social media and the Internet, and community influence health.
- Explain the significance of a holistic approach to nursing care.
- Apply Rosenstock's health belief model and Bandura's theory of perceived self-efficacy to personal health behaviors and health behaviors of others.

- Devise a personal plan for achieving high-level wellness.
- Define and give examples of beliefs.
- Define and give examples of values.
- Cite examples of nursing philosophies.
- Discuss the impact of beliefs and values on nurses' professional behaviors.
- Explain how nurses and organizations educating and employing nurses can use a philosophy of nursing.
- Identify personal beliefs, values, and philosophies as they relate to nursing.

Suppose you were building a house. You would want the most solid, safe, and structurally sound building that you could afford. You would want your house to be built on firm ground, set on a foundation of cinderblocks and concrete. You would want to know that this structure would hold up in high wind, heavy snow, blazing heat, and driving rains. Because of what you are asking of your house—that is, for it to be a place to eat, sleep, be with your family, and protect you from the elements— some parts of your house would be similar to almost all houses: a foundation, framing, walls, windows, rooms, and a good roof. Because you have planned your house and built your house well, it will provide for you what you need from it.

Anything built well must have a solid foundation for support. Your car has a structure—the chassis—that

keeps you safe and gives your car form. Humans have a skeleton that gives us shape and makes us recognizable. The underlying structure tells us something about the function of the object.

The same holds true for a profession; its foundational principles tell us something about what nursing is and what nursing does. These principles are always in place, even when you are not aware of them. Much like the foundation of your house or your own skeleton, you do not have to think about its doing its work—it is simply there.

The foundation of nursing—its bones—is its basic concepts, the ideas that are essential to understanding professional practice. These concepts are person, environment, and health. Each concept has subconcepts, which are other ideas that are related to the larger concept, but

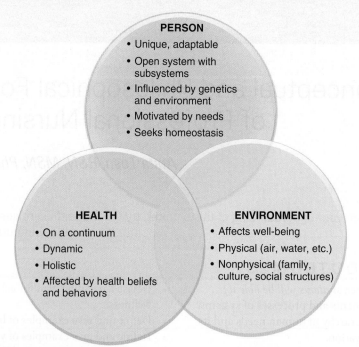

PERSON
- Unique, adaptable
- Open system with subsystems
- Influenced by genetics and environment
- Motivated by needs
- Seeks homeostasis

HEALTH
- On a continuum
- Dynamic
- Holistic
- Affected by health beliefs and behaviors

ENVIRONMENT
- Affects well-being
- Physical (air, water, etc.)
- Nonphysical (family, culture, social structures)

Fig. 8.1 This is the foundation of nursing—its concepts and subconcepts basic to the profession.

which are also related to nursing (Fig. 8.1). Everything professional nurses do is in response to one of these basic interrelated concepts. You do not say, "I am going to check on Mrs. Bruce's homeostasis." But in fact when you check her fluid intake and urine output after her major surgery, you are addressing an element of her *person* (homeostasis—her fluid balance), her *health* (she is in a vulnerable state), and her *environment* (her intravenous line patency, her availability of water), in the context of nursing. You as a nurse are guided by beliefs, values, and a philosophy, which work together to shape your practice.

This is a simple example, but one that will give you an idea of how nursing's concepts are at work in nursing actions. In this chapter we will explore how these concepts relate to each other and to nursing. By the end of this chapter, these abstract ideas will have more meaning to you as you begin to think about your own philosophy of nursing.

UNDERSTANDING SYSTEMS: CONNECTIONS AND INTERACTIONS

An understanding of systems will guide you in understanding the connections and interactions among nursing's basic concepts. A system is a set of interrelated parts that come together to form a whole that performs a function (von Bertalanffy, 1968). General systems theory was developed in 1936 by biologist Ludwig von Bertalanffy, who believed that a common framework for studying several similar disciplines would allow scientists and scholars to organize and communicate findings, making it easier to build on the work of others. Each part of a system is a necessary or integral component required to make a complete, meaningful whole. These parts are input, throughput, output, evaluation, and feedback (von Bertalanffy, 1968).

Components of Systems

Input is the first component of a system—the raw material, such as information, energy, or matter—that enters a system and is transformed by it. For a system to work well, input should contribute to achieving the purpose of the system.

Throughput is the second component of a system. Throughput consists of the processes a system uses to convert raw materials (input) into a form that can be used, either by the system itself or by the environment (also called the *suprasystem*). **Output** is the end result or product of the system. Outputs vary widely, depending on the type and purpose of the system.

Evaluation is the fourth component of a system. **Evaluation** means measuring the success or failure of

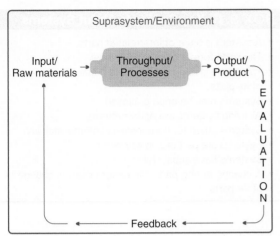

Fig. 8.2 Major components of a general systems model.

the output and consequently the effectiveness of the system. For evaluation to be meaningful in any system, outcome criteria against which performance or product quality is measured must be identified.

Feedback, the final component of a system, is the process of communicating what is found in evaluation of the system. Feedback is the information given back into the system to determine whether the purpose, or end result, of the system has been achieved. Fig. 8.2 depicts the components of systems and illustrates how they relate to one another.

Examples of Systems

A simple example helps clarify the components of systems. In a school of nursing system, the raw material, or input, consists of students, faculty, ideas, the desire to learn, and knowledge. For high-quality input, students need to be ready to learn, and the faculty should be knowledgeable and well prepared to teach. The processes (throughput) whereby ideas, knowledge, and skills are transmitted must be clear and understandable. In this example, throughput consists of learning experiences such as readings, lectures, discussions, labs, and clinical experiences. The output, or product, of the system is well-educated graduates. For evaluation of the output, the National Council Licensure Examination (NCLEX®) is a good measure of how well the system worked. The passing rate of those taking the NCLEX® on their first try provides feedback to the faculty and administrators. If a high percentage of graduates pass on the first try, the system has achieved its purpose. If not, changes need to

be made in the input or in the system itself—for example, setting higher admission standards, hiring more talented faculty, and/or designing more effective courses and curricula.

Systems are usually complex and consist of several parts called *subsystems*. Consider a hospital as a system, for example. Technically, it is a system for providing health care, but the success of the system depends on the functioning of many **subsystems**. The subsystems include many departments: nursing, medicine, imaging, informatics, laboratory, and environmental services, among others. Each of these subsystems is a system itself. All the subsystems function collaboratively to make the health care system—the hospital—work.

Open and Closed Systems

Continuing with the example, the hospital and all its subsystems are open systems. An **open system** promotes the exchange of matter, energy, and information with other systems and the environment. The larger environment outside the hospital is called the **suprasystem**. A **closed system** does not interact with other systems or with the surrounding environment. Matter, energy, and information do not flow into or out of a closed system. There are few totally closed systems. Even a completely balanced aquarium, for example, often thought of as approaching a closed system, needs light, air, and additional water and nutrients from time to time.

Two more points are essential to a basic understanding of systems. First, the whole is different from and greater than the sum of its parts (its subsystems). Anyone who has ever been in a hospital, for example, knows that what happens there is different from and more than the sum of the following equation: nurses + pharmacy + physicians + environmental services = hospital. The second point involves synergy. **Synergy** occurs when all the various subsystems work together to create a result that is not independently achievable. Synergy in the hospital occurs when the people who compose the subsystems collaborate to work with patients and their families, combining efforts to create an outcome that no single group could accomplish alone.

Dynamic Nature of Systems

The final point to be made about systems is that change in one part of the system creates change in other parts. If the hospital admissions office, for example, decided to admit patients only between the hours of 8:00 and 10:00 a.m., that decision would result in changes in the nursing units, environmental services, business office, operating suites, laboratories, and other hospital subsystems. If that change were implemented without prior communication to the other subsystems and coordinated planning, it would likely create chaos in the system.

The exchange of energy and information within open systems and between open systems and their suprasystems is continuous. The dynamic balance within and between the subsystems, the system, and the suprasystems helps create and maintain homeostasis, also known as *internal stability.*

All living systems are open systems. The internal environment is in constant interaction with a changing environment external to the organism. As change occurs in one environment, the other environment is affected. For example, walking into a cold room (change in the external environment) affects a variety of physiologic and psychological subsystems of a person's internal environment. These, in turn, affect a person's blood flow, ability to concentrate, and feeling of comfort, for example (changes in internal environment).

Application of the Systems Model to Nursing

Nurses work within systems every day. Using the hospital example, nurses work within the hospital as a system, the department of nursing's system, within a particular unit's system, and with colleagues in what may be an informal but important system. All are open systems interacting with one another and the environment. If nurses are to work effectively in such complex systems, they need to have an understanding of how systems operate.

At the individual patient level, the openness of human systems makes nursing intervention possible. Understanding systems helps nurses assess relationships among all the factors that affect patients, including the influence of nurses themselves. Nurses who understand systems view patients holistically, including the physiologic subsystems (such as metabolism and the respiratory system) and suprasystem (such as family, culture, and community). These nurses appreciate the influence of change in any part of the system. For instance, when a patient with diabetes has pneumonia (change in subsystem), the infection increases the blood glucose level (metabolic system) and may result in hospitalization. Hospitalization may in turn adversely affect the patient's

> **BOX 8.1   Key Concepts About Systems**
>
> - A system is a set of interrelated parts.
> - The parts form a meaningful whole.
> - The whole is different from and greater than the sum of its parts.
> - Systems may be open or closed.
> - All living systems are open systems.
> - Systems strive for homeostasis (internal stability).
> - Systems are part of suprasystems.
> - Systems have subsystems.
> - A change in one part of a system creates change in other parts.

role in the family and community (change in suprasystem). Key concepts of systems are summarized in Box 8.1. With this brief introduction to systems as a foundation, we can now examine the three basic concepts that are fundamental to the practice of professional nursing: person, environment, and health.

PERSON: AN OPEN SYSTEM WITH HUMAN NEEDS

The term person is used to describe each individual woman, man, and child. There are various approaches to the study of person. This chapter briefly examines the concept of people as systems with human needs.

As mentioned previously, each individual is an open system with numerous subsystems that make up the whole person. For example, the physiologic subsystem is composed of the circulatory, musculoskeletal, respiratory, gastrointestinal, genitourinary, and neurologic subsystems; the psychological, social, cultural, and spiritual subsystems combine with the physiologic subsystem to comprise the whole person. Each person is unique—different from all other people who have been and ever will be. This uniqueness is determined genetically, environmentally, and experientially and is the basis for holistic nursing care—that is, nursing care that takes all the aspects of the person into consideration.

Certain personal characteristics are determined at conception by the genes received from one's biologic parents, such as eye, skin, and hair color; height; sex; and a variety of other features. The environment determines other characteristics. The availability of loving and nurturing parents or parental substitutes, availability of sufficient nutritious foods, cultural beliefs, degree

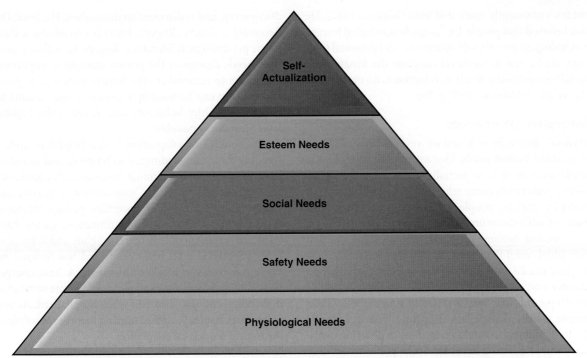

Fig. 8.3 Maslow's hierarchy of needs. Understanding this hierarchy helps nurses prioritize their care. (Maslow AH: A theory of human motivation, Psychological Review 50(4):370-396, 1943.)

of educational opportunities, adequacy of housing, quality and quantity of parental supervision, and safety are all examples of environmental factors that influence how a person develops.

Human Needs

In addition to having unique personal characteristics, people have inborn needs. *Human need* refers to something—food, air, social interaction—required for a person's well-being. In 1954 psychologist Abraham Maslow published *Motivation and Personality*. In this classic book, Maslow rejected earlier ideas of Sigmund Freud, who believed that people are motivated by unconscious instincts, and Ivan Pavlov, who believed humans were driven by conditioned reflexes. Instead, Maslow presented his human needs theory and explained that human behavior is motivated by intrinsic needs. He identified five levels of needs and organized them into a hierarchic order, as shown in Fig. 8.3.

Maslow's Hierarchy of Needs

According to Maslow, the most basic level of needs consists of those necessary for physiologic survival: food,

oxygen, rest, activity, shelter, and sexual expression. These needs are common to all human beings.

The second level of needs is safety and security. These include physical and psychological safety and security needs. Psychological safety and security include having a reasonably predictable environment with which one has some familiarity and relative freedom from fear and chaos.

The third level of needs consists of love and belonging. To a greater or lesser extent, each person needs close, intimate relationships; social relationships; a place in the social structure; and group affiliations.

Next in Maslow's hierarchy is the need for self-esteem. This includes the need to feel self-worth, self-respect, and self-reliance.

Self-actualization is the highest level of needs. Self-actualized people have realized their maximum potential; they use their talents, skills, and abilities to the fullest extent possible and are true to their own nature. People do not stay in a state of self-actualization but may have "peak experiences" during which they realize self-actualization for some period. Maslow believed that many people strive for self-actualization but few consistently reach that level (Maslow, 1987). He also believed that people are "innately motivated toward psychological growth, self-awareness, and personal freedom. As he saw it, we never outgrow the innate need for self-expression and self-development, no matter how old we are" (Hoffman, 2008, p. 36).

Assumptions About Needs

Maslow's hierarchy is based on several basic assumptions about human needs. One assumption is that basic needs must be at least partially satisfied before higher order needs can become relevant to the individual. For example, starving people will not be concerned with issues of self-esteem until their hunger is satisfied.

A second assumption about human needs is that individuals meet their needs in different ways. One person may need 8 or 9 hours of sleep to feel rested, whereas another may require only 5 or 6 hours. Each individual's sleep needs may vary at different stages of life. Older people usually require less sleep than younger people do. Individuals also eat different diets in differing quantities and at differing intervals. Some prefer to eat only twice a day, whereas others may snack six or eight times a day to meet their nutritional needs. Sexual energy also varies widely from person to person. A broad range of individual factors determines the frequency with which normal adults desire sexual activity.

Although sleep, food, and sex are considered examples of basic human needs, the manner in which these needs are met, as well as the extent to which any one of them is considered a need, varies according to each individual. It is therefore extremely important to determine a person's perceptions of his or her own needs to be able to provide appropriate, individualized nursing care. If a patient is uncomfortable eating three large meals, such as those served in most hospitals, nurses can help that person by saving parts of the large meals in the refrigerator on the nursing unit and serving them to the patient between regularly scheduled meals. This is a simple example of what is meant by the term *individualized nursing care,* which recognizes each individual's unique needs and tailors the plan of nursing care to take that uniqueness into consideration.

Adaptation and Human Needs

Another aspect of human needs is the nature of individuals to change, grow, and develop. Carl Rogers, a well-known psychologist, built his theory of personhood based on the idea that people are constantly adapting, discovering, and rediscovering themselves. His book *On Becoming a Person* (Rogers, 1961) is considered a classic in psychological literature. Rogers' idea that a person's needs change as the person changes is important for nurses to remember. The human potential to grow and develop can be used by nurses to assist patients to change unhealthy behaviors and to reach the highest level of wellness possible.

The concept of **adaptation** is also helpful in understanding that people admitted to hospitals and removed from their customary, familiar environments commonly become anxious. Even the most confident person can become fearful when in an uncertain, perhaps threatening, situation. Under these circumstances, nurses have learned to expect people to regress slightly and to become more concerned with basic needs and less focused on the higher needs in Maslow's hierarchy. A "take-charge" professional person, for example, may become somewhat demanding and self-absorbed when hospitalized. As you will see in Chapter 9, several nursing theorists based their theoretical models on adaptation.

Homeostasis

When a person's needs are not met, homeostasis is threatened. Remember that homeostasis is a dynamic balance achieved by effectively functioning open systems. It is a state of equilibrium, a tendency to maintain internal stability. In humans, homeostasis is attained by coordinated responses of organ systems that automatically compensate for environmental changes. When someone goes for a brisk walk, for example, heart rate and respiratory rate automatically increase to keep vital organs supplied with oxygen. When the individual comes home and sits down to read, heart rate and breathing slow down. No conscious decision to speed up or slow down these physiologic functions has to be made. Adjustments occur automatically to maintain homeostasis.

Individuals, as open systems, also endeavor to maintain balance between external and internal forces. When that balance is achieved, the person is healthy, or at least resistant to illness. When environmental factors affect a person's homeostasis, the person attempts to adapt to the change. If adaptation is unsuccessful, disequilibrium may occur, setting the stage for the development of illness or disease. How individuals respond to stress is a major factor in the development of illness. Stress and illness are discussed more fully in Chapter 13, and you may wish to review that information now.

ENVIRONMENT: THE SUPRASYSTEM IN WHICH PERSONS LIVE

The second major concept basic to professional nursing practice is environment, or the suprasystem. **Environment** includes all the circumstances, influences, and conditions that surround and affect individuals, families, and groups. The environment can be as small and controlled as a premature infant's isolette or as large and uncontrollable as the universe. Included in environment are the social and cultural attitudes that profoundly shape human experience.

The environment can either promote or interfere with the homeostasis and well-being of individuals. As seen in Maslow's hierarchy of needs, there is a dynamic interaction between a person's needs, which are internal, and the satisfaction of those needs, which is often environmentally determined.

Nurses have always been aware of the influence of environment on people. Florence Nightingale, in particular, stressed the role of a healthful environment in restoration and preservation of health and prevention of disease and injury. Concerns about the health of the public have led governmental entities at local, state, and national levels to establish standards and regulations that ensure the safety of food, water, air, cosmetics, medications, workplaces, and other areas in which health hazards may occur. Environmental systems to be discussed in this section are family systems, cultural systems, social systems, and community systems.

Family Systems

The most direct environmental influence on a person is the family. Families have all types of configurations, from dual-parent homes with children to single parents raising their children on their own; single adults with networks of close friends who constitute their family; extended families with several generations under one roof; or couples without children. These are just a few examples of the many family structures. Families are defined as the patient defines family and do not necessarily involve "blood relatives." The way the family functions with and within the environment and the dynamics among various members of the family constitute the **family system.** The quality and amount of parenting provided to infants and growing children constitute a major determinant of health. Children who are nurtured when young and vulnerable, who are allowed to grow in independence and self-determination, and who are taught the skills they need for social living have a foundation for growing into strong, productive, autonomous adults. Some strong, productive, autonomous adults, however, come from disadvantaged backgrounds where the nurturing was limited. The family background can shape one's adulthood but is not determinative.

Nuclear and Extended Families

For most of the history of humankind, immediate and extended families were relatively intact units that lived together or lived within close proximity to one another. In the **extended family,** children were nurtured by a variety of relatives, as well as by their own parents. Extended family members also cared for elderly people and those with disabilities. This closeness was affected profoundly by industrialization, which fostered urbanization. When families ceased farming, which was a family endeavor, and moved to cities where fathers worked in factories, the first dilution of the influence of extended family began. The **nuclear family** (parents and their children) moved away from former sources of nurturing, as older relatives such as grandparents, aunts, and uncles often stayed in rural areas.

During World War II, more women began to work, taking them out of the home and away from young children for hours each day. The increased geographic mobility of families since World War II has changed the extent and nature of relationships of extended family members because nuclear families may live across the continent or the world from their relatives. Currently, technologies such as text messaging, FaceTime, Skype, and other social media are changing the relationships of extended family members yet again. These technologies can allow family members who are geographically separate to interact more intensely and frequently than was possible a decade ago. For some families, technology allows extended family members to serve as important sources of advice and support without being physically present; however, access to these technologies varies widely among the population of the United States.

Single-Parent Families

Although the majority of children in the United States lives in two-parent households, the percentage of children living in single-parent households increased dramatically over the past 50 years. According to the U.S. Census Bureau (2016), 23% of all households with children were single-parent households, and most of those were headed by women. For comparison, in 1960, 8% of households were single-parent households. In 2016, 39.8% of all births were to single women (Centers for Disease Control and Prevention [CDC], 2018), a statistic explaining in part the current high percentage of single-parent homes in the United States. Life is challenging for single parents who must earn a living for the family and fulfill the nurturing roles in the family. Bearing these multiple roles alone over long periods can be extremely stressful, even exhausting, to single parents.

The examples given here represent only a few ways families influence the well-being of individuals: there are many others. A complete nursing assessment includes information about a patient's family and home environment. This information is particularly important when a modification of the home environment is needed, especially when a person is returning home with a disability or a limitation in his or her mobility. Importantly, a complete assessment should include screening for intimate partner violence (also known as domestic violence) or, in the case of children, for signs of neglect and abuse. Signs of abuse in both adults and children may not be obvious, and victims often are not forthcoming in the health care setting about being abused and by whom. Abuse and neglect are not uncommon, and careful assessment and the development of a trusting professional relationship may be of benefit in helping persons who have been abused disclose their experience.

Cultural Systems

People are deeply entrenched in their culture and may not even recognize the effect of their culture on their lives. Culture consists of the attitudes, beliefs, and behaviors of social and ethnic groups that have been perpetuated through generations. Patterns of language, clothing, eating habits, activities of daily living, attitudes toward those outside the culture, health beliefs and values, spiritual beliefs or religious orientation, and attitudes toward children, women, men, marriage, education, work, and recreation all are influenced by culture.

Significant changes have occurred in the United States in the past several decades related to culture. The United States was once known as a "melting pot," referring to the assimilation of persons of varying nationalities, cultures, and languages into one homogeneous culture. Recently, however, the melting pot is being replaced with the "salad bowl" metaphor to describe the multiculturalism predominating in the United States today. Multiculturalism has several definitions. The most common usage, however, refers to those with "culturally distinct identities" retaining their cultural identity and enjoying full access to a society's constitutional principles and prevailing shared values (UNESCO, n.d.).

According to the Pew Research Center (2017), as of 2017 more than 13% of people living in the United States were foreign born. The United States has become a multicultural society, with immigrants coming from almost every country in the world. Because basic beliefs about health and illness vary widely from culture to culture, nurses need to develop cultural competence to meet the needs of culturally diverse patients. For example, many Mexican American and Mexican immigrant families observe 40 days of recovery in the postpartum period—*la cuarentena* (*cuarenta dias* or quarantine)—when traditional behaviors related to diet, clothing, sexual abstinence, bathing, and management of the environment are practiced, and social support is intense. This culturally entrenched practice may be misunderstood and even trivialized by providers, leading women to conceal their traditions (Waugh, 2010).

Effective nurses learn to be aware of and to respect cultural influences on patients. Whenever possible, they defer to patients' cultural preferences. They recognize that some cultural groups attribute illness to bad fortune. Individuals from cultures with these beliefs do not see themselves as active participants in their own health status. This attitude is a challenge for nurses who value the collaboration of patients in their own health care planning.

The challenge for nurses in an increasingly diverse world is to understand the risks of ethnocentrism—that is, making judgments, often negative, about another's culture relative to one's own. It is tempting to dismiss a cultural tradition or belief because it is not part of one's own experience. Moreover, it is also easy to be blind to one's own deeply entrenched cultural beliefs. In other words, our own traditions may seem strange to others. Astute nurses realize that integration of a patient's cultural health beliefs into planning patient-centered care can make a strong impact on that patient's desire and ability to improve his or her health.

Understanding the relationship between culture and health is the basis for "transcultural nursing," a field of nursing practice initiated by nurse-anthropologist

Madeleine Leininger. Additional discussion of the influence of culture on nursing practice can be found in Chapter 13.

Social Systems

In addition to being influenced by family and cultural systems, individuals are influenced by the social system in which they live. Social institutions such as families, neighborhoods, schools, churches, professional associations, civic groups, and recreational groups may constitute a form of social support. Social support also includes such factors as family income; presence in the home of a spouse; proximity to neighbors, children, and other supportive individuals; access to medical care; coping abilities; and educational level.

Social Change

Holmes and Rahe (1967) published a study of the relationship of social change to the subsequent development of illness. They found that people with many social changes that disrupt social support, such as death of a loved one, divorce, job changes, moving, or unemployment, were much more likely to experience illness in the following 12 months than people with few social changes. Both positive and negative changes created the need for social readjustment. In 1995 this study was updated, and the Recent Life Changes Questionnaire (Table 8.1) was devised to reflect more accurately contemporary concerns (Miller and Rahe, 1997). Numerous other researchers have found additional evidence that social support has a direct relationship to health.

TABLE 8.1   Recent Life Changes Questionnaire

The following 74 potential life changes inquire about recent events in a person's life. A 6-month total equal to or greater than 300 Life Change Units (LCUs) or a 1-year total equal to or greater than 500 LCUs, is considered indicative of high recent life stress.

Life Change Event	Life Change Units	Life Change Event	Life Change Units
Health		Retirement	52
An injury or illness that:		Loss of job:	
Kept you in bed 1 week or more or sent you to the hospital	74	Laid off from work	68
Was less serious than above	44	Fired from work	79
Major dental work	26	Correspondence course to help you in your work	18
Major change in eating habits	27		
Major change in sleeping habits	26	**Home and Family**	
Major change in your usual type and/or amount of recreation	28	Major change in living conditions	42
		Change in residence:	
		Move within the same town or city	25
Work		Move to a different town, city, or state	47
Change to a new type of work	51	Change in family get-togethers	25
Change in your work hours or conditions	35	Major change in health or behavior of family member	55
Change in your responsibilities at work:		Marriage	50
More responsibilities	29	Pregnancy	67
Fewer responsibilities	21	Miscarriage or abortion	65
Promotion	31	Gain of a new family member:	
Demotion	42	Birth of a child	66
Transfer	32	Adoption of a child	65
Troubles at work:		A relative moving in with you	59
With your boss	29	Spouse beginning or ending work	46
With co-workers	35	Child leaving home:	
With persons under your supervision	35	To attend college	41
Other work troubles	28	Because of marriage	41
Major business adjustment	60	For other reason	45

Continued

TABLE 8.1   Recent Life Changes Questionnaire—cont'd

Life Change Event	Life Change Units	Life Change Event	Life Change Units
Change in arguments with spouse	50	Vacation	24
In-law problems	38	New close, personal relationship	37
Change in the marital status of your parents:		Engagement to marry	45
		Girlfriend or boyfriend problems	39
Divorce	59	Sexual difficulties	44
Remarriage	50	"Falling out" of a close personal relationship	47
Separation from spouse:			
Because of work	53	An accident	48
Because of marital problems	76	Minor violation of the law	20
Divorce	96	Being held in jail	75
Birth of grandchild	43	Death of a close friend	70
Death of spouse	119	Major decision regarding your immediate future	51
Death of a family member:			
Child	123	Major personal achievement	36
Brother or sister	102		
Parent	100	**Financial**	
		Major change in finances:	
Personal and Social		Increased income	38
Change in personal habits	26	Decreased income	60
Beginning or ending school or college	38	Investment and/or credit difficulties	56
Change of school or college	35	Loss or damage of personal property	43
Change in political beliefs	24	Moderate purchase	20
Change in religious beliefs	29	Major purchase	37
Change in social activities	27	Foreclosure on a mortgage or loan	58

From Miller MA, Rahe RH: Life changes scaling for the 1990s, *J Psychosom Res* 43 (3):279–292, 1997. Reprinted with permission.

Social Support

Social support is a commonly used, but rarely defined, term. In its largest sense, social support means that a person belongs to a social network, feels loved and cared for, and can count on people for assistance. Social support can be perceived, meaning that individuals recognize that support has been given or is available if needed in the future. *Received support* refers to the actual helpful (supportive) actions that are offered. Social support works in four ways. *Emotional support* comes in the form of concern for, affection, love, caring, encouragement, and conveying a sense of value to the person being supported. *Companionship* is a form of support that gives the supported person a sense of belonging and provides people with whom to share social activities. *Informational support* is advice and guidance, the sharing of useful information. *Material support,* also called tangible support, refers to financial help, providing material goods and/or services. Individuals vary in

their need and desire for social support. When assessing patients, nurses need to remember that the patient, not the nurse, should determine the adequacy of his or her social support. For patients who need and desire increased informational support as a form of social support, nurses can be excellent sources of knowledge and direction. Nurses can inform patients about resources for patients and families with specific diagnoses (e.g., cancer support groups, Crohn disease support groups, rare chromosomal disorder support group), parenting classes, religious groups, bereavement and loss support groups, formal and informal educational groups, and self-help groups. These groups may have local meetings or may have a strong online presence as a means of emotional support, companionship, and tangible support.

Poverty

Poverty means living with deprivation and the scarcity of necessities such as food and adequate housing. The United

States is one of the wealthiest nations in the world (International Monetary Fund, 2018; Investopedia, 2017). The poverty level in the United States, however, is high relative to the nation's overall wealth: in 2016 the poverty rate was 12.7% (U.S. Census Bureau, 2017). The U.S. Department of Health and Human Services determines the poverty level annually. In 2018 the poverty threshold was a total income of $12,140 or less for a single person and $25,100 or less for a family of four in the 48 contiguous U.S. states plus the District of Columbia. Alaska and Hawaii have higher costs of living; therefore the poverty threshold income level is somewhat higher (U.S. Department of Health and Human Services: HHS poverty guidelines, 2018).

People living in poverty have diminished access to health care for a variety of reasons. Lack of money means inadequate nutrition and lack of basic health care, adversely affecting the health status of all family members. Specific challenges faced by families at or near poverty levels are food insecurity and hunger; poor transportation; inability to pay mortgage or rent; and inability to pay for utilities such as natural gas, water, and electricity. The World Health Organization (WHO, 2018) now considers poverty to be one the most influential determinants of health.

Understanding and appreciating the complex societal forces that contribute to poverty can be challenging for nurses. Some even blame the poor for their situation. Misconceptions can lead to stereotyping and insensitivity to the feelings and concerns of the poor, further alienating them from the health care system. Many nursing students have had limited exposure to poverty and may not fully realize the enormous implications of being poor. One student shared her experience:

Before I did my community health rotation, I thought that poor meant that someone had to shop for clothes at a "big box" store rather than the mall. Then I made a home visit to a nice woman I had met in the high-risk obstetric clinic. She was pregnant and had the early stages of cervical cancer. She told me that to find her house, I would see a mobile home that looked too run down for anybody to live in. She told me to go past it to the next one that looked even worse, and that was where she lived. I kind of didn't believe her, but she was right. One of the bedrooms was a chicken wire and cardboard addition to the side of the house that her teenage son had built. What surprised me was how neat and clean she had tried to make her house, and her children all sat in a line very quietly and responded to my questions politely. This lady's quiet dignity in this horrible poverty really humbled me, and I cried in my car all the way home.

Community, National, and World Systems

The health status of people is also influenced by the larger systems in which they live. The types and availability of jobs, housing, schools, and health care, as well as the overall economic well-being, profoundly affect the citizens in a community. Nurses can be instrumental in improving the community systems. Identifying health needs and bringing these to the attention of community planners, offering screening programs, serving on health-related committees and advisory boards, and lobbying political leaders can bring about positive change in a community. Nurses have also become politically active by running for elected offices at local, state, and national levels. They can energetically support political candidates who have sound environmental platforms. More information about political activism in nursing is provided in Chapter 15.

From a broad perspective, environment also includes the nation and the world. A seemingly isolated incident such as an earthquake in Nepal or an outbreak of Ebola in West Africa can have worldwide health repercussions. Nurses can contribute to a healthier world environment by supporting, promoting, and, when possible, participating in humanitarian responses to national and international disasters.

Nurses' Potential Impact on the Environment/Suprasystem

Individual nurses, in the interest of ecological health, can engage in a variety of environmentally sound practices in their personal lives and encourage others to do the same. Most of these simply require paying attention to some of your regular habits—turning off unused lights and computers, recycling household trash and hazardous materials such as batteries and paint, avoiding insecticides and unnecessary use of pest-control chemicals, staying abreast of product and toy recalls, buying energy-efficient appliances and automobiles, carpooling, walking or biking when possible, and using public transportation. Furthermore, nurses need to pay attention to the environmental impact of corporations and avoid buying from or investing in companies that engage in environmentally unsound practices.

Because nurses are interested in the health of the public, they should look for ways to organize their workplaces to contribute to a healthier environment. Health care facilities are among the largest producers of waste in the nation. Even as nurses work to promote health, that very work creates all types of pollution, including biohazardous waste, which ultimately adversely affects health. The World Health Organization now sponsors a series of 25 online training modules covering a wide variety of issues related to health care waste, including definitions, sources and characteristics of health care waste, impact of this waste, occupational health and safety, and many others (WHO, 2018).

A decade ago, hospitals were a major source of mercury pollution, and in fact two of the WHO health waste modules (no. 19 and no. 20) address the issue of mercury. This highly toxic substance, once used in thermometers, blood pressure measuring devices, and other medical devices, ultimately flowed into the environment, where it contaminated water. Through the oceans' food chain, mercury in contaminated water becomes concentrated in the bodies of predator fish such as tuna and swordfish, which are eventually consumed by humans. Even in small doses, mercury poses serious health risks to pregnant women and young children. Nurses were instrumental in encouraging their employers to avoid purchasing and using mercury-containing devices and to dispose of them properly when they are discarded. Health Care Without Harm is an organization with the mission to reduce hazardous waste, specifically mercury, produced from health care facilities. This organization encourages nurses to become "environmental health activists." You can learn more about Health Care Without Harm at its website: www.noharm.org.

In other efforts to reduce environmental pollution, some health care facilities have established committees, sometimes called *green teams*, dedicated to identifying and recommending environmentally sound products and procedures. Nurses can volunteer to serve on these committees or to start one. They can recommend recycling, using compact fluorescent light bulbs, using certified organic foods, reusing or repurposing products safely, and using fewer disposable products and fewer products with wasteful packaging. They can educate themselves about reducing carbon emissions and advocate for sustainable policies in their workplaces. You can join the movement of nurses and other health care workers to prevent environmental disease. Health Care Without Harm describes their work as to "transform health care worldwide so that it reduces its environmental footprint, becomes a community anchor for sustainability and a leader in the global movement for environmental health and justice" (Health Care Without Harm, 2018). Refer to their website (https://noharm-uscanada.org/) to learn how the organization is addressing this important mission and how you can help.

HEALTH: A CONTINUUM

Health is the third major concept fundamental to the practice of professional nursing. Health is best viewed as a continuum rather than as an absolute state. Each individual's health status varies from day to day depending on a variety of factors, such as rest, nutrition, and stressors; similarly, illness is not an absolute state. People can have chronic illnesses such as diabetes or seizure disorders and still work; take part in recreational activities; and maintain acceptably healthy, meaningful lives. Fig. 8.4 depicts the illness-wellness continuum.

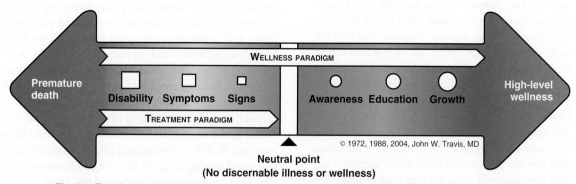

Fig. 8.4 The illness-wellness continuum—a holistic health model. (Copyright 2004 John W. Travis, MD.)

Defining Health

Health "is as hard to define as love or happiness, and even harder to trap and keep" (Zuger, 2008), yet many individuals and organizations have made attempts to define health. More than a half-century ago, WHO defined health as "a state of complete physical, mental, and social well-being and not merely the absence of disease or infirmity" (WHO, 1947, p. 29). This definition was the first official recognition of health as multidimensional. The WHO definition presented a holistic view of health that reflected the interplay among the psychological, social, spiritual, and physical aspects of human life.

A holistic view of health focuses on the interrelationship of all the parts that make up a whole person. Jan Christian Smuts (1926) first introduced the concept of holism in modern Western thought by emphasizing the harmony between people and nature. When health is considered holistically, individual health practices must be taken into account. Health practices are culturally determined and include nutritional habits, type and amount of exercise and rest, how one copes with stress, quality of interpersonal relationships, expression of spirituality, and numerous other lifestyle factors. As a profession, nurses embrace a holistic view of health.

Parsons (1959) defined health as an individual's optimum ability to perform his or her roles and tasks effectively. This definition focused on the roles individuals assume in life and the impact health or illness has on the fulfillment of those roles. A few examples of roles that are familiar may include the student role, the parent role, the provider role, and the friend role. One's health influences how well and the extent to which people carry out their roles in life.

Health has been described as the opposite of illness (Dunn, 1959). In his classic text *High-Level Wellness,* Dunn (1961) described health as a continuum with high-level wellness at one end and death at the other. He described high-level wellness as functioning at maximum potential in an integrated way within the environment. An example of maximizing the potential for health under extreme conditions occurred in Chile, where miners were trapped deep in a collapsed mine for 70 days from August to October 2010. Believed to be dead for 17 days, the men were discovered alive by rescuers with a narrow-bore hole, which became the way that food, water, letters from families, Bibles, and other materials were delivered. Under horribly hot and dark conditions, these men supported each other, got exercise, and kept to a routine for more than 2 months as a rescue operation was implemented. The world celebrated as, one by one, they were brought to the surface, surprisingly vigorous and in good health. Only one miner, the oldest and who also had silicosis (lung fibrosis from inhaling silica dust), needed oxygen as he emerged. After short hospitalizations for observation, all the men returned to their families. Using Dunn's definition, and considering the environment in which these men were confined, they may have attained high-level wellness.

Pender and colleagues (2006) described health promotion as "approach behavior," whereas prevention is "avoidance behavior" (p. 5). This may be a useful concept for nurses to keep in mind when seeking to help patients expand their positive potential for health.

A National Health Initiative: *Healthy People*

Healthy People is a remarkable national initiative to improve the health of the nation. National objectives are introduced every 10 years, providing the agenda for improving the health of Americans. The *Healthy People* initiative was an unprecedented cooperative effort that grew out of the 1979 U.S. Surgeon General's report on health promotion and disease prevention titled *Healthy People.* That report laid the foundation for a national prevention agenda. Federal, state, and territorial governments, as well as hundreds of private, public, and not-for-profit organizations and concerned individuals, worked together for the first time ever. These partnerships resulted in *Healthy People 2000,* an effort designed to stimulate a national disease prevention and health promotion agenda to improve significantly the health of all Americans in the last decade of the 20th century. On September 6, 1990, former U.S. Secretary of Health and Human Services Louis W. Sullivan released a report to the United States titled *Healthy People 2000.* He reported that progress on priority areas was mixed, but enough success was achieved to continue the project.

The third phase of the project, *Healthy People 2020,* was launched in December 2010. It was developed by the Healthy People Consortium, a huge alliance of national membership organizations and state health, mental health, substance abuse, and environmental agencies. *Healthy People 2020* addresses a set of forty-two topic areas that are significant to the health of the public.

Each topic area is assigned to one or more government agencies, which are responsible for developing, monitoring, and periodically reporting on progress toward objectives. The initiative has partners from all sectors (U.S. Department of Health and Human Services: Healthy People 2020, 2018). *Healthy People 2030* is currently being developed (U.S. Department of Health and Human Services: Planning for Healthy People 2030).

Healthy People offers a simple but powerful idea: provide health objectives in a format that enables diverse groups to combine their efforts and work as a team. It is a road map to better health for all and can be used by many different people, states, communities, professional organizations, and groups to improve health. Partners across groups are encouraged to integrate *Healthy People* objectives into their programs, special events, publications, and meetings. When federal, state, and local health entities combine their efforts, improvements in the health of citizens can be made. However, convincing individual Americans to change their lifestyles, even when doing so would result in improved health, remains a challenge. Changing health beliefs and health behaviors is a slow process. You can learn more about *Healthy People 2020* and *Healthy People 2030* online at https://www.healthypeople.gov/.

Another effort to improve health, the Institute for Alternative Futures, founded in 1977, has created the *Public Health 2030* project and published a report in 2014 with recommendations for making sure that public health agencies continue to fulfill their mission to protect the health of the public. Challenges to public health include chronic disease and obesity, climate change, and cuts in spending at the state and federal levels. This report notes that 70% of the variance in individuals' health is explained by socioeconomic and environmental determinants, whereas only 15% to 20% of longevity can be attributed to clinical care. This report makes a compelling case for addressing other determinants of health than simply access to health care (Institute for Alternative Futures, 2014).

Health Beliefs and Health Behaviors

Health is affected by health beliefs and health behaviors. Health behaviors include those choices and habitual actions that promote or diminish health, such as eating habits, frequency of exercise, use of tobacco products and alcohol, sexual practices, and adequacy of rest and sleep (Fig. 8.5). Much is known about health-promoting

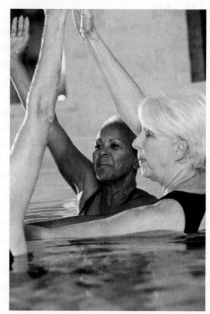

Fig. 8.5 People of all ages are recognizing the benefits of regular exercise. (Photo used with permission from iStockphoto.)

behaviors, and this information has been available to the public for many years. Yet people do not easily change behaviors even when they know they should. Several theories help explain why people change their health behaviors—or why they do not.

Health Beliefs Model

Rosenstock (1966, 1990) was one of the first scholars interested in determining why some people change their health behaviors whereas others do not. For example, when the surgeon general's report on smoking first came out in 1960, some people immediately quit smoking. Over the years, evidence condemning smoking has accumulated and been widely communicated, yet many intelligent people still smoke. Rosenstock wondered why. He formulated a model of health beliefs that illustrates how people behave in relationship to health maintenance activities and has worked to refine it for three decades. Rosenstock's health beliefs model included three components:

1. An evaluation of one's vulnerability to a condition and the seriousness of that condition
2. An evaluation of how effective the health maintenance behavior might be
3. The presence of a trigger event that precipitates the health maintenance behavior

Using Rosenstock's health beliefs model, smokers choose to participate in a stop-smoking program depending on their perception of smoking-related heart disease and their personal susceptibility to it. If, because of family history, they believe that they are susceptible to heart disease and that it may cause premature death, and if they believe that not smoking will substantially reduce that risk, they are likely to participate in the program. If, however, the stop-smoking program is at an inconvenient location, scheduled at an inconvenient time, or not affordable, they are less likely to participate. If a sibling who also smokes has a massive heart attack, they may be motivated to attend the stop-smoking program despite the inconvenience and cost. The illness of their sibling is what Rosenstock called *a cue to action*, or a trigger event. A trigger event propels a previously unmotivated individual into changing health behaviors.

Self-Efficacy and Health-Related Behaviors

Albert Bandura (1997), a cognitive psychologist, developed an approach designed to assist people to exercise influence over their own health-related behaviors. He observed that whether people considered altering detrimental health habits depended on their belief in themselves as having the ability to modify their own behavior. He labeled this belief "perceived self-efficacy." High belief in one's self-efficacy leads to efforts to change, whereas low perceived self-efficacy leads to a fatalistic lack of change.

Bandura identified four components needed for an effective program of lifestyle change: information, skill development, skill enhancement through guided practice and feedback, and creating social supports for change (Bandura, 1992). Using Bandura's model, a man wishing to stop smoking needs knowledge of the potential dangers of smoking; guidance on how to translate concern into action; extensive practice and opportunities to perfect new, nonsmoking skills; and strong involvement in a social network supportive of nonsmoking.

Locus of Control and Health-Related Behaviors

The locus of control concept proposed that people tend to be influenced by either an internal or external view of control. People who believe that their health is internally controlled—that is, by what they themselves do—are said to have an internal locus of control. Those who believe their health is determined by outside factors or chance are said to have an external locus of control. A number of

studies have hypothesized that internally controlled people tend to see themselves as responsible for their own health status and are therefore more amenable to change. Research findings have been inconsistent, however.

Nurses and Health Beliefs Models

Many other models of health beliefs and health behaviors exist, ranging from simple to complex. Identifying the key to motivating people to improve their health choices and behaviors remains a mystery. No single theory of behavior has yet fully explained the way people make decisions about their own health, nor is a single theory likely to. However, nurses should recognize the following:

- Health is relative, constantly changing, and affected by genetics, environment, behaviors, personal beliefs, and cultural beliefs.
- Health affects the entire person—physically, socially, psychologically, and spiritually.
- Individuals' health beliefs are powerful and influence how they respond to efforts to change their health behaviors.
- Individuals needing or desiring change may lack knowledge, motivation, sense of self-efficacy, and support to implement change.
- Increased knowledge does not always help change health behavior, which may persist in spite of increased knowledge.
- Various models of health beliefs can be used to assess individual, family, and group readiness to change.
- Change is often incremental and usually very slow. Multiple interventions may be necessary to bring about behavior change, and even then only modest changes may result.
- Patients, health care providers, and population-focused entities such as public health programs mutually share the burden of action.

"Dr. Google" and the Influence of the Internet

In early 2012 the Canadian newspaper *Edmonton Journal* ran a headline that read: "Dr. Google not always best source, Edmonton parents advised" (Withey, 2012). This newspaper feature described the challenges of sorting through the numerous studies and health information "floating around" on the Internet. One mother cited in this article bemoaned the amount of health information and opinions available online, describing it as "crippling."

In 2017 more than 4.1 billion people—54.4% of the world's population—were Internet users; in the United States alone, 345 million people were Internet users—more than 95% of the population (Internet World Stats, 2018). Virtually every aspect of life has a presence on the Internet. People shop; make travel and restaurant reservations; and check out and download music, movies, and books. Social media dominates the Internet to the extent that "friend" and, occasionally, "unfriend" are commonly understood as verbs. In addition, the venerable *Oxford Dictionary* has added words such as "listicle," "hyper-connected," "binge-watch," and "tech-savvy" that reflect the language that has sprung up around digital technology and viewing habits (OxfordDictionaries.com, 2018).

With tens of thousands of health information websites and social media platforms where individuals post their own health experiences and opinions with just a few clicks, Americans have access to more information than has ever before been available to consumers. With this additional information, patients are demanding to be equal partners in making health care decisions once decided only by the professionals they consulted. Health care providers encounter patients every day who come to appointments with printed results of online research and advice or with links or apps on smartphones, and which include widely divergent information that can be hard for patients to decipher. Some of it is excellent; some is, at best, worthless; some is reckless; and some is dangerous.

"Cyberchondria" is a new word that some use to refer to the propensity of certain people to believe that they suffer from a variety of diseases they read about on the Internet, a form of hypochondria. *Cyberchondria* literally means "online concern about health" and may not necessarily be a negative phenomenon if the use of the Internet does not result in an escalation of anxiety or stress. Box 8.2 contains some information to improve the likelihood of obtaining valid health information from online sources.

Nurses can help their patients determine which sites are useful and provide sound information and

---

BOX 8.2   Assessing Health-Related Sites on the Internet

- Determine who sponsors the site. This should be disclosed on the site itself.
- Be skeptical. Evaluate the source to determine whether there is self-interest on the part of the sponsor. Example: a drug company promoting one of its products.
- Make sure the author's name is clearly indicated, including credentials. Is the author qualified on this topic? For whom does the author work?
- What is the purpose of the site—to inform or to sell something? This is a very important distinction to make.
- Does the site include a date and information about its last revision?
- Is there editorial review of the content by a reputable authority or professional peers?
- Does the material consist of scientific information rather than testimonials?
- Determine who operates the website. University, government, and reputable medical organization sites may be more objective and less commercial than those run by companies or individuals trying to make a profit.
- Is the information unbiased, and are you referred to other sources that can validate it?

- For chat rooms and message boards, go online and "lurk" before getting involved. Monitor conversations and read posts before deciding whether you want to participate.
- Determine whether the group has a moderator who controls those who monopolize the site or make commercial pitches. A moderated board will usually monitor inappropriate behavior and offensive language.
- For interactive sites, be sure to read and understand the privacy policy.
- Until you are confident about the quality of information, cross-check it with print and electronic sources, and discuss it with your health care provider.
- Use the U.S. Department of Health and Human Services' Healthfinder site to find online support groups (www.healthfinder.gov). Note that the .gov indicates a site operated by the government. Its content is typically of high quality.
- Be highly suspicious of reports of "miracle" cures. Rumors and unsupported claims are rampant on the Internet and can cause tremendous harm. Remember that a claim that is too good to be true usually is.

Adapted from Chase M: Health journal: a guide for patients who turn to the Web for solace and support, *Wall Street Journal,* Sept. 17, 1999, p. B1; Beyea SC: Evaluating evidence found on the Internet, *AORN J* 72 (5):906–910, 2000; and Ahmann E: Supporting families' savvy use of the Internet for health research, *Pediatr Nurs* 26 (4):419–423, 2000.

safe advice. Sharing legitimate websites and guidelines for assessing the quality of information is a way to help patients become better consumers of online health data. This means that nurses themselves must be knowledgeable and stay up-to-date on both helpful and unhelpful websites specific to their practice setting and patient population. Nurses also should be supportive of patients when they question traditional advice, citing the Internet as their source. This means that they have an interest in their health and are asserting their autonomy in managing at least some aspects of their own care. These conversations are opportunities to correct misinformation, if needed, and you may even learn something yourself. Visit Evolve for WebLinks related to the content of this chapter (http://evolve.elsevier.com/Black/professional).

Devising a Personal Plan for High-Level Wellness

Each individual nurse has a personal definition of health, certain health beliefs, and individual health behaviors. How nurses view health behaviors in their own lives affects nursing practice, both directly and indirectly. The personal health practices of nurses play a direct role in their effectiveness in counseling patients on health-related matters. Patients are more likely to adopt health-related behaviors such as exercising regularly and maintaining a healthy weight when the caregiver promoting these behaviors also engages in them. Yet nurses' own health behaviors are far from exemplary. In fact, in 2008 one study reported that in a sample of 760 nurses across six regions in the United States, 54% self-reported as being overweight or obese, and 76% do not talk about weight management with their patients (Miller et al., 2008).

Nurses have a professional responsibility to model positive health behaviors in their own lives and, like everyone, have a personal responsibility to take care of their health to the best of their ability. The American Nurses Association (ANA) has a *Healthy Nurse, Healthy Nation Grand Challenge* (https://www.nursingworld.org/practice-policy/work-environment/health-safety/healthy-nurse-healthy-nation/) that encourages nurses to identify and act on personal and workplace health risks (ANA, 2018). Being or becoming a healthy role model may require some effort. If you are not the positive role model for health that you would like to be, Box 8.3 can help you get started.

BOX 8.3 Self-Assessment: Developing a Personal Plan for High-Level Wellness

Nurses' personal health behaviors send a powerful message to consumers of nursing care. Are you in a position to demonstrate that you practice what you preach? By answering the following questions, you can assess how well you are meeting your responsibilities in this area of nursing.

1. I weigh no more than 10 pounds over or under my ideal weight.
   T F
2. I eat a balanced diet, including breakfast, each day.
   T F
3. Of the total calories in my diet, less than 30% come from fat.
   T F
4. I exercise aerobically at least three times each week.
   T F
5. I get at least 7 hours of sleep each night.
   T F
6. I do not smoke or use any other form of tobacco.
   T F
7. I use alcohol in moderation (or not at all) and take mood-altering medication only when prescribed by my physician.
   T F
8. I identify and control the sources of stress in my life.
   T F
9. I have a balanced lifestyle, with work and diversional activities both playing important roles.
   T F
10. I have friends, neighbors, and/or family members who are sources of social support for me.
    T F
11. I practice responsible sex.
    T F

Directions for scoring: If you could not honestly answer "True" to all 11 questions, you need to set goals to enable you to do so.
1. On a piece of paper, begin your personal plan for high-level wellness. Write down at least two things you can do to address each "False" answer you gave to the self-assessment questions.
2. Share your health goals with one other person in your class. Make a contract with that person to serve as your "health coach."
3. Review your progress with your health coach at least once a week for the remainder of the term.
4. Begin your quest for high-level wellness today!

NURSING: FORMING THE MEANINGFUL WHOLE

Nursing integrates concepts from person, environment, and health to form a meaningful whole. See Fig. 8.1 for a depiction of the relationships among nursing's major concepts and how they overlap. This overlap creates nursing's sphere of interest and influence. This is termed the *holistic approach* to nursing.

Holistic Nursing

Holistic nursing care nourishes the whole person—that is, the body, mind, and spirit. Not surprisingly, the root for *nurse* and *nurture* is the same Latin word, *nutrire*, which means "to nourish." Eight factors contribute to a holistic approach to nursing:

1. Nursing is an example of an open system that freely interacts with, influences, and is influenced by external and internal forces.
2. Nursing is the provision of health care services that focuses on assisting people in maintaining health, avoiding or minimizing disease and disability, restoring wellness, or achieving a peaceful death.
3. Nursing involves collaborating with patients and their families to help them cope with and adapt to situations of disequilibrium in an effort to regain homeostasis.
4. Nursing is integrally involved with people at points along the health-illness continuum.
5. Nursing care is provided regardless of diagnosis, individual differences, age, beliefs, gender, sexual orientation, or other factors. As a profession, nursing supports the value, dignity, and uniqueness of every person and takes his or her culture and belief system into consideration.
6. Nurses require advanced knowledge and skills; they also must care about their patients.
7. Nursing requires concern, compassion, respect, and warmth, as well as comprehensive, individualized planning of care, to facilitate patients' growth toward wellness.
8. Nursing links theory and research in an effort to answer difficult questions generated during nursing practice.

With an understanding of nursing's major concepts as a backdrop, it is important to examine the relationship of nurses' attitudes, beliefs, values, and philosophies to the way they practice. It is also useful for readers to explore philosophies of nursing developed by individuals, by divisions of nursing in hospitals, and by schools of nursing; and for readers to begin to develop their own philosophies of nursing.

BELIEFS: GUIDING NURSING BEHAVIORS

Certain beliefs have evolved during the development of professional nursing. Specific statements of beliefs have been published for more than half a century. The most recent code was generated by the members of the ANA and published in the *Code of Ethics for Nurses with Interpretive Statements* (ANA, 2015). Statements such as the *Code* exist to affirm the beliefs of the profession and to guide the practice of nursing.

A **belief** represents the intellectual acceptance of something as true or correct. Beliefs can also be described as convictions. Groupings of beliefs form codes and creeds. Beliefs are opinions that may be, in reality, true or false. They are based on attitudes that have been acquired and verified by experience. Beliefs are generally transmitted from generation to generation, are stable, and are resistant to change.

Beliefs are organized into **belief systems** that serve to guide thinking and decision making. Individuals are not necessarily aware of how their beliefs interrelate or how their beliefs affect their behavior.

Although all people have beliefs, relatively few have spent much time examining their beliefs. In nursing, it is important to know and understand one's beliefs, because the practice of nursing often challenges a nurse's beliefs. Although this conflict may create temporary discomfort, it is ultimately good because it forces nurses to consider their beliefs carefully. They have to answer the question: "Is this something I really believe, or have I accepted it because some influential person [such as a parent or teacher] said it?" Reproductive choice and abortion, advance directives, the right to die, the right to refuse treatment, and similar issues confront all members of contemporary society. Professional nurses must develop and refine their beliefs about these and many other issues. This is often difficult to do, but the self-awareness that follows grappling with your beliefs helps you to identify when your own opinions may be influencing the way you view a patient's situation rather than accepting the patient's point of view.

Beliefs are exhibited through attitudes and behaviors. Simply observing how nurses relate to patients, their

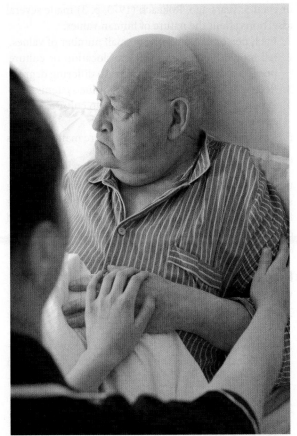

Fig. 8.6 Professional nurses maintain a posture of acceptance and calm, even when patients appear to be angry or upset. This man may simply be very sad or anxious. (Photo used with permission from iStockphoto.)

families, and nursing peers reveals something about those nurses' beliefs. Every day nurses meet people whose beliefs are different from, or even diametrically opposed to, their own. Effective nurses recognize that they need to adopt nonjudgmental attitudes toward patients' beliefs. A nurse with a **nonjudgmental** attitude makes every effort to convey neither approval nor disapproval of patients' beliefs and respects each person's right to his or her beliefs (Fig. 8.6).

An example of differences in beliefs that directly affect nursing is the position taken by some religious groups that all healing should be left to a divine power. For members of such groups, seeking medical treatment, even lifesaving measures such as blood transfusions, insulin for diabetes, or chemotherapy for cancer, is not condoned. From time to time, there have been

news reports of parents who are charged with criminal acts because they did not take a sick child to a physician. According to the advocacy group Children's Healthcare Is a Legal Duty (CHILD), about 300 children have died in this country over the past 25 years after parents withheld medical care because of religious beliefs (Johnson, 2009). After an 11-year-old girl died of untreated diabetic ketoacidosis in Wisconsin (Sataline, 2008), her parents were charged with reckless endangerment despite their claim that the charges violated their constitutional right to religious freedom. In October 2009, both parents were convicted of second-degree reckless homicide, sentenced to 10 years of probation, and ordered to spend 30 days in jail in each of the first 6 years of probation (Fitzsimmons, 2009). Currently a rancorous debate related to childhood vaccinations has been featured in the media, with individuals on both sides of the issue having strong opinions and beliefs. Issues such as this have an impact on patients, families, health care providers, public health authorities, and the court system and often create a frenzy of media coverage.

By virtue of the fact that you are becoming a nurse, you have some set of beliefs about the value of health care. Think about your beliefs about issues related to blood administration, vaccines, and/or parental decisions regarding seeking or avoiding health care institutions. What feelings might you have if assigned to work with a family whose beliefs differ from yours? Even in your imagination, you may be able to see how difficult it can be to maintain a nonjudgmental attitude toward the beliefs of patients.

Three Categories of Beliefs

People often use the words *beliefs* and *values* interchangeably. Even experts disagree about whether they differ or are the same. Although they are related, beliefs and values are differentiated in this chapter and discussed separately.

Theorists studying belief systems have identified three main categories of beliefs:
1. Descriptive or existential beliefs are those that can be shown to be true or false. An example of a descriptive belief is "The sun will come up tomorrow morning."
2. Evaluative beliefs are those in which there is a judgment about good or bad. The belief "Advanced life support for a 90-year-old is immoral" is an example of an evaluative belief.

3. Prescriptive (encouraged) and proscriptive (prohibited) beliefs are those in which certain actions are judged to be desirable or undesirable. The belief "Every citizen of voting age should vote in every election" is a prescriptive belief, whereas the belief "People should not have sex outside of marriage" is a proscriptive belief. These two types of beliefs are closely related to values.

VALUES

Values are the freely chosen principles, ideals, or standards held by an individual, class, or group that give meaning and direction to life. A value is an abstract representation of what is right, worthwhile, or desirable. Values define ideal modes of conduct and reflect what the individual or group endorses and tries to emulate. Values, like beliefs, are relatively stable and resistant to change.

Although many people are unaware of it, values help them make small day-to-day choices, as well as important life decisions. Just as beliefs influence nursing practice, values also influence how nurses practice their profession, often without their conscious awareness. Diann B. Uustal, EdD, RN, is a prominent contemporary nurse who has written and spoken extensively about values and ethics. Dr. Uustal noted in her early work, "Everything we do, every decision we make and course of action we take is based on our consciously and unconsciously chosen beliefs, attitudes and values" (Uustal, 1985, p. 100). Uustal also asserted, "Nursing is a behavioral manifestation of the nurse's value system. It is not merely a career, a job, an assignment; it is a ministry" (Uustal, 1993, p. 10). She wrote that nurses must give "caring attentiveness and presence" to their patients and that to do otherwise "is equivalent to psychological and spiritual abandonment" (Uustal, 1993, p. 10). Notably, Dr. Uustal has survived two severe accidents that left her in pain every day; however, she is now a triathlon coach and world record setter in swimming for her age group. She is also the 2013 winner of the Growing Bolder Inspiration Award (Growing Bolder: Rebranding Aging, 2018).

Nature of Human Values

Values evolve as people mature. An individual's values today are undoubtedly different from those of 10,

or even 5, years ago. Rokeach (1973, p. 3) made several assertions about the nature of human values:

1. Each person has a relatively small number of values.
2. All human beings, regardless of location or culture, possess basically the same values to differing degrees.
3. People organize their values into value systems.
4. People develop values in response to culture, society, and even individual personality traits.
5. Most observable human behaviors are manifestations or consequences of human values.

Values influence behavior; people with unclear values may lack direction, persistence, and decision-making skills. Professional nurses must have clear values because the work of nursing requires direction, persistence, and excellent decision-making skills. A number of professional nursing values are listed in Box 8.4.

Process of Valuing

Valuing is the process by which values are determined. There are three identified steps in the process of valuing: choosing, prizing, and acting.

1. *Choosing* is the cognitive (intellectual) aspect of valuing. Ideally, people choose their values freely from all alternatives after considering the possible consequences of their choices.
2. *Prizing* is the affective (emotional) aspect of valuing. People usually feel good about their values and cherish the choices they make.
3. *Acting* is the kinesthetic (behavioral) aspect of valuing. When people affirm their values publicly by acting on their choices, they make their values part of their behavior. A real value is acted on consistently in behavior.

All three steps must be taken, or the process of valuing is incomplete (Uustal, 2009). For example, a professional nurse might believe that learning is a lifelong process and that nurses have an obligation to keep up with new developments in the profession. This nurse would choose to take continuing education beyond the minimum required for relicensure and appreciate the consequences of the choice. He or she might even publicly affirm this choice and feel good about it. If the nurse follows through consistently with behaviors such as reading journals, attending conferences, and seeking out other learning opportunities, continuing to learn can be seen as a true value in his or her life.

BOX 8.4 Professional Nursing Values

- Accountability and responsibility for own actions
- Altruism
- Balancing cure and care
- Benevolence
- Caring as a foundation for relationships
- Collaborative multidisciplinary practice
- Compassion
- Competence
- Concern
- Continuous improvement of service
- Cooperative work relationships
- Courage
- Dependability
- Empathy
- Ethical conduct
- Flexibility
- Focus on patient-defined quality of life
- Health promotion
- Holistic, person-centered care
- Honesty and authenticity in communication
- Humaneness
- Humility
- Illness prevention
- Individualized patient care
- Integrity—personal and professional
- Involvement with families
- Kindness
- Knowledge
- Listening attentively
- Nonjudgmental attitude
- Objectivity
- Openness to learning
- Partnerships with patients
- Patient advocacy
- Patient education
- Presence (being fully present)
- Promotion of health
- Promotion of patient self-determination and patient preferences
- Providing care regardless of patient's ability to pay
- Quality care—physical, emotional, spiritual, social, intellectual
- Reliability
- Respect for each person's dignity and worth
- Responsibility
- Responsiveness
- Sensitivity
- Sharing decision making
- Sharing self through nursing interventions
- Stewardship; responsible use of resources
- Subordination of self-interest
- Support of fellow nurses
- Teamwork
- Trust in self, others, and the institution

Courtesy Diann B. Uustal, personal communication, 2006.

Values Clarification

Nurses, as well as people in other helping professions, need to understand their values. This is the first step in self-awareness, which is important in maintaining a nonjudgmental approach to patients.

Considering your reactions to the following statements can help in beginning to identify some nursing values you hold:

1. Patients should always be told the truth about their diagnoses.
2. Nurses, if asked, should assist terminally ill patients to die.
3. Severely impaired infants should be kept alive, regardless of their future quality of life.
4. Nurses should never accept gifts from patients.
5. A college professor should receive a heart transplant before a homeless person does.
6. Nurses should be role models of healthy behavior.

As you react both emotionally and intellectually to these statements, something about your personal and professional values is revealed. Determining where you stand on these and other nursing issues is an important step in clarifying your values. A variety of values clarification exercises have been developed to stimulate self-reflection and help people understand their values. Box 8.5 contains a values clarification exercise you may want to complete to assist you further in understanding the valuing process.

Values Undergirding *Nursing's Social Policy Statement*

Professional groups, such as nursing, have a collective identity that is fostered by professional organizations. The ANA sets forth the values that undergird the

BOX 8.5   Clarifying Your Values

Once you have identified a value, it is important to assess its significance to you and to clarify your willingness to act on the value. The following clarifying questions are organized based on the steps of the valuing process and can help you answer questions about what you value. First, identify a value (or values) that is (are) important to you. Write your value(s) below:

_____

_____

_____

_____

   Next, use the questions below to assess the importance of a belief or attitude and to determine whether it is a value. Rephrase the questions to suit your own style of conversation.

Choosing Freely
1. Am I sure I have thought about this value and chosen to believe it myself?
2. Who first taught me this value?
3. How do I know I am "right"?

Choosing Among Alternatives
1. What other alternatives are possible?
2. Which alternative has the most appeal for me and why?
3. Have I thought much about this value/alternative?

Choosing After Considering the Consequences
1. What consequences do I think might occur as a result of my holding this value?

2. What "price" will I pay for my position?
3. Is this value worth the "price" I might pay?

Complement to Other Values
1. Does this value "fit" with my other values, and is it consistent with them?
2. Am I sure this value does not conflict with other values I deem important to me?

Prize and Cherish
1. Am I proud of my position and value? Is this something I feel good about?
2. How important is this value to me?
3. If this were not one of my values, how different would my life be?

Public Affirmation
1. Am I willing to speak out for this value?

Action
1. Am I willing to put this value into action?
2. Do I act on this value? When? How consistently?
3. Is this a value that can guide me in other situations?
4. Would I want others who are important to me to follow this value?
5. Do I think I will always believe this? How committed to this value am I?
6. Am I willing to do anything about this value?
7. How do I know this value is "right"? Are my values ethical?

From Uustal DB: *Clinical ethics and values: issues and insights in a changing healthcare environment*, East Greenwich, RI, 1993, Educational Resources in Healthcare. Reprinted with permission.

profession through the document *Nursing's Social Policy Statement: The Essence of the Profession*, last revised in 2010 (ANA, 2010). This document is published from time to time and is designed to serve as a resource for nurses in various practice settings, in education, and in research. It guides nursing practice and informs others, including the public, about nursing's social responsibility. The social policy statement sets forth several underlying values and assumptions on which the statement is based:

- Humans manifest an essential unity of mind, body, and spirit.
- Human experience is contextually and culturally defined.
- Health and illness are human experiences. The presence of illness does not preclude health, nor does optimal health preclude illness.

- The interaction between the nurse and patient occurs within the context of the values and beliefs of the patient and the nurse.
- Public policy and the health care delivery system influence the health and well-being of society and professional nursing.

   Chapter 7 contains more about values and their relationship to nursing practice.

PHILOSOPHIES AND THEIR RELATIONSHIP TO NURSING CARE

Philosophy is defined as the study of the principles underlying conduct, thought, and the nature of the universe. A simple explanation of philosophy is that it entails a search for meaning in the universe. You may have learned about philosophers such as Plato, Aristotle, Hypatia, Bacon, Kant, Hegel, Kierkegaard, Nietzsche, Descartes, Arendt, and others in general education courses. These philosophers were searching for the underlying principles of reality and truth. Nursing philosophies and theories often derive from or build on the concepts identified by these and other philosophers.

Philosophy begins when someone contemplates, or wonders about, something. If a group of friends sometimes sits and discusses the relationship between men and women and ponders the differences in men's and women's natures and approaches to life, one might say that they were developing a philosophy about male and female ways of being. It is important to remember that philosophy is not the exclusive domain of a few individuals identified as "philosophers"; everyone has a personal philosophy of life that is unique.

People develop personal philosophies as they mature, usually without being aware of it. These philosophies serve as blueprints or guides and incorporate each individual's value and belief systems. Nurses' personal philosophies interact directly with their philosophies of nursing and influence professional behaviors.

Branches of Philosophy

Before examining professional philosophies, consider the discipline of philosophy itself. Philosophy has been divided into specific areas of study. This section reviews six branches: epistemology, logic, aesthetics, ethics, politics, and metaphysics.

1. **Epistemology** is the branch of philosophy dealing with the theory of knowledge itself. The epistemologist attempts to answer such questions as "What can be known?" and "What constitutes knowledge?" Epistemology attempts to determine how we can know whether our beliefs about the world are true.
2. **Logic** is the study of proper and improper methods of reasoning. In logic, the nature of reasoning itself is the subject. Logic attempts to answer the question, "What should our thinking methods be in order to reach true conclusions?" Chapter 11 presents a method of logical thinking that nurses use to plan and implement effective patient care, called *the nursing process.*
3. **Aesthetics** is the study of what is beautiful. It attempts to answer the question, "Why do we find things beautiful?" Painting, sculpture, music, dance, and literature are all associated with beauty. Judgments about what is beautiful, however, differ from individual to

individual and culture to culture. For example, Eastern music may be difficult to appreciate by Western listeners and vice versa.
4. **Ethics** is the branch of philosophy that studies standards of conduct. It attempts to answer the question, "What is the nature of good and evil?" Moral principles and values make up a system of ethics. Behavior depends on moral principles and values. Ethics, therefore, underlies the standards of behavior that govern us as individuals and as nurses. **Bioethics** is a term describing the branch of ethics that deals with biologic issues. Bioethics and nursing ethics are complex areas of study that are explored in Chapter 7.
5. **Politics,** in the context of a discussion of philosophy, means the area of philosophy that deals with the regulation and control of people living in society. Political philosophers study the conditions of society and suggest recommendations for improving these conditions. They work to answer the question, "What makes good governments?"
6. **Metaphysics** is the consideration of the ultimate nature of existence, reality, human experience, and the universe. Metaphysicians believe that through contemplation we can come to a more complete understanding of reality than science alone can provide. They ask the question "What is the meaning of life?" and explore the fundamental nature of all reality.

Philosophies of Nursing

Philosophies of nursing are statements of beliefs about nursing and expressions of values in nursing that are used as bases for thinking and acting. Most philosophies of nursing are built on a foundation of beliefs about people, environment, health, and nursing. Each of these four foundational concepts of nursing is discussed in some detail earlier in this chapter.

Individual Philosophies

If asked, most nurses could list their beliefs about nursing, but it is doubtful that many have written a formal philosophy of nursing. They are influenced daily, however, by their unwritten, informal philosophies. It is useful to go through the process of writing down one's own professional philosophy and revising it from time to time. Comparing recent and earlier versions can reveal professional and personal growth over time. It is also helpful to read one's philosophy of nursing from time to time to make sure daily behaviors are consistent with

---

BOX 8.6   Developing Your Own Philosophy of Nursing

This is an example of one nurse's philosophy of nursing. Read it carefully, and then use the following guide to develop your own philosophy.

- I believe that the essence of nursing is caring about and caring for human beings who are unable to care for themselves. I believe that the central core of nursing is the nurse-patient relationship and that through that relationship I can make a difference in the lives of others at a time when they are most vulnerable.
- Human beings generally do the best they can. When they are uncooperative, critical, or otherwise unpleasant, it is usually because they are frightened; therefore I will remain pleasant and nondefensive and try to understand the patient's perception of the situation. I pledge to be trustworthy and an advocate for my patients.
- I realize that my cultural background affects how I deliver nursing care and that my patients' cultural backgrounds affect how they receive my care. I try to learn as much as I can about each individual's cultural beliefs and preferences and individualize care accordingly.
- My vision for myself as a nurse is that I will provide the best care I can to all patients, regardless of their financial situation, social status, lifestyle choices, or spiritual beliefs. I will collaborate with my patients, their families, and my health care colleagues and work cooperatively with them, valuing and respecting what each brings to the situation.
- I am individually accountable for the care I provide, for what I fail to do and to know. Therefore I pledge to remain a learner all my life and actively seek opportunities to learn how to be a more effective nurse.

- I will strive for a balance of personal and professional responsibilities. This means I will take care of myself physically, emotionally, socially, and spiritually so I can continue to be a productive caregiver.

Use This Guide to Write Your Own Your Philosophy of Nursing

Purpose: To write a beginning philosophy of nursing that reflects the beliefs and values of _____

_____

_____ [your name and date]

I chose nursing as my profession because nursing is ____

_____.

I believe that the core of nursing is _____

_____.

I believe that the focus of nursing is _____

_____.

My vision for myself as a nurse is that I will _____

_____.

To live out my philosophy of nursing, every day I must remember this about:

My patients: _____

_____

My patients' families: _____

_____

My fellow health care professionals: _____

_____

My own health: _____

_____

---

deeply held beliefs. Box 8.6 contains one nurse's philosophy of nursing and contains a guide for you to develop your own philosophy.

Collective Philosophies

Although few individuals write down their nursing philosophies, it is common for hospitals and schools of nursing to express their collective beliefs about nursing in written philosophies. In fact, both hospitals and schools of nursing are required by their accrediting bodies to develop statements of philosophy. Philosophical statements should be relevant to the setting. They are intended to guide the practice of nurses employed in that setting. Examining some of these statements clarifies what constitutes a collective philosophy of nursing.

Philosophy of nursing in a hospital setting or school of nursing. When considering applying for a professional nursing position in a hospital or health care agency, it is a good idea to ask for a copy of the philosophy of nursing of that institution or to find it online. Read it carefully, and make sure you accept the beliefs and values it contains, because they will influence nursing care in that setting.

An important point about philosophies of nursing is that they are dynamic; they change over time. When a collective philosophy is written, it reflects the existing values and beliefs of the particular group of people who wrote it. When the group members change, the philosophy may also change. Therefore, once a collective philosophy is written, it should be "revisited" regularly and modified to reflect accurately the group's current beliefs about nursing practice.

DEVELOPING A PERSONAL PHILOSOPHY OF NURSING

Your philosophy of life, whether or not you can articulate it, is the basis of your day-to-day behavior. It consists of the principles that underlie your thinking and conduct. Developing a philosophy of nursing is not merely an academic exercise required by accrediting bodies.

Having a written philosophy can help guide nurses in the daily decisions they must make in nursing practice.

Writing a philosophy is not a complex, time-consuming task—it simply requires that you write down your beliefs and values about nursing, answering the questions: "What is nursing?" and "Why do I practice nursing the way I do?" Whether individual or collective, a philosophy should provide direction and promote effectiveness.

CONCEPTS AND CHALLENGES

- *Concept:* Knowledge of systems and human motivation can be used to understand nursing's major concepts. Persons are unique open systems who are motivated by needs.

    Challenge: Maslow's hierarchy of needs consists of five levels that range from basic physiologic needs, which are common to all people, to self-actualization, which is attained by few. This is a useful framework to understand human motivation.

- *Concept:* Environment consists of all the circumstances, influences, and conditions that affect an individual. The physical environment and family, cultural, social, and community systems all affect one's health.

    Challenge: In addition to understanding the effects of the environment on an individual's health, nurses recognize that health affects the way one interacts with his or her environment.

- *Concept:* The Internet has become a significant source of health information, the quality of which varies widely.

- *Challenge:* In a respectful way and with appreciation for patients' desire to be involved in their own care,

nurses need to help patients filter useful from poor information they gather from websites.

- *Concept:* Nursing integrates person, environment, and health into a meaningful whole in an open system.

- *Challenge:* This holistic integration of person, environment, and health does not explain patients' health experiences but rather gives nurses a way of considering the wide variety of factors that affect persons' health at any one time.

- *Concept:* Beliefs and values influence how nurses practice their profession and form the basis of one's philosophy of nursing.

    Challenge: Identifying one's beliefs and values will help shape one's philosophy of nursing, which in turn shapes and guides practice.

- *Concept:* As they develop and progress professionally, nurses are likely to change their views about patients, care, and nursing, and their values and beliefs may change.

    Challenge: Philosophies are not static; they are changed and adapted as nurses mature and become more experienced.

IDEAS FOR FURTHER EXPLORATION

1. Consider your own family system. What are the family equivalents of inputs, throughputs, subsystems, suprasystems, outputs, evaluation, and feedback? Does your family tend to be an open or a closed system?

2. Describe Maslow's hierarchy of needs, and place yourself on the hierarchy today, on your first day of college, and when you were in middle school. Were you at a different level each time? Consider what factors—internal and external—may have been

involved in your placement at each of these times. If possible, compare and discuss your findings with at least one other person.

3. What are the factors that influence your personal health behaviors? Make a list of your health behaviors, including those that promote health and those that do not. Think about the reasons you continue both healthy and less-than-healthy behaviors. Identify factors that could influence you to make decisions that support good health.

4. Select a chronic or acute illness or health condition, and do an online search. Examine websites generated by your search, assessing them for accuracy and safety. What items on the site do you consider safe, and why? Why do you consider others as not safe?

5. Conduct an assessment of your community in terms of one of the following factors that affect health: availability of jobs, quality of public education, availability of health services, environmental hazards, and quality of air and water. What is the effect of this factor on the health of the community's citizens? What can you do to improve the health of your community?

6. Find out what your state and community are doing to link their health objectives to those of the *Healthy People* initiatives.

7. Name two of your health-related values. How did these become your values? Describe how you expect these values to influence your nursing practice.

8. Read "Developing Your Own Philosophy of Nursing" in Box 8.6. Then identify at least 10 of that nurse's professional values, using the list in Box 8.4, "Professional Nursing Values." Can you identify other values that are not listed?

9. Obtain the philosophy statement of the faculty of your school of nursing. What concepts are included? Which beliefs do you agree with and disagree with? (Your school may have a vision and mission statement rather than a philosophy. Although they are not usually as detailed, they can be useful in identifying a school's priorities.)

10. Using the work sheet in Box 8.6, write a beginning personal philosophy of nursing. Share your philosophy with one other person.

11. How does articulating one's philosophy of nursing influence a nurse's practice? What if a nurse has never thought about a philosophy?

REFERENCES

American Nurses Association (ANA): *Code of ethics for nurses with interpretive statements*, Washington, DC, 2015, American Nurses Publishing.

American Nurses Association (ANA): *Healthy Nurse, Healthy NationTM* (website). 2018. Available at: https://www.nursingworld.org/practice-policy/work-environment/health-safety/healthy-nurse-healthy-nation/.

American Nurses Association (ANA): *Nursing's social policy statement: the essence of the profession*, Washington, DC, 2010, American Nurses Publishing.

Bandura A: A social cognitive approach to the exercise of control over AIDS infection. In DiClemente RJ, editor: *Adolescents and AIDS: A Generation in Jeopardy*, Newbury Park, CA, 1992, Sage Publications.

Bandura A: *Self-Efficacy: Exercise of Control*, New York, 1997, WH Freeman.

Beyea SC: Evaluating evidence found on the Internet, *AORN J* 72(5):906–910, 2000.

Centers for Disease Control and Prevention (CDC): Births: final data for 2016, *CDC Natl Vital Stat Rep* 67(4), 2018.

Dunn HL: High-level wellness for man and society, *Am J Public Health* 49(6):786–792, 1959.

Dunn HL: *High-Level Wellness*, Thorofare, NJ, 1961, Slack.

Fitzsimmons EG: Wisconsin couple sentenced in death of their sick child, *New York Times*, Oct 7, 2009. A–16.

Growing Bolder: Rebranding aging. *Diann Uustal*, 2018 (website). 2018. Available at: www.growingbolder.com/diann-uustal-892799/.

Health Care Without Harm: *Mission* (website). 2018. Available at: https://noharm-uscanada.org/content/us-canada/mission-and-goals.

Hoffman E: The Maslow effect: a humanist legacy for nursing, *Am Nurs Today* 3(8):36–37, 2008.

Holmes TH, Rahe RH: The social readjustment rating scale, *J Psychosom Res* 11(2):213–218, 1967.

Institute for Alternative Futures: Public health 2030: a scenario exploration (website). 2014. Available at: http://www.altfutures.org/projects/public-health-2030/.

International Monetary Fund: World economic outlook database (website). April 2018. Available at: https://www.imf.org/external/pubs/ft/weo/2017/01/weodata/index.aspx.

Internet World Stats: Usage and population statistics: world internet usage and population statistics (website). 2018. Available at: https://www.internetworldstats.com/stats.htm.

Investopedia: The world's top 10 economies (website). 2017. Available at: https://www.investopedia.com/articles/investing/022415/worlds-top-10-economies.asp.

Johnson D: Trials for Parents Who Chose Faith Over Medicine, *New York Times*, 2009. A–23.

Maslow AH: *Motivation and Personality*, ed 3, New York, 1987, Harper & Row.

Miller MA, Rahe RH: Life changes scaling for the 1990s, *J Psychosom Res* 43(3):279–292, 1997.

Miller SK, Alpert PT, Cross CL: Overweight and obesity in nurses, advanced practiced nurses, and nurse educators, *J Am Acad Nurse Pract* 20(5):259–265, 2008.

OxfordDictionaries.com: *New words added to today include binge-watch, cray, and vape* (website). 2018. Available at: http://blog.oxforddictionaries.com/press-releases/new-words-added-oxforddictionaries-com-august-2014/.

Parsons T: Definitions of health and illness in light of American values and social structure. In Jaco EG, editor: *Patients, Physicians and Illness*, New York, 1959, Free Press, pp 165–187.

Pender NJ, Murdaugh C, Parsons MA: *Health Promotion in Nursing Practice*, ed 5, Upper Saddle River, NJ, 2006, Prentice-Hall Health.

Pew Research Center: Key finding about U.S. immigrants (website). 2017. Available at: http://www.pewresearch.org/fact-tank/2017/05/03/key-findings-about-u-s-immigrants/.

Rogers C: *On Becoming a Person*, Boston, 1961, Houghton Mifflin.

Rokeach M: *The nature of human values*, New York, 1973, Free Press.

Rosenstock IM: Why people use health services, part II, *Milbank Mem Fund Q* 44(3):94–124, 1966.

Rosenstock IM: The health belief model: explaining health behavior through expectancies. In Glans K, Lewis FM, Rimer BK, editors: *Health behavior and health education: theory, research, and practice*, San Francisco, 1990, Jossey-Bass, pp. 39–62.

Sataline S: A child's death and a crisis for faith, *Wall Street Jour*, June 12, 2008. D–1.

Smuts JC: *Holism and evolution*, New York, 1926, Macmillan.

UNESCO: *Learning to live together: multiculturalism* n.d. (website). Available at: http://www.unesco.org/new/en/social-and-human-sciences/themes/international-migration/glossary/multiculturalism/.

U.S. Census Bureau: The majority of children live with two parents, Census Bureau finds (website). 2016. Press Release Number: CB16–192. Available at: https://www.census.gov/newsroom/press-releases/2016/cb16-192.html.

U.S. Census Bureau: 2017 current population survey, annual social and economic supplement (CPS ASEC) (website). 2017. Available at: https://www.census.gov/search-results.html?q=poverty+status&page=1&stateGeo=none&searchtype=web&cssp=SERP.

U.S. Department of Health and Human Services: *Healthy People 2020* (website). 2018. Available at: https://www.healthypeople.gov/.

U.S. Department of Health and Human Services: *Planning for Healthy People 2030* (website). 2018. Available at: https://www.healthypeople.gov/2020/About-Healthy-People/Development-Healthy-People-2030.

U.S. Department of Health and Human Services: HHS poverty guidelines (website). 2018. Available at: https://aspe.hhs.gov/poverty-guidelines.

Uustal DB: *Caring for Yourself, Caring for Others: The Ultimate Balance*, ed 2, East Greenwich, RI, 2009, Educational Resources in Healthcare.

Uustal DB: *Clinical Ethics and Values: Issues and Insights in a Changing Healthcare Environment*, East Greenwich, RI, 1993, Educational Resources in Healthcare.

Uustal DB: *Values and Ethics in Nursing: From Theory to Practice*, East Greenwich, RI, 1985, Educational Resources in Nursing and Holistic Health.

von Bertalanffy L: *General Systems Theory: Foundations, Development, applications*, New York, 1968, George Braziller.

Waugh LJ: Beliefs associated with Mexican immigrant families' practice of La Cuarentena during postpartum recovery, *J Obstet Gynecol Neonat Nurs* 40:732–741, 2010.

Withey E: *Dr. Google Not Always Best Source, Edmonton Parents Advised, Edmonton J* (website). 2012. Available at: www.edmontonjournal.com/life/Google+always+best+source+Edmonton+parents+advised/6288462/story.html.

World Health Organization (WHO): *Constitution*, Geneva, 1947, World Health Organization.

World Health Organization (WHO): The determinants of health (website). 2018. Available at: http://www.who.int/hia/evidence/doh/en/.

World Health Organization (WHO): Water sanitation health (website). 2018. Available at: http://www.who.int/water_sanitation_health/facilities/waste/training_modules_waste_management/en/.

Zuger A: Healthy right up to the day you're not, *New York Times*, Sept 30, 2008. F–3.

9

Nursing Theory: The Basis for Professional Nursing

Anita Tesh, PhD, RN

To enhance your understanding of this chapter, try the Student Exercises on the Evolve site at http://evolve.elsevier.com/Black/professional.

LEARNING OUTCOMES

After studying this chapter, students will be able to:
- Define *philosophy, conceptual frameworks, theory,* and *middle-range theory.*
- Consider how selected nursing theoretical works guide the practice of nursing.

- Understand how nursing philosophy or theory shapes the curriculum in schools of nursing.
- Delineate the role of nursing theory for different levels of nursing education.
- Describe the function of nursing theory in research and practice.

Theory is a word often used in daily conversation, such as "I have a theory about that" or "In theory, this should work." The word *theory* in this context means the person has some idea about a phenomenon and the way this phenomenon works in the world. When people say, "I have a theory…" about a certain phenomenon or situation, they are demonstrating something about their own distinct orientation or way of seeing the world. The word *theory* is derived from the Latin and Greek word for "a viewing" or "contemplating."

Nursing as a profession has a distinct theoretical orientation to practice. This means that the practice of nursing is based on a specific body of knowledge built on theory. This body of knowledge shapes and is shaped by how nurses see the world. Parsons (1949) described theory as important because it makes a distinction between what we know and what we need to know. The word **theory** has many definitions, but generally it refers to a group of related concepts, definitions, and statements that describe a certain view of nursing

phenomena (observable occurrences) from which to describe, explain, or predict outcomes (Chinn and Kramer, 1998). Theories represent abstract ideas rather than concrete facts. New theories are always being generated, although some theories are useful for many years. When new knowledge becomes available, theories that are no longer useful are modified or discarded. You will be reading about Sister Callista Roy's adaptation model, one that has "stood the test of time" since the 1970s; its use expanded from its origins as a curriculum framework for bachelor of science in nursing (BSN) education to its current use as an organizing framework for nurses (Alligood, 2011).

So why is theory important? First, nursing as a profession is strengthened when nursing knowledge is built on sound theory. As seen in Chapter 3, one criterion for a profession is a distinct body of knowledge as the basis for practice. Nursing began its transition from a vocation to a profession and academic discipline in the 1950s (Bond et al., 2011). Nursing has knowledge distinct from, although related to, other disciplines such as medicine, social work, sociology, and physiology, among others. The development of nursing knowledge is the work of nurse researchers and scholars. The evolution of the profession of nursing depends on continued recognition of nursing as a scholarly academic discipline that contributes to society. In today's research environment where theory is developed and tested, interdisciplinary collaboration is now considered a critical approach to the development of knowledge. Use of nursing theory in other disciplines is not yet common, however (March and McCormack, 2009). Even in our own discipline, unfortunately, nursing theory is underused in supporting research. A recent study demonstrated that nursing theory was used infrequently in research published in nursing journals between 2002 and 2006: only 460 of 2184 research articles (21%) published in seven top nursing research journals used nursing theory (Bond et al., 2011).

Second, theory is a useful tool for reasoning, critical thinking, and decision making (Alligood, 2018). The ultimate goal of nursing theory is to support excellence in practice. Nursing practice settings are complex, and a large amount of information (data) about each patient is available to nurses. Nurses must analyze this information to make sound clinical judgments and to generate effective interventions. From organization of patient data to the development and evaluation of interventions, theory provides a guide for nurses in developing effective care. Box 9.1 shows how theory guides nursing practice.

Several words are used to describe abstract thoughts and their linkages. From the most to least abstract, these include *metaparadigm, philosophy, conceptual model* or *framework,* and *theory. Metaparadigm* refers to the most abstract aspect of the structure of nursing knowledge (March and McCormack, 2009). The **metaparadigm** of nursing consists of the major concepts of the discipline—person, environment, health, and nursing—discussed in Chapter 8 and will be addressed again in Chapter 11. In the past two decades, caring has been added as a major concept of the discipline central to nursing knowledge development and practice. Simply stated, these five concepts comprise the metaparadigm of nursing; that is, these are the **concepts** (abstract notions or ideas) of most importance to nursing practice and research. Nursing philosophies, models, and theories contain most or all of these concepts.

BOX 9.1 Nursing Theory and the Professional Nurse

Theory guides the professional nurse in:
1. Making sound clinical judgments based on evidence by
   a. Determining which data are important
   b. Organizing, analyzing, and understanding connections in patient data
2. Planning appropriate nursing interventions
3. Evaluating outcomes of interventions

A **philosophy** is a set of beliefs about the nature of how the world works. A nursing philosophy begins to put together some or all concepts of the metaparadigm. For instance, Florence Nightingale, whose work will be considered in more detail later in this chapter, wrote *Notes on Nursing: What It Is and What It Is Not,* in which her basic philosophy of nursing is described in detail. A **conceptual model** or **framework** is a more specific organization of nursing phenomena than philosophies. As the words *model* or *framework* imply, models provide an organizational structure that makes clearer connections between concepts.

Theories are more concrete descriptions of concepts embedded in propositions. **Propositions** are statements that describe linkages between concepts and are more prescriptive; that is, they propose an outcome that is testable in practice and research. For example, Peplau's (1952/1988) book *Interpersonal Relations in Nursing* contains a theory describing very specific elements of effective interaction between the nurse and patient. Using concepts from nursing's metaparadigm, Peplau created a theory delineating elements of excellent and effective practice in psychiatric nursing. She linked abstract concepts such as health and nursing to create a concrete, useful theory for practice. Peplau's theory will be described later in this chapter.

The **primary source**—the original writings of the theorist—is the best source for in-depth understanding of the theory. In the original writings, the theorist will describe exactly what he or she is thinking and how the concepts go together. Articles written by other scholars can be helpful in explaining and interpreting primary sources. Explanatory or interpretive articles introduce students to the historical development of the philosophy, model, or theory and specify **criteria** (standards) by which to analyze, critique, and evaluate them. Articles such as these were first published in the early 1980s with a completely different purpose than the theorists' original articles. Explanatory or interpretive articles are written to contribute to the general understanding of nursing theory and theoretical developments in nursing in a unique but complementary way. Undergraduate and graduate students, faculty, and practicing nurses have found that these explanatory and interpretive articles on nursing theory make a significant contribution to their knowledge and understanding of nursing science in its own right. Many of the articles and books cited in this chapter were texts written to clarify, describe, and interpret theorists' work.

In this chapter, four types of nursing theoretical works will be presented: philosophies, conceptual models, theories, and middle-range theories. Selected works from each of these four types provide a broad overview of theory within the discipline of nursing. This introduction is designed to help you develop a beginning understanding of nursing theory on which to build as you pursue your nursing education and career in the profession of nursing.

PHILOSOPHIES OF NURSING

Chapter 5 provided several definitions of nursing, and Chapter 8 introduced nursing philosophy and discussed its function in nursing practice and educational institutions. A philosophy provides a broad, general view of nursing that clarifies values and that expands on the definition of nursing to answer broad disciplinary questions, such as "What is nursing?" "What is the profession of nursing?" "What do nurses do?" "What is the nature of human caring?" "What is the nature of nursing practice and the development of practice expertise?" Three philosophies representing different positions in the development of nursing theory are presented here. Table 9.1 contains questions that represent the different views of the same patient situation among nurses who subscribe to the philosophies of Florence Nightingale, Virginia Henderson, and Jean Watson, whose work is presented here.

Nightingale's Philosophy

Florence Nightingale was born in 1820, in Florence, Italy. Her father was William Edward Nightingale, a wealthy English landowner; her mother was Frances Smith Nightingale, who considered it her responsibility

TABLE 9.1 **Three Philosophies of Nursing: Three Different Responses to the Same Patient Situation**	
Florence Nightingale	What needs to be adjusted in this environment to protect the patient?
Virginia Henderson	What can I help this patient do that he would do for himself if he could?
Jean Watson	How can I create an environment of trust, understanding, and openness so that the patient and I can work together in meeting his or her needs?

to find suitable husbands for her daughters. Florence was close to her father, and he undertook the responsibility for her education, teaching her a classical curriculum of Greek, Latin, French, German, Italian, history, philosophy, and mathematics. At 25 years old, after deciding to remain unmarried, Florence announced her decision to go to Kaiserswerth, Germany, to study nursing, over the strong objections of her parents. At that time, nursing was considered the pursuit of working-class women. Her persistence in the face of her parents' opposition proved to be a sustained characteristic over the course of her life. This trait enabled her to accomplish work that most women of the time would have had neither the education nor willingness to achieve.

Nightingale's work represents the beginning of professional nursing as we know it today. In *Notes on Nursing: What It Is and What It Is Not* (1969; originally published in 1859), Nightingale explained her philosophy of health, illness, and the nurse's role in caring for patients. Importantly, she made a distinction between the work of nursing and the work of physicians by identifying health rather than illness as the major concern of nursing. Her writing about nursing reflected the sociohistorical context in which she lived, making a distinction between the work of nursing and the work of household servants, who were common in her day and often cared for the sick.

Nightingale's unique perspective on nursing practice focused on the relationship of patients to their surroundings. She set forth foundational principles for nursing, which remain relevant to nursing practice today. For example, her description of the importance of observing the patient and accurately recording information and her principles of cleanliness still shape hospital-based nursing practice today. Nightingale focused the profession on what has become known as the metaparadigm of nursing: person (patient), health (as opposed to illness), environment (how the environment affects health and recovery from illness), and nursing (as opposed to medicine).

Using Nightingale's Philosophy in Practice

Nightingale believed that the health of patients was related to their environment. She recognized the importance of clean air and water and of adequate ventilation and sunlight and encouraged the arrangement of patients' beds so they were in direct sunlight. In her writing, she described both the necessity of a balanced diet and the nurse's responsibility to observe and record what was eaten. Cleanliness of the patient, the bed linens, and the room itself was essential. Nightingale recognized the problem of noise in hospital rooms and halls, which foreshadowed the attention given to excess noise in inpatient settings in recent years. Rest is important in the restoration of health; Nightingale believed the sudden disruption of sleep was a serious problem. The relationship of health to the environment seems obvious today, but for nursing in the second half of the 19th century, Nightingale's work was radically different.

Nightingale recognized nursing's role in protecting patients. Nurses were newly responsible for shielding patients from possible harm by well-meaning visitors who may provide false hope, discuss upsetting news, or tire the patient with social conversation. Nightingale even suggested the nurse's responsibility for patients did not end when the nurse was off duty. This view underpins the system of primary nursing found in some settings today. Interestingly, Nightingale suggested that patients might benefit from visits by small pets, an idea that has been incorporated today in both long-term and some acute care settings.

The nurse whose practice is guided by Nightingale's philosophy is sensitive to the effect of the environment on the patient's health or recovery from illness. This philosophy provided the foundational work for theory development that proposed changing patients' environments to effect positive changes in their health. Nightingale promoted the view that nurses' primary responsibility was to protect patients by careful management of their surroundings.

Henderson's Philosophy

Virginia Henderson, whose photo is featured in Professional Profile Box 9.1 of this chapter, was born in 1897 in Kansas City, Missouri, and was named for her mother's home state to which her family returned when Henderson was 4 years old. Although she received an excellent education from a family friend who was a schoolmaster and from her father who was a former teacher, Henderson did not receive a traditional education that awarded a diploma, which delayed her entry into nursing school. During World War II, she studied under Annie Goodrich at Teachers College, Columbia University, where, after numerous interruptions, she received her bachelor's and master's degrees. By the time she died in 1996, Virginia Henderson was internationally known and regarded by many as "the Florence Nightingale of the 20th century."

Virginia Henderson's work first was published 100 years after Nightingale, at a time when efforts to clarify nursing as a profession emphasized the need to define nursing. Henderson's philosophical approach to nursing is contained in her comprehensive definition: the "unique function of the nurse … is to assist the individual, sick or well, in the performance of those activities contributing to health or its recovery (or a peaceful death) that he would perform unaided if he had the necessary strength, will or knowledge" (Henderson, 1966, p. 15). Although Henderson was recognized for many contributions to nursing throughout her long career, her early work remains particularly noteworthy and relevant, defining nursing and specifying the role of the nurse in relation to the patient. Henderson's relationship with one of her former students, who recognizes the ongoing contributions of Henderson's work to nursing, is described in Professional Profile Box 9.1.

Henderson's philosophy linked her definition of nursing that emphasized the functions of the nurse with a list of basic patient needs that are the focus of nursing care. She proposed an answer to questions similar to those addressed by Nightingale a century earlier: "What is the nursing profession?" and "What do nurses do?" Henderson described the nurse's role as that of a substitute for the patient, a helper to the patient, or a partner with the patient.

Henderson identified 14 basic needs (Box 9.2) as a general focus for patient care. She proposed that these needs shaped the fundamental elements of nursing care. The function of nurses was to assist patients if they were unable to perform any of these 14 functions themselves. Although these needs could be categorized as physical, psychological, emotional, sociologic, spiritual, or developmental, thoughtful analysis reveals that they represent a holistic view of human development and health.

PROFESSIONAL PROFILE BOX 9.1

Remembering Virginia Henderson

Although I had known Virginia Henderson from the time I was a graduate student at Yale, geography later brought us more closely together. Knowing her family lived in Virginia (mine was in Connecticut), whenever I traveled by car from North Carolina to Connecticut I called and asked if she wanted a ride back home with me, because I could drop her off in Virginia en route to North Carolina. Six times we made the 8-hour ride together. Our conversations were wide-ranging because we were both world travelers. We talked much about politics; most about nurses—"see a nurse before you go to a doctor" as a solution to health care cost, quality, and access problems; some about patients—"give them their records" as a most important patient education tool; and some about our large extended families. I was introduced to two of Virginia Henderson's sisters when they were all in their 90s. Four brothers and a sister had predeceased them, but Frances (Fanny) had maintained the old family homestead so all who could come were welcomed to stay. Come they did for over two generations of reunions, weddings, funerals, and holidays, especially Christmas.

What was most amazing to me about our time together was that Virginia Henderson never said anything to me about our profession that she had not written down somewhere for all nurses to read. Yale's School of Nursing asked me to address the topic of her writing in their Bellos Lecture the year they celebrated her 90th birthday. I read her textbook, *Principles and Practice of Nursing,* sixth edition, and discovered any number of conversations I had experienced with her over the years. In preparing the *Virginia Henderson Reader: Excellence in Nursing,* I discovered even more. Her

writings are conversational—that is, completely without the jargon of the medical and nursing professions. Her description of nursing is best used by nurses to tell patients what can be expected—to paraphrase: I am here to help you do what you would do for yourself if you had the strength, will, or knowledge, and to do so for you to become free of my help as rapidly as possible. It is quite reassuring for a patient to know what the nurse is going to do.

Virginia Henderson's writings are timeless. The information in *The Nature of Nursing* and *Basic Principles of Nursing Care* is as relevant today as the day the books were written. *The Nature of Nursing* is the most important document written about nurses and nursing in the 20th century, because it provided evidence of effective and efficient nursing. If you read her work, you can have a conversation with her too.

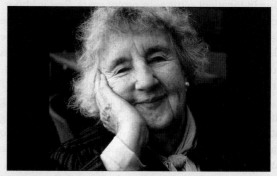

Virginia Henderson

Edward J. Halloran, PhD, RN, FAAN

Courtesy Edward J. Halloran

BOX 9.2   Henderson's 14 Basic Needs of the Patient

1. Breathe normally.
2. Eat and drink adequately.
3. Eliminate body wastes.
4. Move and maintain desirable position.
5. Sleep and rest.
6. Select suitable clothes—dress and undress.
7. Maintain body temperature within normal range by adjusting clothing and modifying the environment.
8. Keep the body clean and well groomed and protect the integument (skin).
9. Avoid dangers in the environment and avoid injuring others.
10. Communicate with others in expressing emotions, needs, fears, or opinions.
11. Worship according to one's faith.
12. Work in such a way that there is a sense of accomplishment.
13. Play or participate in various forms of recreation.
14. Learn, discover, or satisfy the curiosity that leads to normal development and health and use the available health facilities.

Data from Henderson, V. (1966). *The nature of nursing: a definition and its implications for practice, research, and education.* New York: Macmillan.

The first nine needs emphasize the importance of care of the physical body: breathing, eating and drinking, elimination, movement and positioning, sleep and rest, suitable clothing, maintenance of suitable environment for the body temperature, cleanliness, and avoidance of danger or harm. Next she included psychosocial needs such as communication and spirituality, including worship and faith. She concluded with three developmental needs: the need for work and the sense of accomplishment; the need for play and recreation; and the need to learn, discover, and satisfy curiosity. Henderson believed that all 14 basic needs are amenable to nursing care. They continue to be used today in philosophical statements of schools and departments of nursing.

Using Henderson's Philosophy in Practice

Nurses whose practice is consistent with Henderson's philosophy adopt an orientation to care from the perspective of the 14 basic needs. Henderson's clarity about the role and function of the nurse is a strength of her work. This philosophy is easily applied to a variety of patient care settings, from brief outpatient encounters in which a limited number of needs are addressed to a complex setting such as intensive care where patients are extremely vulnerable. Henderson used her definition of nursing and the basic needs approach in her well-known case study of a young patient who had undergone a leg amputation. Using this case, Henderson (1966) demonstrated how the nurse's role changes on a day-to-day, week-to-week, and month-to-month basis in relation to the patient's changing needs and the contributions of other health care providers.

Watson's Philosophy

Jean Watson is a more recent contributor to the evolving philosophy of nursing. Born in West Virginia, she earned her BSN degree from the University of Colorado in 1964, her master of science (MS) from the University of Colorado in 1966, and her doctor of philosophy (PhD) from the University of Colorado in 1973. Six years later, she published her first book, *The Philosophy and Science of Caring*. In this initial work, she called for a return to the earlier values of nursing and emphasized the caring aspects of nursing. Watson's work is recognized as human science. Caring as a theme is reflected in her other professional accomplishments, such as the Center for Human Caring at the University of Colorado in Denver, where nurses can incorporate knowledge of human

BOX 9.3 Watson's 10 Caritas Processes

1. Embrace altruistic values and practice loving kindness with self and others.
2. Instill faith and hope and honor in others.
3. Be sensitive to self and others by nurturing individual beliefs and practices.
4. Develop helping-trusting-caring relationships.
5. Promote and accept positive and negative feelings as you authentically listen to another's story.
6. Use creative scientific problem-solving methods for caring decision making.
7. Share teaching and learning that addresses the individual needs and comprehension styles.
8. Create a healing environment for the physical and spiritual self which respects human dignity.
9. Assist with basic physical, emotional, and spiritual human needs.
10. Open to mystery and allow miracles to enter.

From Jean Watson, Caritas Processes refined from Inova Health. © Copyright 2018 Watson Caring Science Institute, Boulder, CO. Available at www.watsoncaringscience.org.

caring as the basis of nursing practice and scholarship. Watson proposed 10 factors that she initially labeled as "carative" factors, a term she contrasted with *curative* to differentiate nursing from medicine. The term *Caritas Processes* has replaced *carative factors* as Watson's work has continued to be refined. Recently these processes taken together were found to be a measure of the concept of caring (DiNapoli et al., 2010). Watson's Ten Caritas Processes are listed in Box 9.3.

Watson's work (1979, 1988, 1999) addressed the philosophical question of the nature of nursing as viewed as a human-to-human relationship. She focused on the relationship of the nurse and the patient, drawing on philosophical sources for a new approach that emphasized how the nurse and patient change together through transpersonal caring. She proposed that nursing be concerned with spiritual matters and the inner knowledge of nurse and patient as they participate together in the transpersonal caring process. She equated health with harmony, resulting from unity of body, mind, and soul, for which the patient is primarily responsible. Illness or disease was equated with lack of harmony within the mind, body, and soul experienced in internal or external environments (Watson, 1979). Nursing is based on human values and interest in the welfare of others and is concerned with health promotion, health restoration, and illness prevention.

Using Watson's Philosophy in Practice

Watson's caritas processes guide nurses who use transpersonal caring in practice. Caritas processes specify the meaning of the relationship of nurse and patient as human beings. Nurses are encouraged to share their genuine selves with patients. Patients' spiritual strength is recognized, supported, and encouraged for its contribution to health. In the process of transpersonal relationships, nurses develop and encourage openness to understanding of self and others. This leads to the development of trusting, accepting relationships in which feelings are shared freely and confidence is inspired. Even a core element of practice such as patient teaching can be carried out in an interpersonal manner true to the philosophy and nature of the caring relationship.

The nurse guided by Watson's work has responsibility for creating and maintaining an environment supporting human caring while recognizing and providing for patients' primary human requirements. In the end, this human-to-human caring approach leads the nurse to respect the overall meaning of life from the perspective of the patient. Watson's (1988) work formalized the theory of human caring from this philosophy. Key aspects of nursing's metaparadigm evident in Watson's work are environment (one that supports human caring), person (both the patient and the nurse), health (in terms of health promotion and illness prevention), and nursing (what nurses contribute to the encounter with the patient). Importantly, Watson's work on caring has contributed another aspect to the metaparadigm of nursing, because caring itself is now considered by many scholars to be a central concept of the discipline of nursing.

Clinical Example: Watson's Philosophy of Caring

Understanding how philosophy guides practice can be hard, but an example drawn from a nurse's clinical practice may help.

Anna, a hospice nurse, was working with a patient who was very ill with lung cancer and who had received both chemotherapy and radiation with the hope of achieving a long remission. The patient, a 60-year-old woman named Mavis, was what some people would refer to as a "character"—full of opinions that she would share with anyone who came close, still smoking, still cursing. Mavis' cancer did not respond to the various therapies and metastases developed in her brain, causing occasional seizures. Mavis was terminally ill. Her abrasive personality did not allow many people to get near her, but she was very fond of Anna, who understood Mavis in a way that few did. They connected on a deep level, and, although they never talked in great depth about Mavis' impending death, Mavis revealed that one of her unfulfilled plans was to be baptized. She did not remember her baptism from childhood and did not want to die without having that memory.

Although nothing in the nursing texts says it is a good idea to take a terminally ill patient into the cold of January to church for an immersion baptism, it was Anna's human-to-human caring approach that allowed her to respect the meaning of this event from Mavis' point of view.

On a bitterly cold night with a howling wind, Mavis was baptized by a friend who was a minister, her family in attendance, her turban covering her bald head. Mavis told Anna that she was free to die now. Within days she took to her bed. On one of her final days, the family called Anna frantically because Mavis had called for her all day. The on-call nurse covering the weekend simply could not console her, and Mavis' cries for her hospice nurse made the family muster the courage to call Anna on her day off. Anna, knowing Mavis as she did, responded, and when she arrived at the bedside, she asked Mavis what she could do to help her. Mavis' response was what Anna knew as "vintage Mavis": "I just wanted to see if you would come." Anna said simply, "I am here." Mavis lapsed into a peaceful coma that evening. Her last words had been to Anna.

Anna practiced nursing with the philosophy that human-to-human relationships are primary in professional practice. In the confines of this deeply caring relationship, Mavis found acceptance and peace from her nurse and was guided into a calm death. Although the nurse whose guiding philosophy is based on human relationships must set clear professional boundaries, this philosophical approach to the practice of nursing raises the possibility of exquisite experiences between humans that transcend the nurse-patient relationship, just as Anna and Mavis experienced.

CONCEPTUAL MODELS OF NURSING

Conceptual models (or conceptual frameworks) are the second type of theoretical work that provides organizational structures for critical thinking about the processes of nursing (Alligood, 2014; Fawcett and DeSanto-Madeya, 2013). These are broad conceptual structures that provide comprehensive, holistic perspectives of nursing by describing the relationships of specific concepts. Models are less abstract and more formalized than the philosophies just discussed in this chapter; models are more abstract, however, than theories of nursing, which will be discussed later. Theories are built from conceptual models much as buildings are constructed from blueprints. The blueprints show the general relationships between parts of the building and are adaptable; conceptual models provide a preliminary view of the relationship between concepts of nursing that can be used to build theory.

Three conceptual models will be presented in the following section. These models represent different decades in the development of nursing theory; they are models developed by Dorothea Orem, Imogene King, and Sister Callista Roy. The focus and perspective of each model are discussed, followed by a brief overview of how that model guides nursing practice. Table 9.2 contains questions that represent how the same patient situation is viewed differently by nurses whose practices are based on the models of Orem, King, or Roy.

Orem's Self-Care Model

Dorothea Orem, born in 1914 in Baltimore, Maryland, first received her diploma in nursing in the 1930s, soon followed by a BS in nursing education in 1939. Six years later, she earned an MS in nursing education (Sitzman and Eichelberger, 2004). Working as a nurse in a number of roles, Orem first published her concept of self-care in 1959. She continued to develop her conceptual model over several decades, with the sixth edition of her work *Nursing: Concepts of Practice* published in 2001. Over the years, Orem formalized three interrelated theories: the theory of

self-care, theory of self-care deficit, and theory of nursing system. Her model focuses on the patient's self-care capacities and the process of designing nursing actions to meet the patient's self-care needs. In this model the nurse prescribes and regulates the nursing system on the basis of the patient's self-care deficit, which is the extent to which a patient is incapable of providing effective self-care. An underlying assumption of Orem's model is that "ordinary people in contemporary society want to be in control of their lives" (Pearson et al., 2005, p. 104). Nursing is needed in the presence of an actual or potential self-care deficit (Orem, 2001) when patients cannot provide their own care adequately. Orem's work is widely used in nursing education and practice, providing a comprehensive system for nursing practice in a variety of clinical settings.

Orem and Nursing Practice

In Orem's model, appropriate care for the patient is developed through a series of three operations: diagnostic, prescriptive, and regulatory. To determine the patient's ability to provide effective self-care, the nurse initiates a diagnostic operation that begins with the establishment of the nurse-patient relationship. This includes contracting with the patient to explore current and potential self-care demands. Factors such as age, gender, and developmental status, as well as sociocultural and environmental factors, are examined in relation to universal, developmental, and health requirements and related self-care actions of the patient. In other words, the patient's baseline ability to provide adequate self-care is assessed by the nurse to determine the extent to which the patient is limited in providing his or her own effective care. These limitations are self-care deficits.

Prescriptive operations occur when therapeutic self-care requisites (based on deficits) are determined and the nurse reviews various methods, actions, and priorities with the patient. This is a planning stage in which the nurse confirms with the patient the nurse's assessment of the patient's needs and begins to formulate a plan of care. In regulatory operations, the nurse designs, plans, and produces a system for care (Berbiglia, 2014). Systems of care range from wholly compensatory, which is the most comprehensive form of care for patients with few (if any) abilities to provide care for self, to supportive-educative, in which the patient has the ability to provide effective self-care but needs to work with the nurse to further develop these abilities or acquire additional information to promote self-care (George, 2002).

TABLE 9.2 **Three Models of Nursing: Three Different Responses to the Same Patient Situation**	
Dorothea Orem	What deficits does this patient have in providing his or her own self-care?
Imogene King	What goals can we set together to restore the patient to health?
Callista Roy	How can I modify this patient's environment to facilitate his or her adaptation?

King's Interacting Systems Framework and Theory of Goal Attainment

Imogene King was born in 1923 and received her basic nursing education from St. John's Hospital School of Nursing in St. Louis, Missouri, in 1945. Three years later she completed her BS in nursing education from Saint Louis University; in 1957 she earned her master of science in nursing (MSN) degree from Saint Louis University. In 1961 she completed her doctor of education (EdD) degree from Teachers College, Columbia University, in New York City. Much of her career was spent in academic settings, including Ohio State University, Loyola University, and the University of South Florida (Johnson and Webber, 2005).

Although King first published early forms of her theoretical work in 1971, *A Theory for Nursing: Systems, Concepts, Process,* published 10 years later in 1981, contained her first claim to a nursing theory (King, 1981). This complex theory focused on people, their interpersonal relationships, and social contexts, with three interacting systems: personal, interpersonal, and social. Within each of these three systems, King identified concepts that provide a conceptual structure describing the processes in each system. Significantly, the focus of the nurse is on phenomena of importance to the patient; unless attention is paid to concerns of the patient, mutual goal setting is unlikely to happen (Sieloff et al., 2006).

King's interacting systems form a framework to view whole people in their family and social contexts: the personal system identifies concepts that provide an understanding of individuals, personally and intrapersonally (within the person); the interpersonal system deals with interactions and transactions between two or more people; and the social system presents concepts that consider social contacts, such as those at school, at work, or in social settings. King's work is unique because it provides a view of people from the perspective of their interactions (or communications, both verbal and nonverbal) with other people at three levels of interacting systems.

Using King's Model in Practice

When using King's work, nurses focus on goal attainment for and by the patient. The traditional steps of the nursing process—assessment, planning, goal setting, intervention, and evaluation—are augmented in several ways. The steps of the process describe the type of action the nurse is taking, and at each step the nurse gathers and uses information to provide care. Like the nursing process, King's model is not linear: steps occur simultaneously as the nurse and patient work to identify goals and the best means to attain those goals.

The focus of nursing care is guided by concepts at each of the system levels. For example, the personal system leads the nurse to pay close attention to the patient's perceptions; the interpersonal system guides the nurse to explore the patient's roles and the stresses in each role; and the social system cues the nurse to consider influences on the patient's decision making. In this model, for instance, the nurse providing care for a young woman who is a mother will recognize that the patient's maternal role will influence her decisions regarding her health, keeping the best interests of her children in addition to her own health in mind as she makes health-related decisions.

Interaction with the patient is an important component of King's goal attainment model. Nurses are aware of their communication with patients, identifying steps from the first encounter to the attainment of the specified goal. King describes these steps as a progression from perception, judgment, action, reaction, and interaction to transaction (King, 1981). These steps involve increasing involvement between the nurse and the patient, requiring a deep understanding of the goals of the patient within the various contexts of the patient's life to plan and provide effective nursing care. King emphasized the importance of joint goal setting by nurse and patient, reminding nurses that this relationship involves mutuality. King's process provided a structure for the nurse to monitor the relationship's progress. King specified clearly that the goal of nursing is attaining or regaining health.

Roy's Adaptation Model

Sister Callista Roy was born in Los Angeles, California, in 1939. Her first degree was a bachelor of arts in nursing from Mount St. Mary's College in Los Angeles. She then earned a master's degree in pediatric nursing and sociology, followed by a PhD in sociology from the University of California, Los Angeles. She is a member of the order of Sisters of Saint Joseph of Carondelet. Roy is currently on the faculty of the William F. Connell School of Nursing at Boston College. Although the Roy adaptation model has been in use for 35 years, Sr. Roy continues to update, revise, and refine it for use in practice, research, theory, and administration (Roy and Zhan, 2006; Roy and Andrews, 2008).

Roy first presented her model as a conceptual framework for a nursing curriculum in 1970 (Pearson et al., 2005). In 1976 she published *Introduction to Nursing: An Adaptation Model* and followed with a second edition in 1984 (Roy, 1976; Roy, 1984). Roy updated all of her writing in a comprehensive text in 1999 (Roy and Andrews, 1999). Her model is widely used for education, research, and nursing practice today. She focused on the individual as a biopsychosocial adaptive system and described nursing as a humanistic discipline that emphasizes the person's adaptive or coping abilities. Roy's work is based on **adaptation** and adaptive behavior, which is produced by altering the environment. According to Roy, the individual and the environment are sources of stimuli that require modification to promote adaptation in the patient. Roy viewed the person as an adaptive system with physiologic, self-concept, role function, and interdependent modes.

Roy's model provides a comprehensive understanding of nursing from the perspective of adaptation. When the demands of environmental stimuli are too high or the person's adaptive mechanisms are too low, the person's behavioral responses are ineffective for coping. Effective adaptive responses promote the integrity of the individual by conserving energy and promoting the survival, growth, reproduction, and mastery of the human system. Nursing promotes the patient's adaptation and coping, with progress toward integration as the goal (Phillips, 2002).

Using Roy's Model in Practice

The nurse using Roy's model focuses on the adaptation of the patient and on the environment. Adaptation, specifically patients' adaptation behavior and stimuli in the internal and external environments, is assessed and facilitated. Based on these assessments, the nurse develops nursing diagnoses to guide goal setting and interventions aimed at promoting adaptation. Simply stated, the nurse modifies the environment to facilitate patient adaptation.

Observable behavior is recognized and understood in the context of Roy's physiologic, self-concept, role function, and interdependent modes. Descriptions of

the behaviors included in each mode provide the nurse with a means of making evaluative judgments about the patient's progress toward the goal of adaptation (Phillips, 2002). Roy's model is extensively used in nursing practice and has been described comprehensively in the literature (Wood, 2014; Phillips, 2002; Roy and Andrews, 1999).

Clinical Example: Roy's Adaptation Model

A clinical example of Roy's model will help you understand her work in a real-world context.

Mr. Elderd was referred to a home health agency for wound management. He had a very large open wound on his forehead as a result of a wide excision of several deep basal cell carcinomas, a form of skin cancer. Dean, his nurse, was surprised to see that the wound extended completely to Mr. Elderd's skull. Mr. Elderd was out of work as a result of this wound, saw friends infrequently, and was somewhat depressed. His wife, although well meaning, spent hours each day fixing him high-calorie "treats" because she liked to cook and found it was a good way to release her own anxiety about her husband's condition.

Dean's nursing practice was shaped by Roy's adaptation model. In his initial assessment of the home environment, he noticed the cleanliness of the home, the evidence of supportive family and social ties, adequacy of income, availability of good nutrition, and other indicators of health. What Dean did not understand was why Mr. Elderd's wound was not healing. After Dean's assessment, he believed that there was some "missing link" in Mr. Elderd's adaptive abilities, but he was not sure whether the ineffective coping was psychological, environmental, or physiologic.

Dean visited Mr. Elderd daily for 3 weeks and, although the wound did not become infected, it showed little evidence of closure. Dean expressed his concern to Mr. Elderd and decided to ask Mr. Elderd again some questions related to his basic health practices, including nutrition, activity, sleep, and elimination. Mr. Elderd commented almost offhandedly that he was sleeping fine except that he had to get up to go to the bathroom several times each night. His wife chimed in from the kitchen, "But that's no different than from the day. He is always going to the bathroom. I told him to quit drinking so much water all the time!" Dean, being an experienced nurse and seeking ways to assist patients with all forms of adaptation, realized the likely problem. He called Mr. Elderd's physician and asked for an order to draw a blood chemistry, including glucose. Dean's suspicion was correct: Mr. Elderd had undiagnosed type 2 diabetes. Mrs. Elderd's stream of cookies and other treats from the kitchen aggravated the problem to the point that Mr. Elderd was experiencing polyuria and polydipsia, both signs of diabetes. With aggressive blood glucose level management with an oral hypoglycemic drug, a drastic change in diet, and increasing exercise, Mr. Elderd's wound began to heal almost immediately. He did not require a skin graft as had been feared.

The use of Roy's adaptation model allowed Dean to see Mr. Elderd's situation as a function of a variety of maladaptive coping efforts. Correcting the diabetic problem became the foundation for Mr. Elderd's eventual healing and resumption of his usual life activities.

THEORIES OF NURSING: FROM GRAND TO MIDDLE RANGE

Nursing theories are the third type of theoretical work in the structure of nursing knowledge to be reviewed in this chapter. Fawcett and DeSanto-Madeya (2013) classified theories according to their breadth and depth. For example, a **grand theory** is a broad conceptualization of nursing phenomena, whereas a **middle-range theory** is narrower in focus and makes connections between grand theories and nursing practice (Parker, 2006). Theories are less abstract than models and usually propose specific outcomes. Three theories are presented here that are well known and commonly used to shape nursing practice. Table 9.3 contains questions that represent the differing foci of care of nurses whose practices are shaped by the theories of Hildegard Peplau, Ida Orlando, and Madeleine Leininger.

Peplau's Theory of Interpersonal Relations in Nursing

Peplau, born in 1909, was one of the earliest nurse theorists who recognized the importance of the work of nursing rather than continuing to define and delineate nursing (Pearson et al., 2005). After receiving her basic nursing training at the Pottstown, Pennsylvania, Hospital School of Nursing in 1931, Peplau studied interpersonal psychology at Bennington College in Vermont, receiving a bachelor of arts degree. Later she received a master's of arts degree in teaching and supervision of

TABLE 9.3   Three Theories of Nursing: Three Different Responses to the Same Patient Situation

Hildegard Peplau	Within the relationship with my patient, how can I best help him or her understand his or her health problems and develop new, healthier behaviors?
Ida Orlando	How can I best figure out what my patient needs through my interaction with him or her?
Madeleine Leininger	What are the best ways to provide care to my patient that are culturally congruent?

psychiatric nursing, followed by an EdD from Teachers College, Columbia University, in New York City. Although Peplau's first book, *Interpersonal Relations in Nursing*, was published in 1952, it was published again in 1988, reflecting both the value of her work and nursing's continuing focus on interpersonal relationships. Peplau drew from developmental, interactionist, and human needs theories in developing her work (Pearson et al., 2005), which grew from her interest in nursing care of psychiatric patients. Peplau believed, however, that all nursing is based on the interpersonal process and the nurse-patient relationship (Forchuk, 1993).

Peplau's theory is based on the premise that the relationship between patient and nurse is the focus of attention, rather than the patient only as the unit of attention (Forchuk, 1993, p. 7). Nursing care occurs within the context of the patient-nurse relationship. The goals of a therapeutic interpersonal relationship are twofold: first is the survival of the patient; second is the patient's understanding of his or her health problems and learning from these problems as he or she develops new behavior patterns. As the nurse assists the patient in developing new behavior patterns, the nurse also grows and develops a greater understanding of the effect of universal stressors on the lives and behaviors of individual patients (Pearson et al., 2005).

Using Peplau's Theory in Practice

Although Peplau's theory grew from her experience as a psychiatric nurse, her work is applicable to a wide variety of practice settings. Peplau describes a four-pronged process similar to the nursing process by which the nurse assists the patient in achieving personal growth.

Completion of this process involves six roles by the nurse: counselor, resource, teacher, technical expert, surrogate, and leader (Pearson et al., 2005). Depending on the setting, the nurse will spend more or less time in each of these roles. For instance, a nurse in a critical care unit will likely spend more time as a technical expert and less time as a counselor, whereas a nurse on a postpartum unit may act as a surrogate, guiding a new mother into independent care of her newborn infant, with less time spent as a leader.

Peplau's theory is complex. Its importance lies in the focus on what happens between the nurse and patient in a therapeutic relationship. Furthermore, Peplau was visionary in recognizing the importance of the relationship between nurse and patient, publishing her ideas early and continuing to refine and expand her work over several decades.

Orlando's Nursing Process Theory

Ida Orlando was born in New York in 1926 and, like many early nurse theorists, received her basic nursing education in a diploma program. She attended nursing school at the New York Medical College School of Nursing, and in 1951 she graduated with a BS in public health nursing from St. John's University in Brooklyn, New York. Three years later, she completed her MSN from Columbia University. Her early practice settings included maternity, medicine, and emergency department nursing (Gess et al., 2006).

Orlando first proposed her theory of effective nursing practice in 1961 in her first book, *The Dynamic Nurse-Patient Relationship: Function, Process, and Principles.* She later revised it as a nursing process theory (Orlando, 1990). Her work actually proposed both: it is a theory about how nurses process their observations of patient behavior and about how they react to patients based on inferences from patients' behavior, including what they say. Orlando's early research revealed that processing observations as specified in her theory led to effective nursing practice and good outcomes.

Orlando's theory is specific to nurse-patient interactions. The goal of the nurse is to determine and meet patients' immediate needs and to improve their situation by relieving distress or discomfort. Orlando emphasized deliberate action (rather than automatic action) based on observation of the patients' verbal and nonverbal behavior, which leads to inferences. Inferences are confirmed or disconfirmed by the patient, leading the nurse to identify the patient's needs and provide effective nursing care.

Using Orlando's Theory in Practice

In terms of nursing practice, Orlando's theory specified how patients are involved in nurses' decision making. When used in practice, Orlando's theory guides interactions to predictable outcomes, which are different from outcomes that occur when the theory is not used. Nurses individualize care for each patient by attending to behavior, confirming with the patient ideas and inferences the nurse draws from interactions, and identifying pressing needs.

Use of Orlando's theory improves the effectiveness of the nurse by allowing the nurse to get to the "bottom line" more quickly when observing, listening to, and confirming with patients. Therefore use of this theory saves time and energy for both the patient and the nurse.

Leininger's Theory of Culture Care Diversity and Universality

Born in 1924 in Sutton, Nebraska, Madeleine Leininger received her diploma in nursing at St. Anthony's School of Nursing in Denver, Colorado, followed by a BS in biologic science from Benedictine College in Atchison, Kansas, 2 years later. She received her MSN from Catholic University in Washington, D.C., in 1954 and her PhD in anthropology from the University of Washington in Seattle in 1965 (Reynolds and Leininger, 1993).

The work of Madeleine Leininger (1978, 1991) in **cultural care** grew out of her early nursing experiences. She observed that children of different cultures had widely varying behaviors and needs. After discussing the parallels between nursing and anthropology with the noted anthropologist Margaret Mead, Leininger pursued doctoral study in cultural anthropology. Through her doctoral work she became more convinced about the relationship of cultural differences and health practices. This led her to begin developing a theory of cultural care for nursing. Leininger's work is formalized as a theory rather than as a conceptual model. It has stimulated the formation of the Transcultural Nursing Society, transcultural nursing conferences, newsletters, and the *Journal of Transpersonal Nursing*, as well as the awarding of master's degrees in the specialty area known as transcultural nursing.

The goal of transcultural nursing involves more than simply being aware of different cultures. It involves planning nursing care based on knowledge that is culturally defined, classified, and tested—and then used to provide care that is culturally congruent (Leininger, 1978). Leininger described theory as a creative and systematic way of discovering new knowledge or accounting for phenomena in a more complete way (Leininger, 1991). She encouraged nurses to use creativity to discover cultural aspects of human needs and to use these findings to make culturally congruent therapeutic decisions. Her theory is broad because it considers the impact of culture on all aspects of human life, with particular attention to health and caring practices. Leininger's theory has become increasingly relevant as global migration continues and societies become more diverse.

Using Leininger's Theory in Practice

Leininger specified caring as the essence of nursing, and nurses who use Leininger's theory of cultural care in their practices view patients in the context of their cultures. Practice from a cultural perspective begins by respecting the culture of the patient and recognizing the importance of its relationship to nursing care. Use of the "sunrise model" (Fig. 9.1) guides the assessment of cultural data for an understanding of its influence on the patient's life (Leininger, 1991). The nurse plans nursing care, recognizing the health beliefs and folk practices of the patient's culture, as well as the culture of traditional health services. To this end, nursing care is then focused on culture care preservation, accommodations,

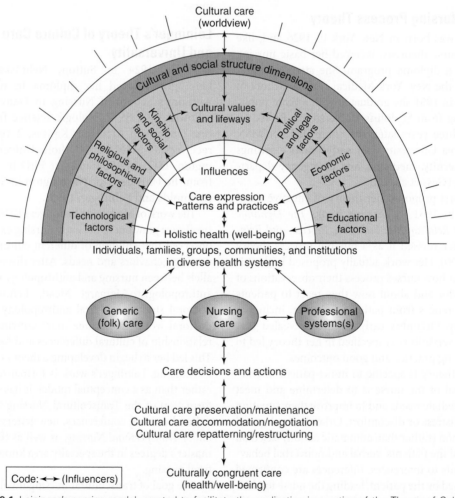

Fig. 9.1 Leininger's sunrise model, created to facilitate the application in practice of the Theory of Culture Care Diversity and Universality. (Courtesy Dr. Madeleine Leininger.)

or repatterning, depending on the patient's need. The nursing outcome of culturally congruent nursing care is health and well-being for the patient.

Clinical Example: Leininger's Theory of Culture Care Diversity and Universality

No matter how expert a nurse is in clinical practice, sometimes failure to recognize and appreciate cultural differences can undermine even the best intentions. The following case is an example of what happens when this occurs.

Jan, a nurse with many years of experience providing care for patients with human immunodeficiency virus (HIV) in a large urban hospital, decided that she would move to a less chaotic environment. Jan applied for a job with an agency providing nursing care in the homes of low-income rural women with HIV. Jan had grown up and gone to college in a city in the northeast; her new home was in a rural county in the Deep South.

Almost immediately Jan ran into some unanticipated situations that posed problems for her. She complained at team meetings that her patients were always late for their appointments. Members of the team, each of whom had grown up nearby, explained to her that this was not unusual behavior and that she should plan "waiting time" into her daily schedule. Jan was always surprised when the rest of the team reported good visits and outcomes with their patients, and almost all seemed to be caught up with their work consistently. Jan always felt like she was running behind. She began to question her nursing skills, her knowledge, and time management behaviors that had served her well in her previous work. Jan described herself as a "fish out of water." She decided that she would spend her "waiting time" by sitting in her car and catching up on paperwork until the patient arrived home.

One day she was invited by the patient's grandmother to wait inside but she declined, saying she would wait in the car and "get some work done." Her patient arrived home after 20 minutes or so and Jan met with her, reporting to the team later that day that she had a productive visit with the patient in which several care goals were addressed. Jan's satisfaction with the visit was short-lived. Her patient called, demanding that she be assigned another nurse because "Jan insulted my grandma." In this community where being invited into the home was considered an honor, Jan's decision to instead wait in the car was interpreted as rude and uncaring. No amount of discussion dissuaded the patient from her insistence that she have a new nurse who "knew how to act." The care team met with Jan, but they too, as products of the culture, did not understand at first that Jan did not mean to be insulting or rude. Because the other members of the team were deeply acculturated, they knew the meaning behind the grandmother's invitation: Jan was an honored, trusted guest who was welcomed in their home.

Jan soon realized that her feelings of being a "fish out of water" in this setting were accurate; in fact, she did not understand the culture and was not eager to learn about the cultural norms that so disturbed her. Importantly, she recognized that this prevented her from providing the effective patient care that she desired. She left the position and moved to a more urban area in which she knew the cultural terrain.

Although this was a sad chapter in Jan's professional life, she grew from the experience in her understanding of the substantial influences of culture and its effects on the nurse-patient relationship.

Middle-Range Theories of Nursing

Middle-range theories are those that are neither overly broad nor narrow in scope, usually incorporating a limited number of concepts and focus on a specific aspect of nursing. Middle-range theories are more focused than the theories described earlier and typically merge practice and research. These theories are based in empirical research and are often embedded within a larger theory. Sometimes middle-range theories are developed from theory from disciplines other than nursing. Some well-known middle-range theories include Swanson's Caring Theory, which was developed from her work with couples experiencing miscarriage (Swanson, 1991). Mishel's Uncertainty in Illness Theory was developed from studying men with prostate cancer who were "watchfully waiting" for disease progression rather than seeking aggressive treatment (Mishel, 1988). Jezewski's Cultural Brokering Theory was developed from her qualitative research on the politically and economically powerless or those who were vulnerable as a function of advanced disease (Jezewski, 1995). You can see how close to practice each of these theories are; they were each developed from a specific population and grew from the theorists' research and experiences.

More recently, Dobratz (2011) published a description of a new middle-range theory of Psychological Adaptation in Death and Dying. Dobratz had noted that

presented in this chapter has been critiqued, analyzed, and evaluated. Application of these works in your practice with specific patient groups is an opportunity to further develop and test middle-range theories.

As you engage in theory-based practice, remember to provide feedback to nurse researchers and theorists concerning your experiences. You can do this through a variety of social media sites, blogs, and microblogs, where you will find groups of nurses using, discussing, and refining the theoretical works that have been discussed in this chapter. The Internet can be a powerful tool to keep you involved with nurses in practice far removed from your own location and practice setting. You can also assist these scholars and the discipline of nursing by developing manuscripts and submitting your experiences for publication, joining the many nurses who have discovered the benefits of theory-based practice.

Theory-Based Research

Great strides have been made in nursing research since the 1970s (Alligood, 2018). The expansion of graduate nursing education at the master's level and the proliferation of PhD and DNP programs have played a major role, as more nurses than ever before are equipped with the knowledge and skills to conduct research and implement its use in practice. Nursing research tests and refines the knowledge base of nursing. Ultimately, research findings enable nurses to improve the quality of care and understand how evidence-based practice influences improved patient outcomes.

Research is vital to the future of nursing, and theory is integral to research. Historically, an emphasis on method has overshadowed the subject of nursing research. In addition, many nurses have continued to use theories developed to address phenomena of interest in other disciplines—theories that do not view persons holistically or provide a nursing perspective. However, nurse researchers remain committed to the vital role of nursing theory in their research for knowledge development in their own discipline. These nurses are meeting the challenge of using nursing theory to structure nursing research that tests theory or that develops theory through the interpretation of data using qualitative techniques. You will be reading more about this in the following chapter.

CONCEPTS AND CHALLENGES

- **Concept:** Nursing philosophies, models, theories, and middle-range theories offer many perspectives on nursing, varying in their levels of abstraction and their definitions of four major concepts known as nursing's metaparadigm: person, environment, health, and nursing.
  Challenge: Theory development is not a mysterious activity restricted to a few nursing scholars. It is an activity that combines education, knowledge, and skill. Theories provide an excellent basis for practice.
- **Concept:** As nurses develop theories and test theories of nursing, the discipline moves forward in the development of its unique knowledge base.
  Challenge: The use of theory in practice creates opportunity for the best outcomes for patients because a guiding framework that makes sense supports care.
- **Concept:** Nurses at every level of educational preparation make scholarly contributions to the development and use nursing knowledge by questioning, reading, studying, networking, and writing about nursing practice.

- **Challenge:** Nurses can get caught up in the tasks of their practice and forget that nursing has a specific knowledge base and theoretical orientation that shapes their practice.
- **Concepts:** Nurses in practice settings have invaluable insights and observations, thereby contributing to the knowledge base for nursing. Nursing theorists' early work grew out of their clinical observations and experiences.
  Challenge: Theorists rely on practicing nurses to test clinical interventions and explore the usefulness of their theories.
- **Concept:** Nurse theorists whose works were reviewed in this chapter, as well as others too numerous to include, have made significant contributions to the development of the unique body of nursing knowledge.
  Challenge: The development of theories continues. Nurses in practice add to the development and refinement of theory by being willing to write about their experiences and perspectives and to communicate with the researchers who continue to expand, clarify, and refine original theories.

IDEAS FOR FURTHER EXPLORATION

1. Which philosophy/conceptual framework/theory/middle-range theory introduced in this chapter appeals to you the most? Which ones describe nursing similar to the way you think about nursing? What is it about these theories that makes sense to you?
2. In thinking about the different examples of philosophy, conceptual frameworks, theories, and middle-range theories, which will be the most useful to help you organize your thoughts for critical thinking and decision making in nursing practice?
3. Describe the use of nursing theory for nurses at your current level of nursing education and how you can begin to shape your practice even during early clinical experiences.
4. Explain why theory development is important to the profession of nursing.

REFERENCES

Alligood MR: *Nursing theorists and their work*, ed 9, St. Louis, 2018, Elsevier.

Alligood MR: Philosophies, models and theories: critical thinking structures. In Tomey AM, Alligood MR, editors: *Nursing theory: utilization and application*, ed 5, St. Louis, 2014, Mosby, pp 40–62.

Alligood MR: The power of theoretical knowledge, *Nurs Sci Q* 24(4):304–305, 2011.

Berbiglia V: Orem's self-care deficit theory in nursing practice. In Alligood MR, Tomey AM, editors: *Nursing theory: utilization and application*, ed 5, St. Louis, 2014, pp 222–244.

Bevis EO, Watson J: *Toward a caring curriculum: a new pedagogy for nursing*, New York, 1989, National League for Nursing.

Bevis EO, Watson J: *Toward a caring curriculum: a new pedagogy for nursing*, Boston, 2000, Jones & Bartlett.

Bond AE, Eshah NF, Bani-Kaled M, et al.: Who uses nursing theory? A univariate descriptive analysis of five years' research articles, *Scand J Caring Sci* 25:404–409, 2011.

Chinn P, Kramer M: *Theory and nursing: a systematic approach*, ed 5, St. Louis, 1998, Mosby.

DiNapoli PP, Turkel M, Nelson J, Watson J: Measuring the caritas processes: caring factor survey, *Int J Human Caring* 14(3):16–21, 2010.

Dobratz MC: Life closure with the Roy adaptation model, *Nurs Sci Q* 27:51–56, 2014.

Dobratz MC: Toward development of a middle-range theory of psychological adaptation in death and dying, *Nurs Sci Q* 24:370–376, 2011.

Fawcett J, DeSanto-Madeya S: *Contemporary nursing knowledge: analysis and evaluation of nursing models and theories*, ed 3, Philadelphia, 2013, FA Davis.

Forchuk C, Hildegard E: *Peplau: interpersonal nursing theory*, Newbury Park, Calif, 1993, Sage Publications.

George JB: *Nursing theories: the base for professional nursing practice*, ed 5, Norwalk, Conn, 2002, Appleton & Lange.

Gess T, Dombro M, Gordon SC, et al.: Part one: twentieth-century nursing: Wiedenbach, Henderson, and Orlando's theories and their applications. In Parker ME, editor: *Nursing theories and nursing practice*, ed 2, Philadelphia, 2006, FA Davis.

Henderson V: *The nature of nursing: a definition and its implications for practice, research, and education*, New York, 1966, Macmillan.

Jezewski MA: Evolution of a grounded theory: conflict resolution through cultural brokering, *Adv Nurs Sci* 17(3):14–30, 1995.

Johnson BM, Webber PB: *An introduction to theory and reasoning in nursing*, ed 2, Philadelphia, 2005, Lippincott Williams & Wilkins.

King IM: *A theory for nursing: systems, concepts, process*, New York, 1981, John Wiley & Sons.

Leininger M: *Transcultural nursing: concepts, theories, and practices*, New York, 1978, John Wiley & Sons.

Leininger M: *Culture care diversity and universality: a theory of nursing*, New York, 1991, National League for Nursing.

Lewis S, Rogers M, Naef R: Caring-human science philosophy in nursing education: beyond the curriculum revolution, *Int J Human Caring* 10(4):31–37, 2006.

March A, McCormack D: Nursing theory-directed healthcare, *Holist Nurs Pract* 23(2):75–80, 2009.

Mishel MH: Uncertainty in illness, *Image J Nurs Sch* 20(4):225–232, 1988.

Nightingale F: *Notes on nursing: what it is and what it is not*, New York, 1969, Dover Publications (originally published in 1859).

Orem D: *Nursing: concepts of practice*, ed 6, St. Louis, 2001, Mosby.

Orlando I: *The dynamic nurse-patient relationship: function, process and principles*, New York, 1990, National League for Nursing (originally published in 1961).

Parker M: *Nursing theories and nursing practice*, Philadelphia, 2006, FA Davis.

Parsons T: *Structure of social action*, Glencoe, Ill, 1949, The Free Press.

Pearson A, Vaughan B, FitzGerald M: *Nursing models for practice*, Edinburgh, United Kingdom, 2005, Butterworth Heinemann.

Peplau HE: *Interpersonal relations in nursing*, New York, 1952/1988, GP Putnam's Sons.

Phillips KD, Harris R: Roy's adaptation model in nursing practice. In Alligood MR, Tomey AM, editors: *Nursing theory: utilization and application*, ed 5, St Louis, 2014, Mosby, pp 263–284.

Phillips KD: Roy's adaptation model in nursing practice. In Alligood MR, & Tomey AM, editors: *Nursing Theory: Utilization and Application*, ed 2, St Louis, 2002, Mosby, pp 289–314.

Reynolds CL, Leininger M: *Madeleine leininger: cultural care diversity and universality theory*, Newbury Park, Calif, 1993, Sage Publications.

Roy Sr C: *Introduction to nursing: an adaptation model*, Old Tappan, NJ, 1976, Prentice Hall.

Roy Sr C: *Introduction to nursing: an adaptation model*, ed 2, Englewood Cliffs, NJ, 1984, Prentice Hall.

Roy Sr C, Andrews HA: *The roy adaptation model*, ed 2, Norwalk, Conn, 1999, Appleton & Lange.

Roy Sr C, Andrews HA: *The roy adaptation model*, ed 3, New York, 2008, Pearson.

Roy Sr C, Zhan L: Sister Callista Roy's adaptation model and its applications. In Parker ME, editor: *Nursing theories and nursing practice*, ed 2, Philadelphia, 2006, FA Davis.

Sieloff CL, Frey M, Killeen M: Part two: Applications of King's theory of goal attainment. In Parker ME, editor: *Nursing theories and nursing practice*, ed 2, Philadelphia, 2006, FA Davis, pp 244–267.

Sitzman K, Eichelberger LW: *Understanding the work of nurse theorists: a creative beginning*, Sudbury, Mass, 2004, Jones & Bartlett.

Swanson KM: Empirical development of a middle range theory of caring, *Nurs Res* 40:161–166, 1991.

Watson J: *Nursing: the philosophy and science of caring*, Boston, 1979, Little, Brown.

Watson J: *Nursing: human science and human care*, New York, 1988, National League for Nursing.

Watson J: *Postmodern nursing and beyond*, Edinburgh, UK, 1999, Churchill Livingstone/Saunders/Harcourt Health Sciences.

Watson J: Caring science theory—10 caritas processesR. (website), 2018. Available at: https://www.watsoncaring-science.org/jean-bio/caring-science-theory/.

Wood AF: Nursing models: normal science for nursing practice. In Alligood MR, Tomey AM, editors: *Nursing theory: utilization and application*, ed 5, St Louis, 2014, Mosby, pp 13–39.

10

The Science of Nursing and Evidence-Based Practice

Beth Perry Black, PhD, RN, FAAN

ⓔ To enhance your understanding of this chapter, try the Student Exercises on the Evolve site at http://evolve.elsevier.com/Black/professional.

LEARNING OUTCOMES

After studying this chapter, students will be able to:

- Differentiate among bench, clinical, and translational science.
- Describe the historical development of the scientific method.
- Give examples of inductive and deductive reasoning.
- Discuss the limitations of the scientific method when applied to nursing.
- Differentiate between problem solving and research.

- List the steps in the research process.
- Discuss contributions nursing research has made to nursing practice and to health care.
- Describe the relationship of nursing research to nursing theory and practice.
- Identify sources of support for nursing research.
- Discuss the roles of nurses in research at various levels of education.
- Define *evidence-based practice*.

The word *science* comes from the Latin word *scire*, "to know," and refers to knowledge gained by systematic study—research. Although science and research can be imposing concepts, they actually form the base of the discipline and profession of nursing. The purpose of this chapter is to help you understand nursing's scientific base—the science of nursing—and the links among nursing practice, research, and science. Many of you who are studying this chapter are working toward completion of a bachelor's degree of science in nursing (BSN); each of you is using nursing science to shape your practice.

Mature professions have a strong scientific base, which both defines and is defined by the purposes of a profession. Florence Nightingale, whose work is detailed in Chapter 2, advanced the practice of nursing by both defining it clearly and providing scientific evidence of the outcomes of excellent nursing care in the Crimea. Fig. 10.1 shows her careful documentation of the improvement in morbidity and mortality rates among soldiers in Bulgaria and the Crimea over a course of a year. In the mid-20th century, scholars and researchers realized that nursing could achieve a high level of professional status only to the extent that the discipline was based on a scientific body of knowledge unique to nursing. As a result, nursing researchers began developing knowledge unique to nursing, and nursing theorists began developing theories and testing them. Theory and research are the foundations of scientifically based nursing practice.

At the same time, nurses realized that professionalization of patient care practices was also needed. Until that time, nurses relied on traditional techniques to manage common patient problems. More unusual problems were often managed by trial and error or intuition. However,

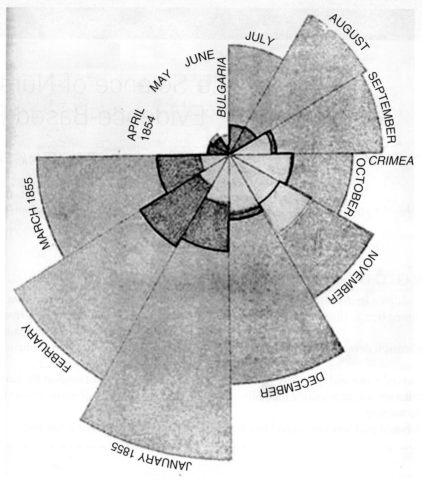

Fig. 10.1 Florence Nightingale's careful detailing of mortality statistics in the Crimean War demonstrated the effectiveness of nursing care in 1855. The area of each wedge is proportional to the statistic being represented. The wedges closest to the center (appearing as yellow) represented deaths from wounds; the largest wedges (appearing as green) represented deaths from contagious diseases such as cholera and typhus; and middle wedges (brown) represented deaths from other causes. (Originally from Nightingale's book *Notes on Matters Affecting the Health, Efficiency and Hospital Administration of the British Army*, published in 1858.)

these were no longer acceptable ways to care for patients. The momentum toward evidence-based practice was developing, which required nurses to base their care and activities on research-based knowledge, in addition to their clinical expertise and patient preferences. The development of evidence-based practice necessitates a strong link between the work of nurse researchers and nurses in practice. The development of the nursing process became a means of adapting a scientific framework to the management of patient care so that nurses were no longer depending on hit-or-miss techniques but were shaping care in direct response to the individual needs of the patient. The nursing process is presented in depth in Chapter 11.

Furthermore, the American Nurses Credentialing Center (ANCC) Magnet Recognition Program, described in Chapter 3, includes in its Magnet Model a requirement for "New Knowledge, Innovation, and Improvements" (Wise, 2009). Inclusion of this requirement for hospitals seeking to attain Magnet status underscores the importance for nursing to be responsible for the development, maintenance, and application of its own professional scientific knowledge base. The Magnet Model requires that initiatives and leadership for nursing research reside with clinical nurses, not nurse managers or others in administrative positions.

SCIENCE AND THE SCIENTIFIC METHOD

Science is research based on one or more past scientific achievements or accomplishments that are acknowledged by the scientific (academic) community as providing a foundation for further study or practice (Kuhn, 1970). Good science—that which contributes to the knowledge bases of a discipline—requires that research be based on the previous work of others in the same academic discipline or be related to work of others from other disciplines. This is a safeguard to ensure that knowledge development is based on sound principles and theory rather than simply the product of a creative idea that is not based on any known science. Sound science and creativity are not mutually exclusive; creativity has led to many interesting and useful research developments that in turn guide nursing practice.

Science has three distinct divisions: natural, social, and formal sciences. Natural sciences include disciplines such as biology, chemistry, and physics. Social sciences such as economics, sociology, anthropology, and history are focused on aspects of the human experience. Formal sciences include logic, systems theory, statistics, and mathematics and are concerned with formal systems—sets of axioms, definitions, and rules—to create knowledge.

Each academic discipline has its own specific scientific community, meaning that nurse researchers and scholars acknowledge and judge scientific developments in nursing. Common to research in all disciplines, however, is the use of an orderly, systematic way of thinking about and solving problems. This systematic way of thinking is traditionally known as the **scientific method,** used by scientists for centuries to discover and test facts and principles. The history of the development of the scientific method is complex; however, Sir Francis Bacon (1561–1626) is widely considered the father of today's scientific method.

The traditional form of "doing science" requires standardized experimental designs with hypotheses, measurable variables and outcomes, and statistical analyses. This form of inquiry is sometimes referred to as **quantitative research,** because variables are measurable (quantifiable). This type of research requires that subjectivity and bias are minimized. *Bias* refers to the systematic distortion of a finding from the data, often resulting from a problem with the sample—that is, the persons being studied. For instance, if you wanted to test an intervention focusing on the benefits of early mobility after abdominal surgery, your sample should include a wide age range of patients. If you included, for instance, only young patients—who, because of their age, are likely to be in otherwise good health and thus are likely to get out of bed soon after surgery—your results may be biased; that is, they show more benefit than the intervention actually delivers because your sample is narrowly confined to younger patients. You introduced bias through your sampling strategy.

Because nursing is interested in human phenomena (events or circumstances) that might not be best studied using traditional quantitative research techniques, a significant number of noted researchers in nursing use a different approach to explore human responses in health and illness. This approach is known as **qualitative research,** because there are no variables being manipulated; rather, qualities of the human experience are described and interpreted. Manipulation of variables is not a goal in this type of research; the systematic and detailed description and interpretation of phenomena are the goals.

Qualitative research, also known as *naturalistic inquiry* or *interpretivism,* relies on data collection techniques such as narrative interviews and participant observation, among others. These techniques are known as "field work," where the researcher spends much time in the setting where the phenomenon occurs. Examples of phenomena studied by qualitative researchers include women's responses to intimate partner violence, fatigue related to human immunodeficiency virus infection, women's experiences of pregnancy when the fetus has been diagnosed with a serious defect, and the adjustment by elders to living in a skilled nursing facility. Qualitative methods are commonly used in the social sciences, where measurement of phenomena may not be possible or even acceptable in terms of understanding the human experience. Several types of inquiry are commonly identified with naturalistic inquiry; ethnography, phenomenology, and grounded theory are the most familiar.

A combination of quantitative and qualitative methodologies is known as **mixed-methods research,** a means of examining phenomena of interest using a variety of data collection techniques and analyses. Regardless of type of methods, all good research has a theoretical basis and is carried out in a systematic, disciplined way that furthers the development of a discipline's knowledge base.

Basic, Clinical, and Translational Science

Traditionally, scientists divided scientific knowledge into two categories: pure and applied. **Pure science** or pure research, sometimes referred to as bench science, summarizes and explains the universe without regard for whether the information is immediately useful. When Joseph Priestley discovered oxygen in 1774, he did not have an immediate use for that information. Therefore that discovery could be classified as pure science—that is, information gathered solely for the sake of obtaining new knowledge. **Applied science** is the practical application of scientific theory and laws. Applied science is usually referred to as clinical science now—taking to the patient's bedside those findings that may be useful in curing, managing, or preventing diseases or managing symptoms. For instance, when Priestley discovered oxygen more than 240 years ago, he had no idea that one day this elemental substance would be used as a therapy under pressure (as hyperbaric oxygen therapy) in the treatment of air emboli, decompression sickness, myonecrosis (gangrene), and other wounds.

More recently, however, scientists have recognized the importance of a third type of research—**translational research**—that serves as a conduit between the "bench and the bedside." Translational research takes the findings in the laboratories and develops them for use at the bedside. In turn, translational research takes the findings from clinical research done at the bedside to ask new questions and to direct new research at the bench level.

In 2006 the National Institutes of Health (NIH), an agency of the U.S. Department of Health and Human Services and the largest source of public funding for health-related research, launched an initiative known as the NIH Common Fund. The Common Fund supports "short-term, goal-driven strategic investments" that are "transformative, catalytic, synergistic, cross-cutting (across NIH centers and institutes), and unique" (NIH, 2018). The Common Fund has supported a series of high-impact programs across the NIH in an effort to enhance the way that American biomedical research is conducted, making it more streamlined and flexible in responding to the health needs of society, while still maintaining the high standards required of excellent scholarship and science.

Inductive and Deductive Reasoning

Research requires the use of one of two kinds of logic: inductive reasoning or deductive reasoning. In **inductive reasoning,** the process begins with a particular experience and proceeds to generalizations. Repeated observations of an experiment or event enable the observer to draw general conclusions. For example, a researcher may be interested in the experiences of women who participated in centering, a form of group prenatal care. After interviewing 25 women who had this form of care and finding a generally positive response, inductive reasoning may lead the researcher to infer that this is an acceptable intervention for pregnant women, based on the responses from this small sample of women. Note that the research did not address the effectiveness of centering prenatal care, but determined that at least for this sample of women, their responses to centering were generally positive. This type of inferential reasoning leads to the development of probabilities but not certainties, unless every single woman who received centering prenatal care was included in the research—a study that would be impossible to conduct.

One of the important uses of research that uses an inductive approach is that inferences are made that lead to further research. For instance, the researcher studying centering prenatal care finds that most women experienced this form of care as acceptable, but also that several mentioned they would appreciate some one-to-one time with a provider to discuss more personal matters. From the findings in the original study, the researcher can develop an intervention and test it against the usual standards of care. In this case three different forms of care could be tested: centering only, centering with provider time (based on the responses of several women in the original qualitative study), and usual care as typically provided in the clinical setting. Note that the research still is focused on the acceptability of care, not the effectiveness of care. The extent of acceptability can be measured and have meaningful results.

Scientists also use **deductive reasoning,** a process in which conclusions are drawn by logical inference from given premises. Deductive reasoning proceeds from the general case to the specific. For example, if the premises "All pregnant women benefit from centering prenatal care" and "Ms. Foster is a pregnant woman" are accepted, the conclusion "Ms. Foster will benefit from centering prenatal care" can be drawn. It may be entirely possible, however, that Ms. Foster, although pregnant and needing prenatal care, may have specific needs not amenable to centering care and will not benefit from receiving care in a group setting. In deductive reasoning, the premises used must be correct or the conclusions will not be. The faulty premise in this example is that "All pregnant women will benefit from centering prenatal care."

Conclusions drawn through deductive processes are called *valid* rather than *true*. *Valid* is a term meaning "soundly founded," whereas *true* means "in accordance with the fact or reality" (Flexner et al., 1980). It is possible for a conclusion to be solidly founded without being true for everyone. There is a subtle but real difference between the words *valid* and *true*. For example, the premise that women benefit from centering care may be valid; this is soundly founded in the original findings of the researcher who interviewed 25 women. What is not true, however, is that *all* women benefit from centering care. The premise is valid but not true in all cases.

As seen by these examples, neither inductive nor deductive processes alone are adequate. If scientists used only deductive logic, experience would be ignored. If they used only inductive logic, relationships between facts and principles could be overlooked. A combination of both types of reasoning processes in science unifies the theoretical and the practical, which is the basis for the scientific method and research.

Limitations of the Strict Definition of Scientific Method in Nursing

The traditional scientific method used by quantitative researchers has considerable value, and it has been used by nurse researchers to address a wide range of nursing problems. However, the scientific method as implemented exclusively with quantitative techniques has limitations when applied to phenomena of interest to nursing.

The first and most obvious drawback is that health care settings are not comparable with laboratories. Certain phenomena of interest to nurses are not amenable to study in a laboratory setting and in fact are not amenable to study in tightly controlled circumstances. For instance, in the discussion of inductive/deductive logic regarding centering prenatal care, measurement of women's experiences and reactions to this method of care is not possible in the laboratory setting by conventional measures. The phenomenon of pregnancy care may be of great interest to perinatal nurses; however,

the systematic examination of this intervention and the measurement of outcomes may not be a particularly good fit with the laboratory setting. Women's reaction to this form of care is a human response that occurs in real-world settings. Research techniques associated with qualitative research may be more appropriate to the aims of this research. Note that the term *naturalistic inquiry* is sometimes used in place of *qualitative research* to refer to the examination of phenomena that occur in the "real world" as opposed to the laboratory setting or in research where variables are controlled.

Second, human beings are far more than collections of parts to be dissected and subjected to examination or experimentation. A criticism of methodology that relies solely on measuring attributes of people is that it is "reductionistic"; that is, the richness of human experience is reduced to variables that can be measured. Conversely, a strength of nursing is its holistic view of patients. Because humans are complex organisms with interrelated parts and systems, the scientific method loses much of its usefulness in the examination of complex human phenomena.

A third limitation of the scientific method as the only approach to solving patient problems is its claim to objectivity (freedom from bias); it fails to consider the meaning of patients' own experiences—that is, their subjective view of reality. Nurses are keenly aware, however, that patients' perceptions of their experiences (subjective data) are just as important as objective data and may have significant effects on their health behaviors. Again referring to the centering prenatal care example, assume that a well-designed, reliable, and valid instrument (such as a questionnaire) can measure Ms. Foster's satisfaction with this form of care. One month after giving birth, her satisfaction scores are higher than they were when she was pregnant, thus it appears that she is satisfied from the centering care. However, this approach fails to take into consideration the complex changes one undergoes when becoming a mother, and Ms. Foster's higher scores may represent something completely different from her satisfaction with her care—her happiness in being a new mother or her relief that she is not pregnant anymore. There may be many reasons she is now scoring higher on satisfaction with this form of prenatal care. The questionnaire by itself may not capture in its entirety the nuances of the experience of Ms. Foster's centering prenatal care in light of her new motherhood.

NURSING RESEARCH: IMPROVING CARE OF PATIENTS

If you are a college or university student, you may have been introduced to research through your basic psychology or sociology courses, or you may have participated in professors' research on your campus. Although sometimes these projects involve interesting experiments, in some cases the only type of research to which you may have been exposed used surveys or questionnaires to collect data. This kind of introduction to research may lead you to wonder what research has to do with your ability to care for patients.

The rest of this chapter describes some basic concepts of nursing research. The purpose is to introduce nursing research, demonstrate its merit, and provide a basic vocabulary. The ultimate goal is for nurses to participate in the research process and apply research findings to clinical practice. This is a key component of what is known as evidence-based practice.

Nursing research is the systematic investigation of phenomena related to improving patient care. Ideas for nursing research often arise from nurses' clinical observations. Although a research topic may be new and innovative, much can be gained from choosing research problems that are connected to work already done, thereby building the body of knowledge of nursing. A problem may be amenable to being addressed by research if these criteria are met:

1. A conceptual framework exists or can be constructed from research that already has been done; that is, the researcher's ideas about the problem fit logically and align with what is already known about the topic.
2. The proposed research project is based on related research findings published in professional peer-reviewed journals or is supported by similar ongoing research in other settings or disciplines, thereby building nursing knowledge.
3. The proposed research is carefully designed so that the results will be applicable in similar situations or will generate hypotheses for further research and testing.

In addition to building nursing knowledge, studies building on previous work are more likely to receive financial support. Research can be expensive and sometimes requires funding beyond what one nurse, hospital, or university can supply. Small projects such as survey research may not be prohibitively expensive, especially if the sample (the persons in the study) is not large or if the survey can be completed online. Many hospitals and professional nursing organizations have funds available for small projects to encourage nurses in practice to do research.

Nurses who want to do large, expensive research studies will find it necessary to obtain outside (external) funding or compete with other aspiring researchers for limited internal (from within the agency) funding. Therefore to receive funding, nurses must do research that interests others, has demonstrated significance, and has support from reviewers who examine the proposed research for the specific funding agency and make recommendations about whether or not to fund it.

Furthermore, research that is not based on or is not related to previous foundational work may have inadvertent violations of human participants' rights. In other words, it is hard to justify asking people to participate in research if there is no real connection to previous work or theory that supports the idea that an intervention works or a problem is significant. Researching or testing an intervention in humans just to see whether it works or that "seemed like a good idea" ignores potential shortcomings or may fail to anticipate problems if adequate foundational work is not done before instituting the research. In fact, such research will not receive approval from a federal human participants' review board if significant linkages with previous research are not demonstrated. This review board (commonly known as the institutional review board) approval must occur before any research involving humans is undertaken.

Thus, although nursing research may be broadly defined as anything that interests nurses and helps them provide better care, controversy exists over what can legitimately be included. When considering a research question, nurse researchers consider the practical issues of background and financial support. An important source of funding and support for nursing research is the NIH's National Institute of Nursing Research (NINR), which in 2020 will celebrate its 35th year of existence. NINR notes that nursing research functions to "build the scientific foundation for clinical practice; prevent disease and disability; manage and eliminate symptoms caused by illness; and enhance end-of-life and palliative care" (NINR, 2016). To advance the science of health, NINR has identified four strategic areas in which it will invest. These highlights from the NINR Strategic Plan are included in Box 10.1.

Research is different from **problem solving.** Problem solving is specific to a given situation and is designed for immediate action, whereas research is **generalizable** or transferable to other situations and deals with long-term solutions rather than immediate ones. For example, Mrs. Abney, an 80-year-old woman with Alzheimer's disease, is a resident in a skilled nursing facility and is often found wandering

the halls unable to find her way back to her room. This is distressing to her and time consuming for the nursing staff who help her find her way "home." A nurse notices that Mrs. Abney has no difficulty recognizing her daughter, so she tapes a photograph of the daughter to Mrs. Abney's door. Now Mrs. Abney can find her room easily. She is less agitated, and the nursing staff time can be spent elsewhere.

Mrs. Abney's case is an example of problem solving, an effective intervention in one set of circumstances that has immediate application. However, the solution that worked for Mrs. Abney may not work for all confused patients. In fact, it may not continue to work for Mrs. Abney as her cognitive abilities decline further. Remember that nursing research was developed in response to the professional and scientific mandate that nursing care be based on evidence and not simply on trial and error. Occasionally, creative problem solving such as that of Mrs. Abney's nurse is required on a per-case, situational basis. But this sort of trial-and-error problem-solving approach is not adequate to base one's professional practice in a substantial and sustained way. Table 10.1 contrasts research and problem solving.

BOX 10.1   National Institute of Nursing Research: Strategic Plan

The mission of the National Institute of Nursing Research (NINR) is to promote and improve the health of individuals, families, communities, and populations. The Institute supports and conducts clinical and basic research and research training on health and illness across the life span to build the scientific foundation for clinical practice and to improve persons' quality of life in all stages of life, and spanning populations and settings. NINR seeks to advance nursing science by supporting research on the science of health, which focuses on the promotion of health and quality of life.

The current areas of scientific focus by NINR are:

- Symptom science: Promoting personalized health strategies
- Wellness: Promoting health and preventing illness
- Self-management: Improving quality of life for individuals with chronic conditions
- End-of-life and palliative care: The science of compassion.

From the National Institute of Nursing Research: *The NINR strategic plan: Advancing science, improving lives.* Bethesda, MD, 2016. National Institutes of Health (NIH). Available at https://www.ninr.nih.gov/sites/files/docs/NINR_StratPlan2016_reduced.pdf.

EVIDENCE-BASED PRACTICE: EVIDENCE, EXPERTISE, PATIENT PREFERENCE

The best efforts of nurse researchers are pointless unless nurses make use of their research findings to improve patient care in their day-to-day practices. Patients have become more knowledgeable consumers of health care, and nurses must ensure that they provide the latest and best available care. One way to ensure positive patient outcomes is through evidence-based practice.

TABLE 10.1   Comparison of Research and Problem Solving

Characteristic	Research	Problem Solving
Type of problems addressed	Significant number of people affected or significant impact on smaller number of people	Situation specific
Conceptual basis	Theoretical framework; keys to researching the problem found in previous research	Often none; trial and error
Knowledge base needed	Extensive review of literature to determine latest thinking and research	Practical knowledge, common sense, and experience
Scope of application	Generalizable or transferable to similar situations	Useful in immediate situation; may or may not be useful in other situations

Evidence-based practice (EBP) is defined as an approach to the delivery of health care that "integrates the best evidence from [research] studies and patient care data with clinician expertise and patient preferences and values" (Melnyk et al., 2009, p. 49). The development of EBP is credited to the work of Archie Cochrane, a British epidemiologist. His work ultimately was reflected in the development of the Cochrane Library, which holds the *Cochrane Database of Systematic Reviews*. Systematic reviews are important means of reviewing data collectively across a number of studies. Clinicians and scholars recognized that practice was improved when critical appraisal of the best evidence is the foundation for practice (Cleary-Holdforth and Leufer, 2008).

In nursing, EBP requires that you be aware of research that supports specific interventions (Alfaro-LeFevre, 2006; Melnyk et al., 2009). Basing one's practice on published work or reliable texts is an element of critical thinking and a good means of improving clinical judgment. Focusing on evidence of effective interventions is a good means of preventing one's practice from deteriorating into routine or traditional care based on what has always been done without concern for advances in care. Taking continuing education courses, attending professional conferences, reading journals, and maintaining membership in professional organizations are good ways of staying current and keeping aware of new evidence of best practices.

Evidence-based practice, however, requires more than simply knowing what the research shows. Clinician expertise and patient preferences are equally important in determining best practices. Sometimes nurses do not realize the importance of these two prongs of the requirement for practice to be evidence based. The issue of patient preference became an important one in the early days of human immunodeficiency virus (HIV) antiretroviral treatments, which at the time were very complicated regimens that sometimes required patients to set an alarm clock to wake themselves in the middle of the night to take their scheduled medications. These were very effective medications; there was a great deal of scientific research to demonstrate they worked to decrease the patient's viral load and extend survival. Furthermore, infectious disease providers had tremendous expertise in managing HIV and prescribing effective medication regimens.

So what happened? Many patients simply could not follow the complex routines these regimens required. It

was not that they did not want to get better; it was simply that the regimens altered the way they lived their lives so much that sustaining these complex schedules was untenable. This reality led to the development of drugs in which doses could be given at longer intervals and some drugs could be given in combination. Research evidence, clinician expertise, and patient preference for more manageable treatment regimens meant that HIV could be managed much more effectively. Patient preference had been the "missing link" in the equation.

Questions regarding best practices are raised daily by nurses in direct patient care roles. Nurses in practice commonly question procedures and routines, asking whether there is a better way to achieve the outcomes of patient care. Most nurses in bedside practice are not equipped to study those questions; however, answers may already be available in the nursing literature. An important focus of professional nursing education is to learn how to seek out and critique research findings to implement best practices in one's own nursing practice. One way to streamline the process of examining research literature is a process known as PICO, an acronym for a four-step process: *P*—population of interest, *I*—intervention, *C*—comparison, *O*—outcome (Cleary-Holdforth and Leufer, 2008). Often *T*—time is added to the acronym. By using PICOT as a framework, you can eliminate research that is not specific enough to the particular problem or intervention you are interested in. Table 10.2 details the elements of the PICOT process with an example of pain management in preschool children after uncomplicated abdominal surgery. By using the PICOT format, evidence addressing pain management in other populations could be eliminated, such as pain management in elderly patients after hip fracture. PICOT is a way of focusing your search for evidence.

Some research carries more weight than others in terms of immediate change in practice. Well-executed randomized controlled trials, long considered the gold standard in research, carry much weight in determining a change in practice; however, descriptive or qualitative studies may inform practice. This means that the findings from a descriptive study may suggest that further research needs to done or an intervention needs to be developed and tested. For example, suppose a hospice nurse notes that the families of terminally ill patients appear to become increasingly anxious about pain symptoms in the evenings, evidenced by an increase in

TABLE 10.2   PICOT as a Tool for Evaluating Interventions

You are concerned by the lack of adequate pain management for preschool children on your pediatric surgery unit:

P	Population of interest (patient group with which you want to intervene)	Children aged 2–5 after uncomplicated abdominal surgery
I	Intervention (a new idea or practice that you are interested in implementing)	Quiet environment; presence of a parent or other family member; scheduled pain medicine administration rather than as needed (PRN)
C	Comparison (what is already being done)	No accommodations in environment; parental presence is common; pain medication given on PRN basis as evidenced by child crying or parent report that child is in pain
O	Outcome (the goal of interventions with the population)	Patients will have better pain management, which allows them improved sleep, increased mobility, and faster healing
T	Time (the time frame in which the patient problem is relevant)	For 48 hours postsurgery

BOX 10.2   Sigma Theta Tau International Position Statement on Evidence-Based Nursing

As a leader in the development and dissemination of knowledge to improve nursing practice, the Honor Society of Nursing, Sigma Theta Tau International, supports the development and implementation of evidence-based nursing. The society defines EBN [evidence-based nursing] as an integration of the best evidence available, nursing expertise, and the values and preferences of the individuals, families, and communities who are served. This assumes that optimal nursing care is provided when nurses and health care decision-makers have access to a synthesis of the latest research, a consensus of expert opinion, and are thus able to exercise their judgment as they plan and provide care that takes into account cultural and personal values and preferences. This approach to nursing care bridges the gap between the best evidence available and the most appropriate nursing care of individuals, groups, and populations with varied needs.

The society, working closely with key partners who provide information to support nursing research and EBN around the world, will be a leading source of information on EBN with an integrated cluster of resources, products, and services that will foster optimal nursing care globally. The society, along with its strategic partners, will provide nurses with the most current and comprehensive resources to translate the best evidence into the best nursing research, education, administration, policy, and practice.

From Sigma Theta Tau International (STTI): *Position statement on evidence-based nursing,* 2005. Available at https://www.sigma-nursing.org/why-sigma/about-sigma/position-statements-and-resource-papers/evidence-based-nursing-position-statement.

phone calls to the on-call nurse after 7 p.m. Interestingly, the patients do not seem to be reporting increased pain. The hospice nurse consults the research literature and finds numerous descriptions of this same phenomenon described several times, but no tested interventions are reported. The nurse, who happens to be a graduate student in a local school of nursing, has identified an interesting topic for her doctor of nursing practice (DNP) project—identifying ways to decrease families' anxiety so that they may spend quality time with their family member.

Sigma, formerly Sigma Theta Tau International, has a long history of support of nursing research and dissemination of research findings. This association has adopted a position statement on evidence-based nursing (EBN) that demonstrates the importance of EBP to its members. Although this position statement was written in 2005, it still appears on the Sigma website as one of their active positions. Note that this statement refers to EBN, as opposed to evidence-based practice. This reflects early discussion about semantic differences between EBN and EBP. *EBP* is now typically used in nursing, which is consistent with other practice disciplines; you can read this position statement in Box 10.2. Drs. Bernadette Melnyk and Ellen Fineout-Overholt have written extensively about EBP in nursing. The *American Journal of Nursing (AJN),* starting in November 2009, published a series of articles every 2 months, "Evidence-Based

Practice: Step by Step," from the Arizona State University College of Nursing and Health Innovation's Center for the Advancement of Evidence-Based Practice. The purpose of this series was to give nurses in practice the tools they need to implement EBP and remains applicable to today's nurses (Melnyk et al., 2009).

THE RESEARCH PROCESS

The **research process** used by nurses is the same process used in any other scientific endeavor; nursing research, however, focuses on patients' responses amenable to nursing care. Research starts with a problem: an observation that something related to practice or patients' responses needs to be addressed. This may be a newly recognized problem that needs an innovative solution. The problem may have been addressed by researchers previously, but the research is insufficient or the findings are inconsistent, unclear, or conflicting. When the need for more information exists, or information is unclear or conflicting, research is the means to resolve, clarify, or inform.

Whether using quantitative or qualitative techniques or mixed methods, all research must be rigorously planned, carefully implemented, and analyzed meticulously. Therefore most research follows a formal order known as the research process. Students in BSN programs often take a semester-long course in nursing research in which both qualitative and quantitative methods are described, so this chapter will attempt only a brief introduction to the research process. Steps in the research process will be presented briefly and include the following:

1. Identification of a researchable problem
2. Review of the literature
3. Formulation of the research question or hypothesis
4. Design of the study
5. Implementation of the study
6. Drawing conclusions based on findings
7. Discussion and/or clinical implications
8. Dissemination of findings

Identification of a Researchable Problem

Researchable problems generally come from three sources: clinical situations, the literature, or theories. The word *researchable* is used specifically, because not all problems are researchable; sometimes a problem may occur too infrequently or pose such ethical challenges that conducting research on the problem is not feasible. Clinical situations are rich sources for researchable problems, and nurses are in a prime position for identifying problems and issues for research. For instance, a common issue among nurses in gerontologic settings is the propensity for some elderly patients to wander and risk getting lost or injured. There are several issues related to this problem, including characteristics of patients who tend to wander, time of day this occurs, staffing issues, and medications. Is the nurse seeking to identify patients at high risk for wandering, or is the nurse more interested in preventing nighttime wandering, specifically? A nurse who has identified a clinical problem that may be amenable to research will have a number of questions to consider while formulating the research. Streamlining the problem into a researchable question is a primary goal early in the research process.

Second, sometimes researchers become interested in a problem because someone else has published research findings about the problem from their own study. The researchers may decide to **replicate** (repeat) the published study or may design a similar one to test part of the original study in a new way. For example, suppose that the nurses in the previous scenario read an article in a professional journal reporting findings from a research study testing an innovative intervention to minimize wandering among elderly patients, and the intervention was found to be effective. In a discussion at their staff meeting about the article, one of the nurses suggests that this approach may not work on this unit for several reasons. The nurses decide to consult with a nurse researcher at the local university to discuss replicating the study on their unit to determine whether, in fact, this innovative intervention will work under the conditions in place here or to determine what prevents the intervention from working.

The third source of research problems—theory—relates to testing theoretical models. In Chapter 9, you read about several types of nursing theory that have been developed. Theoretical models are designed to predict patients' responses to nursing actions; whether a model actually does predict patients' responses can be tested through research. The researcher can create certain conditions and determine whether, in fact, the events happen as predicted by the theoretical model. Again consider the nurses on the gerontology nursing unit. Suppose that one of the nurses who has a psychiatric nursing background noted that some psychiatric patients will wander, but using Peplau's theory of interpersonal relations as the basis for their psychiatric practice, the nurses on the unit found that patients who formed excellent relationships with their primary nurses were the least likely to wander. The gerontology nursing staff decided to test this theory in their elderly patients, using Peplau's theoretical model as a basis for their intervention, predicting that the formation of a trusting relationship between patient and primary nurse would result in less nighttime wandering among patients without cognitive impairment.

Review of the Literature

Once a problem is identified, researchers must review the current literature to see what has been published about the topic. A review of the literature (ROL) is comprehensive and covers all relevant research and supporting documents to support the research. Completing a thorough ROL requires a great deal of searching and detective work, made much easier with sophisticated search engines and tools. A major study with many parts requires huge review efforts, usually involving multiple investigators (researchers) in the work to make sure that the literature review is comprehensive and reflects the current state of the science. A research librarian can be extremely helpful in determining search terms to ensure that the literature review is thorough and comprehensive.

The ROL is essential to locate similar or related studies that have already been completed and on which a new study can build. The review is helpful in creating a conceptual framework, or organization of supporting ideas, on which to base the study. The ROL addresses the question, "What have other researchers and theorists written about this problem?" Sometimes the literature review causes the researcher to rethink or reconceptualize the initial problem, especially if the problem has been studied a variety of ways or if findings in other work are unclear, statistically insignificant, or ambiguous.

Nursing as an academic discipline is relatively young in comparison with other disciplines such as medicine, and the humanities and social sciences, such as history, sociology, and anthropology. Because nursing has a holistic view of patients and problems, and the nursing literature may not be sufficiently broad, often the ROL has to include research outside of the discipline of nursing. For instance, if a researcher is interested in a phenomenon such as perinatal loss, an ROL must include

what has been written in nursing about the phenomenon of perinatal loss, including all aspects such as early and late miscarriage, stillbirth, and elective termination. However, because this is a subject that has many social, ethical, and psychological issues at stake, a thorough ROL would include literature from sociology, anthropology, ethics, and psychology. In addition, the researcher would review literature from the medical field, such as maternal-fetal medicine and reproductive genetics.

As the researcher reviews the literature, he or she will find that other researchers commonly cite some specific papers. These "classics" in research, despite being older papers, have a place in a new ROL. Otherwise, most researchers find that literature published within the past 5 years tends to be adequate. Although reviewing literature can seem tedious, it is a crucial step in ensuring that the planned research will be scientifically sound and theoretically congruent with work that has already been completed.

A caveat is in order here about the use of Internet resources for scholarly work. Although much information is available on the Internet about almost any topic you can imagine, much of this work is not peer reviewed and should be used with caution. The Internet is best used as a tool for disciplined, organized searches of established databases such as CINAHL, Web of Science, PsycINFO, and PubMed. Your school, college, or university may have licenses for these databases so that you have them available to you as a student. These online databases will lead you to peer-reviewed articles that have earned a place in scholarly work. Increasing your ability to use database searches well strengthens your ROL by allowing you increased access to scientific publications that have met the challenges of peer review. When you become a professional nurse, knowing how to gain access to the best research evidence available is an excellent tool in maintaining an up-to-date, informed practice.

Formulation of the Research Question or Hypothesis

Once researchers have identified a research problem, are thoroughly knowledgeable of the relevant literature, and have chosen or created a conceptual framework that helps focus and support the topic, they will formulate the research question. If the researcher is interested in determining and describing certain characteristics of a situation, he or she may simply pose the situation as a question. For example, "What are the characteristics of mothers who have difficulty initiating breastfeeding with their newborns?" is a research question asking about specific characteristics of a population (mothers with breastfeeding difficulties). If comparing the relationship of two or more variables, a different type of question might be asked, such as "What are the relationships among maternal age, number of previous children, and difficulty in initiating breastfeeding?" This question demonstrates that the researcher has some idea that these variables are related (and that the literature supports this idea), but the exact nature of the relationship is not known or hypothesized.

If conducting an experiment, researchers must have a **hypothesis** (educated or informed speculation as to what the outcome will be) so that hypothesis-testing statistics may later be applied. For example, "Younger, inexperienced mothers giving birth for the first time will demonstrate later initiation of breastfeeding than older, experienced mothers who have given birth previously" is a testable hypothesis. The form and content of the research question are key to the development of the rest of the study. Larger, more complex studies will have multiple questions or hypotheses to address.

In the example on breastfeeding, the challenge to the researcher is to define the variables such as "younger" versus "older." The researcher might establish a cutoff in age, defining "younger" as younger than 30 years old and "older" as equal to or older than 30. Defining "experienced" versus "not experienced" might be more challenging: a mother might have previous children but may be breastfeeding for the first time—is she experienced or not? Researchers have to define their variables in a way that makes sense and is consistent with what has been shown in the literature. In other words, the researcher must be able to defend how the variables are defined.

Design of the Study

Once the research questions are identified or hypotheses are generated, the researcher then designs the study. Numerous forms of research designs exist, but experimental and nonexperimental designs are the two major categories. If the purpose of the research is to determine the effect of an intervention or to compare the responses of participants to two or more differing treatments, for example, the research will have an **experimental design.** If not, the research will have a **nonexperimental design.** The main difference between experimental

and nonexperimental research is whether the researcher manipulates, influences, or changes the participants in any way by the testing of an intervention or medication or other substance.

True experimental designs provide evidence of a cause-and-effect relationship between actions. For example, testing the hypothesis "Patients who receive preoperative anxiolytics need less pain medication in the first 24 hours postoperatively than those who do not" could provide evidence of a significant relationship between preoperative anxiolytics and perception of pain. Experimental designs require quantitative measures to determine whether there are statistically significant differences between the conditions being tested. Nurses Doing Research Box 10.1 features the work of Robin Knobel, PhD, RN, who tested a simple intervention of preventing the loss of body heat in preterm infants in the delivery room, a major cause of morbidity in these vulnerable patients. From her nursing practice, she noticed the importance of and challenges in keeping very small newborns warm. She used this interest to develop a program of research on thermoregulation in preterm infants. Nurses Doing Research Box 10.2 contains a description of the research of Diane Berry, PhD, ANP-BC, FAANP, FAAN, whose work involves the management of diabetes, overweight, and obesity that disproportionately affect ethnic minority families.

Sometimes it is impossible to conduct a true experimental study with human beings because to do so might endanger them in some way. In those instances, modified experimental studies are used. In this case, a new intensive form of preparation for discharge home might be compared with the usual form of discharge teaching. Because discharge teaching is standard care and an expected nursing action, denying discharge teaching to patients would be unethical and inappropriate. The experimental design could, however, test a new intervention against the usual care received by patients who are preparing for discharge home.

Nonexperimental designs are sometimes referred to as "descriptive" or "exploratory" research because the investigator is seeking to increase the knowledge base about a nursing phenomenon by doing careful, disciplined research. There are many types of nonexperimental designs: surveys, descriptive comparisons, evaluation studies, and historical-documentary research, among others. Nonexperimental designs may be either quantitative or qualitative, or they may use a combination of both.

NURSES DOING RESEARCH BOX 10.1

Addressing the Problem of Hypothermia in Premature Infants

As a neonatal nurse practitioner, I became aware of the problem of hypothermia (low body temperature) in premature infants. Infants can become very cold in the delivery room (DR), leaving the warm maternal environment. They are then taken to neonatal intensive care units (NICUs), further increasing exposure to cold. Unlike full-term infants, preterm infants, especially those weighing less than 1000 g (2.2 lb), cannot generate their own heat by nonshivering thermogenesis; lacking insulating body fat, their temperature falls. A tiny infant transferred to our NICU from a smaller hospital had a temperature of 91° F. The baby died 2 weeks later.

I began to examine hypothermia in our NICU. In a medical record review of 100 patients, I found that 93% of infants less than 1000 g had rectal temperatures less than 36.4° C on admission, a cold temperature for even full-term infants. I reviewed the literature, finding a small study in which researchers reduced evaporative heat loss in the DR by wrapping preterm infants in an occlusive material. I replicated this study with a sample of 88 infants less than 29 weeks' gestation. While still wet, they were placed up to their necks in a polyurethane bag and were then resuscitated normally (top photo). Infants placed in bags were less likely to be hypothermic on admission to the NICU (44% vs. 70%, $p < 0.01$) and had higher mean admission temperatures than those not placed in bags (36.5° C vs. 36° C, $p < 0.003$). Neonatal Resuscitation Program standards now suggest that an infant younger than 28 weeks be placed up to the neck in a polyethylene bag.

During my PhD program, I continued to study temperature in infants less than 1000 g, measuring central and peripheral temperature in 10 infants for the first 12 hours after birth to determine whether they exhibited peripheral vasoconstriction in response to cold body temperatures. Infants should constrict vessels in their feet once their core becomes cold. Nine of the ten infants did not exhibit peripheral vasoconstriction; thus their peripheral temperatures tended to be higher than their central temperatures. A preterm infant's neural control over blood flow to control body temperature may be immature during this period.

More recently, I worked with a team examining infants less than 1000 g for the first 2 weeks after birth. Our purpose was to describe the trajectory of maturing neural control over blood flow to control body temperature. We measured central and peripheral body temperature every minute for 14 days to determine when small infants are able to consistently exhibit peripheral vasoconstriction in response to cold body temperatures, keeping their central body temperature warmer than their peripheral temperature. We used an infrared camera to look at temperature over the entire body surface daily. This is a novel technology that can measure body temperature for any pixel in a picture of the infant, creating a thermal image (bottom photo) that allowed us to compare simultaneous temperatures in central and peripheral areas. This study provided interesting data related to maturation of neural control of body temperature between different gestational ages and over postnatal age.

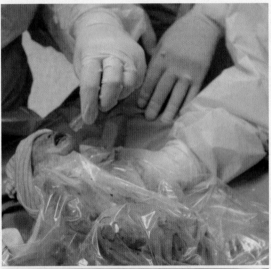

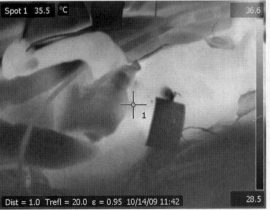

Robin Knobel, PhD, RN, FAAN.
Professor, University of South Carolina
College of Nursing

Courtesy Robin Knobel.

NURSES DOING RESEARCH BOX 10.2

Understanding How Overweight and Obesity Affect Ethnic Minority Families Disproportionately

I started nursing school when I was 16 years old at the Sisters of Charity Hospital School of Nursing and Canisus College in Buffalo, New York, and graduated with a diploma and became a registered nurse at 19 years old. I worked as a registered nurse in cardiology for years and eventually went back to school to earn a bachelor's of science from Lenoir Rhyne College in Hickory, North Carolina. I then moved to Boston, Massachusetts, to work in cardiology at New England Medical Center. It was during this time that I started to wonder why so many patients with cardiology problems were overweight and had type 2 diabetes and witnessed the ethnic disparities between those who could afford care and had insurance and those who could not.

I decided that to help answer those questions, I needed to go back to school. I was fortunate to go to Boston College in Chestnut Hill, Massachusetts, for my master of science in nursing (MSN) and adult nurse practitioner and doctor of philosophy (PhD) degrees. My dissertation focused on women who were successful at long-term weight loss and maintenance, and I used qualitative methods to interview women about what they thought they needed to be successful at weight loss and maintenance. My dissertation gave me insight into what women needed to ensure weight loss and maintenance. After completing my dissertation, I was accepted at Yale University to do a postdoctoral fellowship ("postdoc") in self and family management.

During my postdoc I developed and pilot tested a nutrition and exercise education and cognitive-behavioral theory intervention focusing on parents and children in inner-city New Haven. My travels next took me to the University of North Carolina at Chapel Hill where I have developed and worked with interdisciplinary teams developing research and interventions that focus on developing community-based nutrition and exercise education and cognitive-behavioral theory for parents and children struggling with overweight, obesity, type 2 diabetes mellitus, and gestational diabetes mellitus. I have developed

long-standing partnerships with school systems, federally qualified public health centers, and community-based clinics focusing on ethnic minority families in the United States and most recently in Mexico. The basic intervention focuses on nutrition and exercise education and cognitive-behavioral theory.

A "program of research" refers to a sustained focus on a particular area of interest. My program of research on management of weight and type 2 diabetes mellitus is currently moving toward an intervention that features the use of a multimodal web-based platform, which gives participants convenient, affordable access through computer, tablet, and smartphone technologies. Although I have been doing this research for a number of years, I still find it enjoyable and fulfilling—and I know that it makes a positive difference for those persons struggling with diabetes and management of their weight.

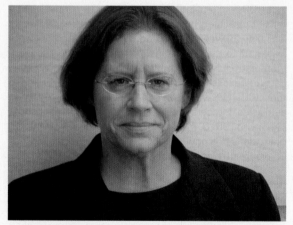

Diane Berry, PhD, ANP-BC, FAANP, FAAN.

Professor and Assistant Dean for Research, University of North Carolina at Chapel Hill School of Nursing

Courtesy Diane Berry.

Nurses Doing Research Box 10.3 features the work of Cheryl Woods-Giscombé, PhD, PMHNP, whose descriptive research of African American women has resulted in a clearer understanding of the stresses of the Superwoman Role that pose challenges to their health. Like Drs. Knobel and Berry, whose work was described

earlier, Dr. Woods-Giscombé's early experiences shaped the direction of her research career.

Whether the researcher chooses an experimental or nonexperimental design influences the data collection process. The data collection process includes selection of data collection instruments, design of the data collection

NURSES DOING RESEARCH BOX 10.3

Understanding How Stress and Coping Contribute to Psychological and Physical Health Outcomes in African American Women

I was always perplexed by health disparities and the contribution of stress to health behaviors and overall well-being. I learned in health classes that African Americans had disproportionately high rates of chronic illness and experienced a shorter life span, yet I never heard any explanation for these disparities. In eighth grade I set the goal of earning my doctor of philosophy (PhD) degree in psychology. My grandmother, a licensed practical/vocational nurse, reminded me that as a young child I had wanted to be a nurse; as a teenager, I did not yet connect nursing with a career in psychology.

As an undergraduate psychology major, I witnessed a psychiatric intake interview with an elderly African American woman admitted to the hospital for "psychotic symptoms." As the only other African American in the room among a team of well-intentioned medical personnel, I thought that no one seemed to "get her." The patient seemed overwhelmed by us. The medical team's labeling of her behavior as bizarre overshadowed her humanity; her explanation of her religious faith was interpreted as delusional. Yet to me she was not so different from other older African American women I knew: optimistic and faithful, yet worn down by chronic stress and familial commitments. I realized then that communication gaps and limited understanding of sociocultural context could not only limit the delivery of health care but also contribute to worsening symptoms and disparities.

While working on my PhD in psychology, I collected data for a clinic-based study that allowed me to observe the work of a nurse practitioner (NP). After a short time of observing how the NP engaged with her patients, their positive responses, and the NP's delight and commitment to providing the best interpersonal and clinically sound strategies to promote health, I was sold! I became a nurse and a psychiatric NP to achieve my career goal of being a national leader in health disparities research and having a clinical practice focusing on the influence of stress on mental and physical health outcomes and on culturally relevant stress management interventions.

Currently my research incorporates sociohistorical and biopsychosocial perspectives to investigate how stress and coping strategies contribute to psychological and physical health outcomes. My Multi-Dimensional Stress Model and Superwoman Schema (SWS) Conceptual Framework show how race- and gender-related factors specifically influence stress, coping, and health inequities among African American women. The SWS Conceptual Framework posits that African American women are at increased risk of health disparities as a result of perceived obligations to remain silent about feelings of distress in order to project an image of strength for their families and communities. These obligations may result from sociohistorical patterns of marginalization, oppression, and stress exposure related to African American women's interconnected race, gender, and socioeconomic status and contribute to the development of resilience, fortitude, and a sense of invulnerability.

The potential contributions of nursing to science and evidence-based health care are practically limitless. I am so proud to be a nursing scholar!

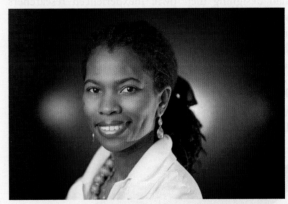

Cheryl Woods-Giscombé, PhD, PMHNP.

Associate Professor of Nursing, University of North Carolina at Chapel Hill

Courtesy Cheryl Woods-Giscombé.

protocol, the data analysis plan, participant selection and informed consent, and institutional review plans.

Data Collection Instruments

When designing a study, researchers must consider how the **data** will be collected. Data collection instruments, sometimes called *data collection tools*, range from simple survey forms to complex gene sequencing instruments. The selected instrument used must be **reliable,** or consistently accurate. A reliable instrument is one that yields the same values dependably each time the instrument is used to measure the same thing. The tool must also be valid, which means that it must measure what it is supposed to be measuring. The ideal instrument is highly reliable and provides a valid measure of the condition under study, such as weight, temperature, depression, or anxiety.

If body temperature is being measured, a thermometer is an obvious data collection tool—meaning that it is known to be a valid measure of temperature—and a scale is the appropriate (valid) measure for weight. Importantly, a valid measure may not be reliable. A scale that varies widely between measurements is not reliable; anyone who has stepped on and off a scale several times to (eventually) get it to show an acceptable weight understands what "unreliable" means (Fig. 10.2). The scale is a valid tool to measure weight; its fluctuation, however, means that it is not reliable.

When measuring psychological phenomena such as anxiety or depression, or constructs (conditions) such as satisfaction or quality of life, researchers face a challenge to determine the best data collection tool. To minimize measurement errors, beginning researchers should choose instruments with established reliability and validity that have been published and widely used rather than designing their own. Inexperienced researchers will occasionally make the mistake of designing a questionnaire they believe is a valid measure of the construct they want to study; doing this, however, constitutes a serious flaw in the research and must be avoided.

Data Collection Protocol

Another aspect of designing the study is deciding on the data collection protocol. The quality of the data depends on strict adherence to the protocol. If, for example, the protocol calls for administering a questionnaire to patients with cancer 2 days after their first cycle of chemotherapy, the data collectors must be sure to give the questionnaire to all participants on time. The protocol for data collection must be explicit and used by everyone who is collecting data for the study. Data collected in the wrong way or at the wrong time introduce errors into the study.

Data Analysis Plan

It may seem premature to decide how the data will be analyzed before they are even collected, but careful planning for the analysis is important. The research design is developed with data analysis in mind. The analysis must be part of the planning process, because the data and the protocols for collecting them depend on how the data will be analyzed. Unless the nurse researcher is an expert in statistics or a statistician is on the research team, consultation with a statistician well versed in human research is recommended in designing the data analysis plan, which answers the question, "What will we do with the data once we collect them?"

Qualitative analysis, notably, begins immediately with the collection of data, because the data themselves often drive the shape and design of the research. Qualitative analysis is a difficult and exacting procedure requiring extensive training. Although some researchers believe that qualitative research may be easier to execute than quantitative research, in fact they are similar in the disciplined approach to data analysis required to produce usable, meaningful results.

Participant Selection

A key part of planning research is determining specifically the population to be studied. The individuals enrolled in a study are participants (formerly "subjects"). If the researchers plan to study pain management in patients with traumatic injuries in the emergency department, for example, they have to decide the specific type and severity of traumatic injury and will likely consider the age, gender, ethnicity, and geographic location of the patients, as well as a variety of other factors, in planning the participant selection. Qualitative studies use different sampling strategies; that is, the participants are selected for study in a different manner than is typically used in quantitative studies. Qualitative researchers often use a strategy

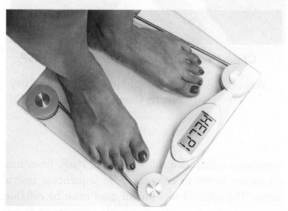

Fig. 10.2 A scale may not always be an accurate way to measure your weight.

known as "purposeful sampling"; potential participants are selected for the study specifically rather than randomly, as is sometimes used in quantitative studies. These participants exhibit a trait or have had an experience that the researcher is studying.

Informed Consent and Institutional Review

Next, researchers who want to enroll humans in their study must protect the rights of participants. This involves the use of the informed consent process, which includes having participants sign an **informed consent** document detailing the study and what participation in the research means. Any risks must be explained. A basic principle of informed consent is that participation in research is *always voluntary*—no one may be pressured in any way to enroll in the study or to continue in the study once enrolled. **Confidentiality** (privacy) of participants must be ensured. Considering Culture Box 10.1 addresses the difficulties of enrolling participants in research when they do not speak English.

A related step when studying humans is the submission of the proposal to the institution, such as a hospital or clinic, where the research will take place, for review by a federally approved board known as an institutional review board (IRB). An IRB is composed of individuals from the community and different academic disciplines and exists to ensure that research is well designed and does not violate the policies and procedures of the institution or the rights of the participants. Only after the IRB approves the proposal can the study begin. Persons conducting research or assisting with the management of data must demonstrate evidence that they have

⊕ CONSIDERING CULTURE BOX 10.1

The Challenge of Informed Consent: When the Participant Does Not Speak English

Researchers studying humans must protect the rights of their participants by asking them to sign a detailed consent form that describes the study and what participation in the study means. With an increasing number of potential participants who may not know English or for whom English is a second language, what measures would researchers need to consider when a potential participant may not fully understand the consent form? What are the risks to these persons? How can these risks be minimized? How might researchers ensure that these participants do not feel pressured to participate?

taken an online course on the protection of the rights of human participants (www.citiprogram.org). The protection of the rights of participants is the primary consideration of all research involving humans. Modification of any aspect of the research requires that the IRB be notified and approval procured before the change is implemented.

Implementation of the Study

Up until this point, only planning has taken place. Careful planning is, however, the key to a successful study. In the implementation phase, the actual study is conducted. The two main tasks during this phase are data collection and data analysis.

Data Collection

Data (research-generated information) should be collected only by persons (usually research assistants) thoroughly familiar with the study. All research assistants should understand the purpose of the data and the importance of accuracy and careful record keeping. No matter who is collecting the data, the integrity of the project is ultimately the responsibility of the primary researcher.

Data Analysis

If all goes well, data are analyzed exactly as proposed. In analyzing data, most researchers use the same statistician with whom they consulted in planning the study. The researcher works closely with the statistician in interpreting, as well as analyzing, the data. The nurse researcher is in charge, however, and he or she has the final word on what interpretations are made from the data.

Analyzing the findings of qualitative research presents formidable challenges for several reasons. First, the data sets are huge, often consisting of lengthy dialogues between researchers and participants. Next, dialogues must be transcribed verbatim, yielding long transcripts. The investigator then faces the task of organizing the transcripts, identifying themes, and arranging the themes into meaningful patterns. Software is available to assist in this process; however, nothing substitutes for contemplation in determining the nuances of meanings in narrative data.

Findings, Discussion, and Clinical Implications

In writing the research report, the findings directly related to the research question are presented first.

Findings are presented objectively—without value judgments. The findings must speak for themselves. Accurate presentation of the facts is the only requirement. After findings related to the research question are reported, unexpected findings can be reported. The researchers address the question, "What do these findings mean?" In discussion sections, researchers can be more reflective about the findings, discussing what was anticipated versus what was found in the study, suggesting alternative explanations for their findings and further research to clarify findings.

Researchers are always alert to the implications of their studies. Implications are suggestions for actions that can be taken as a result of the research findings in the future. Every good study raises more questions than it answers. In nursing studies there may be indications for modifications in nursing education or nursing practice. Nearly every study has implications for further research, and if the findings turn out as expected, almost all studies should be carefully replicated. Replication can answer these and other questions: What needs to be known to develop more confidence in the findings? Will the research instrument produce similar results in a similar population in a different geographic location? Will the procedure be effective with patients having a slightly different diagnosis, condition, or type of surgery? Will age make a difference? Will cultural beliefs make a difference? What else do we need to know to improve the care of patients?

Dissemination of Findings

Findings from a research study must be disseminated so that others can learn from the work that was done. Dissemination refers to the process of publication and presentation of findings. Most funding agencies want to know in advance how the researcher plans to disseminate findings, because letting others know about the findings is essential. The two major vehicles for dissemination of knowledge are articles published in professional journals and presentations given at conferences. Prominent nursing research journals include *Research in Nursing & Health (RINAH)*, *Nursing Research (NR)*, *Journal of Nursing Scholarship* (published by Sigma), *Nursing Inquiry*, *Journal of Advanced Nursing*, *Advances in Nursing Science (ANS)*, and the *Western Journal of Nursing Research*. These journals are not specific to any particular type of nursing but publish articles of wide interest in nursing. Professional nursing organizations

are likely to have their own research journals targeting specific interests, such as *JOGNN: Journal of Obstetric, Gynecologic, & Neonatal Nursing*, published by the Association of Women's Health, Obstetric and Neonatal Nurses (AWHONN), and *Journal of the Association of Nurses in AIDS Care (JANAC)*, published by the Association of Nurses in AIDS Care (ANAC).

A review process, called peer review, is the method most journals use to determine whether to publish a research report. During peer review, a manuscript is circulated, usually anonymously, to a review panel consisting of two to three experts in the area of study. Reviewers evaluate its scientific soundness, appropriateness of design, and accuracy and recommend that it be published, that it be revised and then resubmitted with changes, or that it be rejected. Most research that is carefully conceived, conducted, and presented can get published, although the researcher must be persistent and resilient in taking criticism and revising manuscripts.

A somewhat easier, yet still discriminating, route to dissemination is presentation at one or more of the numerous nursing research conferences. Many research conferences also use the peer-review process. In general, however, the proportion of abstracts (summaries of research) selected for presentation at conferences is higher than the proportion of manuscripts chosen for publication. In addition to oral presentation of research papers, conferences offer the opportunity for nurses to present their findings in poster sessions, especially appropriate when work is preliminary or still in progress. Posters allow for brief explanations of the research method and findings in written form, usually a 3- × 4-foot poster that is professionally designed. Poster presentations are often the first way that students doing research disseminate their findings.

Whether research is published or presented at conferences, it is important to disseminate research results to other nurses, who may choose to use the results either to improve patient care practices or to replicate the study.

THE RELATIONSHIP OF RESEARCH TO THEORY AND PRACTICE

Relationships among nursing research, practice, and theory are circular. As mentioned earlier, research ideas are generated from three sources: (1) clinical practice, (2) literature, and (3) theory.

Questions about how best to deal with patient problems regularly arise in clinical situations. As shown in the earlier example of Mrs. Abney, the elderly woman who could not find her room, problems often can be "solved" for the present. However, when the same questions recur, long-term answers may be needed. Research develops solutions that can be used with confidence in different situations.

Published articles about nursing research often generate interest in further studies. If there is published research on a particular nursing care problem, other researchers may be stimulated to investigate the subject further and refine the solutions. This is how nursing knowledge builds.

Nursing theorists also generate research ideas. They piece together postulates or premises that explain what has been discovered. The explanation is tested via research to determine whether it is robust or strong enough to be useful. If so, there may be more implications for applications in clinical practice. Nursing research journals are filled with clinical studies that have made a difference in patient care. A few examples of changes in nursing practice stimulated by research include decreasing light and noise in critical care units to prevent sleep deprivation; using caps on newborns to decrease heat loss and stabilize body temperature; and proper positioning of patients after chest surgery to facilitate respiration.

Nursing research findings not only improve patient care but also affect the health care system itself. For example, research studies have demonstrated the cost effectiveness of nurses as health care providers. This is discussed further in Chapter 14.

A final point about the influence of research on practice is a reminder about the relationship of research and professionalism. In Chapter 3, you learned about the characteristics of professions. One of the hallmarks of a mature profession is a scientific body of knowledge that is expanded through research. Nursing research enhances the status of nursing as a profession by expanding nursing's scientific knowledge base. Researchers in other disciplines can then use the sound research produced by nurse researchers as part of a foundation for their own work.

FINANCIAL SUPPORT FOR NURSING RESEARCH

Nursing research is expensive, and support takes many forms. It can include encouragement, consultation, computer and library resources, money, and release time from researchers' regular teaching responsibilities. Each of these forms of support is important, but none alone is adequate. Early in the development of nursing research, encouragement was often the only support available, and not all nurse researchers had that. Gradually over the years, more sources of funding have been identified, but financial support can still be difficult to obtain, particularly for new researchers.

Many other federal agencies accept proposals that meet their funding guidelines when submitted by qualified nurse researchers. These include the 27 centers and institutes of the NIH, including NINR. Competition with researchers from other disciplines is strong, however, and generally only experienced nurse researchers are successful in obtaining funding from these sources.

Nursing associations also fund nursing research. The American Nurses Foundation, Sigma, and many clinical specialty organizations provide research awards, even for beginning researchers. State and local nursing associations sometimes have seed money for pilot projects. Universities, schools of nursing, and large hospitals also may provide small amounts of research funds. In general, however, finding adequate funding for large-scale studies continues to be a problem faced by researchers.

ADVANCING THE PROFESSION THROUGH THE USE OF RESEARCH

The American Nurses Association's *Code of Ethics,* Provision 7.3, states: "The nursing profession should engage in scholarly inquiry to identify, evaluate, refine, and expand the body of knowledge that forms the foundation of its discipline and practice. ... All nurses working alone or in collaboration with others can participate in the advancement of the profession through the development, evaluation, dissemination, and application of knowledge in practice" (American Nurses Association, 2015). Ideally, every nurse should be involved in research, but practically, as a minimum, all nurses should use research to support and improve their practices. EBP requires staying informed about current research literature, especially studies done in one's own specific area of clinical practice.

As shown in Table 10.3, in addition to using research to improve practice, all professional nurses can contribute to one or more aspects of the research process. From the time nurses begin their basic nursing education, they become consumers of research. BSN-prepared

TABLE 10.3 Levels of Educational Preparation and Participation in Nursing Research

Level of Preparation	Level of Research Participation
Nursing student	Learning about research; doing honors projects or assisting in laboratories
Bachelor of science in nursing (BSN)	Identifies problems that can be studied; may do data collection for research studies
Master of science in nursing (MSN)	Replicates earlier research; beginning independent research
Doctor of nursing practice (DNP)	Connect research to practice; do research in collaboration with a PhD-prepared colleague
Doctor of philosophy (PhD)	Generate and test theory; establishing independent research career with external funding (e.g., National Institutes of Health, foundation grants)

Note: Nurses at all levels are assumed to be consumers of research.

nurses can read, interpret, and evaluate research for use in supporting their EBN practice. Through clinical practice they can identify nursing problems that need to be investigated. They can also participate in the implementation of scientific studies by helping principal researchers collect data in clinical settings or elsewhere. These beginning researchers must know enough about the purpose of the research to follow the research protocols explicitly or know when it is necessary to deviate from the protocol for a patient's well-being. BSN-prepared nurses also can help disseminate research-based knowledge by sharing useful research findings with colleagues.

The master's-prepared nurse may be ready to work with experienced nurse researchers to replicate studies that have been previously conducted. Researchers cannot be sure that their findings are valid until studies are repeated with similar results. Nurse researchers have

learned that it is not necessary (or even desirable) to generate a totally new and disconnected idea to do research. As mentioned earlier, to be most useful, research must be based on a conceptual framework and related to previous research.

Depending on education, clinical and research experiences, and interests, some nurses at the master's level are better prepared to conduct research than others. In addition to education and experience, a crucial factor is the support system the nurse has available. To do research, nurses need time, money, consultation, and participants. With rich resources in a research environment, master's degree–prepared nurses can and do make vital research contributions.

Nurses with doctor of philosophy (PhD) or other doctoral degrees (e.g., doctor of nursing practice [DNP], doctor of education [EdD], doctor of public health [DrPH]) are more favorably positioned to receive research funding than are nurses without doctorates. Researchers across the United States in all professions and academic disciplines compete for a limited pool of research dollars available each year. Only those nurses with strong academic and experiential backgrounds and the best proposals succeed in obtaining federal funding. Currently, only nurses with PhDs may receive funding from the NIH, although other funding sources are open to nurses with other doctoral degrees.

Research in nursing provides the avenue for creative, scholarly endeavors driven by a desire to improve the care for patients. Professional Profile Box 10.1 contains a description of the work and career of Claudia Christy, MSN, RN, CCRC, whose work demonstrates ways other than conducting studies that nurses can be involved in the development and implementation of research. You will find research to be an important part of your professional practice both as a consumer of research and as an adherent to evidence-based practice. And someday you may confront a question or situation in practice so compelling that you respond by starting your own research career to improve patient outcomes by improving nursing practice.

A Career Helping Others with Their Research

After earning my bachelor of science degree in nursing (BSN) with a major in nursing at Villa Maria College in Erie, Pennsylvania, I first worked as a staff nurse in a surgery intensive care unit in Pittsburg, Pennsylvania, but within a short time I moved to Chapel Hill, North Carolina, to work in the cardiothoracic intensive care unit.

To be truthful, I got into clinical research by accident for my first position as a cardiology research nurse, an experience in which I learned—unfortunately—what the term *soft money* means. It means that funding for research is not permanent or guaranteed, and after 1½ years, we lost our funding. But even after learning what it meant to be working on soft money, I knew I wanted to continue working as a clinical research nurse. Soon hired as a pediatric intensive care unit (PICU) research nurse, I managed all aspects of a research study (screening for participants, completing the informed consent process, collecting data, responding to queries, negotiating budgets, and eventually closing out the study).

Most recently, I was a research nurse consultant with North Carolina Translational and Clinical Sciences Institute (NC TraCS). I facilitated a study group for persons interested in preparation for the clinical research certification examination—and 29 people who participated in the study group passed the examination. I am a member of the Association of Clinical Research Professionals (ACRP) and have been a Certified Clinical Research Coordinator (CCRC) for 10 years.

I have done many local and national presentations on the protection of the rights of human subjects in research. Through the ACRP I met Eva Mozes Kor, a survivor of Mengele's experiments at Auschwitz, touring Auschwitz with her during the 65th anniversary of its liberation. This relationship fueled my passion for research ethics.

Being a nurse is a real asset in my role as a research nurse. One of the PICU researchers asked me, "When did you quit being a real nurse?" I responded, "I am still a nurse." The role of the nurse is not limited to bedside patient care. There are other ways to be a nurse! In both roles, the first priority is protection—of your patient or your research participant.

Because I am a nurse, I can review a medical record to see if someone qualifies for a study, understand the participant's disease process, and recognize adverse events. As a research nurse I have to *assess* the situation, participant, or protocol; *plan* how the study would be implemented; *implement* the study; and *evaluate* the extent to which it is being implemented correctly. That sounds like the nursing process to me. Critical thinking is central in the role of the research nurse.

While completing my master of science in nursing (MSN), I developed an interest in four areas—research, ethics, legal, and quality. As a clinical research nurse, I found a role where I could be involved in all four.

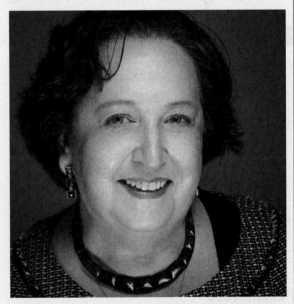

Claudia Christy, MSN, RN, CCRC.

Courtesy Claudia Christy.

CONCEPTS AND CHALLENGES

- *Concept:* Nursing research is defined as the systematic investigation of phenomena of interest to nursing with the goal of improving care.

  Challenge: Nurses must value research as an important means of optimizing patient outcomes, in addition to clinician expertise and patient preferences, in having practices that are evidence based.

- *Concept:* The scientific method is a systematic, orderly process of solving problems. It has been used for centuries and is applicable in many different situations.

  Challenge: There are several types of research—laboratory (bench) research and bedside (clinical) research are two traditional types. Translational research is a means of connecting more efficiently the work that is generated in laboratories and directly within patient populations, a connection that is not always easy to make.

- **Concept:** For safety and ethical reasons, there are limitations on research with human participants.

  Challenge: It can be difficult to determine all of the ways that research may pose a threat to participants; therefore all research involving humans must go through a process of approval by an institutional review board.

- **Concept:** The major steps in the research process are identification of a research problem, review of the literature, formulation of the research question, design of the study, implementation, drawing conclusions based on findings, discussion of implications, and dissemination of findings.

  Challenge: Assessing research for its usefulness requires that nurses recognize the presence of

each of these steps. Well-executed research has followed these steps carefully.

- **Concept:** Nursing research is related to and informed by nursing theory and nursing practice and in turn influences them.

  Challenge: The relationship among theory, research, and practice can be difficult to understand; however, each depends on the others for clarity and direction.

- **Concept:** Nurses of all educational backgrounds are consumers of research and have a role in carrying out research either directly through the implementation of a study or through the use of research in informing practice.

  Challenge: Envisioning oneself as a nurse researcher can pose a challenge; however, the use of research must be a priority for students and nurses to continue to advance the profession and discipline of nursing.

IDEAS FOR FURTHER EXPLORATION

1. Define *inductive* and *deductive reasoning*. Why is neither adequate to advance knowledge alone? Are you more likely to change practice using research that uses an inductive or a deductive approach to reasoning?

2. Go to your college or university library or online site and determine what nursing research journals are available to you. Scan through some recent issues and notice the types of studies reported. Compare them with studies done 20 years ago. What similarities and differences do you note?

3. Read a research article on a topic of interest to you. See whether you can identify each of the steps in the

research process. Is the article one that makes you consider practicing in a different way?

4. Find out what research is being done in your school of nursing or patient care setting. Talk to the nurses who are involved in the research for their perspectives about their role in the study and what the research will accomplish.

5. Consider what it means to have your nursing practice based in evidence. What are the implications for a new nurse who lacks the clinical expertise that is required for EBP? Can a nurse without much experience have a practice that is evidence based?

REFERENCES

Alfaro-LeFevre R: *Applying the nursing process: a tool for critical thinking*, Philadelphia, 2006, Lippincott Williams & Wilkins.

American Nurses Association: *Code of ethics*, Washington, DC, 2015, American Nurses Publishing (website). Available at: www.nursingworld.org/provision-7.

Cleary-Holdforth J, Leufer T: Essential elements in developing evidence-based practice, *Nurs Stand* 23(2):42–46, 2008.

Flexner SB, Stein J, Su PY, editors: *The Random House dictionary*, New York, 1980, Random House.

Kuhn TS: The structure of scientific revolutions. In ed 2, Nurath O, editor: *International Encyclopedia of Unified Science*, vol. 2. Chicago, 1970, University of Chicago Press.

Melnyk BM, Fineout-Overhold E, Stillwell SB, et al.: Igniting a spirit of inquiry: An essential foundation for evidence-based practice, *Am J Nurs* 109(11):49–52, 2009.

National Institutes of Health: *Office of strategic coordination: the common fund*, (website). Available at: www.commonfund.nih.gov, 2018.

National Institute of Nursing Research (NINR): *The NINR strategic plan: advancing science, improving lives*, Bethesda, Md, 2016, National Institutes of Health (NIH) (website). Available at: https://www.ninr.nih.gov/sites/files/docs/NINR_StratPlan2016_reduced.pdf.

Wise N: Maintaining magnet status: establishing an evidence-based practice committee, *AORN* 90(2):205–213, 2009.

11

Developing Nursing Judgment through Critical Thinking

Beth Perry Black, PhD, RN, FAAN

ⓔ To enhance your understanding of this chapter, try the Student Exercises on the Evolve site at http://evolve.elsevier.com/Black/professional.

LEARNING OUTCOMES

After studying this chapter, students will be able to:

- Define *critical thinking,* and describe its importance in nursing.
- Contrast the characteristics of "novice thinking" with those of "expert thinking."
- Explain the purpose and phases of the nursing process.

- Explain the differences between independent, interdependent (collaborative), and dependent nursing actions.
- Describe evaluation and its importance in the nursing process.
- Define *clinical judgment in nursing practice,* and explain how it is developed.
- Devise a personal plan to use in developing sound clinical judgment.

Almost every encounter a nurse has with a patient is an opportunity for the nurse to assist the patient to a higher level of wellness or comfort. A nurse's ability to think critically about a patient's particular needs and how best to meet them will determine the extent to which a patient benefits from the nurse's care. A nurse's ability to use a reliable, consistent cognitive approach is crucial in determining a patient's priorities for care and in making sound clinical decisions in addressing those priorities. This chapter explores important and interdependent aspects of thinking and decision making in nursing. Some of these aspects include critical thinking, the nursing process, and clinical judgment.

CRITICAL THINKING: CULTIVATING INTELLECTUAL STANDARDS

Defining *critical thinking* is a complex task that requires an understanding of how people think through problems.

Educators and philosophers struggled with definitions of critical thinking for several decades. Two decades ago, the American Philosophical Association published an expert consensus statement (Box 11.1) describing critical thinking and attributes of the ideal critical thinker. This expert statement, still widely used, was the culmination of 3 years of work by Facione and others who synthesized the work of numerous persons who had defined critical thinking. More recently, Facione (2013) noted that giving a definition of critical thinking that can be memorized by the learner is actually antithetical to critical thinking. This means that the very definition of critical thinking does not lend itself to simplistic thinking and memorization.

The Paul-Elder Critical Thinking Framework (Paul and Elder, 2015) is grounded in this definition of critical thinking:

Critical thinking is that mode of thinking—about any subject, content, or problem—in which the thinker

BOX 11.1 Expert Consensus Statement Regarding Critical Thinking and the Ideal Critical Thinker

We understand critical thinking (CT) to be purposeful, self-regulatory judgment that results in interpretation, analysis, evaluation, and inference, as well as explanation of the evidential, conceptual, methodological, criteriological, or contextual considerations upon which that judgment is based. CT is essential as a tool of inquiry. As such, CT is a liberating force in education and a powerful resource in one's personal and civic life. While not synonymous with good thinking, CT is a pervasive and self-rectifying human phenomenon. The ideal critical thinker is habitually inquisitive, well-informed, trustful of reason, open-minded, flexible, fair-minded in evaluation, honest in facing personal biases, prudent in making judgments, willing to reconsider, clear about issues, orderly in complex matters, diligent in seeking relevant information, reasonable in the selection of criteria, focused in inquiry, and persistent in seeking results that are as precise as the subject and the circumstances of inquiry permit. Thus educating good critical thinkers means working toward this ideal. It combines developing CT skills with nurturing those dispositions that consistently yield useful insights and that are the basis of a rational and democratic society.

From American Philosophical Association: *Critical thinking: a statement of expert consensus for purposes of educational assessment and instruction,* The Delphi report: Research findings and recommendations prepared for the committee on pre-college philosophy, 1990, Newark, ERIC Document Reproduction Services, pp 315–423.

improves the quality of his or her thinking by skillfully taking charge of the structures inherent in thinking and imposing intellectual standards upon them.

Paul and Elder (2015) describe the "well-cultivated critical thinker" as one who does the following:

- Raises questions and problems and formulates them clearly and precisely
- Gathers and assesses relevant information, using abstract ideas for interpretation
- Arrives at conclusions and solutions that are well reasoned and tests them against relevant standards
- Is open-minded and recognizes alternative ways of seeing problems and has the ability to assess the assumptions, implications, and consequences of alternative views of problems
- Communicates effectively with others as solutions to complex problems are formulated

We live in a "new knowledge economy" driven by information and technology that changes quickly. Analyzing and integrating information across an increasing number of sources of knowledge require that you have flexible intellectual skills. Being a good critical thinker makes you more adaptable in this new economy of knowledge (Lau and Chan, 2012). An excellent website on critical thinking can be found at http://philosophy.hku.hk/think/ (OpenCourseWare on critical thinking, logic, and creativity).

So what does this have to do with nursing? The answer is simple: excellent critical thinking skills are required for you to make good clinical judgments. You will be responsible and accountable for your own decisions as a professional nurse. The development of critical thinking skills is crucial as you provide nursing care for patients with increasingly complex conditions. Critical thinking skills provide you with a powerful means of determining patient needs, interpreting physician orders, and intervening appropriately. Box 11.2 presents an example of the importance of critical thinking in the provision of safe care. The nurse in this example takes several sources of data about her patient, uses her clinical expertise, advocates for her patient, and thus gets the patient help for a serious postoperative complication.

CRITICAL THINKING IN NURSING

You may be wondering at this point, "How am I ever going to learn how to make connections among all of the data I have about a patient?" This is a common response for a nursing student who is just learning some of the most basic psychomotor skills in preparation for practice. You need to understand that, just like learning to give injections safely and maintaining a sterile field, you can learn to think critically. This involves paying attention to how you think and making thinking itself a focus of concern. A nurse who is exercising critical thinking asks the following questions: "What assumptions have I made about this patient?" "How do I know my assumptions are accurate?" "Do I need any additional information?" and "How might I look at this situation differently?" Schneider (2015) noted that "basic nursing care encompasses a responsibility for correct interpretation of assessment data using critical thinking" (p. 60).

Nurses just beginning to pay attention to their thinking processes may ask these questions after nurse-patient interactions have ended. This is known

BOX 11.2 Using Critical Thinking Skills to Improve a Patient's Care

Ms. George has recently undergone bariatric surgery after many attempts to lose weight over the years have failed. She is to be discharged home on postoperative day 2, as per the usual protocol. Although she describes herself as "not feeling well at all," the physician writes the order for discharge and you, as the nurse who does postoperative discharge planning for the surgery practice, meet with Ms. George to go over dietary guidelines that should help her lose weight successfully. You note that Ms. George does not seem as comfortable or pleased with her surgery as most patients with whom you have worked in the past.

Ms. George has to wait 3 hours for her husband to drive her home, and you note that she continues to lie on the bed passively, and her lethargy is increasing. You take her vital signs, and note that her temperature is 37.8° C and her pulse is 115. You listen to her chest, and note that it is difficult to appreciate breath sounds because of the patient's body habitus. Ms. George points to an area just below her left breast where she notes pain with inspiration. You call her physician to report your findings; she responds that Ms. George's pain is "not unusual" with her type of bariatric surgery and that her slightly increased temperature is "most likely" related to her being somewhat dehydrated. She instructs you to have Ms. George force fluids to the extent that she can tolerate it and take mild pain medication for postoperative pain. You ask the surgeon to consider delaying Ms. George's discharge home, but she refuses.

You give Ms. George acetaminophen as ordered, but her pain on inspiration continues. Her temperature remains at 37.8° C, and her pulse is 120. You measure her O_2 saturation with a pulse oximeter, and it is 91%. Her respirations are 26 and somewhat shallow. Her surgeon does not respond to your page, so you call the nursing supervisor, explaining to him that you are concerned with Ms. George's impending discharge. Because Ms. George's surgeon has not been responsive to your concerns, you call the hospitalist (a physician who sees inpatients in the absence of their attending physician), who orders a chest x-ray study. Ms. George has evidence of a consolidation in her left lower lobe, which turns out to be a pulmonary abscess in its early stages. She is treated on intravenous antibiotics for 5 days, and the abscess eventually has to be aspirated and drained.

Your critical thinking skills and willingness to advocate for your patient prevented an even worse postoperative course. You recognized that Ms. George's lethargy was unusual, and the location and timing of her pain were of concern. You also realized that although her temperature appeared to be stable, she had been given a pain medicine (acetaminophen) that also reduces fever, so in fact, a temperature increase may have been masked by the antipyretic properties of the acetaminophen. You demonstrated excellent clinical judgment in measuring her O_2 saturation, noting that her respiratory rate and pulse were consistent with decreased oxygenation. Furthermore, you sought support through the nursing "chain of command" when you engaged the nursing supervisor, who supported you in contacting the hospitalist. The specific, detailed information that you were able to provide the hospitalist allowed him to follow a logical diagnostic path, determining that Ms. George did indeed have a significant postoperative complication. Two days later, Ms. George reports that she is "feeling much better" and is walking in the hallways several times a day.

as **reflective thinking,** an active process valuable in learning and changing behaviors, perspectives, or practices. Nurses can also learn to examine their thinking processes during an interaction as they learn to "think on their feet." This is a characteristic of expert nurses. As you move from novice to expert, your ability to think critically will improve with practice. In Chapter 5 you read about Dr. Patricia Benner (1984; Benner et al., 1996), who studied the differences in expertise of nurses at different stages in their careers, from novice to expert. So it is with critical thinking: novices think differently from experts. Box 11.3 summarizes the differences in novice and expert thinking.

Critical thinking is a complex, purposeful, disciplined process that has specific characteristics that make it different from typical problem solving. Critical thinking in nursing is undergirded by the standards and ethics of the profession. Consciously developed to improve patient outcomes, critical thinking by the nurse is driven by the needs of the patient and family. Nurses who think critically are engaged in a process of constant evaluation, redirection, improvement, and increased efficiency. Be aware that critical thinking involves far more than stating your opinion; critical thinking is not the same as being critical. You must be able to describe how you came to a conclusion and support your conclusions with explicit data and rationales. Becoming an excellent

---

BOX 11.3   Novice Thinking Compared with Expert Thinking

Novice Nurses

- Tend to organize knowledge as separate facts. Must rely heavily on resources (e.g., texts, notes, preceptors). Lack knowledge gained from actually doing (e.g., listening to breath sounds).
- Focus so much on actions that they may not fully assess before acting.
- Need and follow clear-cut rules.
- Are often hampered by unawareness of resources.
- May be hindered by anxiety and lack of self-confidence.
- Tend to rely on step-by-step procedures and follow standards and policies rigidly.
- Tend to focus more on performing procedures correctly than on the patient's response to the procedure.
- Have limited knowledge of suspected problems; therefore they question and collect data more superficially or in a less focused way than more experienced nurses.
- Learn more readily when matched with a supportive, knowledgeable preceptor or mentor.

Expert Nurses

- Tend to store knowledge in a highly organized and structured manner, making recall of information easier.

- Have a large storehouse of experiential knowledge (e.g., what abnormal breath sounds sound like, what subtle changes look like).
- Assess and consider different options for intervening before acting.
- Know which rules are flexible and when it is appropriate to bend the rules.
- Are aware of resources and how to use them.
- Are usually more self-confident, less anxious, and therefore more focused than less experienced nurses.
- Are comfortable with rethinking a procedure if patient needs require modification of the procedure.
- Have a better idea of suspected problems, allowing them to question more deeply and collect more relevant and in-depth data.
- Analyze standards and policies, looking for ways to improve them.
- Are challenged by novices' questions, clarifying their own thinking when teaching novices.

From Alfaro-LeFevre R: *Critical thinking in nursing: a practical approach,* ed 2, Philadelphia, 1999, Saunders. Reprinted with permission.

---

critical thinker is significantly related to increased years of work experience and to higher education level; moreover, nurses with critical thinking abilities tend to be more competent in their practice than nurses with less well-developed critical thinking skills (Chang et al., 2011). Box 11.4 summarizes these characteristics and offers an opportunity for you to evaluate your progress as a critical thinker.

An excellent continuing education (CE) self-study module designed to improve your ability to think critically can be found online at http://ce.nurse.com/course/ce168-60/improving-your-ability-to-think-critically/. (Note that there is a modest fee for this course.) Continuing one's education through lifelong learning is an excellent way to maintain and enhance your critical thinking skills. The website http://ce.nurse.com has more than 500 CE opportunities available online and may be helpful to you as you seek to increase your knowledge base and improve your clinical judgment. Being intentional about improving your critical thinking skills ensures that you bring your best effort to the bedside in providing care for your patients.

THE NURSING PROCESS: A UNIVERSAL INTELLECTUAL STANDARD

Critical thinking requires systematic and disciplined use of universal intellectual standards (Paul and Elder, 2015). In the practice of nursing, the **nursing process** represents a universal intellectual standard by which problems are addressed and solved. The nursing process is a method of critical thinking focused on solving patient problems in professional practice. The nursing process is "a conceptual framework that enables the student or the practicing nurse to think systematically and process pertinent information about the patient" (Huckabay, 2009, p. 72). This process combines the "art of nursing" (creativity) with systems theory and the scientific method to produce high level care for your patients that is both interpersonal and interactive (Doenges et al., 2013).

You engage in problem solving daily. Suppose your favorite band is performing in a nearby city the night before a big exam in pathophysiology. Your exam counts as 35% of your final grade. But you have wanted to see this band since you were 15, and you do not know when you

BOX 11.4 Self-Assessment: Critical Thinking

Directions: Listed below are 15 characteristics of critical thinkers. Mark a plus sign (+) next to those you now possess, mark IP (in progress) next to those you have partially mastered, and mark a zero (0) next to those you have not yet mastered. When you are finished, make a plan for developing the areas that need improvement. Share it with at least one person, and report on progress weekly.

Characteristics of Critical Thinkers

_____ Inquisitive/curious/seeks truth
_____ Self-informed/finds own answers
_____ Analytic/confident in own reasoning skills
_____ Open-minded
_____ Flexible
_____ Fair-minded
_____ Honest about personal biases/self-aware
_____ Prudent/exercises sound judgment
_____ Willing to revise judgment when new evidence
warrants
_____ Clear about issues
_____ Orderly in complex matters/organized approach
to problems
_____ Diligent in seeking information
_____ Persistent
_____ Reasonable
_____ Focused on inquiry

will have another chance. You are faced with weighing a number of factors that will influence your decision about whether to go see the band: your grade going into the exam; how late you will be out the night before the exam; how far you will have to drive to see the band; and how much study time you will have to prepare for the exam in advance. You are really conflicted about this, so you decide to let another factor determine what you will do: the cost of the ticket. When you learn that the only seats available are near the back of the venue and cost $120.00 each, you decide to stay home and get a good night's sleep before the big exam; the next day you make a grade of 98% on the exam. You then realize that because you made such a good grade on this exam, you will have much less pressure when studying for the final exam at the end of the semester. You have identified a problem (not a particularly serious one, but one with personal significance), considered various factors related to the problem, identified possible actions, selected the best alternative, evaluated the success of the alternative selected, and made adjustments to the solution

based on the evaluation. This is the same general process nurses use in solving patient problems through the nursing process.

For individuals outside the profession, nursing is commonly and simplistically defined in terms of tasks nurses perform. Many students get frustrated with activities and courses in nursing school that are not focused on these tasks, believing that the tasks of nursing *are* nursing. Even within the profession, the intellectual basis of nursing practice was not articulated until the 1960s, when nursing educators and leaders began to identify and name the components of nursing's intellectual processes. This marked the beginning of the nursing process. In today's evolving health care environment, the use of the nursing process streamlines the processes of care that are entered into the electronic health record (EHR). Furthermore, the use of the nursing process provides a means of determining the economic contributions of nursing to patient outcomes, so nursing care can be cost effective yet still be consistent with the goals and perspectives of the profession (Doenges et al., 2013).

In the 1970s and 1980s, debate about the use of the term *diagnosis* began. Until then, diagnosis was considered to be within the scope of practice of physicians only. Although nurses were not educated or licensed to diagnose medical conditions in patients, nurses recognized that there were human responses amenable to independent nursing intervention. Using diagnoses gave nurses a universal terminology, "standardizing the 'what' and 'how' of the work of nursing" (Doenges et al., 2013, p. 10). A nursing diagnosis, then, is "a clinical judgment about individual, family or community responses to actual or potential health problems or life processes which provide the basis for selection of nursing interventions to achieve outcomes for which the nurse has accountability" (NANDA-I, 2012). These responses could be identified (diagnosed) through the careful application of specific defining characteristics. On its website, NANDA-I notes that "Nursing diagnoses communicate the professional judgments that nurses make every day to our patients, colleagues, members of other disciplines, and the public" (NANDA-I, 2018).

In 1973 the National Group for the Classification of Nursing Diagnosis published its first list of nursing diagnoses. This group later became known as NANDA, founded in 1982, and is now known as **NANDA International, Inc.** (NANDA-I; NANDA was the acronym for the now obsolete name North American Nursing Diagnosis Association). Its mission is to "facilitate the development, refinement, dissemination and use of standardized nursing diagnostic terminology" with the goal to "improve the health care of all people" (NANDA-I, 2012). NANDA-I's 2015–2017 edition of *Nursing Diagnoses: Definitions and Classifications* contains 235 diagnoses approved for clinical testing, with 25 new diagnoses and 13 revised diagnoses. Diagnoses are retired if it becomes evident that their usefulness is limited or outdated, such as the former diagnosis "disturbed thought processes."

The development of the concept of nursing diagnosis was an effort to standardize the language of care by nurses. This is part of what has become a larger issue of the development of standardized nursing languages (SNLs) that describe what nurses do. Other SNLs include the Clinical Care Classification (CCC), Nursing Interventions Classifications (NIC), Nursing Outcomes Classifications (NOC), the Omaha System–Community Health Classification System (OS), and the Perioperative Nursing Data Set (PNDS) (Doenges et al., 2013). Your exposure and experience with these SNLs will vary depending on the location and setting where you practice.

A diagnosis is approved for use by NANDA-I based on up-to-date evidence and the guidance from researchers, expert diagnosticians, and educators. Each diagnosis has standard diagnostic indicators such as defining characteristics of the patient problem, related factors, and risk factors. Here is a simple example of how an approved nursing diagnosis may be used:

Two days after a surgery for a large but benign abdominal mass, Mr. Stevens, 55 years old, 104 kg (229 lb), is not able to cough up the significant secretions he has accumulated in his airway. He is having some dyspnea and has audible wheezes. Your diagnosis is that Mr. Stevens has ineffective airway clearance, based on NANDA-I's taxonomy, because you have determined that the risk factors and physical signs and symptoms associated with this diagnosis apply to him.

A more detailed discussion of nursing diagnosis is located in the next section of this chapter.

The nursing process as a method of addressing clinical problems is taught in schools of nursing across the United States, and many states refer to it in their nursing practice acts. Ideally, the nursing process is used as a creative approach to thinking and decision making in nursing. Because the nursing process is an integral aspect of nursing education, practice, standards, and practice acts nationwide, learning to use it as a mechanism for critical thinking and as a dynamic and creative approach to patient care is a worthwhile endeavor. The nursing process has sometimes been the subject of criticism among nurses. In recent years, some nursing leaders have questioned the use of the nursing process, describing it as linear, rigid, and mechanistic. They believe that the nursing process contributes to linear thinking and stymies critical thinking. Despite reservations among some nurses about its use, the nursing process remains the cornerstone of nursing standards, legal definitions, and practice and, as such, should be well understood by every nurse.

STEPS OF THE NURSING PROCESS

Like many frameworks for thinking through problems, the nursing process is a series of organized steps, the purpose of which is to impose some discipline and critical thinking on the provision of excellent care. Identifying specific steps makes the process clear and concrete but can cause nurses to use them rigidly. Keep in mind that this is a process, that progression through the process may not be linear, and that it is a tool to use, not a road map to follow rigidly. More creative use of the nursing process may occur by expert nurses who have a greater repertoire of interventions from which to select. For example, if a newly hospitalized patient is experiencing a great deal of pain, a novice nurse might proceed by asking family members to leave so that the patient could rest in a quiet environment. An expert nurse would realize that the family may be a source of distraction from the pain or may be a source of comfort in ways that the nurse may not be able to provide. The expert nurse, in addition to assessing the patient, is willing to consider alternative explanations and interventions, enhancing the possibility that the patient's pain will be relieved.

Phase 1: Assessment

Assessment is the initial phase or operation in the nursing process. During this phase, information or data about the individual patient, family, or community are gathered. Data may include physiologic, psychological, sociocultural, developmental, spiritual, and environmental information. The patient's available financial or material resources also need to be assessed and recorded in a standard format; each institution will have its distinct method of collecting and recording assessment data.

Types of Data

Nurses obtain two types of data about and from patients: subjective and objective. Subjective data are obtained from patients as they describe their needs, feelings, strengths, and perceptions of the problem. Subjective data are often referred to as symptoms. Examples of subjective data are statements such as, "I am in pain" and "I don't have much energy." The only source for these data is the patient. Subjective data should include physical, psychosocial, and spiritual information. Subjective data can be very private. Nurses must be sensitive to the patient's need for confidence in the nurse's trustworthiness when collecting subjective data.

Objective data are the other types of data that the nurse will collect through observation, examination, or consultation with other health care providers. These data are measurable, such as pulse rate and blood pressure, and include observable patient behaviors. Objective data are often called *signs*. An example of objective data that a nurse might gather is the observation that the patient, who is lying in bed, is diaphoretic, pale, and tachypneic, clutching his hands to his chest.

Objective data and subjective data usually are congruent; that is, they usually are in agreement. In the situation just described, if the patient told the nurse, "I feel like a rock is crushing my chest," the subjective data would substantiate the nurse's observations (objective data) that the patient has signs consistent with a heart attack (myocardial infarction). Occasionally, subjective and objective data are in conflict. In this example, the patient may deny having chest pain (subjective data) despite evidence of signs of a myocardial infarction, including characteristic changes associated with a heart attack on the patient's electrocardiogram (objective data). A stark example of incongruent subjective and objective data unfortunately well known to labor and delivery nurses is that of a pregnant woman in labor who describes ongoing fetal activity (subjective data); however, there are no fetal heart tones (objective data), and it is determined that the fetus has died in utero. Incongruent objective and subjective data require further careful assessment to ascertain the patient's situation more completely and accurately. Sometimes incongruent data reveal something about the patient's concerns and fears—such as the fear of a heart attack or that one's baby will be stillborn. To get a clearer picture of the patient's situation, the nurse should use the best communication skills he or she possesses to increase the patient's trust.

Methods of Collecting Patient Data

A number of methods are used when collecting patient data. The patient interview is a primary means of obtaining both subjective and objective data. The interview typically involves a face-to-face

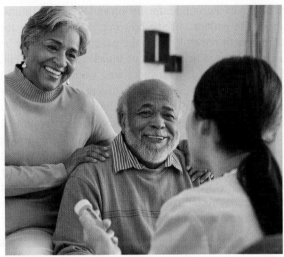

Fig. 11.1 A face-to-face interview with a patient is a primary means of collecting data and requires good interviewing skills, observation, and listening. (Photo used with permission from iStockPhoto.)

interaction with the patient that requires the nurse to use the skills of interviewing, observation, and listening (Fig. 11.1). Many factors influence the quality of the interview, including the physical environment in which the interaction occurs. If the patient is not in a private room, the open exchange of information may not occur easily. Sometimes the presence of family members constrains the flow of information from a patient, especially when dealing with sensitive or private issues. Similarly, if an interview takes place in a cold, noisy, or public place, the type of data obtained may be affected by environmental distractions. Internal factors related to the patient's condition may influence the amount and the type of data obtained. For example, when interviewing a patient who is experiencing shortness of breath, the verbal data obtained in the interview may be limited, but careful observation and attentive listening can yield much information about the patient's condition.

Physical examination is the second method for obtaining data. Nurses use physical assessment techniques of inspection, auscultation, percussion, and palpation to obtain these data, in addition to technology such as a bladder scan to detect urinary retention. A third method of obtaining data is through consultation. Consultation is discussing patient needs with health care providers who are directly involved in the care of the patient. Nurses also consult with patients' families to obtain background information and their perceptions about the patients' needs; however, it is necessary for the nurse to remember that the patient's family may be unaware of certain concerns or situations of the patient. For example, an 18-year-old young woman is brought to the emergency department's urgent care facility for dysuria (pain on urination). While her mother is out of the room, she tells you that she had intercourse 2 days earlier, a useful piece of history in determining the patient's likely medical diagnosis of a urinary tract infection. You note that she has waited until her mother is absent before telling you this important piece of information; recognizing that this is sensitive and private information, you do not mention it in front of the patient's mother.

Organizing Patient Data

Once patient data have been collected, they must be sorted or organized. A number of methods have been developed to assist nurses in organizing patient data. Abdellah's 21 nursing problems, Henderson's 14 nursing problems, Yura and Walsh's (1983) human needs approach, and Gordon's (1976) 11 functional health patterns are commonly used frameworks for collecting and organizing patient data. Contemporary nursing theorists continue to develop other organizing frameworks, including those of Madeleine Leininger, Sister Callista Roy, Dorothy Orem, and others that you read about in Chapter 9.

Confidentiality of Patient Data

A word of caution is needed concerning patient data. Earlier it was noted that patients confide personal information to nurses if they believe the nurse is trustworthy. It can seem obvious when to avoid sharing sensitive information with patients' families. However, nurses must limit the sharing of information to only the other providers directly involved in the patient's care. Nurses must respect patients' privacy rights and should never discuss patient information with anyone who does not have a work-related need to know. This is not only an ethical issue but also a legal issue. Patients' privacy is protected by federal law (see Health Insurance Portability and Accountability Act of 1996 [HIPAA] in Chapter 6). Conversations about patients in public places or consulting with other providers on a cell phone in a hallway or elevator are other ways in which patients' privacy is breached.

Ensuring patients' privacy is complicated in that vast amounts of patient data are stored digitally and retrieved relatively easily. Although the issues of confidentiality and access to digital data have yet to be fully resolved, each nurse should be entrusted never to violate a patient's privacy by revealing patient information except to other members of that patient's treatment team on a need-to-know basis.

Phase 2: Analysis and Identification of the Problem

During the data-gathering phase of the nursing process, nurses obtain a great deal of information about their patients. These data must first be validated and then compared with norms to sort out data that might indicate a problem or identify a pattern. Next, the data must be clustered or grouped so that problems can be identified and their cause discerned. Knowledge from the science of nursing, biologic sciences, and social sciences enables nurses to observe relationships among various pieces of patient data. This process is known as data analysis and results in the identification of one or more problems that are amenable to nursing intervention. The problems are often then characterized as nursing diagnoses.

Here is an example of how a nurse will take information from a variety of sources, analyze it, and adjust the plan of care accordingly:

Ms. Wills is a 62-year-old woman with a 4-year history of stage 4 breast cancer who is admitted to your unit for paracentesis to remove the large volume of ascites that has accumulated in her abdomen, making it very uncomfortable for her to breathe and move. Ms. Wills is a good historian: she tells you in detail about her cancer diagnosis and treatments, her abundant family support, her religious faith, and her decision to enter hospice care after the cancer was found to have metastasized to her brain.

Ms. Wills' hospice nurse calls to check on her and gives you some important information: although Ms. Wills is receiving end-of-life care, she insists that her cancer will be cured because she and others have been praying for a cure. The hospice nurse shares this information because she believes that you need to know this may be a factor in Ms. Wills' care. You read part of the patient's medical record and note that it is consistent with Ms. Wills' account of her illness. The paracentesis removes 4 L of ascites. Afterward, Ms. Wills tells you that she feels so much better that she plans to contact her hospice nurse and tell her she will not be needing their services any longer because she is cured. Ms. Wills' physician believes that she needs a psychiatric consultation because he believes that she is "in denial" about still having cancer.

What had appeared to be a short admission for the management of a common occurrence (ascites) may have become a bit more complicated when Ms. Wills—the excellent historian who chronicled her cancer progression in such detail—makes a statement that may have surprised you had you not been given specific information about Ms. Wills' hope for a cure from her hospice nurse. This is the type of behavior you may see in certain settings, and although it seems inconsistent and even alarming, having the right information about a patient can be very useful in analyzing the patient's responses.

Distinctions between Medical and Nursing Diagnosis

Nursing diagnosis is different from medical diagnosis and was never intended to be a substitute. Rather than focusing on what is wrong with the patient in terms of a disease process, a nursing diagnosis identifies the problems the patient is experiencing as a result of the disease process, that is, the **human responses** to the illness, injury, or threat.

An important difference between nursing diagnosis and medical diagnosis is that nursing diagnoses address patient problems that nurses can treat within their scope of practice. Proponents of nursing diagnosis argue that it does little good for nursing diagnoses to include "appendicitis," because appendicitis is a medical diagnosis requiring surgery, and nurses do not perform surgery. A nursing diagnosis for a patient after an appendectomy might be "ineffective airway clearance" (as was the case with Mr. Stevens). Because it is within the scope of practice in all states for nurses to provide comfort measures and to assist patients to cough and deep breathe, this would be an appropriate nursing diagnosis that is remedied by nursing interventions. The medical diagnosis becomes a platform from which nursing diagnoses are developed: a patient with a new medical diagnosis of diabetes will have some very specific nursing diagnoses and interventions based on the requirements of the medical condition (diabetes) that caused the patient to seek care.

The use of nursing diagnosis does not have universal support among various constituencies of the discipline and profession. Critics believe that the language of nursing diagnosis obscures rather than clarifies patient problems. This causes confusion between disciplines involved in care of patients. Suppose a patient has a simple postoperative ileus. This is a medical diagnosis, but its management has important implications for nursing. The nursing diagnosis "gastrointestinal motility, dysfunctional, related to decreased motor activity status post–abdominal surgery," with its accompanying "comfort, impaired, related to intolerance of medications," is a long way of saying that the patient has an ileus, has not been moving around, is in pain, and is not tolerating his medications. This more streamlined description of the patient's clinical condition is recognizable across disciplines, and the implications for nursing management remain the same. In 2008 the American Association of Colleges of Nursing (AACN) issued an executive summary, *The Essentials of Baccalaureate Education for Professional Nursing Practice,* which is described in Chapter 4. This summary emphasizes patient-centered care in interprofessional teams, which requires excellent communication across disciplines. Particular emphasis is placed on the translation of evidence into practice. Nursing diagnosis is not mentioned among the nine essentials. The complete summary can be found on the AACN website (http://www.aacnnursing.org).

Despite a new focus on evidence-based practice, the need for interdisciplinary collaboration, and interprofessional teamwork, many schools of nursing still teach NANDA-I nursing diagnoses, and many advanced practice nurses use them in their own practices. NANDA-approved nursing diagnoses consist of six components (NANDA-I, 2003, pp. 263–264):

1. *Label:* Concise term or phrase that names the diagnosis
2. *Definition:* Term or phrase that clearly delineates meaning and helps differentiate from similar diagnoses
3. *Related factors:* Factors that precede, are associated with, or relate to the diagnosis
4. *Defining characteristics:* Subjective and objective features
5. *Desired outcomes/evaluation criteria:* What the patient and you set as goals and how you will measure progress toward those goals
6. *Actions/interventions:* What the patient and you will do to reach the goals for care

---

BOX 11.5   Writing Nursing Diagnoses

P = Problem (NANDA-I diagnostic label)
E = Etiology (causal factors)
S = Signs and symptoms (defining characteristics)

All nursing diagnoses must be supported by data, which NANDA-I refers to as defining characteristics (i.e., signs and symptoms).

Accurate diagnosis of human responses is very important. Effective interventions depend on an accurate diagnosis. Lunney (2008) wrote an appeal to nurses in practice and education to address this issue of diagnostic accuracy. Lunney based the appeal on research findings that there is a need for more diagnostic consistency among nurses, that the issue of accuracy will always be present because of the complexities of nursing, and that EHRs make the issue of accuracy of diagnosis even more significant. Paans and colleagues (2011) found four domains of factors that affect nurses' accurate documentation of diagnoses: (1) nurses themselves as effective diagnosticians; (2) how nurses are educated about nursing diagnoses; (3) the complexity of a patient's situation; and (4) the degree to which a hospital's policy and environment supports the use of nursing diagnosis.

A format formerly used to write the diagnostic statement, called the PES format (problem, etiology, signs/symptoms), was developed by Marjory Gordon (1987), a founder of NANDA-I. Once commonly used, NANDA-I no longer uses this format and now refers to the component parts of the nursing diagnosis as related factors and defining characteristics. Several countries and nursing publications, however, still use the PES format, which is shown in Box 11.5 so that you can become familiar with it when you run across it in journals and settings that still use this format. NANDA-I continues to work to align its mission for a nursing diagnostic system to the demands of today's health care environment.

Prioritizing Nursing Diagnoses

After diagnoses are identified, the nurse must put them in order of priority. Two common frameworks are used to establish priorities. One of these considers the relative danger to the patient. With use of this framework, diagnoses that are life threatening are the nurse's first priority. Next are those that have the potential to cause

harm or injury. Last in priority are those diagnoses that are related to the overall general health of the patient. Thus a diagnosis of "ineffective airway clearance" would be dealt with before "sleep pattern disturbance," and "sleep pattern disturbance" would have priority over "knowledge deficit."

Another framework used to prioritize diagnoses is Maslow's (1970) hierarchy of needs (refer to Chapter 8, Fig. 8.3). When this framework is used, there is an inverse relationship between high-priority nursing diagnoses and high-level needs. In other words, highest priority is given to diagnoses related to basic physiologic needs. Diagnoses related to higher-level needs such as love and belonging or self-esteem, although important, have priority only after basic physiologic needs are met.

Except in life-threatening or other emergency situations, nurses should take care to involve patients in identifying priority diagnoses. Because varied sociocultural factors have a great impact on the manner in which patients prioritize problems, nurses must be aware of these factors and take them into consideration when planning patient care. The nurse's own cultural perspective must not take priority over that of the patient in determining priorities. For example, many maternity nurses are very strong proponents of breastfeeding and consider it one of their priorities to assist new mothers to establish effective breastfeeding patterns. However, for some women, breastfeeding is not a cultural norm or a desirable behavior of new motherhood. Although it may be difficult to understand for the maternity nurse who has expertise in the benefits of breastfeeding, imposing the nurse's cultural and professional perspective on the patient is unacceptable and can lead to diminished effectiveness of nursing care in other domains in which the new mother needs assistance.

Phase 3: Planning

Planning is the third phase in the nursing process. Planning begins with identification of patient goals and determination of ways to reach those goals. Goals are used by the patient and the nurse to guide the selection of interventions and to evaluate patient progress. Bloom's taxonomy (as described by Spring, 2010) in Box 11.6 provides a simple description of domains of learning that drive the development of patient goals: psychomotor, cognitive, and affective goals.

BOX 11.6 Bloom's Taxonomy

A taxonomy is a classification system. Bloom, an educator, described types of learning in terms of domains of educational activities. This taxonomy is helpful for nursing:

- **Psychomotor domain:** Involves physical movement and increasingly complex activities in the motor-skill arena. Learning in this domain can be assessed by measures such as distance, time, and speed.
  - *Nursing goal:* Patient will move from bed to chair three times today without assistance.
- **Cognitive domain:** Involves knowledge and intellectual skills. Cognitive skills range from simple recall to complex tasks such as synthesis and evaluation.
  - *Nursing goal:* Maternity patient will list five signs of illness in her newborn infant by the time she is discharged.
- **Affective domain:** Involves the emotions, such as feelings, values, and attitudes.
  - *Nursing goal:* Pregnant patient will describe willingness to consider breastfeeding her newborn infant.

Setting nursing goals using Bloom's taxonomy is a simple way to address the three important domains of the patient's needs. A single patient is likely to have goals in each of these domains.

Modified from American Philosophical Association: *The Delphi report: research findings and recommendations prepared for the Committee on Pre-college Philosophy,* Milbrae, Calif, 1990, The California Academic Press.

This taxonomy identified domains of educational activities well suited to nursing.

Just as nursing diagnoses are written in collaboration with the patient, goals should also be agreed on by both nurse and patient unless collaboration is impossible, such as when the patient has an altered mental status, is a young child, or is incapacitated in some way, or if the nurse and patient do not speak the same language. In the event of a cognitive problem, family members or significant others can collaborate with the nurse. In the case of the nurse whose patient speaks another language, a qualified medical interpreter can be instrumental in helping the nurse collaborate with the patient; in fact, it is not acceptable to use a patient's family members or friends to interpret. Goals give the patient, family, significant others, and nurse direction and make them active partners.

Writing Patient Goals and Outcomes

The terms *goal* and *objective* are often used interchangeably. Note that the word *objective* is used differently here than its earlier use, when it was used as an adjective describing observable and measurable data. In terms of outcomes, the word *objective* is a noun and means a goal or specific aim of intervention. Goals or objectives are statements of what is to be accomplished and are derived from the diagnoses. Because the problem or diagnosis is written as a patient problem, the goal should also be stated in terms of what the patient will do rather than what the nurse will do. The goal begins with the words *the patient will* or *the patient will be able to.* The goal sets a general direction, includes an action verb, and should be both attainable and realistic for the patient.

Outcome criteria are specific and make the goal measurable. Outcome criteria define the terms under which the goal is said to be met, partially met, or unmet. Each diagnosis has at least one patient goal, and each patient goal may have several outcome criteria. Effective outcome criteria state under what conditions, to what extent, and in what time frame the patient is to act. For the postoperative patient who had an abdominal procedure, a sample patient goal with outcome criteria might be, "The patient will be able to walk 3 blocks a day with a cane within 1 month after hip replacement surgery." It is easy to see that this goal is written in terms of what the patient will do (walk), is measurable (3 blocks), gives conditions (with a cane), and has a specified time frame for accomplishment (1 month after surgery).

Establishing a time frame for patient goals to be met is important. **Short-term goals** may be attainable within hours or days. They are usually specific and are small steps leading to the achievement of broader, long-term goals. For example, "The patient will limit his smoking to a half-pack per day within a week" is a short-term goal, and the time limit for accomplishment can be brief, perhaps a week or 10 days. **Long-term goals,** however, usually represent major changes or rehabilitation. A goal such as "The patient will stop smoking entirely" may take months or perhaps even years to accomplish, and the time frame should be set accordingly. Setting realistic goals in terms of both outcomes and time is extremely important. Frustration and discouragement can occur when goals are unrealistic in outcomes or time.

The nurse can be a good resource for helping patients in determining accessible goals. For example, assume that your patient is a young man with a severe compound fracture of his thigh and several torn ligaments in his knee from a single-car automobile accident. The injury will require several orthopedic surgeries. To complicate matters, he has a nosocomial (hospital-acquired) infection in his surgical site. One day, he mentions to you that his goal is to run a marathon within a year. Running a marathon is a worthy goal and is reachable eventually for this young man. It is immaterial whether you believe he can reach his goal; however, as his nurse on the orthopedic and trauma unit, you recognize the importance of setting short-term goals right now that will improve his health and better the chances of achieving his goal of running a marathon. Your care plan should reflect the short-term, attainable goals (such as walking with a walker the length of the hallway twice a day) that he needs to reach in the meantime that will move him toward his long-term, personal goal.

Cultural congruency is an important consideration in setting patient goals and selecting interventions. A culturally congruent intervention is one that is developed within the broad social, cultural, and demographic context of the patient's life. The patient is more likely to benefit from an intervention that is tailored to his or her specific sociocultural needs and interests. Although cultural congruency is an important element to effective intervention, the nurse must take care not to stereotype patients or assume that "all _____" (fill in the blank) like the same things, will react the same way, or respond to the same intervention. In Considering Culture Box 11.1, you will be introduced to a research report explaining the importance of having culturally appropriate educational materials to prepare African American women for their breast biopsies. Read the paper carefully, and then address the questions.

Selecting Interventions and Planning Care

After short- and long-term goals are identified through collaboration between nurse and patient, the nurse develops a plan of care that contains actions designed to assist the patient in achieving a stated goal. Every goal has a specific intervention, which may be carried out by a registered nurse (RN) or delegated to other members of the nursing staff.

The nursing care plan is part of the whole plan of care by the health care team. Nursing interventions are designed to treat the patient's response to an illness

---

⊕ CONSIDERING CULTURE BOX 11.1

Challenge: Culturally Appropriate Interventions—Impact of Culture on Nursing Interventions

From the Association of Black Nursing Faculty website (www.abnf.net): "The purpose of the Association of Black Nursing Faculty, Inc. (ABNF) is to form and maintain a group whereby Black professional nurses with similar credentials, interests, and concerns may work to promote certain health-related issues and educational interests for the benefit of themselves and the Black community."

An example of the interests and work that have developed from the ABNF is found in The ABNF Journal, published six times each year. Volume 17, issue 1 in 2006 was dedicated to the issue of breast cancer in African American women. The research article "Getting Ready: Developing an Educational Intervention to Prepare African American Women for Breast Biopsy" describes the efforts to produce intervention materials for African American women preparing to undergo breast biopsies. African American women are more likely to die of breast cancer than are White American women, although fewer Black women than White women have a diagnosis of breast cancer. This is a source of great concern in the African American community and among researchers, who are trying to determine why this is the case.

In the Implications section at the end of the article, the authors refer to the cultural appropriateness of study materials to be used in an intervention. As you read this article, consider these questions:

1. In addition to ethnicity, can you think of other ways that interventions should be made culturally appropriate?
2. What might happen if an intervention is not culturally appropriate?
3. Who determines what is and is not culturally appropriate?

You can find the article here: Bradley PK, Berry A, Lang C, Myers RE: Getting ready: developing an educational intervention to prepare African American women for breast biopsy, ABFN J 17(1):15–19, 2006.

---

or medical treatment, whereas the physician or an advanced practice nurse will prescribe treatments for the specific illness or disease. Nursing interventions can and should begin before diagnostic testing or surgery, common reasons why patients are admitted to inpatient units. For example, before surgery patients are taught about pain management and pulmonary care that they will face after surgery. These activities are designed to manage pain and prevent postoperative respiratory problems caused by immobility. They are appropriate because prevention of complications resulting from immobility is a nursing responsibility. Nurses may consult with other health care providers, such as the dietitian, physical therapist, or pharmacist, to adequately prepare their patient for upcoming surgery or other invasive procedures.

Types of nursing interventions. Nursing interventions are of three basic types: independent, dependent, or interdependent. Independent interventions are those for which the nurse's intervention requires no supervision or direction by others and are within their scope of practice as defined by their state nursing practice act. Nurses have the knowledge and skills to carry out independent actions safely. An example of an independent nursing intervention is teaching a patient how to breastfeed her newborn infant.

Dependent interventions require instructions, written prescriptions, or supervision of another health professional with prescriptive authority. These actions require knowledge and skills on the part of the nurse but may not be done without explicit directions. An example of a dependent nursing intervention is the administration of medications. Although a physician or advanced practice nurse must prescribe medications in inpatient settings, it is the responsibility of the nurse to know how to administer them safely and to monitor their effectiveness. The nurse also must question prescriptions he or she thinks are inconsistent with safe care or are not within accepted standards of care.

The third type, interdependent (or collaborative) interventions, includes actions in which the nurse must collaborate or consult with another health professional before carrying out the action. One example of this type of action is the nurse implementing prescriptions or treatments that have been written by a physician in a protocol. Protocols define under what conditions and circumstances a nurse is allowed to treat the patient, as well as what treatments are permissible. They are used in situations in which nurses need to take immediate action without consulting with a physician, such as in an emergency department, a critical care unit, or a home setting.

Writing the Plan of Care

Once interventions are selected, a written plan of care is devised, often in the EHR. Some health care agencies use individually developed plans of care for their patients. The nurse creates and develops a plan for each patient. Others use standardized plans of care that are based on common and recurring problems. The nurse then individualizes these standard plans of care. An advantage of using standardized plans is that they can decrease the time spent in generating a completely new plan each time a patient is seen. These plans are easily generated in the EHR, with the nurse making selections from menus to individualize the plan to the particular patient. The amount of time needed to update and document these plans is then minimized.

Because of the decreasing average length of stay for patients in health care facilities, the increasing focus on achieving timely patient outcomes in the specific time frame permitted by reimbursement systems, and the emphasis by accrediting bodies on multidisciplinary care, many agencies have adopted the use of multidisciplinary plans of care known as critical pathways, collaborative care plans, or care maps. Critical pathways have been replaced with other types of multidisciplinary care plans in some settings. Multidisciplinary care plans are written in collaboration with physicians and other health care providers and establish a sequence of short-term daily outcomes that are easily measured. This type of care planning facilitates communication and collaboration among all members of the health care team. It also permits comparisons of outcomes between treatment plans, as well as among health care facilities. As with the nursing process, unyielding adherence to the critical path without considering a patient's idiosyncratic responses can negatively affect patient outcomes and is a detriment to successful nursing care.

The development of appropriate plans of care depends on the nurse's ability to use critical thinking. Nurses must be able to analyze information and arguments, make reasoned decisions, recognize many viewpoints, and question and seek answers continuously. At the same time, nurses must be logical, flexible, and creative and take initiative while considering the holistic nature of each patient.

Phase 4: Implementation of Planned Interventions

Implementation, the fourth phase or operation of the nursing process, occurs when nursing orders are actually carried out. Most people think of nursing as "doing something" for or to a patient. Notice, however, that in using the nursing process, nurses do a great deal of thinking, analyzing, and planning before the first actual nursing action takes place.

Professional nurses understand the crucial nature of the first three phases of the nursing process in ensuring that safe and appropriate care occurs. Nurses who forgo these essential phases and move immediately into action are not providing care in a responsible, professional manner. Patients feel a greater sense of trust in nurses who are providing care when dependent, independent, and interdependent orders are planned and carried out in an orderly, competent manner. Common nursing interventions include such actions as managing pain, preventing postoperative complications, educating patients, and monitoring certain aspects of the patient's physiologic care. As the nurse carries out planned interventions, he or she is continually assessing the patient, noting responses to nursing interventions, and modifying the care plan or adding nursing diagnoses as needed. Documentation of nursing actions is an integral part of the implementation phase.

Let's refer back to the case of Ms. Wills, who appears to believe after her paracentesis that she is cured of cancer and no longer needs hospice care; remember that her physician believes that she needs a psychiatric consultation.

You have done a thorough assessment of Ms. Wills and have no reason to believe, given what you have noted about her from both her objective and subjective data, that she has developed a psychiatric problem. You do know, however, that she has been praying a lot for a cure and that as a person of faith, she wants to trust that this will happen. You also know that she had in fact agreed to enter hospice care rather than to continue to seek medical treatment. Furthermore, you know that she truly feels better after having a gallon or more of fluid removed from her abdomen. As you are doing her 4 p.m. assessment, she says, "I feel so good, I'm going to call my hospice nurse right now." Without judgment or further questioning, you sit at her bedside, take her hand and simply say, "It must feel so good to have all that fluid gone." Ms. Wills says with a sigh, "You can't imagine. I just wish it was that easy to drain away all the cancer." You ask Ms. Wills if she would like for you to help her call her hospice nurse to tell her how much better she feels.

You acted in a very caring, very professional way by addressing the specific reason Ms. Wills feels

better—the fluid removal—without confronting her with harsh fact that her cancer was not gone. You correctly surmised that she in fact knew that. Helping her call her hospice nurse is a good way to help connect Ms. Wills to her substantial supportive network in hospice. The simple act of affirming her relief without judgment or trying to correct a momentarily hopeful thought gave you time to assess that Ms. Wills in fact does understand her situation. Sometimes the intervention itself becomes a means of assessment. You can tell Ms. Wills' physician after your assessment that you do not recommend a psychiatric consultation. (You will read about SBAR communication—situation, **b**ackground, **a**ssessment, **r**ecommendation—in Chapter 12.)

Phase 5: Evaluation

Evaluation is the final phase of the nursing process. In this phase the nurse examines the patient's progress in relation to the goals and outcome criteria to determine whether a problem is resolved, is in the process of being resolved, or is unresolved. In other words, the outcome criteria are the basis for evaluation of the goal. Evaluation may reveal that data, diagnosis, goals, and nursing interventions were all on target and that the problem is resolved.

Evaluation may also indicate a need for a change in the plan of care. Perhaps inadequate patient data were the basis for the plan, and further assessment has uncovered additional needs. The nursing diagnoses may have been incorrect or placed in the wrong order of priority. Patient goals may have been inappropriate or unattainable within the designated time frame. It is possible that nursing actions were incorrectly implemented.

Evaluation is a critical phase in the nursing process and one that is often slighted. The best nursing care plan is one that is evaluated frequently and changed in response to the patient's condition. Sometimes a care plan will reflect all the most common nursing interventions used to treat specific diagnoses; it is not enough, however, to continue to do the "right things" if the patient is not improving in the expected manner. If, on evaluation, the problem is not resolving in a timely way or will not resolve at all, the nursing care plan must be revised to reflect the necessary changes.

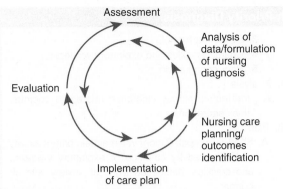

Fig. 11.2 The nursing process is a dynamic, nonlinear tool for critical thinking about human responses.

THE DYNAMIC NATURE OF THE NURSING PROCESS

The next morning Ms. Wills is leaving for home with her daughter after a restful night. She asks you if there is anything she can do to keep her ascites from coming back, such as limiting her fluid intake. Even as she is preparing to walk out the door, you understand that she is still your patient and has a specific need for knowledge. You tell her that the fluid—ascites—is happening because of the cancer and that there is really no way to prevent it from recurring. You also assure her, "We are always here to take care of you if you need us again."

A good plan is a flexible, responsive one; however, a care plan is only as effective as the nurse who carries it out.

Although the phases in the nursing process are discussed separately here, in practice they are not so clearly delineated, nor do they always proceed from one to another in a linear fashion. The nursing process (Fig. 11.2) is dynamic, meaning that nurses are continuously moving from one phase to another and then beginning the process again. Often a nurse performs two or more phases at the same time—for instance, observing a wound for signs of infection (assessment) while changing the dressing on the wound (intervention) and asking the patient the extent to which pain has been relieved by comfort measures (evaluation).

Now that you have read about the phases of the nursing process, we will look back at the scenario in which you tried to determine whether you should go see your favorite band. The problem that was identified was the choice between studying for a pathophysiology exam or going to see the band. Data, both objective (the schedule of the exam and the concert, the distance to be driven, the percentage of the final grade the exam represents, the cost of the ticket, the location of the available seats) and subjective (the long-term desire to see your favorite band, your hope to make a good grade on the exam), were gathered. Selection was made and implemented, and an evaluation of the implementation was carried out when you got your grade on your exam. Problem solving is something each person does every day. The use of the nursing process provides professional nurses with a patient-centered framework with which to solve clinical problems to optimize the opportunity for excellent patient outcomes.

An example of using the nursing process in a high-priority clinical situation is described in Box 11.7. This case study demonstrates how using the nursing process becomes so natural that experienced nurses go through the phases fluidly and automatically. Although no responsible nurse would take the time to write out this care plan in advance of acting on a diagnosis of "ineffective airway clearance," you should understand that the nursing process is exactly the same for those high-priority nursing situations that require immediate action and those that will evolve over time.

DEVELOPING CLINICAL JUDGMENT IN NURSING

Becoming an effective nurse involves more than critical thinking and the ability to use the nursing process. It depends heavily on developing excellent **clinical judgment.** Clinical judgment consists of informed opinions and decisions based on empirical knowledge and experience. Nurses develop clinical judgment gradually as they gain a broader, deeper knowledge base and clinical experience. Extensive direct patient contact is the best means of developing clinical judgment.

Critical thinking and clinical reasoning used in the nursing process are both important aspects of clinical judgment. A nurse who has developed sound clinical judgment knows what to look for (e.g., elevation of temperature in a surgical patient), draws valid conclusions about possible alternative meanings of signs and symptoms (e.g., dehydration, atelectasis, postoperative infection), and knows what to do about it (e.g., assess for

BOX 11.7 Nursing Process Case Study of a High-Priority Diagnosis

You have just received a report from the day shift about Mr. Burkes. You were told that he had been admitted with a diagnosis of cancer of the tongue and that he had a radical neck dissection yesterday. He has a tracheostomy and requires frequent suctioning of his secretions. He is alert and responds by nodding his head or writing short notes.

When you enter his room, you note that he is apprehensive and tachypneic and is gesturing for you to come into the room. You auscultate his lungs and note coarse crackles and expiratory wheezes. You can see thick secretions bubbling out of his tracheotomy. He has poor cough effort.

Based on these data, you realize that a priority nursing diagnosis is ineffective airway clearance. You immediately prepare to perform tracheal suctioning. As you are suctioning, you watch the patient's nonverbal responses and note that he is less apprehensive when the suctioning is completed. You also auscultate the lungs and note that there are decreased crackles and that the expiratory wheezes are no longer present. Mr. Burkes writes "I can breathe now" on his note pad.

I. Assessment
   A. Subjective data
      1. None because of inability to speak
   B. Objective data
      1. Tracheostomy with copious, thick secretions
      2. Tachypnea
      3. Gesturing for help
      4. Coarse crackles and expiratory wheezes
      5. Poor cough effort

II. Analysis
   A. Ineffective airway clearance related to copious, thick secretions

III. Plan
   A. Short-term goal: Patient will maintain patent airway as evidenced by absence of expiratory wheezes and crackles, decreased signs of anxiety, and air hunger.
   B. Long-term goal: Patient will have patent airway as evidenced by his ability to clear the airway without the use of suctioning by the time of discharge.

IV. Implementation
   A. Assess lung sounds every hour for crackles and wheezes.
   B. Suction airway as needed.
   C. Elevate head of bed to 45 degrees.
   D. Teach patient abdominal breathing techniques.
   E. Encourage patient to cough out secretions.

V. Evaluation
   A. Short-term goal: Achieved as evidenced by decreased crackles and absent wheezes when auscultating the lungs; patient appears less anxious, indicated by writing that he "can breathe now"
   B. Long-term goal: Will be evaluated before discharge

dehydration, listen to breath sounds, check incision for redness and drainage, seek another opinion, notify the surgeon). Developing sound clinical judgment requires recalling facts, recognizing patterns in patient behaviors, putting facts and observations together to form a meaningful whole, and acting on the resulting information in an appropriate way.

Knowing the limitations of your expertise is an important aspect of clinical judgment. Most nurses have an instinctive awareness of when they are approaching the limits of their expertise and will consult with other professionals as needed. Your state's nursing practice act, health agency policies, school of nursing policies, and the profession's standards of practice all provide guidance in making the decision about nursing actions within your scope of practice. Nursing students, whether new to nursing or RNs in baccalaureate and master's programs, must consider policies and standards in determining their scope of practice in any given nursing situation.

Box 11.8 contains a list of nine key questions to consider as you seek to improve your clinical judgment. Because the goal of nursing is to provide the best care to patients based on research and clinical evidence, the development of excellent clinical judgment is a professional responsibility. As you work to gain clinical experience and improve your own clinical judgment, these questions will help focus your thinking.

Nurses are responsible for developing sound clinical judgment and are accountable for their decisions and nursing practice that arises from those decisions. Your current level of clinical judgment can always be improved, and you may want to devise a personal plan for improving your own clinical decision making. Working thoughtfully through the self-assessment in Box 11.9 will help you begin.

BOX 11.8 Clinical Judgment: Nine Key Questions

1. What major outcomes (observable beneficial results) do we expect to see in this particular patient, family, or group when the plan of care is terminated? Example: The patient will be discharged without complications, able to care for himself, 3 days after surgery. Outcomes may be addressed on a standard plan, or you may have to develop these outcomes yourself. Make sure any predetermined outcomes in standard plans are appropriate to your patient's specific situation.

2. What problems or issues must be addressed to achieve the major outcomes? Answering this question will help you prioritize. You may have a long list of actual or potential health problems needing to be structured to set your priorities.

3. What are the circumstances? Who is involved (e.g., child, adult, group)? How urgent are the problems (e.g., life-threatening, chronic)? What are the factors influencing their presentation (e.g., when, where, and how did the problems develop)? What are the patient's values, beliefs, and cultural influences?

4. What knowledge is required? You must know problem-specific facts (e.g., how problems usually present, how they are diagnosed, what their common causes and risk factors are, what common complications occur, and how these complications are prevented and managed), nursing process and related knowledge and skills (e.g., ethics, research, health assessment, communication, priority setting), and related sciences (e.g., anatomy, physiology, pathophysiology, pharmacology, chemistry, physics, psychology, sociology). You must also be clearly aware of the circumstances, as addressed in question 3 above.

5. How much room is there for error? In the clinical setting, there is usually minimal room for error. However, it depends on the health of the individual and the risks of interventions. A healthy, young postoperative patient with no chronic illnesses may tolerate early mobility after surgery better than an elderly person with a history of multiple chronic problems requiring numerous medications. Although their orders for postoperative ambulation may be identical and your commitment to their safe care exactly the same for these two patients, excellent clinical judgment based on your assessments allows you to conclude that the young patient is safe walking in the hallway with a family member, whereas the elderly patient needs your assistance and guidance during early ambulation.

6. How much time do I have? Time frame for decision making depends on (1) the urgency of the problems (e.g., there is little time in life-threatening situations, such as cardiac arrest) and (2) the planned length of contact (e.g., if your patient will be hospitalized for only 2 days, you have to be realistic about what can be accomplished, and key decisions need to be made early).

7. What resources can help me? Human resources include clinical nurse educators, nursing faculty, preceptors, experienced nurses, advanced practice nurses, peers, librarians, and other health care professionals (e.g., pharmacists, nutritionists, physical therapists, physicians). The patient and family are also valuable resources (usually they know their own problems best). Other resources include texts, articles, other references, computer databases, decision-making support, national practice guidelines, and facility documents (e.g., guidelines, policies, procedures, assessment forms).

8. Whose perspectives must be considered? The most significant perspective to consider is the patient's point of view. Other important perspectives include those of the family and significant others, caregivers, and relevant third parties (e.g., insurers).

9. What is influencing my thinking? Identify your personal biases and any other factors influencing your critical thinking and therefore your clinical judgment.

From Alfaro-LeFevre R: *Critical thinking in nursing: a practical approach,* ed 2, Philadelphia, 1999, Saunders. Reprinted with permission.

BOX 11.9   Self-Assessment: Developing Sound Clinical Judgment

Answer the following questions honestly. When finished, make a list of the items you need to work on in your quest to develop sound clinical judgment and review it often. Seek opportunities to practice activities you have identified that you need.

1. Use high-quality references and resources.
   - Do I look up new terms when I encounter them to make them part of my vocabulary?
   - Do I familiarize myself with normal findings so that I can recognize those outside the norm?
   - Do I use research findings and base my practice on scientific evidence?
   - Do I learn the signs and symptoms of various conditions, what causes them, and how they are managed?
2. Use the nursing process.
   - Do I always assess before acting, stay focused on outcomes, and make changes as needed?
   - Do I always base my judgments on fact, not emotion or speculation?
3. Assess systematically.
   - Do I have a systematic approach to assessing patients to decrease the likelihood that I will overlook important data?
4. Set priorities systematically.
   - Do I evaluate both the problem and the probable cause before acting?
   - Am I willing to obtain assistance from a more knowledgeable source when indicated?
5. Refuse to act without knowledge.
   - Do I refuse to act when I do not know the indication, why it works, and what risks there are for harm to this particular patient?

6. Use resources wisely.
   - Do I look for opportunities to learn from others, such as teachers, other experts, my colleagues, and continuing education?
   - Do I seek help when needed, being mindful of patient privacy?
7. Know standards of care.
   - Do I know facility policies, professional standards, school policies, and state board of nursing rules and regulations with regard to my legal scope of practice?
   - Do I know the clinical agency's policies and procedures affecting my particular patients?
   - Do I attempt to understand the rationales behind policies and procedures?
   - Do I follow policies and procedures carefully, recognizing that they are designed to help me use good judgment?
   - Do I recognize that no workplace policy or procedure can override my state's limits on scope of practice?
8. Know technology and equipment.
   - Do I routinely learn how to use patient technology such as intravenous pumps, patient monitors, and other equipment?
   - Do I learn how to check equipment for proper functioning and safety?
9. Give patient-centered care.
   - Do I always remember the needs and feelings of the patient, family, and significant others?
   - Do I value knowing my patients' health beliefs and values within context of their own culture?
   - Am I willing to "go the extra mile" for patients?
   - Do I demonstrate the belief that every patient deserves my very best efforts?

Modified from Alfaro-LeFevre R: *Critical thinking in nursing: a practical approach,* ed 2, Philadelphia, 1999, Saunders, pp. 88–92. Used with permission.

CONCEPTS AND CHALLENGES

- *Concept:* In nursing, critical thinking is a purposeful, disciplined, active process that improves clinical judgment and thereby improves patient care.
  Challenge: Critical thinking is a skill that can be learned and requires that one continues to "think about thinking" to sustain high-level critical thinking ability.
- *Concept:* The nursing process is a systematic problem-solving framework that ensures that care is developed in an organized, analytic way.

   Challenge: Properly used, the nursing process is cyclic and dynamic rather than rigid and linear.
- *Concept:* Consistent, comprehensive, and coordinated patient care results when all nurses use the nursing process effectively.
  Challenge: Nurses may initially find that using the nursing process feels awkward or slow. With experience, however, most find that it becomes a natural, organized approach to patient care.

- *Concept:* Both the scientific basis of nursing and professionalism are advanced when nurses resolve patient problems through development of sound clinical judgment.

Challenge: Sound clinical judgment is developed when nurses use critical thinking, apply the nursing process, stay current with developments in practice and research, understand their scope of practice, and acquire substantial clinical experience.

IDEAS FOR FURTHER EXPLORATION

1. Describe the characteristics of critical thinkers, and explain why critical thinking is important in nursing.
2. List at least four ways in which novice thinking and expert thinking differ, and give an example that illustrates each.
3. Describe the phases in the nursing process, and explain the activities of each phase.
4. Describe the debate related to the use of nursing diagnosis. Which side do you agree with and why?

5. Describe what is meant by the statement, "The nursing process is a cyclic process."
6. Using what you learned about yourself from Self-Assessment: Developing Sound Clinical Judgment (see Box 11.9), set short-term goals for improvement in each of the nine areas. Make a checklist to take to your next clinical experience, and consciously work on improving your clinical judgment.

REFERENCES

Alfaro-LeFevre R: *Critical thinking in nursing: a practical approach*, ed 2, Philadelphia, 1999, Saunders.

American Association of Colleges of Nursing (AACN): *The essentials of baccalaureate education for professional nursing practice*, Washington, DC, 2008, American Association of Colleges of Nursing.

American Philosophical Association: *Critical thinking: a statement of expert consensus for purposes of educational assessment and instruction*, The Delphi report: research findings and recommendations prepared for the committee on pre-college philosophy, 1990, *ERIC Document Reproduction Services* pp, 315–423.

Benner P: *From novice to expert*, Menlo Park, Calif, 1984, Addison-Wesley.

Benner P, Tanner CA, Chesla CA: *Expertise in nursing practice: caring, clinical judgment, and ethics*, New York, 1996, Springer.

Bradley PK, Berry A, Lang C, et al.: Getting ready: developing an educational intervention to prepare African American women for breast biopsy, *ABFN J* 17(1): 15–19, 2006.

Chang MJ, Chang Y-J, Kuo S-H, et al.: Relationships between critical thinking ability and nursing competence in clinical nurses, *J Clin Nurs* 20:3224–3232, 2011.

Facione PA: Critical thinking: what it is and why it counts, (website), 2013. Available at: https://spu.edu/depts/health-sciences/grad/documents/CTbyFacione.pdf.

Doenges M, Moorhouse MF, Murr AC: *Nursing diagnosis manual: planning, individualizing, and documenting client care*, Philadelphia, 2013, FA Davis.

Gordon M: Nursing diagnosis and the diagnostic process, *Am J Nurs* 76(5):1298–1300, 1976.

Gordon M: *Nursing diagnosis: process and application*, ed 2, New York, 1987, McGraw-Hill.

Huckabay LM: Clinical reasoned judgment and the nursing process, *Nurs Forum* 44(2):72–78, 2009.

Lau J, Chan J: OpenCourseWare on critical thinking, logic, and creativity. (website), 2012. Available at: http://philosophy.hku.hk/think.

Lunney M: Critical need to address accuracy of nurses' diagnoses, *Online J Issues Nurs* 13(3), 2008. (website). Available at: www.nursingworld.org/MainMenuCategories/ANAMarketplace/ANAPeriodicals/OJIN/TableofContents/vol132008/No1Jan08/ArticlePreviousTopic/AccuracyofNursesDiagnoses.aspx.

Maslow AH: *Motivation and personality*, New York, 1970, Harper & Row.

NANDA International (NANDA-I): *Nursing diagnoses: definitions and classification, 2003–2004*, Philadelphia, 2003, NANDA International.

NANDA International (NANDA-I): *Nursing diagnoses: definitions and classification, 2012–2014*, Philadelphia, 2012, Wiley-Blackwell.

NANDA International (NANDA-I): About NANDA International. (website), 2018. Available at: kb.nanda.org.

NANDA International (NANDA-I): Nursing diagnosis frequently asked questions. (website), 2012. Available at: www.nanda.org/NursingDiagnosisFAQ.aspx.

Paans W, Nieweg RMB, van der Schans CP, et al.: What factors influence the prevalence and accuracy of nursing diagnoses documentation in clinical practice? A systematic literature review, *J Clin Nurs* 20(17–18):2386–2403, 2011.

Paul R, Elder L: Paul-Elder critical thinking framework. (website), 2015. Available at: www.louisville.edu/ideasto-action/about/criticalthinking/framework.

Schneider MA: Fundamentals: still the building block of safe patient care, *Nursing* 45(6):60–63, 2015.

Spring H: Learning and teaching in action, *Health Info Libr J* 27:327–331, 2010.

Yura H, Walsh MB: *The nursing process: assessing, planning, implementing, evaluation*, ed 4, Norwalk, Conn, 1983, Appleton-Century-Crofts.

12

Communication and Collaboration in Professional Nursing

Maxine Fearrington, MS, RN-BC

(e) To enhance your understanding of this chapter, try the Student Exercises on the Evolve site at http://evolve.elsevier.com/Black/professional.

LEARNING OUTCOMES

After studying this chapter, students will be able to:

- Describe therapeutic use of self.
- Identify and describe the phases of the traditional nurse-patient relationship.
- Differentiate between social and professional relationships.
- Explore the role self-awareness plays in the ability to use nonjudgmental acceptance as a helping technique.
- Explain the concept of professional boundaries.
- Discuss factors creating successful or unsuccessful communication.

- Evaluate helpful and unhelpful communication techniques.
- Identify strategies in providing care to patients who do not speak English.
- Understand the roles of professional interpreters and translators.
- Identify their own communication strengths and challenges.
- Demonstrate components of active listening.
- Identify key aspects of collaboration.
- Explain the effects of gender, cultural, and generational diversity on nurse-patient and nurse-colleague relationships.

The name Joseph Priestley may be familiar to you; if you were reading carefully, you will remember his name from Chapter 10 as the scientist who discovered oxygen, an example of "pure science." Priestley was an interesting figure in 18th-century England—in addition to being a chemist, he was also a theologian, philosopher, educator, and political theorist. He once wrote, "The more elaborate our means of communication, the less we communicate." Priestley's words have particular relevance now because even as excellent communication is highly valued in health care, the many forms and avenues of communication create opportunities for communication to break down.

In nursing, breakdowns in communication can have significant, even dire consequences. Developing excellent communication skills is important in your education as a nurse, because much of what you do as a professional nurse requires the ability to express yourself clearly and to understand another person. Note that communication does not involve simply being able to talk, but to listen to and engage with another person nonverbally, because much of the way that humans express themselves is through nonverbal communication.

The skill set that includes communication is often referred to as *interpersonal skills.* Nurses interact with many people every day regardless of their role or the setting in which they work. The way in which they relate to patients, families, colleagues, and other professionals and nonprofessionals determines the level of comfort and trust others feel and, ultimately, the success of their

259

interactions. This chapter includes information that can enhance the development of self-awareness, nonjudgmental acceptance of others, communication skills, and collaboration skills, all of which are essential components of effective interpersonal skills in nursing.

THE THERAPEUTIC USE OF SELF

Hildegard Peplau, a pioneer in nursing theory development, first focused on the importance of the nurse-patient relationship in her 1952 book *Interpersonal Relations in Nursing*. She referred to the use of one's personality and communication skills to help patients as the "therapeutic use of self" (Peplau, 1952), a strategy that you can develop with practice. Therapeutic use of self can be helpful to you in relating effectively to patients, patients' families, and other health care professionals.

The Therapeutic Nurse-Patient Relationship: A Traditional Model

The nursing process can begin only after the nurse and patient establish their initial therapeutic nurse-patient relationship. Awareness of the three identifiable phases of the nurse-patient relationship helps nurses to be realistic in their expectations of this important relationship. Each of three phases—orientation, working, and termination—is sequential and builds on previous phases.

The Orientation Phase

The orientation phase, or introductory phase, is the period often described as "getting to know you" in social settings. Relationships between nurses and their patients have some commonalities with other types of relationships. The chief similarity is that there must be trust between the two parties for the relationship to develop. Nurses cannot expect patients to trust them automatically and to reveal their innermost thoughts and feelings immediately.

During the orientation phase, the nurse and patient assess each other. Early impressions made by the nurse are important. Some people have difficulty accepting help of any kind, including nursing care. Putting the patient at ease with a calm, unhurried approach is important during the early part of any nurse-patient relationship.

During the orientation phase, the patient has a right to expect to learn the nurse's name, credentials, and extent of responsibility. The use of simple orienting statements is one way to begin: "Good morning, Mr. Davis. I am Jennifer Carter, and I am your nurse until 7 this evening. I am responsible for your care while I am here."

Developing trust. The orientation phase includes the initial development of trust. Notice the use of the phrase "initial development." Full development of trust is slow and may take months of regular contact. A fact of contemporary nursing practice is that patient interactions may be brief, sometimes lasting only minutes. However, even in the most abbreviated contacts, nurses must orient patients and help them feel comfortable and as trusting as possible.

Certain behaviors help patients develop trust in the nurse. A straightforward, nondefensive manner is important. Answering all questions as fully as possible and admitting to the limits of your knowledge also facilitate trust. Patients accept a simple explanation, such as "I don't know the answer to your question, but I will find out for you," more readily than a thinly veiled, evasive response. Promise to find out the answers to all questions, and report the information to the patient as soon as possible. If you tell a patient that you will check on her at 11:30 a.m., make every attempt to follow through on that promise, even if it means that you send someone else in to explain that you are otherwise occupied and will be in as soon as possible. In addition, and most important, withhold judgments about patients and their situations. Use active listening, and accept the patient's thoughts and feelings without passing judgment on what he or she is telling you.

Listen carefully to your own responses, because it is easy to fall into the habit of using platitudes and clichés in response. Imagine your patient telling you, "I am really worried about my surgery tomorrow." Then imagine yourself responding with, "That's silly, you will be fine," as you take her blood pressure and then leave the room. Even as a student, you recognize the potential harm that this dismissive response will have for the frightened patient awaiting surgery.

Congruence between verbal and nonverbal communication is a key factor in the development of trust. Communicating in a congruent manner requires that nurses be aware of their own thoughts and feelings and be able to share those with others in a nonthreatening manner. Developing an initial understanding of the patient's problem or needs also starts in the orientation phase. Because patients themselves often do not clearly understand their problems or may be reluctant to discuss them, nurses must use their communication skills to elicit the information needed to make a nursing diagnosis. Communication skills useful in nurse-patient interactions are discussed later in this chapter

Tasks of the orientation phase. By the end of a successful orientation phase, regardless of its length, several things will have happened. First, the patient will have developed enough trust in the nurse to continue to participate in the relationship. Second, the patient and nurse will see each other as individuals. Third, the patient's perception of major problems and needs will have been identified. Fourth, the approximate length of the relationship will have been estimated, and the nurse and patient will have agreed to work together on some aspect of the identified problems. This agreement, whether formalized in writing or informally agreed on, is sometimes called a *contract*. An example of a contract that might emerge from the orientation phase of the relationship with a patient with newly diagnosed diabetes is an agreement to work together on the patient's ability to monitor glucose levels and to manage diet using specific guidelines.

The Working Phase

The second phase of the nurse-patient relationship is called the working phase, during which the nurse and patient address tasks outlined in the previous phase. Because the participants in this relationship now know each other in a professional context, a sense of interpersonal comfort in the relationship may be possible.

Nurses should recognize that in the working phase patients may exhibit alternating periods of intense effort and of resistance to change. Continuing the example of the patient with diabetes, the nurse can anticipate that the patient will experience some degree of difficulty in accepting the lifestyle changes that managing diabetes requires. The patient may show progress one week but not be able to sustain improved diet the following week. This "two steps forward and one backward" approach to behavior change is common; it is not a reflection on one's skill as a nurse, nor is it an indictment of the patient's desire to manage his or her own care. This is a phenomenon known as regression, a psychological device that occurs as a reaction to stress and that often precedes positive changes in behaviors.

Making and sustaining change are very difficult. Patience, self-awareness, and maturity are required of nurses during the working phase. Continued building of trust, use of active listening, and other helpful communication responses facilitate the patient's expression of needs and feelings during the working phase.

The Termination Phase

The termination phase includes those activities that enable the patient and the nurse to end the relationship in a therapeutic manner. The process of terminating the nurse-patient relationship begins in the orientation phase when participants estimate the length of time it will take to accomplish the desired outcomes. This is part of the informal contract.

As in any relationship, positive and negative feelings often accompany termination. The patient and nurse feel good about the gains the patient has made in accomplishing goals. They may feel sadness about ending a relationship that has been open and trusting. People tend to respond to the end of relationships in much the same way they have responded to other losses in life. Feelings of anger and fear may surface, in addition to sadness. This is particularly true on the part of the patient who has come to trust and depend on you because you tended to his or her needs at a time of vulnerability.

Feelings evoked by termination should be discussed and accepted. Summarizing the gains the patient has made is an important activity during this phase. The importance of the relationship to both patient and nurse can be shared in a caring manner.

The giving and receiving of gifts at termination have different meanings for different people. The meaning of such behavior should be explored in a sensitive manner with the patient. When a nurse has been involved with a family over a long or intense period, such as in an end-of-life setting, it is common for those families to want to give the nurse a gift as a sign of their appreciation and as a remembrance of the patient who has died. Both the agency's policy on gifts and your clinical faculty should be consulted. Even if you are not allowed to accept a gift, you can acknowledge that you wish you could accept their gift and express your gratitude for their thoughtfulness.

Because termination is often painful, participants are often tempted to continue the relationship on a social basis, and requests for screen names for social media, addresses, phone numbers, and e-mail addresses are not uncommon. The nurse must realize that professional relationships are different from social relationships. This is an issue of professional boundaries that has been

---

BOX 12.1   Differences in Social and Professional Relationships

Social Relationships
- Evolve spontaneously
- Not time limited
- Not necessarily goal directed; broad purpose is pleasure, companionship, sharing
- Centered on meeting both parties' needs
- Problem solving is rarely/occasionally a focus
- May or may not include nonjudgmental acceptance
- Outcome is pleasure for both parties

Professional Relationships
- Evolve through recognized phases; interactions are planned and purposeful
- Limited in time with termination date often predetermined
- Goal directed; systematic exploration of identified problem areas
- Centered on meeting patient's needs; do not address nurse's needs
- Problem solving is a primary focus
- Includes nonjudgmental acceptance
- Outcome is improved health status of patient

---

discussed earlier in this text. Differences between social and professional relationships are outlined in Box 12.1.

During the course of a professional career, every nurse will develop a large number of relationships with patients, each with its own meaning and duration. If nurses can view each new relationship both as an opportunity to assist another human being to grow and change in a positive, healthful way and as a challenge to grow and change themselves, the rewards of nursing will be rich in and of themselves, allowing the nurse to separate from patients gracefully at the natural end of the therapeutic relationship.

Developing Self-Awareness

Self-awareness is basic to effective interpersonal relationships and is especially important in the nurse-patient relationship. Few people, however, recognize their own emotions, prejudices, and biases and how they are perceived by others. With practice, however, most people can become self-aware, thereby increasing their effectiveness in both professional and personal relationships.

Nurses must get their own emotional needs met outside of the nurse-patient relationship. When nurses have strong unmet needs for acceptance, approval, friendship, or even love, they run the risk of allowing these needs to enter into their relationships with patients at the cost of professionalism. Boundaries get blurred, and relationships become social, not professional. Worse, patients can bear the burden of their nurses' emotional needs. This is a particular risk in settings where the nurse takes care of a patient and family over a long period, such as in home health or hospice/palliative care settings, or in long-term care facilities. Patients come to know their nurses well, and details of nurses' lives are sometimes shared as part of conversation over time.

Although it is not necessarily a boundary issue for a patient to learn certain details of nurses' lives, it is always a problem when the nurse comes to depend on patients for his or her own emotional support.

Baca (2011) listed five ways in which self-disclosure becomes problematic: (1) if the nurse's problems or needs are disclosed; (2) if disclosure by the nurse becomes a common, rather than rare, event during interactions with a patient; (3) when the disclosure is unrelated to the patient's problems or experiences; (4) if it takes more than a very short time during an interaction; and (5) when the nurse discloses personal information even if it is clear that the patient is confused by the interaction. Becoming aware of one's needs and making conscious efforts to have those needs met in one's private life keep relationships with patients professional and therapeutic for the patient. When the nurse-patient relationship crosses professional boundaries, role confusion can result, risking harm to both patient and nurse.

Professional Boundaries

Questions of professional boundaries are common in nursing. They were first addressed by Florence Nightingale in the Nightingale Pledge (refer to Box 3.1 to review this statement). The National Council of State Boards of Nursing (NCSBN) detailed the subject of professional boundaries comprehensively in a document available online titled "A Nurse's Guide to Professional Boundaries" (NCSBN, 2014). In this document, the NCSBN defines professional boundaries as "the spaces between the nurse's power and the client's vulnerability. The power of the nurse comes from the professional position and the access to private knowledge about the client"

BOX 12.2 Nurse's Relationship With Patient Results in Disciplinary Action

Tapp v. Board of Registered Nursing, 2002 WL 31820206 P2d-CA

This case involved a California registered nurse at a psychiatric facility in Fresno who was accused of having sexual relations with his former patient after her discharge. The patient was hospitalized for emotional problems related to sex. She was hospitalized on a unit where the nurse worked the night shift. They became friendly; he brought her small gifts, gave her his phone number, and called her during his off-work hours. After she was discharged, they spoke often by phone, and he began to visit her at her apartment. On one occasion, the nurse gave his former patient a tablet of a controlled substance.

One week after her discharge, they began a sexual relationship that lasted for 2 weeks. Shortly after the relationship ended, the patient was readmitted, "suffering adverse effects from the affair" (p. 4). The California Board of Registered Nursing initiated disciplinary proceedings for "acts of unprofessional conduct." An administrative law judge heard testimony, made a determination of misconduct, and recommended that the nurse's license be revoked, but stayed the revocation and recommended that the nurse be placed on probation for 5 years on multiple conditions. The California Board of Registered Nursing disagreed and ordered the revocation of his license. There were subsequent appeals, dismissals, and further appeals.

Nurses must realize that there can be no socialization between themselves and patients, particularly when sexual in nature. The ruling noted that not only was this nurse's behavior with this patient during her hospitalization "highly improper, but his socialization with the patient after her discharge from the hospital, not to mention the fact that he provided the patient with a controlled substance, was ample reason to impose strict disciplinary action" (p. 5).

Abstracted from Nurse's relationship with patient results in disciplinary action, *Nurs Law Regan Rep* 43(8):4–5, 2003.

BOX 12.3 Principles for Determining Professional Boundaries

1. Establishing and maintaining professional boundaries is the nurse's responsibility.
2. The nurse-patient relationship should be helpful while still maintaining professional boundaries and without an emotional investment.
3. Factors such as the care setting, community resources, patient's needs, and type of therapies or treatments need to be considered when establishing those boundaries.
4. Mixing or combining a professional and a personal or business relationship should be avoided.
5. The nurse is responsible for reviewing any deviations outside of those boundaries and modifying behaviors to prevent further deviations.
6. Termination of the professional relationship is the nurse's responsibility and may be difficult to complete as some patients require continuous services.

Modified from National Council of State Boards of Nursing (NCSBN): *Professional boundaries: a nurse's guide to the importance of appropriate professional boundaries,* Chicago, 1996, National Council of State Boards of Nursing.

as excessive personal disclosure by the nurse, secrecy, role reversal, touching, gestures, money or gifts, special attention, social contact, getting involved in a patient's personal affairs, and/or sexual misconduct). Both underinvolvement and overinvolvement can be detrimental to patient and nurse. A quick way of monitoring yourself with regard to boundaries is to ask yourself, "Could I feel comfortable telling a colleague about my interaction with this patient?" If the answer is no, then you are at least on the edge of a boundary violation and need to take corrective measures. Secretive behavior is a signal that a nurse does not feel comfortable or is unwilling to share with trusted others (Baca, 2011). Box 12.2 describes a case in which a nurse was disciplined by his state board of nursing for failing to honor the professional boundaries between a nurse and patient.

Failure to maintain professional boundaries with a patient is an offense reportable to your employer and/or your state board of nursing and violates nursing's code of ethics. This means that students and nurses in practice must have a thorough understanding of professional boundaries. Box 12.3 contains seven principles to guide nurses in determining professional boundaries across

(NCSBN, 2014). Boundary violations occur when "there is confusion between the needs of the nurse and those of the client" (NCSBN, 2014).

According to the NCSBN, nurse-patient relationships can be plotted on a continuum of professional behavior that ranges from underinvolvement (such as distancing, disinterest, neglect) through a zone of helpfulness (the ideal space) to overinvolvement (such the continuum of professional behavior (NCSBN, 2014). You can find a .pdf file of the popular NCSBN publication explaining professional boundaries by following the links at www.ncsbn.org.

Reflective Practice

Nurses care for a diverse array of patients whose values, beliefs, and lifestyles may challenge the nurses' own values. Although nurses sometimes are attracted to patients, conversely, nurses may be repelled by some patients. Nurses who have emotional reactions to patients—positive or negative—sometimes feel guilty or disturbed about these feelings. Being self-aware means recognizing one's feelings and understanding that, although feelings cannot be controlled, behaviors can. Effective nurses conducting themselves professionally take charge of their behavior to prevent their own prejudices, beliefs, and needs from intruding into nurse-patient relationships. This ability arises from self-awareness.

Developing self-awareness requires individuals to engage in personal reflection. This requires taking time to focus on their own thoughts, feelings, actions, and beliefs. Finding the time and space for **reflective practice** can be a challenge to busy students and practicing nurses alike. Reflection can produce discomfort as nurses become aware of the tensions and anxieties within themselves about their everyday activities. Nurses and nursing students may find that their personal values are challenged by the realities of practice. Importantly, nurses may recognize in themselves a desensitization to the needs of their patients because of time constraints, the need to create emotional space, or a personal dislike for a particular patient. It can be hard for you when you recognize that you may have thoughts that are less than kind about patients entrusted to your care. This makes the need for reflection more, not less, important. No human being is immune from emotional responses to others, both positive and negative. Despite the difficulty in coming to terms with your emotional responses to patients and to your work, becoming self-aware allows you to understand your responses and to look past your own negative (and positive) responses to particular patients in order to create and maintain a healthy professional space in which you can provide care most effectively. Box 12.4 contains a model for structured reflection that will be helpful to you reflecting on your practice and becoming more self-aware.

BOX 12.4   Model for Structured Reflection

- Write a description of an experience that seems significant in some way.
- What issue seemed significant to pay attention to?
- How was I feeling and what made me feel that way?
- What was I trying to achieve?
- Did I respond effectively and in tune with my values?
- What were the consequences of my actions on the patient, others, and myself?
- How were others feeling?
- What made them feel that way?
- What factors influenced the way I was feeling, thinking, or responding?
- What knowledge did or might have informed me?
- To what extent did I act with best intentions?
- How does this situation connect with previous experiences?
- How might I respond more effectively given this situation again?
- What would be the consequences of alternative actions for the patient, others, and myself?
- How do I now feel about this experience?
- Am I now more able to support myself and others as a consequence?
- Am I now more available to work with patients/families and staff to help them meet their needs?

From Johns C: *Guided reflection: advancing practice,* Oxford, 2002, Blackwell Science, p. 10. Reprinted with permission of Wiley-Blackwell.

Avoiding Stereotypes

Stereotypes are simplistic, distorted images used to describe or characterize groups. Stereotypes result in prejudices and negative attitudes developed through social and cultural interactions. Even well-educated professionals have stereotypical views of groups of people different from themselves and may hold expectations of those groups based on these distorted images. Stereotypes are established through a lifetime of experiences and negatively affect relationships with people in the stereotyped group. Because stereotypes and prejudices tend to persist despite contrary experiences, they are irrational or illogical beliefs. Stereotypes may be based on ethnicity, gender, nationality, or political affiliation, among others; for instance, portrayals or descriptions of nurses as sex objects, physicians' handmaidens, or not bright enough to attend medical school are all stereotypes that negatively affect the profession of nursing.

A subtle form of stereotyping that affects nursing is related to expectations of others based on one's distorted view of the other. This in turn causes problems relating to patients who are stereotyped. For example, if a nurse expects that elderly people are irritable and demanding, the nurse may seek to avoid caring for elderly patients or may treat their complaints as unimportant: "just another grumpy old person." Moreover, some nurses demonstrate lack of respect to elderly patients, using names such as "sweetie," "dear," and "honey," among others. (These types of names are actually inappropriate in any professional nursing setting—especially with adult patients; these types of names diminish the patient by demonstrating a lack of respect for the patient as a person.)

Professional nurses deliver high-quality care to all patients regardless of the patients' ethnicity, age, sex, gender identity, sexual orientation, religion, lifestyle, or diagnosis. The ANA's Code of Ethics for Nurses requires nurses to do this. Nurses are prone to stereotyping just like anyone else; however, the nature of the nurse-patient relationship requires that nurses become aware of how their stereotypical views of certain patients negatively affect the delivery of care. Every professional nurse's goal is to accept all patients as individuals of dignity and worth who deserve the best nursing care possible.

Becoming Nonjudgmental

Prejudices are simply what the word implies: judging a person in advance of knowing him or her, based on stereotypes and biases. Prejudices are strong and are often outside our awareness, which in turn makes **acceptance** of others difficult. Prejudging others as "good" or "bad," "right" or "wrong," is usually unconscious, hence the need for nurses to examine their prejudices and become aware of when prejudices are operating. **Nonjudgmental acceptance** means that nurses acknowledge all patients' rights to be who they are and to express their uniqueness. Acceptance conveys neither approval nor disapproval of patients and their personal beliefs, habits, expressions of feelings, or lifestyles.

Therapeutic use of self begins with the ability to convey acceptance to patients and requires self-awareness and nonjudgmental attitudes on the part of nurses. Ongoing examination of attitudes toward others is both a lifelong process and an essential part of self-awareness, maturation, and personal growth.

Thinking Differently about Nurses and Patients: Caring and Human Relatedness

Fundamentals of the traditional nurse-patient relationship model as described earlier have been taught and practiced since the middle of the 20th century; however, several assumptions on which it is based no longer hold true in many of today's practice settings. For instance, this older model assumes that the development of the nurse-patient relationship is linear, is incremental, and requires trust-building in the earliest phases of the relationship, and, importantly, it assumes that patients desire relationships with nurses, wish to receive services from them, and will cooperate and comply with those nurses (Hagerty and Patusky, 2003).

Although the traditional nurse-patient relationship is still appropriate in some settings, the assumptions on which it is based are being challenged by the fact that hospitalized patients today are more acutely ill, nurses' workloads have increased, and the time nurses spend with patients may be limited. This raises the question of how we can rethink the nurse-patient relationship and find ways to modify it to suit today's contexts of health care delivery.

Patient-Centered Care

Patient-centered care has been proposed as an approach to alleviating some of the problems that currently trouble the U.S. health care system, such as poor care quality, limited access to care, and dehumanization of care (Hobbs, 2009). In a detailed analysis, Hobbs (2009) found that alleviating vulnerabilities (e.g., feeling alienated, lack of control) experienced by the patient is central to patient-centered care in acute care settings. Furthermore, the process of therapeutic engagement is the key process in alleviating vulnerabilities, and one of the mechanisms by which this occurs is by the nurse's caring presence (p. 55).

Theories of caring and human relatedness provide a powerful basis for practice. Many theorists have written about the nature of the nurse-patient relationship, with several writing about caring as the central concept in nursing, through which effective nursing practice occurs. Swanson (1991) defined caring as "a nurturing way of relating to a valued other, toward whom one feels a personal sense of commitment and responsibility" (p. 165). Five caring processes are germane to nursing practice: (1) knowing, (2) being with, (3) doing for, (4) enabling, and (5) maintaining belief (Swanson, 1991).

Others have written about caring in nursing, including Watson (1988), whose theory is discussed in Chapter 9, and Roach and Maykut (2010), who described the essential elements of comportment central to professional caring.

Hagerty and Patusky (2003) proposed an interesting theory of human relatedness through which to conceptualize the nurse-patient relationship. Each nurse-patient contact holds the potential for connection and goal achievement, as opposed to one step in a lengthy relationship-building process. They also recommended that nurses approach their patients with a sense of the patient's autonomy, choice, and participation (p. 147), putting the relationship on a more equitable basis than the traditional nurse-patient relationship, which gives much of the power to the nurse.

The Quality and Safety Education for Nurses (QSEN) project identified patient-centered care as one of six competencies required of all prelicensure nurses and defines patient-centered care as fully engaging the patient or designee in all care decisions, respecting the values, needs, and preferences of the patient or designee in all care coordination (QSEN, 2012). Communication is a key component in realizing patient-centered care. A basic understanding of communication theory is a necessary component of becoming a more effective communicator and therefore a better nurse.

COMMUNICATION THEORY

Communication is the exchange of thoughts, ideas, or information and is at the heart of all relationships. Jurgen Ruesch (1972), a pioneer communications theorist, defined communication as "all the modes of behavior that one individual employs, conscious or unconscious, to affect another: not only the spoken and written word, but also gestures, body movements, somatic signals, and symbolism in the arts" (p. 16).

Communication begins the moment two people become aware of each other's presence. Communication occurs when one is in the presence of another person, even if no words are spoken. Even when alone, people routinely engage in "self-talk," which is an internal form of communication.

Levels of Communication

Communication exists simultaneously on at least two levels: verbal and nonverbal. Verbal communication

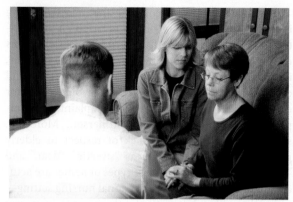

Fig. 12.1 Nonverbal communication consists of grooming, clothing, gestures, posture, facial expressions, tone and volume of voice, and actions. Simply from the visual cues in this picture, you can form an idea of what is happening. (Photo used with permission from iStockPhoto.)

consists of all speech and represents the most obvious aspect of communication. Much of one's message, however, consists of nonverbal communication. Nonverbal communication includes grooming, clothing, gestures, posture, facial expressions, eye contact, tone and volume of voice, and actions, among other things (Fig. 12.1). Words can be used to mask feelings, but individuals are less able to exercise conscious control over nonverbal communication than verbal communication, therefore the nonverbal component may be a more reliable expression of feeling. Nurses must pay attention to nonverbal messages as closely as they do to verbal ones.

Consider this example: A nurse who is helping a patient prepare for a breast biopsy notices that the patient keeps her head turned away, has tears in her eyes, and will not look at the nurse. When the nurse says, "Is there anything you want to talk about or ask?" the patient responds, "No, I'm fine." The sensitive nurse would pay closer attention to her nonverbal communication than to the spoken word. If the nurse pays attention only to the patient's words, her underlying feelings would be ignored. The nurse's job in evaluating this patient's needs is made more difficult by the incongruence between her verbal and nonverbal messages.

When congruent communication occurs, the verbal and nonverbal aspects match and reinforce each other. In incongruent communication, the words and nonverbal communication do not match. Incongruent communication creates confusion in receivers, who are unsure

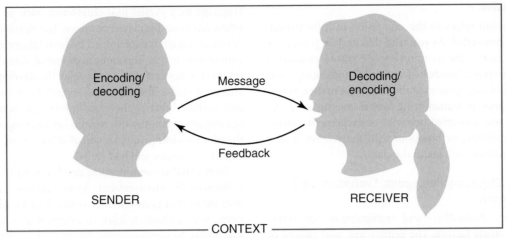

Fig. 12.2 The five major elements of the communication process.

which level of communication they should respond to. Nurses should be alert to incongruent communication for clues to patients' unexpressed feelings. Nurses need to understand that patients are vulnerable, and expressions such as "I'm okay" or "No, I'm fine," despite their incongruent nonverbal cues, do not mean that your patient is lying. It may simply mean that the patient is not ready or willing to share verbally what their nonverbal communication is relaying.

Elements of the Communication Process

Five major elements must be present for communication to occur: a sender, a message, a receiver, feedback, and a context (Ruesch, 1972). The sender is the person sending the message; the message is what is actually said plus accompanying nonverbal communication; the receiver is the person acquiring the message. A response to a message is termed feedback. The setting in which an interaction occurs—including the mood, relationship between sender and receiver, and other factors—is known as the context. All these elements are necessary for communication to occur.

Consider the classroom situation. During a lecture, the professor is the sender, the lecture is the message, and students are the receivers. The professor (sender) receives feedback from the students (receivers) through their facial expressions, alertness, posture, attentiveness, and comments. The atmosphere in the classroom is the context. If the atmosphere is a relaxed one of give-and-take discussion between students and professor,

the feedback is quite different from feedback in a more formal context of professor as lecturer and students as note takers. Fig. 12.2 shows the relationships among the elements of communication.

Operations in the Communication Process

In addition to the five elements of communication, three major operations occur in communication: perception, evaluation, and transmission (Ruesch, 1972).

Perception

Perception is the selection, organization, and interpretation of incoming signals into meaningful messages. In the classroom situation just described, students select, organize, and interpret various pieces of the professor's message or lecture. Each student perceives the information differently; his or her perception is based on a variety of factors such as personal experience, preparation before class, alertness, fatigue, sensitivity to subtleties of meaning, and sociocultural background. This is sometimes referred to as an individual's perceptual screen, through which all incoming messages are filtered.

Evaluation

Evaluation is the analysis of received information. Students will evaluate the content of their professor's lecture—Is it useful? Is it important or relevant? Does it make sense? Is it likely to be on the next test? Each student evaluates the same message (what the sender transmitted) differently.

Transmission

Transmission refers to the expression of information, verbal or nonverbal. As you read this, certain professors of yours may come to mind—those whose nonverbal behaviors spoke "louder than words," indicating their own level of engagement with the subject matter. While the professor is transmitting verbal messages to the students, the nonverbal behavior of excitement, uncertainty, confusion, or boredom with the subject matter also transmits a message to the class.

Factors Influencing Perception, Evaluation, and Transmission

Perception, evaluation, and transmission are influenced by many factors. The gender, age, and culture of the sender and receiver; the interest and mood of both parties; the value, clarity, and length of the message; the presence or absence of feedback; and the context all are powerful influences. Also involved are individuals' needs, values, self-concepts, sensory and intellectual abilities or deficits, and sociocultural conditioning. Clearly, communication is a complex human activity to which nurses must pay careful attention.

THE DEVELOPMENT OF HUMAN COMMUNICATION

Humans learn to communicate through a certain developmental sequence, which begins in infancy. Infants use somatic language to signal their needs to caretakers. Somatic language consists of crying; reddening of the skin; fast, shallow breathing; facial expressions; and jerking of the limbs. The sequence progresses to action language in older infants. Mothers describe knowing the difference in their infants' cries: the "hungry" cry, the "mad" cry, the "pick me up!" cry. Understanding somatic language can be learned with close attention. Action language consists of reaching out, pointing, crawling toward a desired object, or closing the lips and turning the head when an undesired food is offered. Even without a sound, an infant's intention or desire has been clearly communicated. Verbal language develops last, beginning with repetitive noises and sounds and progressing to words, phrases, and complete sentences.

In normal child development, any one or combination of these forms of communication can be used. Somatic language usually decreases with maturity, but, because it is not under conscious control, some somatic language may persist past childhood, such as blushing when one is embarrassed or angry. The development of communication is determined by both inborn and environmental factors. The amount of verbal stimulation an infant receives can enhance or delay the development of language skills. The extent of a caretaker's vocabulary and verbal ability is therefore influential. Some families engage in lengthy discussions on a variety of issues, thereby providing intense verbal stimulation, whereas others are quieter and less verbal.

Nonverbal communication development is similarly influenced by environment. Most families have their own nonverbal gestures such as touch or facial expressions, which children learn to interpret at young ages. The ability to communicate effectively is dependent on a number of factors. The quantity and quality of verbal and nonverbal stimulation received during early development are keys to one's ability to communicate.

CRITERIA FOR SUCCESSFUL COMMUNICATION

Everyone has had the experience of being the sender or receiver of unsuccessful communication. A simple example is arriving for a coffee date with a friend at the wrong time or wrong place because of a problem in communication. Unsuccessful communication in certain social circumstances creates little harm. In nursing situations, however, accurate, complete communication is vitally important. Nurses can achieve successful communication on most occasions if they plan their communication to meet four major criteria: feedback, appropriateness, efficiency, and flexibility.

Feedback

When a receiver relays to a sender the effect of the sender's message, feedback has occurred. It is also a criterion for successful communication. In making the social appointment mentioned earlier, if the receiver of the message had said, "Let's make sure I've got this—12:30 on Tuesday April 4th at the Looking Glass Café for coffee," that feedback would be successful as an effective way to ensure that both persons were at the same place at the same time.

In a nurse-patient interaction, a nurse can give feedback to a patient by saying, "If I understand you correctly, you are saying that you have pain in your lower abdomen every time you stand up." The patient can then either agree or correct what the nurse has said: "No, the pain is there only when I get up in the morning." Effective nurses do not assume that they fully understand what their patients are telling them until they confirm their understanding with the patient.

Appropriateness

Appropriateness refers to the correct "fit" of a reply—that is, when it matches the message, and the size of the reply is neither too lengthy nor too brief. In day-to-day conversation among casual acquaintances passing in a hallway or in public, most people recognize the question "How are you?" as an expression of greeting in brief social interaction and not as a genuine inquiry into one's health and well-being. The individual who launches into a lengthy, detailed description of how his morning has gone has responded inappropriately to the casual question, "How are you?" The reply does not fit the circumstances, and the reply is too expansive for casual discourse. An appropriate response is, "Fine, and how are you?" or other short colloquialism.

Conversely, when you go into a patient's room and ask "How are you?" your intention is to inquire about your patient's health and well-being as a professional interest, and the patient may respond accordingly; however, because this question is so pervasive in everyday discourse, the patient may simply answer, "Fine, how are you?" You will need to ask the question more specifically if your patient responds in that manner. If a patient asks, "When is my doctor coming to see me?" just after the physician has visited the patient, the nurse will be alert to other inappropriate messages by this patient that may signal a variety of problems. In this instance the inappropriate message does not match the context.

Efficiency

Efficiency means using simple, clear words that are timed at a pace suitable to participants. Explaining to an adult that she will have "an angioplasty" tomorrow morning may not result in successful communication. Telling her she will have "an angioplasty, a procedure in which a small balloon is threaded into an artery and inflated to open up the vessel so more blood can flow through," will more likely ensure her understanding. This message would not be an efficient one for a small child, however. Messages must be adapted to each patient's age, verbal level, and level of understanding.

Oversimplification is a risk in trying to adapt one's language style and word choice to a particular patient.

What may seem to be useful simplicity and efficiency may be perceived as "dumbing down" or patronizing language to the patient. One cannot tell with any certainty a patient's communication level, and to assume that a patient cannot understand may also cause problems. For instance, a nurse (the editor of this text) once heard a physician tell a teenager with a urinary tract infection that she had "bugs in [her] bladder." The physician's attempt to make the language efficient and simple was misguided; the young woman took his words at face value and became upset to the point of almost fainting at the thought that she had insects in her body. The nurse immediately intervened, explaining to the patient that sometimes providers refer to bacteria or germs as "bugs"; she had bacteria in her bladder causing an infection. The patient immediately calmed down, asking, "Why didn't he just say that? I need some antibiotics." The physician made a significant misjudgment related to the patient's level of understanding. He came across as patronizing, and the patient was unnecessarily upset by his simplistic explanation. He followed up with the nurse, asking, "What just happened in there?" The nurse explained to him what had gone wrong.

Some examples of patients who require special assistance in evaluating and responding to messages are young children; people with certain mental illnesses, neurologic deficits, or autism spectrum disorders; those with significant developmental delays; and those recovering from anesthesia or receiving pain medication. Although it may seem obvious that people with hearing loss will require special assistance in communication, those with impaired vision do not have the ability to note nonverbal cues, an important element of communication. For efficient communication to occur, nurses must recognize patients' needs and adjust messages accordingly.

Flexibility

Flexibility is the fourth criterion for successful communication. The flexible communicator bases messages on the immediate situation rather than preconceived expectations. When a nursing student who plans to teach a patient about managing diabetes with diet enters the patient's room and finds the patient crying, the student must be flexible enough to regroup and deal with the feelings the patient is expressing. Pressing on with the teaching plan in the face of the patient's distress shows a lack of compassion, as well as inflexibility in communicating.

Nurses can learn to use these four measures of successful communication to enhance their effectiveness with patients. If any of these four criteria are missing, communication can be disrupted and hamper the successful implementation of the nursing process. The following is a true story of what happens when communication breaks down and a rigid reliance on a bureaucratic system prevails. Some details are changed to protect the privacy of the patient and family.

Mr. Lewis came to the local emergency department (ED) accompanied by his wife, who was a nurse. Mr. Lewis, who had advanced cancer, was occasionally confused and had tried to retrieve a Popsicle stick stuck on the roof of his large dog's mouth. In the process, he caught the back of his hand on an upper canine tooth, resulting in a deep gash. Mrs. Lewis had witnessed the accident and gave details to the triage nurse, including her first-person account that the dog did not bite her husband and that his long-term use of high-dose steroids had made his skin fragile and prone to tearing. The nurse noted "dog bite" on her intake form over Mrs. Lewis' objection that the injury was clearly not a bite and that the dog was not at fault. The triage nurse did not acknowledge Mrs. Lewis' account of the accident, continued to get vital signs, and complained about "getting slammed"—meaning that the ED was busy.

Mr. Lewis was soon escorted to the urgent care room, where his wound was cleaned and sutured. Both the nurse practitioner and resident physician asked questions about how the "dog bite" happened, and Mrs. Lewis again protested that it was not a bite and pointed out the lack of tooth marks, crushing, or other signs of a bite. The attending physician told the couple that he had no choice but to report "the bite" to the county emergency medical services (EMS) per protocol, because the triage nurse had documented it as a "dog bite," although the couple had never said it was a bite and the wound was not consistent with a bite. The unit secretary called 911 and asked Mrs. Lewis to tell the dispatcher about the "dog that bit your husband." Mrs. Lewis explained what had happened to the dispatcher, who said that he had no discretion in the matter and that he had to report this to the local police.

Within a half hour of arriving home at 12:30 a.m., Mrs. Lewis received a call from a police officer who said he was "initiating an investigation about the dog attack at this address." At that point, Mrs. Lewis burst into tears in frustration and explained one more time to the police officer that there was no attack, no bite, just an accident by her sick and confused husband. The officer said he had no discretion in the case and had to make a report to animal control, who would have the final say about whether their beloved dog would have to be quarantined or worse. He said he would make his report in a way that was sympathetic to the Lewises, although he could not promise what animal control would do. For more than a week, the Lewises were nervous and upset, and every time the phone rang or someone came to the door they feared it was animal control. Gratefully, they never heard anything else about the matter. But the triage nurse's failure to listen carefully created a cascade of bureaucratic procedure causing avoidable pain for this couple who were already dealing with devastating illness.

Consider the many ways that communication went wrong in this scenario. Identify points where you believe that this cascade of events could have been interrupted.

DEVELOPING EFFECTIVE COMMUNICATION SKILLS

People are not born as good communicators, although it is hard to argue that a screaming infant is not communicating something. Exactly what the baby is communicating, however, needs to be deciphered by an attentive parent or other caregiver. As the baby grows into a toddler, he or she learns that "no" is a particularly useful word. Anyone who has responded to a petulant 2-year-old, however, knows that the child has much to learn about the other side of communication—being a good listener. The child must learn to increase his or her repertoire of responses.

Communication skills can be developed with time and practice. Becoming a better listener, learning a few basic helpful responding styles, and avoiding common causes of communication breakdowns can put you on the path to becoming a better communicator. To begin evaluating your communication skills, refer to the Communication Patterns Self-Assessment in Box 12.5.

Listening

Listening is hard work, yet it is the only way to get to know patients and understand what is important to them. A requirement of successful communication is listening, but too often we hear without listening or engage in a task while not fully listening. (This was a problem with the triage nurse in the earlier example.) **Active listening** involves focusing solely on a person and acknowledging

---

BOX 12.5 Communication Patterns Self-Assessment

Directions: Answer the following true-or-false questions as honestly as possible; then review your answers, and draw at least two conclusions about your habitual communication patterns that you need to work to improve. Check your conclusions for accuracy with a friend who knows your style of communicating well. Then score yourself using the key below.

1. I find it easier to start conversations by talking about myself.
2. I usually listen about as much as I talk.
3. I tend to be long-winded.
4. I rarely interrupt others.
5. When people hesitate or speak slowly, I try to complete their sentences for them.
6. I pay close attention to what others say, as well as to body cues.
7. I find it difficult to make eye contact with the person I am talking with.
8. I can usually tell if someone is angry or upset.
9. I find it difficult to express myself assertively.
10. I expect others to read my mind.
11. I hesitate to interrupt someone to ask for clarification.
12. People often tell me personal things about themselves.
13. I find it is best to change the subject if someone gets too emotional.
14. If I cannot "make things better" for a friend with a problem, I feel uncomfortable.
15. I am comfortable talking with people much older or much younger than I am.
16. I have difficulty saying no.
17. I speak to others the way I like to be spoken to.
18. I get irritated easily.
19. I tend to withdraw from conflict or remain silent.
20. I try to evaluate when someone will be most receptive to my message.

Key: If you answered True to questions 2, 4, 6, 8, 12, 15, 17, and 20, you are on your way to becoming an effective communicator. If you answered True to other questions, select several to improve. Set a realistic goal and seek help from a trusted friend or faculty member.

---

feelings in a nonjudgmental manner. In active listening, the nurse is communicating interest and attention. It is best accomplished without background distractions, such as the television or chatting visitors. Using an intentionally unrushed manner, making good eye contact, nodding, and encouraging the speaker ("Go on" or "Tell me more") also help to communicate interest. Facing the speaker squarely and using an **open posture** (leaning forward, relaxed, arms uncrossed) also communicate interest. Sit, bend, or stoop to place your eye level at that of the patient, and repeat (reflect) what you hear, including feelings, checking to be sure you heard correctly. These indications of interest and active listening will help you focus on patients and tune into the meanings behind their words.

Having someone listen to concerns, even if no problem solving takes place, may be therapeutic. **Venting** is the term used to describe the verbal "letting off steam" that occurs when talking about concerns or frustrations. In today's complex health care system, the risk is high that patients feel ignored or anxious on occasion. Because nurses are available to patients more than any other health care provider, they are likely to hear patients' complaints. It is important that nurses understand these complaints and frustrations as a professional, realizing that they are rarely personally directed at the nurse.

Nurses may have difficulty listening for a variety of reasons. They may be intent on accomplishing a task and be frustrated by the time it takes to be a good listener. They may be planning their own next question or response and not truly hear what the patient is saying. They may be distracted by a colleague, a cell phone, or worries about another patient. Like all people, nurses have their own personal and professional problems that sometimes preoccupy them and interfere with effective listening. No message can be received if the receiver (the nurse) is not listening. In the context of care, being listened to meets the patient's emotional need to be respected and valued by the nurse. Hospitalized patients particularly may feel that their lives are out of control and that they are isolated or invisible. They may need to discuss those feelings with someone who will listen without judgment or defensiveness (Fig. 12.3).

Nurses at all levels find listening a useful and rewarding skill and one that can be used effectively in their own personal and social lives. Nurse managers often use listening as a tool for dealing with staff members' problems and concerns and find that no other intervention is required. Listening is a talent that can be developed; properly used, it can be an essential part of a nurse's communication repertoire.

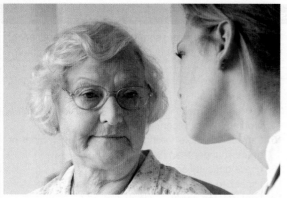

Fig. 12.3 Being an active listener is an important part of communication. Identify behaviors in this photograph that demonstrate active listening by the nurse. (Photo used with permission from iStockPhoto.)

Using Helpful Responding Techniques

A variety of helpful responding techniques demonstrate respect and encourage patients to communicate openly with their nurses. Helpful responses that have already been discussed in this chapter include being nonjudgmental, observing body language, and using active listening. Other useful responses, detailed in the following five sections, include demonstrating empathy, asking open-ended questions, giving information, using reflection, and being silent.

Empathy

Empathy consists of awareness of, sensitivity to, and identification with the feelings of another person. Nurses can empathize with patients even if they have not experienced an event in their own lives exactly like the one the patient is experiencing. If nurses have had a similar or parallel experience, empathy is possible. For example, the feeling of loss is familiar to most nurses, even though they may not personally have lost a close family member. The nurse, however, must avoid the temptation to overidentify with patients when the patient's situation is very similar to one that the nurse has experienced. "I know exactly how you feel" is not helpful in good communication, because human experience varies widely.

Empathy is different from sympathy in that the sympathetic nurse enters into the feeling with the patient, whereas the empathic nurse appreciates the patient's feelings but is not swept along with the feelings. "You

seem upset about the upcoming procedure" is an example of a nursing statement that demonstrates empathy.

If you find yourself overcome by emotions related to a patient, you will need to seek out a colleague to assist you or even replace you in providing care for your patient, because you cannot be effective under these circumstances. You will learn what situations are the most likely to cause you to be emotional and will develop strategies to deal with them. Nurses often "cover" for each other as a matter of collegiality by switching patient assignments or volunteering to work with a particular patient if it is overly burdensome for a colleague.

Open-Ended Questions

An **open-ended question** is one that causes the patient to answer fully, giving more than a "yes" or "no" answer. Open-ended questions are very useful in data gathering and in the opening stages of any nurse-patient interaction. For example, asking a patient, "Are you in pain?" may elicit only a confirming yes. Saying to the patient, "Tell me about your pain" is more likely to elicit information about the site, type, intensity, and duration of the pain, therefore making the nurse-patient interaction more useful.

Giving Information

An essential part of nursing is providing information to patients and their significant others. Giving information includes sharing knowledge that the recipients are not expected to know. Nurses provide information when they tell patients what to expect during diagnostic procedures; inform them of their rights as patients; and teach them about their conditions, diets, or medications.

An important distinction every nurse needs to make is the difference between providing information and giving opinions. Although providing information is a helpful aspect of the nursing role, giving opinions is unhelpful. Instead, nurses should encourage patients to consider their own values and opinions as primary in importance. Nurses are occasionally asked about other providers, especially physicians, with questions such as "Is Dr. Charles a good surgeon?" or "Would you go to see Dr. Adams if you had cancer?" The nurse will need to refocus the patient's question, for instance, responding, "I am wondering if you have a concern about your care." This deflects the question asked of the nurse and returns the focus of the interaction back to the patient.

Reflection

The nurse using **reflection** is serving as a mirror for the patient. Reflection demonstrates understanding and acceptance. It is a method of encouraging patients to think through problems for themselves by directing patient questions back to the patient. Reflection implies respect because the nurse believes the patient has adequate resources to solve the problem without outside assistance. In response to the patient's question, "Do you think I should go through with this surgery?" the nurse can reflect the question: "What *you* think is most important. Do you think you should go through with this surgery?" Note that the patient's exact words are used. Reflection helps clarify the patient's thoughts and feelings and helps the nurse obtain additional information that may assist in developing the plan of care.

Silence

Although silent periods in social conversations may feel uncomfortable, using silence in nurse-patient relationships can be helpful. Using silence means allowing periods of quiet thought during an interaction without feeling pressure to fill the silence with conversation or activity. For example, when a patient has just been given upsetting news, sitting quietly without making any demands for conversation may be the most therapeutic response a nurse can make at that time. Being with patients (presence) is just as valuable as doing for them and conveys respect for the patient's feelings in distressing circumstances.

Nurses have at their disposal many more helpful responding styles to use in their interactions with patients. The five discussed here, once practiced and mastered, can be a foundation on which to build.

Communication across Differing Languages

Nurses in the United States are encountering an increasing number of patients whose command of spoken English may be limited. Because communication is the means by which people connect, speaking different languages poses significant barriers to the formation of a therapeutic relationship. The nursing process becomes additionally complex when assessment and intervention must span two languages.

Spanish is the second most prevalent language spoken in the United States today, and many nurses are achieving increased fluency in Spanish. Some nurses are bilingual, a significant advantage in the context of today's health care system. Most larger health care systems now provide interpreter services for patients on nursing units and in clinics. An **interpreter** is a professional who is fluent in two or more languages or is bilingual and is trained to translate orally from one language to another. A **translator** is a professional who works with written documents, moving words and meaning from one document into another. Patient education materials are usually offered in a variety of languages, although you should not assume that a patient is literate regardless of his or her ability to speak English. Some persons will work to hide their limited reading skills.

Note that the word *professional* is attached to both these definitions. It is tempting to have a patient's family members interpret for you if a family member speaks both English and the patient's primary language; however, this is not good practice and in fact is not within acceptable standards of care. Interpreters have special training in medical language and in how to do this work most effectively. Similarly, it may be tempting to have a colleague translate teaching materials and other patient information into a second language that your colleague speaks. Again, this is not good practice. Translators are specially trained in how to maintain meaning as closely as possible across languages using the written word. The command of a conversational level of a foreign language, such as what one obtains in high school and basic college courses, is not adequate; very specific technical language required in health care settings. Also, fluency in spoken language does not mean that one's written skills are adequate to translate patient materials correctly.

Working with an interpreter takes practice, and you will become more comfortable with over time. You will notice that having a third person present can both enhance and inhibit communication. The helpfulness of having an interpreter with you may allow you to be more relaxed and assured that your patient is getting high-quality care. Some patients may find that having an interpreter present may be inhibiting, especially in relation to very sensitive topics. For instance, some women may feel very shy about discussing issues related to childbirth and reproduction in the presence of a male interpreter, regardless of his professional conduct and demeanor. You may have to make some decisions about issues related to gender on occasion if the interpreter and the patient are not of the same gender. Some patients do not have any problem and welcome the assistance by these trained professionals. Your careful guidance may help your patients feel more comfortable,

PROFESSIONAL PROFILE BOX 12.1
MINIMIZING LANGUAGE BARRIERS: WORKING WITH A MEDICAL INTERPRETER

The goal of the medical interpreter is to facilitate patient care by minimizing language barriers; as a nurse, it is important to know how to best use an interpreter's services so that the patient who speaks limited English may receive proper care. The first step is to call the interpreter. It is obvious: if a patient does not understand the provider, an interpreter must be called. What is less obvious: even if your patient seems to speak English as a second language fairly well, the stress of being sick is likely to inhibit his or her ability to understand you. You will reduce a huge burden for your patient by calling an interpreter.

Your patient may confuse you, however, by using body cues such as nodding in agreement or even verbal cues such as the repetition of words of assent ("yes," "okay") that may lead you to believe he or she understands English well. A quick assessment using open-ended questions might reveal that the patient is only showing respect for you but does not understand the content of the interaction. If the patient cannot answer your open-ended questions, or if a family member offers to interpret, an interpreter should be called to give expert assistance in this situation.

When the interpreter arrives, brief her or him about any delicate situations that might be at play with the patient. For example, if you need to ask about domestic violence or substance abuse, the interpreter should be warned in advance. Once the interpreter has been briefed and you and the interpreter have entered the room together, you should approach the patient as you would any other patient, without hiding behind the interpreter.

Make eye contact with the patient, not the interpreter. Despite the popular image of the triangular positioning of patient-interpreter-provider, to ensure adequate facilitation of the conversation, the interpreter should be positioned behind you or behind the patient. The interpreter's position may change depending on environmental factors such as the availability of space or seating options.

The medical interpreter uses transparency to mitigate communication factors that contribute to health disparities; the ultimate goal is to ensure equal care for those patients for whom English represents a significant barrier. The principle of transparency dictates that anything the nurse says, or other provider or party says, stays within the confines of the patient's room. All of the patient's verbal expressions will, in turn, be repeated to the provider. The interpreter will use the first person to relay the information between the parties. If the interpreter feels the need to intervene, whether to explain a cultural gap or to clarify word choice to either party, she or he will advise both parties that the correction or clarification is taking place.

Your rhythm of speech should be adjusted so that the interpreter can keep pace. This means stopping every few sentences so as not to present too much content for the interpreter to relay at once. If the pace is too fast, the interpreter may indicate the need for a break between sentences. The interpretation should be consecutive, not simultaneous, meaning that the interpreter waits for you or the patient to stop speaking before interpreting your words.

Whenever possible, all applicable paperwork that has previously been translated (consent forms, patient forms, informational brochures) should be gathered before the interpreter arrives. If a form has not yet been translated, the interpreter may use sight translation to read the form aloud to the patient. A form must be completely understood by the patient in order to serve as a legal document.

The expertise of a professional interpreter is essential for carrying out patient-centered care when you and your patient do not speak the same language. Although you may feel awkward at first when working with an interpreter, you will soon realize that the interpreter is a great ally in your nursing practice.

Amanda M. Black, MA
Professional Interpreter and Translator

Courtesy Amanda Black.

especially when they are reminded that you can provide better care when you can communicate more clearly. The Professional Profile Box 12.1 contains information from a professional interpreter on how to best work with an interpreter. Once you have learned about working with an interpreter, use this knowledge to analyze the scenario in Considering Culture Box 12.1.

Communication practices are unique for each individual and vary widely, even for people from the same cultural backgrounds. Nurses must become skilled in assessing various elements of communication: dialect, style, volume, use of touch, emotional tone, gestures, stance, space needs, and eye contact of individual patients. Note that this requires you to recognize your stereotypes

CONSIDERING CULTURE BOX 12.1

The Challenge: When You Don't Speak the Patient's Language

Mrs. Reyes gave birth by cesarean section to her first child, a baby boy she named Carlos, yesterday, and she is recovering well. She speaks Spanish only. On the previous shift, she had received a mild narcotic twice for incisional pain. Her nurse on that shift had learned Spanish through high school and then two semesters in college, so she felt that she was able to communicate very basic information with Mrs. Reyes, who will be your patient today.

When you go in to take care of Mrs. Reyes, you find her lying on her side, weeping brokenheartedly. You know only a few words of Spanish, so you ask her if she has pain, and point to your lower abdomen. She replies, "No, no, *aquí*" and puts her hand on her chest. You are wondering if she is having some problem with breastfeeding or if she is having chest pain, so you take her pulse and blood pressure, which are both a little elevated but within normal limits. You know she is upset, and her pain appears to be emotional. You realize that she has said something about *"mi niño"* [my baby boy] and *"cirugía"* [surgery]; you decide it is time to call in a medical interpreter, because you know that her baby is healthy and is in the newborn nursery.

The interpreter arrives and you explain briefly what you understand Mrs. Reyes to have said. Mrs. Reyes is still crying when you go back in her room with the interpreter, and you tell Mrs. Reyes through the interpreter that the interpreter speaks Spanish and will be assisting you in figuring out what is wrong. Mrs. Reyes begins a very animated narrative to the interpreter who tries to get her to slow down and let her tell you what she (Mrs. Reyes) has said.

Mrs. Reyes tells you through the interpreter that the nurse on the previous shift had awakened her to sign a paper giving permission for a doctor to "do surgery—to cut" on her baby, and now she is afraid something is wrong with the baby and no one has told her. You realize the nurse had gotten Mrs. Reyes to sign a consent form for circumcision, a common procedure in newborn male infants, and that the nurse had not explained it properly, nor had she used an interpreter to help. You explain through the interpreter, carefully, about circumcision and Mrs. Reyes calms down quickly, because she understands what circumcision is. You realize that a serious, preventable communication problem has occurred.

As you think about this situation, address these questions:
1. What were the errors that occurred in this situation?
2. How could they have been avoided?
3. What are the ethical considerations in this situation?
4. What are your next steps in helping manage this situation?
5. What should you do regarding your co-worker?

and biases and to avoid making assumptions about how any individual patient is likely to communicate.

Nurses who are sensitive to culture recognize that even when individuals speak the same language, the sender and receiver may perceive different meanings because of life experiences unique to each person. Patients may be unwilling to share certain information with nurses because of cultural constraints. In turn, nurses may inadvertently offend patients or family members by violating cultural norms concerning touch, space, and eye contact. Because nursing involves much hands-on work, it is imperative that nurses be aware of the impact of cultural issues that may affect patients' responses to their care.

Avoiding Common Causes of Communication Breakdown

Unsuccessful communication can occur for many reasons. A sender may send an incomplete or confusing message. A message may not be received, or it may be misunderstood or distorted by the receiver. Incongruent messages may cause confusion in the receiver. In nursing situations, there are several common causes of communication breakdown. These include failing to see each individual as unique, failing to recognize levels of meaning, using value statements, using false reassurance, and failing to clarify unclear messages.

Failing to See the Uniqueness of the Individual

Failing to see the uniqueness of each individual is a common cause of communication breakdown. This failure is caused by preconceived ideas, prejudices, and stereotypes, illustrated by the following interchange between a 65-year-old patient and a nurse:

Patient: "My back is really hurting today. I can hardly turn over in bed."

Nurse: "I guess we have to expect these little problems when we get older."

This nurse has categorized the patient into a specific group, "older people," and therefore does not respond

THINKING CRITICALLY BOX 12.1

Helpful and Unhelpful Responding Techniques

Directions: Critique both of the following interactions, identifying each helpful and unhelpful response used by the nurse. Describe how you imagine the patient might feel at the close of each interaction. Identify what the nurse has accomplished in each instance.

Mr. Goodman has been admitted to the hospital for coronary bypass surgery. During the admission process, the following interactions might take place.

Interaction One

Nurse: Mr. Goodman, I am Mrs. Scott. Can I get some information about you now?

Patient: Okay.

Nurse: You're here for bypass surgery?

Patient: Yes, that's what they tell me.

Nurse: (Taking blood pressure) Do you have any allergies to foods or medications?

Patient: Not that I know of. I've never been in a hospital before.

Nurse: Well, your blood pressure looks good. (Silence while patient has thermometer in mouth.) This is a really nice room—just remodeled. I know you'll be comfortable here. Will your wife be coming to see you tonight? (Removes thermometer.)

Patient: My wife is sick. She hasn't been able to leave home for 2 years. I don't know what will happen to her while I am here.

Nurse: Gosh, I'm so sorry to hear that. I guess having you back home healthy is what she wants though, isn't it? And you've got a great surgeon. Well, I've got to run now. Check on you later.

Interaction Two

Nurse: Good afternoon, Mr. Goodman. I'm Mrs. Scott, and I'll be your nurse this evening. If this is a good time, I'd like to ask you some questions and complete your admission process.

Patient: Okay.

Nurse: First, I'll get your temperature and blood pressure, and then we'll talk. (Silence while nurse takes vital signs.) Everything looks good. Do you have any allergies to foods or medications?

Patient: Not that I know of. I've never been in a hospital before.

Nurse: Hospitals can be a little overwhelming, especially when you've never been a patient before. Now, would you please tell me in your own words why you are here?

Patient: Well, the doc tells me I have a clogged artery and I need a bypass. I guess they'll open up my heart.

Nurse: What exactly do you know about the surgery?

Patient: Not too much, really. He told me yesterday that I need it right away—and here I am.

Nurse: It sounds like you need some more information about what will happen. Later this evening I will come back, and we'll talk some more. Are you expecting to have visitors tonight?

Patient: No, my wife can't leave home. I don't know what she will do without me while I'm here. This came up so suddenly.

Nurse: I can see that this is a serious concern for you. We can explore some possibilities when I come back this evening. I'll plan to come around 7:15, if that suits you.

Patient: Sure, I can use all the help I can get.

(**B**ackground): Jeremy is a White male born 22 hours ago at 32 weeks' gestation, weighing 1550 g. He has been on CPAP [continuous positive airway pressure] since birth and is now at 40% O_2, up from 35% 8 hours ago. In the past 2 hours, his respiratory rate has increased from 60 to 88 and his O_2 saturation has decreased from 96% to 92%.

(**A**ssessment): My assessment is that Jeremy is developing respiratory failure.

(**R**ecommendation): I recommend that you or one of the neonatal fellows come see him and

that I call for a respiratory therapist to be in the NICU in case Jeremy needs to be intubated.

Nurse Practitioner: I will be there shortly, but in the meantime, call a respiratory therapist to adjust the CPAP as necessary, and I will also order a chest x-ray STAT. Recheck blood gases in 15 minutes.

(**R**eadback—nurse): I will call respiratory therapy and request adjustment to CPAP, and I will confirm that radiology will perform a chest x-ray STAT. I will recheck ABG [arterial blood gases] in 15 minutes.

The information the nurse has communicated is clear, appropriate, and without tangential details that obscure the problem. The nurse practitioner has clear data from a professional registered nurse who has captured the most salient issues related to the care of a premature infant. No time is wasted in filtering out extraneous information such as, "Jeremy's mother came in for a visit this afternoon. She is really worried about him, but she has a lot of family support." Is this helpful information? No, not in this circumstance. However, if Paola was responding to a call from a social worker assigned to the Benton family, this may be useful background information.

Safety is the key issue behind I-SBAR-R as a communication format. This format decreases the inherently unsafe and dysfunctional hierarchy of providers. In his introduction to John Nance's (2009) important book *Why Hospitals Should Fly: The Ultimate Flight Plan to Patient Safety and Quality Care,* Lucian Leape, MD, a physician and professor at the Harvard School of Public Health, noted that "an authoritarian structure that devalues many workers, lacks of a sense of personal accountability, autonomous functioning and major barriers to effective care stymies progress" in creating a safe culture of health care (p. viii). A culture of safety requires teamwork, Leape argued, the "common denominator" in safe cultures, which are "rarely found in health care organizations" (p. viii).

As you gain more experience clinically, develop your critical thinking skills, and improve your clinical judgment, you will become increasingly comfortable in communicating using the I-SBAR-R format.

Effective Use of Electronic Communication Devices

An unprecedented proliferation of ways to communicate exist today: mobile phones; smart phones; e-mail; messaging on apps such as iMessage, WhatsApp, and WeChat; and services such as Skype and FaceTime, among many others. Nurses are often interrupted in their care by the ringing of their mobile phones or unit communication devices, consulting with other staff members even as they care for patients. This behavior is insensitive and sends a message to patients that they and their needs are secondary. The use of e-mail in professional settings can lead to misunderstanding because the facial expression, tone of voice, and other contextual cues are not visible to message recipients and are

therefore subject to misinterpretation (everyone knows someone who appears to be yelling on e-mail because they type in all capital letters). A few commonsense guidelines are useful to prevent the use of communication devices from becoming a barrier to nurse-patient or nurse-colleague communication:

- Give your full attention to the person you are with. Avoid checking your phone for messages while conversing with others.
- If you are interrupted by a call that you must take, go into the hallway to have your conversation; you may need to leave the patient area completely to avoid having your personal business overheard in a professional setting.
- Adopt a courteous tone in e-mail and voicemail messages regardless of how rushed you are; remember that the recipient cannot see your nonverbal communication. Emoticons or emojis, however, are rarely appropriate. If you have to use a ":)" to show that you are not really upset or to take the edge off criticism, you probably need to reword your e-mail rather than resort to smiley faces. Like all communication, they too can be misconstrued or seem incongruent with the message.
- Avoid the use of jargon in verbal and written communication; use acronyms only when you are confident of their universal understanding.
- Keep messages short; include only necessary useful details, but avoid being abrupt.
- When leaving your return phone number in a voicemail, make sure that you enunciate the number slowly and clearly. It is helpful to repeat at the end of your message: "Again, this is [first and last name] at 111-555-4321."
- When receiving a message, read, listen, and evaluate the entire message before reacting. This is particularly important when you are feeling pressed for time or if your first response to the message is one of irritation or anger.

Communication in Today's Multicultural Workplace

Sensitivity to cultural differences in communication is essential in today's culturally diverse workplace. The composition of the health care workforce is being rapidly transformed by the population demographics of the nation. Diversity in age, race, ethnicity, country of origin, gender, gender identity, sexual orientation, and levels of abilities creates opportunities for nurses to develop skill in transcultural communication.

One's culture determines the lens through which most aspects of life are viewed and experienced and includes an individual's health beliefs and practices. Culture also dictates the meaning of work, such as caring for the sick. Some cultures see caring for the sick to be a sacred responsibility, whereas others place care for the sick with no significance beyond an occupation or means of income. The meaning of work in a given culture also affects how people of that culture communicate.

Attention is now being paid to the cultural differences among different generations of nurses, all of whom can be found working side by side. Even when race and ethnicity are similar, the ages of nurses in a single setting may range from early 20s to middle 60s, a 40-year span. This can create interpersonal challenges in the workplace. Although it is risky to make generalizations about groups, anecdotal evidence and research studies reveal differing opinions among age-groups about what is important to them professionally and personally.

Each generation experiences political and historical events and social trends during their formative years that influence their values, and hence become part of a cohort similarly affected by historical and sociocultural events. Known as the sociohistorical context of one's life, these influences cut across racial and ethnic lines. Different age groups may have differing work ethics, means of communication, manners, and views of authority; more superficial issues such as habits of speech, modes of dress, and even hairstyles and music choices can be the source of tension and friction (Siela, 2006).

Three generations currently occupy the workforce. Two-thirds of today's workforce in all occupational groups consists of Baby Boomers, people born between 1946 and 1959; many in this group are now at the age of retirement. Those born between 1960 and 1980 make up Generation X. Generation Y, also known as Millennials, were born between 1981 and 2000. Generation Y overlaps with a newer group born since 1990 known as the Net Generation, or N-Geners, who have grown up with an unprecedented high level of interconnectivity in the digital age.

As you can see in Table 12.1, the characteristics and attitudes of the various groups are different. Professional nurses strive to understand colleagues of different generations and capitalize on the strengths each group brings to the workplace, rather than viewing these varying attitudes toward life and work as problems. Siela offers this insight: "Knowing the characteristics and core values of each generation can help nurses of diverse ages understand colleagues who are much younger or older than they are. However, take care not to stereotype anyone. Each person is a unique individual with distinctive traits, which may or may not be typical of his or her generation as a whole" (2006, p. 47).

Astute nurses use their communication skills throughout their personal and professional lives. Using clear, simple messages and clarifying the intent of others constitute a positive goal in all personal and professional communication.

INTERPROFESSIONAL COLLABORATION: PRESCRIPTION FOR IMPROVED PATIENT OUTCOMES

Interprofessional collaboration is central to excellent patient outcomes (Rose, 2011). **Collaboration** is a complex process that builds on communication. Collaboration in health care settings is far more than simply cooperation, negotiation, or compromise. It implies working jointly with other professionals, all of whom are respected for their unique knowledge and abilities, to improve a patient's health status or to solve an organizational problem. Furthermore, interprofessional collaboration implies interdependency, rather than autonomy, and roles among providers are understood as complementary and require mutual respect and power sharing (Rose, 2011). The Institute of Medicine (IOM; now the National Academy of Medicine) (2003) made interdisciplinary learning a core educational requirement, with the assumption that education across health care disciplines will improve communication, increase collaboration, and decrease errors (Reese et al., 2010).

Interdisciplinary learning provides the setting for professionals to learn specific roles of others in health care and to understand clearly delineated professional contributions of each member of the health care team (Suter et al., 2009). Currently, most health care providers are taught similar core content, skills, knowledge, and values; however, this education occurs in isolation (Angelini, 2011) or "professional silos" (Margalit et al., 2009). In addition, interdisciplinary learning may serve to reduce stereotypes and alleviate misconceptions

TABLE 12.1	Selected Characteristics of a Multigenerational Nursing Workforce	
Baby Boomers (Born 1946–1959)	**Generation X (Born 1960–1980)**	**Generation Y (Millennials) and N-Geners (Born 1981–2000)**
Beginning to experience physical limitations	Ample physical energy; few limitations	High levels of youthful energy
Love-hate relationship with authority; may question rules but generally follow them; comfortable bending rules	Expect authority figures to earn their respect; distrust bureaucracy; desire frequent positive reinforcement and feedback	Not awed by authority figures; relaxed approach to the bureaucracy
Work gives meaning to life; willing to work long hours; will sacrifice for success	Little trust of work environment or loyalty to it; seek to avoid long hours and have fun on the job; desire life-work balance	High expectations of the workplace; may set unrealistic goals; need prolonged job orientation and mentoring; desire life-work balance
Value consensus building	Dislike process; focused on outcomes; want to know how decisions will affect them	Highly collaborative
Enjoy competition; comfortable working in teams and value teamwork	Prefer to work alone; entrepreneurial	Desire to participate in decisions; team players
Generally optimistic; not comfortable with conflict in the workplace; feel indispensable; can be intellectually arrogant; tend to be socially conscious	Generally skeptical; tend to be pessimistic; desire accolades, whether deserved or not; motivated by money and success; seek to start at the top	Optimistic; confident; share feelings with ease; high expectations of selves; impatient to get to the top; may feel unappreciated; desire positive feedback; accept change eagerly
Favor an informal work environment	Informal; flexible; not known for manners, etiquette, or interpersonal skills; accustomed to diversity; irreverent sense of humor; may be perceived as rude	Behave and dress casually; most tolerant of cultural diversity; desire to have fun on the job; value good manners; have best rapport with other generations
Many are technically literate and most are willing to learn	Technically literate	Highly proficient with technology; use the Internet for research and communication; accustomed to multitasking

Compiled from Halfer D, Saver C: Bridging the generation gaps, *Nursing Spectrum (SE ed)* 4(3):28–33, 2008; Siela D: Managing the multigenerational nursing staff, *Am Nurse Today* 1(3):47–49, 2006; Wieck KL: Motivating an intergenerational workforce: scenarios for success, *Orthop Nurs* 26(6):366–371, 2007.

regarding the value of other professional roles (MacDonald et al., 2010). Furthermore, MacDonald and colleagues (2010) found that knowledge of the professional role of others is related to successful interprofessional practice and that the development of this core competency should ideally begin during nurses' basic education. Box 12.6 contains a checklist of key components necessary for effective collaboration. You can check your own readiness for interprofessional collaboration by referring to this list. At this point in your education, you will probably have most of these components mastered.

Successful collaboration entails several steps (Gardner, 2005):

- Identification of those who have stake in the outcome of the collaboration
- Identification of the problem(s) to be solved
- Identification of barriers to creating a solution
- Clarification of the desired outcomes (agree on criteria for success)
- Clarification of the process (How will we approach the task?)
- Identification of who will be responsible for each step in the task
- Evaluation (Have we met our criteria for success?)

Collaboration is a positive process that benefits the people involved, as individuals and as a group; the organization in which they work; and health care

BOX 12.6 Key Components Necessary for Effective Interprofessional Collaboration

- Respect for other collaborators
- Confidence in own knowledge
- Willingness to learn
- Cooperative spirit
- Belief in a common purpose
- Value contributions of other disciplines
- Willingness to negotiate
- Excellent communication skills
- Self-awareness (e.g., biases, values, goals, agendas)
- Tolerance of differing opinions
- Not threatened by conflict
- Knowledge of one's own limits

consumers. Increased feelings of self-worth; a sense of accomplishment; *esprit de corps;* enhanced collegiality and respect; and increased productivity, retention, and employee satisfaction are positive benefits of collaboration (LeTourneau, 2004). Despite these positive benefits and potential for improved patient outcomes, interprofessional collaboration can be difficult to institute. Rice and colleagues (2010) found that even though a well-planned and well-implemented intervention to increase interprofessional communication and collaboration was received with enthusiasm by various stakeholders on general internal medicine units, no changes in behaviors were noted over the year after the intervention. This was attributed to several causes, including deeply entrenched interprofessional hierarchies.

One of the most deeply entrenched hierarchies in health care today is that of nursing in relation to medicine. Weinberg and colleagues (2009) noted that this hierarchy is dominated by physicians, in which they see their role as one of giving orders that nurses carry out; nurses, however, prefer collaborative interactions that are more egalitarian. In their study of the quality of the nurse-physician relationship, Weinberg and colleagues found that 19 of 20 resident physicians reported instances of poor communication or troubled relationships with nurses, which, unfortunately, was not seen as a threat to patient care. The nurses' role was limited, in their opinion, to following the physicians' orders. The findings of this relatively recent research are troublesome in light of the directives by the IOM to foster interprofessional collaboration that would include the disciplines of nursing and medicine.

Recent strategies to increase interprofessional collaboration through interprofessional educational will require what is sometimes called a "sea change"—a reference to Ariel's song in the Shakespeare play *The Tempest.* A sea change is a progressive transformation over time during which the substance of a structure is changed, although its form remains. A hospital may still look like a hospital, but what goes on within that structure will be required to change in response to substantial reform in the health care system. Change is difficult, however, and is usually accompanied by conflict. Conflict resolution requires constructive conflict negotiation skills that can be developed (Gerardi and Morrison, 2005). Examples of these conflict resolution skills include the following:

- Acknowledge the conflict.
- Recognize and affirm that positives can result from conflict.
- Facilitate debate over task issues while redirecting concerns away from the personal level.
- Promote expression of varying perspectives.
- As conflict is worked through, explore alternative positions, taking opportunities to synthesize several ideas to create a new position.
- Be willing to change your position on an issue.
- Share power: elicit everyone's opinions, and look for win-win situations.
- Stay focused on the desired outcome.

A caveat is in order, however. More than a decade ago, David (2000) wrote a powerful treatise on the gender politics of nursing; among her many important arguments, she noted that nurses' ongoing self-deception in terms of the location of power in health care has served to "perpetuate professional mediocrity . . . and preserve the borderline status of nurses" (p. 83). This means that nurses take a secondary role to physicians and others in the health care hierarchy, making true interprofessional collaboration impossible under these conditions. There are no simple fixes for this deeply entrenched view of nursing for which nurses are ultimately responsible. A good first step for you is to consider the negative effects of gender politics on you as a nurse (regardless of your own gender identity) and on the profession of nursing.

You have been exposed to a great deal of material in this chapter—from the therapeutic use of self in one-on-one professional relationships with patients to the effect of gender politics on the profession of nursing. The "take-home message" of this chapter is an important one, however, and one not to be lost in the wide range of topics to which you have been exposed. The message: How you communicate as a professional nurse matters. Whether you are sitting at the bedside consoling a frantic mother of a sick infant, addressing a group of citizens concerned about environmental issues in your community, or writing a letter to your representative in Congress about health care coverage, you are never "not a nurse."

CONCEPTS AND CHALLENGES

- **Concept:** The "therapeutic use of self" means using one's personality and communication skills effectively while implementing the nursing process to help patients improve their health status.
  Challenge: Although it is difficult, nurses can learn new skills to improve their communication.

- **Concept:** In long-term nurse-patient relationships, each phase (orientation, working, and termination) has specific tasks that should be accomplished before progressing to subsequent phases.
  Challenge: Short-term patient contacts in today's streamlined care delivery system also present opportunities for connection and goal achievement.

- **Concept:** Acceptance of others is important for effective nursing practice.
  Challenge: Developing awareness of biases can help nurses to prevent the intrusion of these biases into nurse-patient relationships.

- **Concept:** Professional nurses are aware of the boundaries of the therapeutic relationship and strive to stay within the "zone of helpfulness" at all times.
  Challenge: Boundaries can be difficult to ascertain, especially in the use of social media. Nurses have to be vigilant in identifying professional boundaries and setting limits to prevent crossing a boundary.

- **Concept:** Communication is the core of all relationships; it is both verbal and nonverbal and consists of a sender, a receiver, a message, feedback, and context.
  Challenge: Effective communication meets four major criteria: feedback, appropriateness, efficiency, and flexibility.

- **Concept:** Professional medical interpreters are your best resource in providing care for patients for whom English is their second language or who do not speak English.
  Challenge: Conversational skills in a second language are inadequate in the provision of health care, and asking a family member to interpret is inappropriate and can be unsafe.

- **Concept:** SBAR is an excellent means of communication to transmit important data effectively across health care disciplines and all members of the health care team.
  Challenge: Effective communication both requires and reflects excellent critical thinking and clinical judgment.

IDEAS FOR FURTHER EXPLORATION

1. Explain what is meant by the expression "therapeutic use of self." What challenges, if any, do you anticipate encountering in learning this important communication technique?
2. Describe professional boundaries and what the implications are in crossing professional boundaries.
3. Think about why nonverbal communication may be more reliable than verbal communication. Consider your own nonverbal communication style and what you might be communicating unintentionally.
4. Identify a recent interaction you have had in which communication was incongruent. Analyze the effect of the incongruence on the communication. When are people most likely to use incongruent communication?
5. Think of a person with whom you have experienced difficult communication. Identify the barriers to successful communication between you and the other person, and critique your responses to that person.
6. Think about a collaborative experience you have had with another health care professional. What are the features of that collaboration in which collaboration improved the outcome for the patient? Were there features of the collaboration with which you were uncomfortable?

REFERENCES

Angelini D: Interdisciplinary and interprofessional education: What are the key issues and considerations for the future? *J Perinat Neonatal Nurs* 25(2):175–179, 2011.

Baca M: Professional boundaries and dual relationships in clinical practice, *J Nurs Pract* 7(3):195–200, 2011.

David BA: Nursing's gender politics: reformulating the footnotes, *Adv Nurs Sci* 23(1):83–93, 2000.

Gardner DB: Ten lessons in collaboration, *Online J Issues Nurs* 10(1):1–6, 2005. (website). Available at: www.nursingworld.org/MainMenuCategories/ANAMarketplace/ANAPeriodicals/OJIN/TableofContents/Volume102005/No1Jan05/tpc26_116008.aspx.

Gerardi DS, Morrison F: Managing conflict creatively, *Crit Care Nurs* (Suppl)31–32, 2005.

Hagerty BM, Patusky KL: Reconceptualizing the nurse-patient relationship, *Image J Nurs Sch* 35(2):145–150, 2003.

Halfer D, Saver C: Bridging the generation gaps, *Nursing Spectrum* (SE ed) 4(3):28–33, 2008.

Hobbs JL: A dimensional analysis of patient-centered care, *Nurs Res* 58(1):52–62, 2009.

Institute of Medicine (IOM): *Health professions education: a bridge to quality*, Washington, DC, 2003, National Academies Press.

Johns C: *Guided reflection: advancing practice*, Oxford, 2002, Blackwell Science.

LeTourneau B: Physicians and nurses: friends or foes? *J Healthc Manag* 49(1):12–14, 2004.

MacDonald MB, Bally JM, Ferguson LM, et al.: Knowledge of the professional role of others: a key interprofessional competency, *Nurs Ed Prac* 217:238–242, 2010.

Margalit R, Thompson S, Visovsky C, et al.: From professional silos to interprofessional education: campuswide focus on quality of care, *Qual Manag Health Care* 18:165–173, 2009.

Nance JJ: *Why hospitals should fly: the ultimate flight plan to patient safety and quality care*, Bozeman, MT, 2009, Second River Health Care Books.

National Council of State Boards of Nursing (NCSBN): *Professional boundaries: a nurse's guide to the importance of appropriate professional boundaries*, Chicago, 2014,

National Council of State Boards of Nursing (website). Available at: www.ncsbn.org.

Nurse's relationship with patient results in disciplinary action, *Nurs Law Regan Rep* 43(8):4–5, 2003.

Peplau H: *Interpersonal relations in nursing*, New York, 1952, GP Putnam's Sons.

Quality and Safety Education for Nurses: *Reformulating SBAR to I-SBAR-R*, (website), 2008. Retrieved from: http://qsen.org/reformulating-sbar-to-i-sbar-r/.

Reese CE, Jeffries PR, Scott AE: Learning together: using simulations to develop nursing and medical student collaboration, *Nurse Ed Perspec* 31(1):33–37, 2010.

Rice K, Zwarenstein M, Conn LG, et al.: An intervention to improve interpersonal collaboration and communications: a comparative qualitative study, *J Interprof Care* 24(4):350–361, 2010.

Roach MS, Maykut C, Comportment: A caring attribute in the formation of an intentional practice, *Int J Hum Caring* 14(4):22–26, 2010.

Rose L: Interprofessional collaboration in the ICU: how to define? *Nurs Crit Care* 16(1):5–10, 2011.

Ruesch J: *Disturbed communication: the clinical assessment of normal and pathological communicative behavior*, New York, 1972, WW Norton.

Siela D: Managing the multigenerational nursing staff, *Am Nurse Today* 1(3):47–49, 2006.

Suter E, Arndt J, Arthur N, et al.: Role understanding and effective communication as core competencies for collaborative practice, *J Interprof Care* 23(1):41–51, 2009.

Swanson KM: Empirical development of a middle range theory of caring, *Nurs Res* 40:161–166, 1991.

Watson J: *Nursing: human science and human care*, New York, 1988, National League for Nursing.

Weinberg DB, Miner DC, Rivlin L: "It depends": medical residents' perspectives on working with nurses: a qualitative study shows that residents don't necessarily view nurses as colleagues and collaborators, *Am J Nurs* 109(7):34–43, 2009.

Wieck KL: Motivating an intergenerational workforce: scenarios for success, *Orthop Nurs* 26(6):366–371, 2007.

13

Nurses, Patients, and Families: Caring at the Intersection of Health, Illness, and Culture

Maureen J. Baker, BSN, MSN, PhD

Ⓔ To enhance your understanding of this chapter, try the Student Exercises on the Evolve site at http://evolve.elsevier.com/Black/professional.

LEARNING OUTCOMES

After studying this chapter, students will be able to:

- Differentiate between acute and chronic illness.
- Describe the stages of illness and how patients move among the stages.
- Explain behavioral responses to illness and what influences these behaviors.
- Discuss the influence of culture on illness behaviors.

- Describe the characteristics of the culturally competent nurse.
- Explain the physical, emotional, and cognitive effects of stress.
- Discuss how family functioning is altered during illness.
- Explain the necessity of and strategies for self-care by nurses.

Joyful partners stand at the altar or before a magistrate on their wedding day, vowing to "have and to hold … in sickness and in health …" On a day of robust health and exuberant energy, couples rarely envision the specter of illness as they celebrate their marriage. It is a day of hope and expectation. Sickness, and all it means, has little place at the wedding. Yet as the anniversaries of this beautiful day come and go, the meaning of sickness becomes clearer. A part of life, illness affects not just the sick person, but the people providing care—the spouse, the partner, their children. Illness changes lives (Fig. 13.1). In Chapter 8 you were introduced to systems theory in depth. Remember, a key concept of systems theory is that a change in one part of a system results in changes in other parts. A family is system; a change in one member affects the other members.

Supporting health, managing illness, and addressing the complex changes and human responses to illness are central to nursing. A key characteristic of nursing is the emphasis on viewing patients holistically. Nurses recognize that human beings are complex beings with physical, mental, emotional, spiritual, social, and cultural dimensions. Each of these dimensions may be challenged by illness. A caring nurse considers each of these dimensions in caring for patients, whether supporting their health or helping them manage their responses to illness. In this chapter the stages of illness, illness behaviors, and cultural factors that influence them are explored, as is the impact of illness and culture on patients, families, and nurses. Developing strategies to maintain your own health and learning to develop balance in your life—care of self—is also explored.

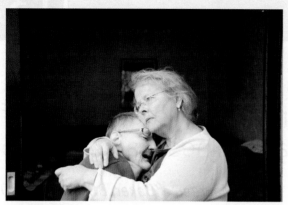

Fig. 13.1 In times of illness, roles in families change. A daughter is caring for and comforting her elderly mother. (Photo used with permission from iStockphoto.)

ACUTE AND CHRONIC ILLNESS

Illness is a highly personal experience. Culture plays a significant role in health beliefs and behaviors; it also determines how individuals and families react to illness. Nurses can be more effective in providing care when they understand some of the factors that affect how people cope with illness.

Acute Illness

Acute illness is characterized by severe symptoms that are relatively short lived. Symptoms tend to appear suddenly, progress steadily, and subside quickly. Depending on the illness, the patient may or may not require medical attention. The common cold is an example of an acute illness that does not usually require a health care provider's attention. Others, such as acute appendicitis, can become life threatening without timely surgical intervention. Unless complications arise, people with acute illness usually return to their previous level of wellness. Some acute illnesses, such as acute myocardial infarction, may lead to chronic conditions, such as congestive heart failure. Another example is a new infection with human immunodeficiency virus (HIV). The initial signs and symptoms of HIV infection occur 2 to 4 weeks after exposure to the virus as a flulike syndrome with fever, malaise, rash, myalgia, and other discomforts. Usually lasting fewer than 10 days, patients believe that the resolution of their acute illness means that they are well, when in fact they are seropositive for HIV. They are chronically ill.

Individuals with sudden, catastrophic injuries, such as a spinal cord injury or major stroke, experience dramatic and extensive changes in an instant. They face physical limitations, significant modifications in daily living, and changes in social roles for which they had no preparation. They face daily challenges that may seem unbearable. They use a variety of coping mechanisms, strategies that differ from person to person.

Chronic Illness

A chronic illness usually develops gradually, requires ongoing medical attention, and may continue for the duration of the individual's life. Hypertension, diabetes, and Parkinson's disease are examples of chronic illnesses; they can be treated but not cured.

Chronic illnesses have a significant social and economic impact, being one of the fastest-growing health problems in the United States. In 2012 almost one of every two adults—117 million people—had at least one chronic illness (Centers for Disease Control and Prevention [CDC], 2015). Factors such as sedentary lifestyles, obesity, and the aging of the population are expected to contribute to a continued increase in the number of chronically ill Americans for the foreseeable future. Arthritis is the most common disabling illness, with 53 million adults having a diagnosis from a care provider of arthritis (as opposed to self-diagnosis). Of these 53 million people, 42% report that their arthritis affects their usual activities. Diabetes is the leading cause of serious disabling conditions, including renal failure, amputations from diabetes-related conditions, and new cases of blindness among adults (CDC, 2015).

Chronic illnesses are caused by permanent changes that leave residual disability. They vary in severity and outcomes, but a state of "normal" health is elusive, although many chronic conditions can be managed successfully. Some chronic illnesses are progressively debilitating and result in premature death, whereas others are associated with a normal life span, even though functioning is impaired. Some chronic illnesses go through periods of remission, when symptoms subside, and exacerbation, when symptoms reappear or worsen.

Chronic illnesses are pervasive and life altering. They lead to altered individual functioning and disruption of family life. Long-term medical management of chronic illness can create financial hardship as well. Patients with chronic illness may need to change the way they live, often making many changes simultaneously. They must begin doing things they are not accustomed to doing and stop doing things they normally do. Patients with diabetes, for example, must begin monitoring their

BOX 13.1 **Types of Illness**	
Acute	**Chronic**
• Sudden onset of symptoms	• Gradual onset of symptoms
• Symptoms progress quickly from mild to severe	• Symptoms may be mild or vague; once illness is resolved may have remissions and exacerbations
• Patient usually returns to former level of functioning	• Illness continues throughout the life span
• Changes often not permanent but may progress to chronic illness	• Changes are permanent and progressive
• Does not usually require long-term behavioral change/treatment	• Requires long-term behavioral change/treatment
• May represent a life crisis	• Often represents a life crisis

blood glucose levels, change their eating habits, and increase their exercise. Box 13.1 presents the similarities and differences between acute and chronic illnesses.

The diagnosis of an acute or chronic illness can be a major life crisis. The emotional reactions of the patient and family sometimes present a greater challenge than dealing with the physical aspects of the disease. Despite the prevalence of emotional responses to illness, most medical and nursing attention is focused on physical aspects of the disease process rather than emotions. Box 13.2 describes how one patient experiences a chronic illness, systemic lupus erythematosus (SLE), and describes its effect on her feelings, family responsibilities, and relationships. As you read her narrative, pay attention to her reaction to her nurses' focus on her physical condition at a time when her emotional responses were her greatest concern. Consider what this narrative says about quality care and if this woman is getting the help that she needs.

Chronically ill people can become acutely ill with something not related to their chronic illness, which will still need management even while the acute condition is being treated. For instance, a 28-year-old man comes to the emergency department (ED) with a severely sprained ankle from a skiing accident. His electronic health record (EHR) indicates that he has HIV, although his viral load is nondetectable because of his strict adherence to his highly active antiretroviral therapy (HAART) regimen. What are the implications for

---

BOX 13.2 Comments of a Patient with a Chronic Disease: Systemic Lupus Erythematosus

If there is one thing I want to say to nurses who work with patients with chronic disease, it is "Be patient and understand our problems and feelings." When I go to the doctor's office or to the hospital, I usually leave feeling guilty because I have been impatient with everyone I saw. Guilt and anger are the two feelings I seem to have had since I was diagnosed with this disease. I alternate between being angry that I got lupus and feeling that I should be grateful for the fact that I have something I can at least live with when others are not so fortunate.

I guess the thing that bothers me most is that the nurses keep telling me what changes I need to make to take better care of myself. They never seem to understand that I am doing the best I can do. I can't possibly get the amount of rest they seem to think I need, and I can't avoid as much stress as they seem to think I should avoid. Both my husband and I work hard at our jobs, and I hate asking him and my sons to take over my responsibilities at home when I am sick, so I wind up compromising. I ask them to help some and I do more than I should. When I get the lecture from the nurses on how I should take better care of myself, I usually just nod and say that I will, even when I know that I probably won't be able to.

---

the ED providers of his HIV status? If you were giving an SBAR (see Chapter 12) update at your end-of-shift handoff to the next nurse, would you include his HIV status in your report?

ADJUSTING TO ILLNESS

Adjusting to illness is a process. Although the responses are different for each person, people who are ill typically progress through somewhat predictable states. Experts from medicine, sociology, psychology, and nursing have described the states that people experience in adjustment to illness as stages—disbelief and denial, irritability and anger, attempting to gain control, depression and despair, and acceptance and participation. Remember that there are many influences on the way a person responds to an illness and that these states are fluid, meaning that the patient will go back and forth between responses. Human responses to illness are rarely if ever linear.

Disbelief and Denial

People have difficulty believing that signs and symptoms are caused by illness. They may believe that the symptoms will go away. Fear of illness often leads to the mistaken belief that the symptoms will subside without treatment and can delay seeking a diagnosis.

Denial is a psychological defense mechanism that people sometimes use to avoid the anxiety associated with illness. People who pride themselves on their vigorous health may downplay the significance of symptoms. If this occurs, they may avoid treatment or attempt inappropriate self-treatment. Extended denial can have serious results, because some illnesses, left untreated, may become too advanced for effective treatment. (Note that the word *denial* is often used in a way that is incorrect. For instance, someone getting very bad news, such as the sudden death of a loved one, may be in shock such that they cannot take in the reality of trauma. "Denial" in this sense works to protect them from being overwhelmed.) A nurse described her own prolonged denial of the significance of a lump in her breast:

> *I thought it would go away. I thought it was anything but cancer. But I would lie awake at night and run my fingers over the lump and in the dark I would know it was growing. I would tell myself, "I will call the doctor in the morning." But when morning came I would make myself believe that the lump was smaller. Then it began to hurt, a little, then a lot. I didn't tell anyone, including my partner. One morning she asked me, "What is that?" and to my horror, I realized that the tumor had broken through my skin and was oozing through my nightgown. She took me to the doctor. I think that my denial will cost me my life. I am a nurse practitioner, and I am dying of breast cancer that could have been treated.*

Irritability and Anger

Some patients get irritable as their ability to function declines, and prolonged irritability may be an indication that the patient is depressed. Anger may be directed at specific people or simply be general—"mad at the world." Anger may also be directed toward others—spouse, family members, co-workers, or health care providers. Anger may be directed inward, and guilt feelings may occur for failing to prevent the illness. This is one nurse's experience of a patient's anger directed at her:

> *I dreaded my daily visits to Mr. Kaman. He had pancreatic cancer and a surgical wound that was really slow to heal. It wasn't that he was mean to me, exactly. It was more like I didn't exist to him, or that he had contempt for me. I just couldn't reach him, which was pretty rare in my experience. At first, I would try to chat with him just to draw him out, but he withdrew further and further. I finally got a response from him one day when I commented on a photograph on his dresser. He responded by lashing out at me for "meddling" and told me to mind my own damn business. I was stunned and apologized (although I didn't know exactly what for). When I told Mrs. Kaman what had happened, she explained that the photo was of their son who had died in an accident a few years ago and that her husband had "never been the same" since. I felt like I at least understood a bit more about Mr. Kaman and felt compassion for him.*

Attempting to Gain Control

In the stage of attempting to gain control, people may consult their health care provider or use over-the-counter medications, folk practices, or home remedies. They are aware that they are ill and usually experience some concern or even fear about the outcome. These fears usually stimulate treatment-seeking behavior as a way of gaining control over the illness, but fears may also lead to further denial and avoidance, such as the nurse with breast cancer in the earlier example. As in her case, family members may become involved, encouraging or insisting that the person to seek treatment or follow medical advice. Here is another nurse's experience:

> *I was admitting a patient to hospice and per routine, I asked about medications. The patient's oncologist had given me a list of medications when he made the referral for this patient, but I wanted to see what else the patient was taking. I knew that sometimes patients took supplements. This patient brought out a bag, literally a paper grocery bag, full of supplements, vitamins, many that he had bought on the Internet that were not adequately labeled. I had no idea what he was taking and neither did he. When I asked him if he was concerned that some of these may be harmful, he laughed and said that he was dying anyway, so what did he have to lose? His husband said that he had tried to talk him out of taking all of these "potions," but in the end, it was not his call to make.*

Depression and Grief

Depression is perhaps the most common mood disorder that occurs with illness. The ability to work is altered, daily activities must be modified, and the sense of well-being and freedom from pain may be lost. Illness results in many types of losses. The difficulty is figuring out the difference between grief—the normal and expected response to any loss, including one's health—and depression, a treatable mental health condition. Immediately after diagnosis, patients may grieve the loss of their previous state of good health. As time goes on and functional limitations add up, persons with chronic illnesses may undergo cycles of depression as remissions and exacerbations occur. Remember that it is beyond the scope of practice for a nurse to diagnose a condition such as depression, which is a psychiatric diagnosis that needs treatment. A careful assessment, however, of the patient's mood states may give the observant nurse an indication that the patient is depressed and can help get him or her the care that he or she needs.

Consider Mr. Kaman's story. How would you assess further to determine if he was grieving or depressed?

Acceptance and Participation

At this point, the patient has acknowledged the reality of illness and may be ready to participate in decisions about treatment. Active involvement and the hope attached to pursuing treatment usually lead to increased feelings of mastery of the illness. Patients with long-term chronic illnesses become experts in their own care and management of their condition. From the nurse practitioner with breast cancer:

> I didn't have time to waste getting mad or angry. My partner was doing that for the both of us. I felt horribly guilty at first, but I couldn't spend time on "what ifs" and wishing that I could have a do-over. I had to focus on what to do next. My oncologist set out a plan of care based on where I am now, not what might have been. He has been great. I am getting radiation and chemotherapy as palliative treatment because I have some metastasis in my spine, and there is no point in going through surgery. I feel pretty well, although I am tired. I am eating well and getting some exercise and taking one day at a time.

Remember that these states are described as a means of describing how patients work through their illness. Patients do not move through these states in a linear way, nor should they be used by the student or nurse to characterize a patient's particular response at any one time. Doing this ignores the complex changes that an illness brings to almost every element of a patient's life. One's response to illness is highly idiosyncratic, and it should be treated as such. Acute illness may be experienced in a very different way from chronic illness.

ILLNESS BEHAVIORS

Although illness is highly subjective and is experienced differently by each individual, a number of factors influence how a particular person will respond. One important factor is the cultural expectation about how people should behave when ill. Children learn the part they are expected to play as an ill person through model-ing—that is, by observing how their parents or significant adults in their lives respond to major and minor illnesses. These responses can vary from stoic, uncomplaining independence to very passive dependence, with many variations in between. Stoicism in the face of illness should not be confused with strength of character—it may simply mean that the sick person is not comfortable sharing his or her symptoms and does not want to appear to be complaining.

Each culture generally requires that certain criteria be met before people can qualify as "sick." Talcott Parsons (1964), a renowned sociologist, identified five attributes and expectations of the sick role that guided the view of illness among White Americans for decades. According to Parsons, the sick White American:

1. Is exempt from social responsibilities
2. Cannot be expected to care for himself or herself
3. Should want to get well
4. Should seek medical advice
5. Should cooperate with the medical experts

In other words, Parsons' definition of the sick role includes behavior that is dependent, passive, and submissive. For decades, Parsons' sick role expectations were taught in medical and nursing schools and guided the way health care providers viewed patients' reactions to pain and illness. This view is no longer adequate, because different cultures have differing sick role expectations. Moreover, patients have become increasingly likely to actively engage in their health and health care, challenge providers, and seek information regarding their care from persons or sources that are not health care providers.

Migration has changed the world and requires that nurses are educated to attain a level of cultural competence. Cultural competence is having "the attitudes, knowledge and skills necessary for providing quality care to diverse populations" (American Association of Colleges of Nursing, 2008). Culturally competent nurses are prepared to provide patient-centered care with a focus on the patient's specific needs that are shaped by culture. Being culturally competent means that nurses are more likely to be attuned to the significant problem of health disparities. Cultural competence does not mean, however, that nurses learn every facet in detail of each culture's practices. In fact, mastering the subtleties of every culture is impossible. Importantly, no normative illness response based on culture exists. *Normative* means that there is one standard by which all others are judged and valued.

A cultural expectation that prevails among some White Americans is that sick people should want to get well and return to their normal activities as quickly as possible, which means that patients should cooperate in the treatment process and, to some extent, become submissive to the demands of their health care providers. (Recall the response of woman with SLE whose nurses demanded more of her than she could do.) People who refuse to take medications as ordered or who refuse to perform prescribed activities, such as adhering to an exercise program or therapeutic diet, are often viewed negatively. Their friends and family members may become irritated at their lack of participation in getting well again. Their providers may refer to them as "noncompliant" or "disengaged." Often what is missing is an understanding of the patient's perception of the illness. Illnesses and their treatments have great meaning to patients. One patient with HIV describes the meaning of taking antiretroviral medications:

> *Every time I look at those pills, I am reminded all over again that I have HIV. Every day I am reminded. I feel good, and I sometimes think that if I just didn't have to take these pills, I wouldn't even think about having HIV. So now and then I skip a dose to take a little vacation from HIV. It's not about the pills, really. It's about what they mean, and about what having HIV means.*

Working with patients with chronic illnesses can be particularly challenging for nurses. The inability to cure disease sometimes leads health care providers to feel hopeless and powerless as they look at their very sick patients and to feel overwhelmed and inadequate at times. Self-aware nurses recognize these feelings and seek to address them outside of the clinical setting where it is safe to "vent" and work through these feelings (reflective practice).

Responses to illness vary widely and are, of course, idiosyncratic. Each person in whom diabetes, for example, is newly diagnosed behaves differently from other people with the same condition. Both internal and external variables affect how an individual acts when ill (Box 13.3). An individual's personality has a great deal of influence on the response to illness. Past experiences with illness and cultural background also influence illness behaviors.

Internal Influences on Illness Behaviors

One's personality is an internal variable that determines, to a large extent, how one manages illness. Personality characteristics the nurse should consider when assessing the person with an illness are dependence/independence, coping ability, hardiness, learned resourcefulness, resilience, and spirituality.

Dependence and Independence

Patients' needs for **dependence** may be unrelated to the severity of their illnesses. Some patients adopt a passive attitude and rely completely on others to take care of them. Others may simply ignore their illness or do not like the idea of being dependent; therefore they try to continue living as independently as they did before becoming sick.

BOX 13.3 Internal and External Influences on Illness Behavior

Internal Influences	External Influences
• Dependence/independence needs	• Past experiences
• Coping ability	• Culture
• Hardiness	• Communication patterns
• Learned resourcefulness	• Personal space norms
• Resilience	• Role expectations
• Spirituality	• Values
	• Reaction to prescribed medications
	• Ethnocentrism

People who perceive themselves as helpless may be more willing to submit to health care personnel and do what they are told. Those who are used to being in charge and see themselves as independent may resent the enforced dependency of hospitalization and illness. These two different attitudes are illustrated in Case Study 13.1.

Both overly dependent and overly independent behavior can be frustrating to nurses, who sometimes become angry with patients who request help with activities they are physically capable of doing themselves. Patients who are too dependent require encouragement to assume more responsibility. Highly independent patients may have problems relying on caregivers and may inadvertently put themselves in danger of falls or other accidents. Independent patients need assistance in recognizing limitations and using available resources to meet his or her needs. For instance, Mr. Johnson in Case Study 13.1 risks a fall and injury by not recognizing that his recent surgery will require him to be temporarily more dependent than he is comfortable with.

CASE STUDY 13.1
Dependence vs. Independence

Example 1: Dependence
Mrs. Pierce has been in the hospital for several days after major abdominal surgery. Even after she progressed to the point at which she could feed herself, turn over in bed, and go to the bathroom unaided, she continued to call for assistance with these activities of daily living. She now calls the nurse every few minutes, making some small request that she is capable of performing for herself. She is communicating to the nurse that she needs a great deal of assistance and is demonstrating overly dependent behavior.

Example 2: Independence
Three hours ago, Mr. Johnson returned to his room after surgery. The nurse found him trying to get out of bed by himself. He did not call to ask for assistance and, although he has some pain even after being medicated, he says that he is used to doing things for himself and does not like asking the nurses for help. Mr. Johnson is demonstrating behavior that is too independent for his current physical status.

Because nurses most often focus on promoting patient independence, they may react negatively to patients who are exhibiting dependent behavior. Keep in mind that these behaviors may be the patient's way of signaling an increased need for security or support. Sometimes independence may not be the desired outcome. For patients with chronic illnesses who must rely on others for assistance in meeting their needs, too much independence may actually be problematic, even dangerous.

Coping Ability

An individual copes with disease or illness in a variety of ways. **Coping** is a term that describes the strategies a person uses to assess and manage demands. With an acute illness, coping is generally short term and leads to a return to the pre-illness state. With chronic disorders, coping behaviors must be used continuously.

Sick people use coping strategies to deal with the negative consequences of the disorder, such as pain or physical limitations. Each individual has a unique coping repertoire that is formed across previous illness episodes, modeling coping by others, and by significant factors in the context of his or her life over which he or she has little or no control, such as poverty, concurrent losses, tenuous employment, and unstable relationships, among others. Higher levels of life stresses are associated with patients' perceptions of severe consequences of illness and less control over the illness (Karademas et al., 2009).

Resourcefulness

Resourcefulness refers to the use of cognitive skills that one uses to adapt to the world around him, often in very creative ways. Throughout life, individuals acquire a number of skills that enable them to cope effectively with stressful situations. Resourceful people may have an attitude of self-mastery that can be particularly helpful in reducing the feelings of despair and helplessness that can accompany the numerous stressors of chronic illness. Note that *resource* does not refer to material belongings but involves the ability to make the most out of what one has.

Resourcefulness can be taught as a form of coping. Self-regulation, problem solving, conflict resolution, and emotion management are examples of the types of educational interventions the nurse may implement.

Past experiences

Some adults may accept being ill fairly easily and will accept care easily. It is unclear why some people more than others simply are able to acquiesce to illness, at least temporarily, and take on the sick role. Some adults, however, who as children received signals from their parents or adult caretakers that "it is weak to be ill" or "one must keep going even when not feeling well" may have difficulty accepting illness and the restrictions that accompany it. Other adults who experienced traumatic hospitalizations as children or who were threatened with injections for misbehaving may see hospitals and nurses as threatening. They are understandably affected by their early negative experiences. Nurses should determine the patient's past experiences with illness and the health care system during a careful admission assessment. These findings can be used to individualize care.

Culture

Culture has been discussed several times throughout this book and chapter, because it is difficult to discuss almost any topic related to health care without mentioning culture. Culture is a pattern of learned behavior and values that are reinforced through social interactions, shared by members of a particular group, and transmitted from one generation to the next. Culture exerts considerable influence over most of an individual's life experiences. Meanings attached to health, illness, and perceptions of treatment are affected to a large degree by a person's culture. Culture determines when one seeks help and the type of practitioner consulted. It also prescribes customs of responding to the sick. Culture defines whether illness is seen as a punishment for misdeeds or as the result of inadequate personal health practices. It influences whether one goes to an acupuncturist, an herbalist, a folk healer, or a traditional health care provider such as physicians and nurse practitioners.

Beginning in the early 1970s, schools of nursing began including cultural concepts in their curricula. Increasing numbers of universities and colleges offered graduate programs in transcultural nursing. The Transcultural Nursing Society was incorporated in 1981, and in 1988 it began certifying nurses in transcultural nursing. Through oral and written examinations and evaluation of educational background and working experiences, a qualified nurse can become a certified transcultural nurse (CTN). More information about this interesting certification can be found at https://tcns.org/tcncertification/.

The Transcultural Nursing Society began publishing the *Journal of Transcultural Nursing* in 1989. In the decades since transcultural nursing was first emphasized in educational programs, the cultural makeup of the U.S. population has undergone rapid change. Census demographers, who study population trends, predict that today's ethnic and racial minorities will outnumber non-Hispanic Whites by 2042. Even sooner, by 2023, they will constitute a majority of the nation's children younger than 18 years of age (Roberts, 2008). These cultural shifts mean that changes in the nursing workforce are needed to deal more effectively with commonalities and differences in patients. Significant disparities exist between the health status of Whites and non-Whites in the United States. For example, the death rate for heart disease is more than 40% higher in African Americans than in the White population. Similarly discouraging disparities exist in death rates for cancer and HIV/acquired immunodeficiency syndrome (AIDS), among other diseases. Although these disparities may partly result from education, poverty, and lifestyle factors, there is a growing recognition among health professionals that racism may play a role. As a result, professional associations such as the American Nurses Association, The Joint Commission, and the federal government have all endorsed standards for culturally appropriate health care services.

The Joint Commission developed and revised accreditation standards for hospitals to incorporate diversity, cultural, language, and health literacy issues into patient care processes. In 2010 The Joint Commission published a monograph, *Advancing Effective Communication, Cultural Competence, and Patient- and Family-Centered Care: A Roadmap for Hospitals,* to set standards for quality, safety, and equity for hospitalized patients. This document is available at http://www.jointcommission.org/assets/1/6/ARoadmapforHospitals-finalversion727.pdf. Some states have passed legislation requiring health care professions to include cultural competence training in their educational and continuing education programs. The profession of nursing is largely White, whereas the nation is racially more diverse than ever before, which underscores the need for culturally competent nurses. Clearly, transcultural nursing is an important field of study, practice, and research and an essential one in today's increasingly diverse society. The Joint Commission and The California Endowment published their recommendations in a document titled *One Size Does Not Fit All: Meeting the Health Care Needs of Diverse Populations* (www.jointcommission.org/assets/1/6/HLCOneSizeFinal.pdf).

The culturally competent nurse. Cultural competence, defined earlier, guides the nurse in understanding behaviors and planning appropriate approaches to patient needs. Conversely, culture will also guide the patient's response to health care providers and their interventions. The U.S. Office of Minority Health defined culturally competent health care as "services that are respectful of and responsive to the health beliefs and practices and cultural and linguistic needs of diverse patient populations" (U.S. Department of Health and Human Services, 2001, p. 131), a definition still being used today. Understanding a patient's cultural background can facilitate communication and support establishing an effective nurse-patient relationship. Conversely, lack of understanding can create barriers that impede nursing care.

The shared values and beliefs in a culture enable its members to predict each other's actions. They also affect how members react to each other's behavior. When nurses work with patients from cultures different from their own and about which little is known, they lack these familiar guidelines for predicting behavior. This can cause anxiety, frustration, and feelings of distrust in both patient and nurse. Some of the issues that can arise when nurses care for patients from other cultures include stereotyping, communication difficulties, misperceptions about personal space, differing values and role expectations, ethnopharmacologic considerations, and ethnocentrism.

Stereotyping. In an effort to predict behavior, nurses may stereotype or make prejudgments about patients from different cultures. It is important that nurses refrain from **stereotyping** members of cultures or ethnic groups that are different from their own. When providing nursing care, one size does not fit all. *Cultural conditioning* is a term that means people are culture bound. They are unconscious of their own innate values and beliefs and assume that all people are basically alike—that is, that all people share their values and beliefs.

It is important to recognize that the health care professions create **cultural conditioning** in their practitioners during school. Nursing is no exception. Nurses tend to hold their knowledge and beliefs about health in high regard and may devalue people who do not possess similar knowledge and beliefs. Individualized planning is always the best basis for care, whatever the patient's culture or ethnic group. Care that is not individualized can result in nonadherence to treatment plans, dissatisfaction with care, and suboptimal outcomes.

Ethnocentrism. Nurses respond to sick people based not only on their formal education but also on their own socialization and culture. All persons can be unaware of their own biases and tend to be ethnocentric. **Ethnocentrism** is the inclination to view one's own cultural group as the standard by which to judge the value of other cultural groups. One nurse describes her embarrassment when a patient challenged her ethnocentric view of eating customs:

> *My patient was from India, and her family brought in the most delicious smelling food. When I went into the room, I was surprised to see them all eating with their fingers. I left right away and brought them some knives and forks. They refused them, nicely. I regret that I mentioned how messy this probably was. My patient asked me, "Do you use a fork when you eat?" I answered, "Of course," and the patient laughed and pointed out that I had a good portion of salad dressing down the front of my scrubs. The patient and her family, on the other hand, were immaculate. I was a little embarrassed, but I learned a good lesson. I didn't have any choice except to laugh too, and apologize.*

The nurse who identifies how personal beliefs and expectations can influence care is better able to recognize and deal with any prejudices that may impede patient care. **Cultural assessment** therefore begins with self-assessment. To begin a cultural self-assessment, examine your own values. The nurse who is frustrated by the difficulty of caring for a patient from a different culture may benefit from taking a few minutes to imagine what it would be like to be hospitalized in a foreign country. Candidly answering the questions in Considering Culture Box 13.1 will help you begin the important process of self-assessment.

Cultural assessment. An important step in meeting the challenge of providing nursing care to diverse patients is the **cultural assessment**. Cultural assessments are used to identify beliefs, values, and health practices that may help or hinder nursing interventions. Dr. Madeleine Leininger, an iconic figure in nursing—anthropologist, theorist, and founder of transcultural nursing—advocated that nurses routinely perform cultural assessments to determine patients' culturally specific needs (Leininger, 1999).

A cultural assessment is really as simple as asking patients their preferences, what they think or believe about their illness, their family structure, who

CONSIDERING CULTURE BOX 13.1

The Challenge of Understanding Your Own Cultural Beliefs—Sociocultural Self-Assessment

Directions: Use your answers to these questions to better understand your own social and cultural beliefs and expectations.

1. To what groups do I belong? What is my cultural heritage? My socioeconomic status? My age-group? My religious affiliation?
2. How do I describe myself? What parts of the description come from the groups to which I belong?
3. What kinds of contact have I had with people from different groups? Do I assume that others have the same values and beliefs that I have?
4. What makes me feel proud about my group affiliations? Am I ethnocentric in my attitudes and behavior? What would I change about my group affiliations if I could? Why?
5. Have I ever experienced the feeling of being rejected by another group? Did this experience heighten my sensitivity to other cultures or cause me to denigrate others different from myself?
6. When I was growing up, what messages did I get from parents and friends about people from groups different from mine? Do these attitudes cause me any difficulty today?
7. What are the major stereotypes I hold about people from different groups? Do these biases help or hinder me in developing cultural sensitivity?
8. To work effectively with people from different cultural groups, what do I need to change about myself?

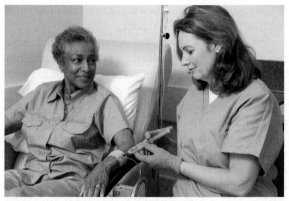

Fig. 13.3 Nurses administering chemotherapy in an outpatient setting often see the same patients over time. A cultural assessment at the onset of treatment can be useful in helping the patient feel accepted and supported as she faces the challenges of having cancer. (Photo used with permission from iStockphoto.)

providers should talk to in making a decision, and what the illness and its treatments mean to them (Fig. 13.3). Numerous cultural assessment instruments have been developed. Some of them require in-depth interviews and comprehensive data gathering, which may prove to be challenging for busy nurses. However, patients often find themselves "a stranger in a strange land" just by virtue of entering the health care setting with its own language, routines, and culture. For a patient who is from a country or culture that diverges greatly from American culture, being hospitalized poses numerous threats to his or her identity. A careful assessment is warranted, and if language is problematic, a professional interpreter should be used (see Chapter 12).

Culturally competent nurses take cultural differences into consideration, are aware of potential "trouble spots" that can occur, usually interpret patient behavior accurately, and recognize problems that need to be managed. They realize that cultural norms must be included in the plan of care to prevent conflicts between nursing goals and patient/family goals. Planning culturally congruent care is the most time-effective way to achieve the desired goals.

In addition, being knowledgeable about other cultures promotes feelings of respect and enhances understanding of attitudes, behaviors, and the impact of illness. The accompanying interview with Dr. Madeleine Leininger provides insights into her vast experience and strongly held beliefs about cultural competence in nursing. Becoming culturally competent is a process. Nurses must remember that continuous learning and sensitivity to and respect for cultural differences are qualities required of culturally competent nurses (Interview Box 13.1).

THE IMPACT OF ILLNESS ON PATIENTS AND FAMILIES

Across all cultures, illness forces change in patients and their families: behavioral and emotional changes, role changes, and unpredictable changes in family dynamics. Illness creates stress and other emotional responses. The

INTERVIEW BOX 13.1

Dr. Madeleine Leininger, Founder of Transcultural Nursing

Interviewer: Dr. Leininger, please tell us what you mean by the term *culturally competent.*

Dr. Leininger: Culturally competent care has been defined as the culturally based knowledge with a care focus that is used in creative, meaningful, and appropriate ways to provide beneficial and satisfying care to individuals, families, groups, or communities or to help people face death or disabilities. I coined this term in 1962 as the goal of my theory of culture care diversity and universality. The term has caught hold today and is being used by many health care providers. It is now used as a requirement for The Joint Commission accreditation and with other organizations as essential to work effectively with cultures and their health care needs.

Interviewer: Please describe how a culturally competent nurse's patient care differs from that of one who is not culturally competent.

Dr. Leininger: A culturally competent nurse demonstrates the following attributes and skills: (1) uses transcultural nursing concepts, principles, and available research findings to assess and guide care practices; (2) understands and values the cultural beliefs and practices of designated cultures so that nursing care is tailor-made or fits individuals' needs in meaningful ways; (3) knows how to prevent major kinds of cultural conflicts, clashes, or hurtful care practices; (4) demonstrates reasonable confidence to work effectively and knowingly with clients of different cultures and can also evaluate transcultural nursing care outcomes.

The nurse who is unable to demonstrate these culturally competent attributes often shows signs of being frustrated and impatient with people of different cultures. Moreover, the nurse who does not practice cultural competencies often shows signs of excessive ethnocentrism, biases, and related problems that impede client recovery and well-being.

Interviewer: How do patients respond differently when nurses take their cultural patterns into consideration when planning and implementing care?

Dr. Leininger: It is most encouraging to observe and listen to clients who have received culturally based nursing care. These clients often exhibit the following behaviors: (1) They show signs of being satisfied and very pleased with nurse's actions and decisions. (2) They make comments such as, "This is the best care I or my family members have received from health care providers." Frequently they say, "How did you know about my values, my culture, and how to use these ideas in my care? You anticipated my needs well." (3) They appreciate the different ways the nurse incorporates their cultural needs.

They express their gratitude to the nurse. (4) Clients appreciate respect for their culture shown by the nurse in care decisions and practices. (5) The clients do not experience racial biases and negative comments about their cultures or familiar life-ways.

Interviewer: With so many cultural groups in this country, knowing all one needs to know about other cultures seems overwhelming. How do you advise nurses to begin the process of becoming culturally competent?

Dr. Leininger: The nurse should first enroll in a substantive transcultural nursing course to learn the basic and important concepts, principles, and practices of transcultural nursing. This knowledge base is essential so the nurse becomes aware of common cultural needs and ways to work with a few cultures that are different. A few cultures are studied in depth, focusing on common and unique cultural features. The most frequently occurring cultures in the nurse's home or local region are studied first, and then one learns about other cultures over time, becoming sensitive and knowledgeable about these cultures. The nurse can greatly increase her or his knowledge of several cultures or subcultures by reading the literature, or by studying specific cultures when caring for people under transcultural mentors. Gradually, the nurse learns several cultures in a general way and a few in depth. As the nurse becomes increasingly knowledgeable about several cultures, comparative knowledge and competencies become evident.

There is no expectation that professional nurses can know all human cultures, as this would be impossible. An open learning attitude and mind with a sincere desire to learn as much as possible about a few cultures will help the nurse in becoming culturally knowledgeable, competent, and sensitive.

Interviewer: What signs can students look for to determine whether their nursing programs are preparing them to provide culturally competent care?

Dr. Leininger: Nursing students will find they are able to provide culturally competent care when (or if) the following signs are evident:

- They consistently know, understand, and respect specific cultures and appreciate commonalities and differences among cultures.
- They feel a sense of confidence, creativity, and competence in their nursing care practices, see how their care fits specific cultures, and accommodate cultural differences in meaningful and creative ways.
- They go beyond common sense to actual use of culture-specific knowledge in patient care as shown in the Sunrise Model (see Chapter 9, Fig. 9.2).

Continued

? INTERVIEW BOX 13.1

Dr. Madeleine Leininger, Founder of Transcultural Nursing—cont'd

- They creatively use the clients' beliefs, values, and patterns along with appropriate professional knowledge and skills that meet clients' needs.
- They prevent racial discrimination practices in nursing and in other places; they avoid cultural imposition, ethnocentrism, cultural conflicts, cultural pain, and related negative practices.
- They value and know how to use Leininger's Culture Care Theory and basic transcultural care concepts, principles, and research findings in their nursing practices

- to provide culturally congruent care for people's health and well-being.
- They appreciate a global perspective of nursing and value transcultural nursing to meet a growing and intense multicultural world.
- They markedly grow in their professional knowledge and sensitivities, developing a global worldview of transcultural nursing. They reach out to help cultural strangers in different living contexts.

Courtesy Dr. Madeleine Leininger.

suddenness and seriousness of an illness affect responses to illness: sudden, severe illness is upsetting in almost all aspects of family life. The personality of the patient before illness affects how he or she may respond: a pessimistic person for whom the glass is always "half empty" is not likely to become an optimist in the face of serious illness. Illnesses that result in enduring lifestyle adjustments have serious effects on the family. Responses to illness are usually affected by the patient's stage of human development. For instance, an elderly widowed family member who has previously enjoyed good health may elect not to seek treatment for cancer, but a younger member with a spouse and children may elect aggressive treatment for the same illness. Religious faith also plays a role in responses to illness.

Severe illnesses that profoundly affect physical appearance and functioning are more likely to result in high levels of anxiety and extensive behavioral changes than are short-term, non–life-threatening illnesses. The impact of a chronic illness is significant and continues for the lifetime of the patient. When planning holistic nursing care, the nurse must take into consideration how the family both influences and is influenced by the illness of a family member.

Impact of Illness on Patients

Illness creates a variety of emotional responses, some of which have been described briefly earlier in this chapter. Among the more common responses are guilt, anger, anxiety, and stress.

Guilt

Guilt is not uncommon when a person becomes ill, particularly if the illness is related to behavioral choices

such as smoking. Guilt may also be associated with the inability to perform usual activities because of illness. A mother who is unable to take care of her children or a father who has to take a lower-paying job because of illness may experience considerable guilt. Some cultures view certain illnesses as shameful and people who have them as guilty of some type of transgression. Nurses who identify and encourage patients to talk about their feelings of guilt may help assuage these uncomfortable feelings that may impede the patient's ability to participate in his or her care.

Anger

Anger is another common emotional response to illness. When patients must make sacrifices to manage their illnesses, such as giving up favorite foods or activities, they may experience anger about the changes. Anger may also be directed toward caregivers for their inability to produce a cure, reduce pain, or prevent negative consequences of the illness. Nurses must be prepared to accept such angry feelings, to refrain from rejecting or avoiding patients who express their fears through anger, and to encourage the adaptive expression of angry feelings. Angry patients can be difficult to deal with, and the nurse must be very careful not to further incite the patient by becoming upset or angry too. In the example of Mr. Kaman earlier in this chapter, the nurse appropriately sought out some explanation from Mrs. Kaman, who was able to help her understand the source of at least some of Mr. Kaman's anger.

Anxiety

Anxiety is a common and universal experience. It is also a common emotional response to illness and hospitalization. **Anxiety** is an ill-defined, diffuse feeling of apprehension and uncertainty. Anxiety occurs as a result of some threat to an individual's selfhood, self-esteem, or identity. A number of threats are associated with illness. Illness may alter the way people view themselves. Some illnesses result in a change in physical appearance. Often, ability to function is affected, altering relationships, work performance, and abilities to meet others' expectations. In addition, there may be concern about pain and discomfort associated with illness or treatment. Because of real and potential threats and changes arising from illness, nurses must develop skills that enable them to help patients recognize and manage anxiety.

Although the responses are similar, anxiety and fear are different. Fear results from specific known causes, whereas anxiety is more unfocused. For example, if you are home alone at night and you hear an unusual noise outside, your heartbeat and respirations may increase, your stomach tightens, and you perspire. The emotion in this situation is fear of an intruder. If you begin to have the same feelings but have heard no noises and cannot identify a source of fear, you may be experiencing anxiety. Both emotions may be present at the same time. The patient who is in the hospital for surgery or invasive testing may experience anxiety about the unknown consequences of the surgery and fear in anticipation of pain, a long recovery, or a diagnosis of a life-limiting illness.

Symptoms of anxiety. Nurses should be familiar with the numerous symptoms of anxiety. They are classified as physiologic, emotional, and cognitive. Signs and symptoms include increased heart rate, respirations, and blood pressure; insomnia; nausea and vomiting; fatigue; sweaty palms; and tremors. Emotional responses include restlessness, irritability, feelings of helplessness, crying, and depression. Cognitive symptoms include inability to concentrate, forgetfulness, inattention to surroundings, and preoccupation.

Responses to anxiety. Responses to anxiety occur on a continuum. The continuum is along four levels of anxiety: mild, moderate, severe, and panic. A mild level is characterized by increased alertness and ability to focus attention and concentrate. There is an expanded capacity for learning at this stage.

A person with a moderate level of anxiety is able to concentrate on only one thing at a time. Commonly, there is increased body movement (restlessness), rapid speech, and a subjective awareness of discomfort.

BOX 13.4 Levels of Anxiety

Mild Anxiety
- Increased alertness, increased ability to focus, improved concentration, expanded capacity for learning

Moderate Anxiety
- Concentration limited to one thing, increased body movement, rapid speech, subjective awareness of discomfort

Severe Anxiety
- Scattered thoughts, difficulty with verbal communication, considerable discomfort, purposeless movements

Panic
- Complete disorganization, difficulty differentiating reality from unreality, constant random movements, unable to function without assistance

---

At the severe level, thoughts become scattered. The severely anxious person may not be able to communicate verbally, and there is considerable discomfort accompanied by purposeless movements such as hand-wringing and pacing.

At the panic level, the person becomes completely disorganized and loses the ability to differentiate between reality and unreality. There are constant random and purposeless movements. The individual experiencing panic levels of anxiety is unable to function without assistance. Panic levels of anxiety cannot be continued indefinitely, because the body will become exhausted, and death may occur if the anxiety is not reduced. Box 13.4 lists the characteristics of each level of anxiety.

Because anxiety is such a common response to illness and hospitalization, nurses often encounter patients who are experiencing mild or moderate anxiety and, occasionally, patients who are severely anxious. When interacting with an anxious patient, the nurse should carefully assess the level of anxiety before attempting to develop the plan of care.

Anxiety tends to be transferred between persons. For this reason, nurses must be aware of and manage personal anxiety so that it is not inadvertently transferred to patients. Conversely, self-awareness is essential to prevent responding to a patient's anxiety by becoming anxious.

Stress

Stress is another internal variable that affects patients. Stress is both a response to illness and an important factor in the development of illness. Because illness and hospitalization involve so many alterations in lifestyle, they tend to cause a great deal of stress.

Stress is an unavoidable and essential part of life. To survive and grow, individuals must cope adaptively with constantly changing demands. The stress related to examinations, for example, motivates most students to grow by studying and learning. Although stress is unavoidable, and even sometimes desirable, some control can be exerted over the number and types of stressors (factors that create stress) encountered, and responses to the stressors can often be managed.

Hospitalized patients are removed from their usual routines and support systems. They lose much of their control because nurses and other care providers make decisions for them. Often, being ill means that they are no longer able to perform activities as they did before the illness occurred. Some patients find themselves in the role of comforting other family members rather than being comforted, to avoid increasing family members' distress. Stress is a common response to all these circumstances.

Differentiating between stress and anxiety. Stress and anxiety have some characteristics in common. The physiologic responses are similar. Anxiety is a response to a real or perceived threat to the individual, whereas stress is an interaction between the individual and the environment. Stress includes all the responses the body makes while striving to maintain equilibrium and deal with demands.

Internal, external, and interpersonal stressors. Selye (1956) defined *stress* as the nonspecific response of the body to any demand made on it. He named this response the *general adaptation syndrome* and identified three stages through which the body progresses while responding to stress.

Stressors trigger the body's stress response. Stressors are agents or stimuli that an individual perceives as posing a threat to homeostasis. Stressors may come from external, interpersonal, or internal sources. External stressors include such things as noise, heat, cold, malfunctioning equipment (such as an intravenous pump that keeps alarming), or organizational rules and expectations. Interpersonal sources of stress include the demands made by others and conflicts with others.

Placing unrealistic expectations on oneself is an example of an internal stressor. For example, a patient with a traumatic injury to his lower extremity begins making plans to take part in a race within a month. Although his rehabilitation advances well, he becomes discouraged and experiences stress because it is not at a pace that he would like, and it becomes clear that racing will not be part of his life in the near future.

Responses to stress. Outward responses to stress are determined by the individual's perception of the stressor. Cognitive appraisal, or the way one thinks about a specific situation, determines the degree to which the situation is considered stressful. Loud music at a concert, for example, might seem less stressful to adolescents than it would to their parents.

Another factor related to the assessment of threat is whether the individual feels capable of handling the threat—that is, whether the person exhibits hardiness. The person who feels capable can be expected to feel less stress than the person who does not generally feel competent.

Stress affects the physical, emotional, and cognitive areas of functioning just as anxiety does. Physically, there can be a feeling of fatigue with muscular tightness and tension. Heart rate and respirations are increased. The person who is under prolonged or serious stress may be unable to sleep or eat, or he or she may sleep or eat excessively in an attempt to avoid or cope with the stress.

Emotionally, people under stress feel drained and unable to care for themselves or others. This can result in social isolation and distancing from others. They experience difficulty enjoying life. They may have feelings of hopelessness and of being out of control. Irritability and impatience often occur.

Cognitively, stress causes decreased mental capacity and problem-solving skills; therefore there is a tendency to have difficulty making decisions. Someone who is under a great deal of stress may be experiencing *distress*—a response to environmental, physical, or cognitive stressors in which the person may find it difficult to function and cope.

Stress and illness. Constant stress plays a role in the development of illness. Recent research has provided better understanding of the links between prolonged stress and body functioning.

The person who is under stress for long periods is at risk for a number of physical problems. The body

---

BOX 13.5 **Breathing Exercises**

1. Sit comfortably with feet on the floor and eyes closed.
2. Inhale slowly and deeply through the nose and fill the lungs completely. As you breathe in, imagine the oxygen flowing to all your cells. Hold your breath while slowly counting to four.
3. Slowly release all the air while thinking the word *calm*. As you breathe out, imagine the air taking all the tension out with it.
4. Repeat the cycle four times. Try to banish all thoughts except those related to your breathing, but do not fight them if other thoughts creep in.
5. When you have completed the exercise, open your eyes slowly and sit for a moment before resuming your regular activities.

BOX 13.6 **Relaxation Exercises**

Get into a comfortable position in a place where you will not be interrupted. First focus on slow, deep breathing. Close your eyes and begin to think about the muscle sensations in your body. Identify where you are feeling tense. Slowly inhale as you stretch; then exhale and allow the tension to flow out.

Neck and Shoulders

- Slowly bend your head forward and backward, then side to side three times. Bring your shoulders up as if you were trying to touch them to your ears. Slowly relax and feel the difference in tension.

Arms and Hands

- Make a tight fist in one hand, and tighten the muscles throughout your arm. Slowly release the muscles from the shoulder to the hand. Repeat with the other arm and hand.

Head

- Make a wide smile, and hold for a count of five. Slowly relax your face muscles and let your jaw go loose. Tightly close your eyes and feel the tension. Slowly give up the tension and allow your eyes to remain gently closed.

Stomach

- Make your abdominal muscles tight by pushing them out as far as possible. Make your abdomen hard and feel the tension. Slowly relax your muscles and notice the difference.

Legs and Feet

- Holding your leg still, curl your toes down to point to the floor. Do first one leg and then the other. As you tighten your muscles, feel the tension. Then slowly relax.
- Sit quietly for a few moments and feel the relaxation in your body before you resume your activities.

---

produces cortisol when a person is under stress. Cortisol, a steroid hormone, can affect both the metabolism and immune response and lead to susceptibility to weight gain and poor healing. Disorders such as hypertension, certain skin disorders, and autoimmune disorders have been termed *stress-related diseases*, because they commonly occur in individuals who have been severely stressed.

Coping with stress. Nurses have a role in helping patients modify their stressors. They should assess patients' abilities to recognize symptoms of stress and their usual methods of coping.

Coping with stress can be direct or indirect. In assisting patients to use direct coping, nurses help patients to identify those situations that can be changed and to take responsibility for changing them. The focus is on using problem-solving skills and planning to eliminate or avoid as many stressors as possible. Completely eliminating stress from one's life is neither possible nor desirable.

In helping patients use indirect coping, nurses' actions are aimed at reducing the affective (feelings) and physiologic (body) disturbances resulting from stress. Patients are taught techniques such as deep breathing, muscle relaxation, and imagery, which help them cope more effectively with stress (Boxes 13.5 and 13.6).

To help patients manage stress, nurses must be skilled in assessing and managing their own personal stress. Nurses who are feeling stressed themselves have difficulty assisting patients in dealing with similar problems.

The statements in Table 13.1 can help you identify your own sources of stress and develop self-awareness so that you can be effective in helping patients deal with their stress.

Coping with stress through education. Patient education is a major part of the practice of nursing, and nurses have a professional responsibility to ensure that their patients' learning needs are met. When patients are competent in the knowledge and skills they need to

TABLE 13.1	**Personal Stress Inventory**			
		Very Often	**Sometimes**	**Rarely or Never**
1. I feel tense and anxious and have some nervous indigestion.				
2. People at home, school, or work make me feel tense.				
3. I eat, drink, or smoke in response to tension.				
4. I have tension or pain in my neck or shoulders.				
5. I have headaches or insomnia.				
6. I have trouble turning off my thoughts long enough to feel relaxed.				
7. I find it difficult to concentrate on what I am doing because I worry about other things.				
8. I use alcohol, tranquilizers, or other medications to relax or sleep.				
9. I feel a lot of pressure at work or school.				
10. I do not feel that my work is appreciated.				
11. My family does not appreciate what I do for them.				
12. I feel I do not have enough time for myself.				
13. I have difficulty saying "no."				
14. I wish I had more friends with whom to share experiences.				
15. I do not have enough time for physical exercise.				

Scoring: Give yourself 2 points for every check in the Very Often column, 1 point for every check in the Sometimes column, and 0 points for every check in the Rarely or Never column. Total the number of points. A score of 20 to 30 represents a high level of stress. If you scored in this range, you should take steps to reduce your stress level. A score from 10 to 19 means that you are experiencing midlevel stress. You should monitor your stress and begin relaxation exercises. A score of 9 or less means that you are experiencing relatively low stress at present.

manage their illnesses, they tend to feel more masterful and less stressed.

As a first step, nurses must identify factors that can create barriers to learning (Box 13.7). One factor is anxiety. Mild anxiety improves learning by increasing the ability to focus on the task. As anxiety increases, however, the ability to listen, focus, and concentrate decreases. Information is not retained, and the patient is unable to make the cognitive connections required for learning to take place.

Physiologic factors may also impede learning. For instance, visual or hearing deficits must be addressed. Unmet physiologic needs, such as fatigue, shortness of breath, hunger, and thirst, decrease the patient's attention to learning. Pain dramatically impairs the ability to learn, and pain medication may make the patient drowsy and unable to focus. Learning requires energy so a fatigued patient may not learn well. Nurses who assess and ensure that patients' physiologic needs are met enhance these patients' readiness to learn.

Patient teaching is an important part of the culture of nursing; however, culture also can influence patients' responses to teaching by nurses. Understanding the meaning of illness in the patient's culture is an early

---

BOX 13.7   Barriers to Patient Learning

- High anxiety
- Sensory deficits (e.g., vision, hearing)
- Pain
- Fatigue
- Hunger/thirst
- Shortness of breath
- Cultural expectations
- Language barriers
- Differing health values
- Low literacy
- Lack of motivation
- Environmental factors (e.g., noise, lack of privacy)

---

step that will help the nurse determine the educational needs of the patient and family and effectively provide culturally congruent patient education. When the nurse works toward a learning goal that is not seen as desirable by a patient, their cultural values may be in conflict. In fact, this is not really a patient goal but a reflection of the nurse's ingrained cultural expectation that patients need or want to be taught.

Self-awareness on the part of the nurse is essential to avoid allowing cross-cultural barriers to occur. In all patient teaching, and especially in a cross-cultural situation, individualizing patient teaching is essential. Learning appropriate greetings and phrases in the patient's language and obtaining the services of an interpreter also show sensitivity to cultural differences. Always show respect for folk remedies and traditions valued by the patient and family and make every effort to incorporate them into the patient's health care treatment plan. Nurses must recognize that low literacy rates are a problem among patients of all cultures. This may require communicating in simple language both orally and with printed materials that the patient can understand.

Lack of motivation and readiness are often significant barriers to education. The patient may still be emotionally upset from an unexpected serious diagnosis and may not be able to focus on learning or simply may not be motivated to learn what the nurse believes is important to teach. Patients with an external locus of control, for example, believe that nothing they can do will make a difference and may not be motivated to learn about their own illnesses. Often nurses believe that simply pointing out what patients need to know is sufficient to motivate them. When nurses help the patients make their own decisions about the knowledge they need, teaching is usually more effective. This approach may require greater effort initially, but it is ultimately more efficient to assess patient motivation and readiness first, before engaging in patient teaching.

The nurse who is preparing to teach should also assess and manage the environment. A setting that is private, comfortable, and free of distractions is beneficial to the learning process. Once barriers have been identified and removed to the extent possible, nurses must plan patient education using sound principles of learning and teaching-learning concepts. Although it goes beyond the scope of this text to review all the complexities of learning, certain basic ideas should be considered. The patient's prior experiences, gender, culture, cognitive style, and motivation are all important determinants of learning. The nurse-teacher's knowledge, flexibility, creativity, communication skills, confidence in the patient's ability to learn, and ability to motivate all facilitate or impede learning. Boxes 13.8 and 13.9 include simple principles of adult learning and teaching-learning concepts that are useful in working with patients.

BOX 13.8 Principles of Adult Learning

- Prior experiences are resources for learning.
  - *Example:* If the patient enjoys gardening, try to link health maintenance suggestions to preventive maintenance of indoor/outdoor plants.
- Readiness to learn is usually related to a social role or developmental task.
  - *Example:* New parents are usually eager to learn how to care for their first infants.
- Motivation to learn is greater when the material is seen as immediately useful.
  - *Example:* The same new parents are more motivated to learn care of the small infant than they are to learn about disciplining toddlers.
- The learning environment must be arranged to facilitate learning.
  - *Example:* The room is quiet and kept at a comfortable temperature, with adequate lighting, privacy, and seating.
- Physical needs are met before the teaching session.
  - *Example:* The patient has his or her reading glasses and/or hearing aid, has been given the opportunity to go to the bathroom, and is relatively pain free.

Impact of Illness on Families

Families are best understood as systems, which means that change in one member changes the functioning of the total family. The entire family system is affected by a member's illness. Whether the ill family member is hospitalized or cared for in the home, illness drastically increases stress in a family and disrupts usual family function.

The most important factor in how a family tolerates stress is the individual and group coping abilities. Families already experiencing difficulties may find that their problems are intensified to the point of disruption when acute or chronic illness occurs.

A sick family member has to give up responsibility to other family members. The family must continue to fulfill its usual functions while dealing with the alterations imposed by the illness or absence of a member. Family members who are able to be flexible and assume different roles, who can share their feelings, and who seek assistance may adjust better to changes than those who are inflexible. Some persons are simply more resilient than others and adapt more easily in stressful situations.

Both acute and chronic illnesses cause changes in family functioning and create stress. Chronic illness can

BOX 13.9 Basics of Teaching Patients and Families

- Identify and remove, if possible, barriers to learning.
- Evaluate what the patient and family already know and what they want to know.
- When possible, frequent, short sessions work better than long ones.
- Goals for each session must be realistic.
- Be respectful of cultural differences, for example, in diet planning.
- Avoid medical jargon, acronyms such as "PRN," and slang.
- The presentation should proceed from simple to complex concepts.
- Present complex concepts only after there is mastery of simpler ones.
- Patients learn best when they are actively engaged.
- Learning is enhanced when multiple senses are used: seeing, hearing, telling, and doing make the best combination.
- Practice, or frequent repetition, reinforces skill acquisition.
- Reinforce learning with return demonstrations of skills.
- When you give feedback, be sure to include positives, as well as negatives.
- Written materials should be at a fourth-grade reading level and, if possible, in the patient's native language to make reading easier for the patient.
- Evaluate patient's understanding of the information presented; provide time to clarify misunderstandings and answer questions.
- Remember to document the teaching session and your evaluation of the outcome.

be particularly stressful because it is never completely cured. Families experience emotional highs and lows as the patient has remissions and exacerbations. They may experience resentment and other negative feelings. Family members may feel angry too—and often will explain that they are angry "at the situation" and not the person who is sick. Guilt often accompanies the anger of family members. If they cannot deal directly with feelings of anger, they may displace them onto nurses by becoming critical and demanding. Similarly, patients may feel guilty about creating hardships for loved ones. They may become convinced that they are no longer essential because others are capably taking over their roles. Family members sometimes withdraw from each other because

they fear that their negative feelings may not be understood and accepted. This mutual withdrawal leads to feelings of isolation for both patients and family members.

Families are often confused or uncertain about how to treat the sick person. They may have problems accepting and responding appropriately to the patients' dependency needs. As discussed earlier, patients may react to illness with either dependent or independent behaviors that sometimes become problematic. Nurses need to monitor whether family members foster dependence, thereby keeping the patient from becoming more independent. Here is a home health nurse's extreme and sad example:

I was taking care of a 45-year-old patient in her own home. She was morbidly obese, weighing over 400 pounds. She had a lot of health problems. I was doing wound care of deep stasis ulcers on her lower legs. I knew it was going to be hard for them to heal. I did a lot of teaching with her and her elderly mother, who seemed to understand that her daughter's healing was going to require that she lose a lot of weight and eat a high-quality diet. Well, we went nowhere fast. No matter what I did, the ulcers got worse and although my patient said that she was trying to lose weight, she did not seem to be making progress. One day I came to her house earlier than usual and her mother was in the kitchen, cooking a tall stack of French toast with syrup for her daughter. She laughed a little about "being caught in the act." I realized that I was caught in the middle of a complex relationship where the mother enjoyed "taking care of" her daughter by providing her with food that wasn't healthy, and that the daughter enjoyed being taken care of. I am not sure that "enjoyed" is the right word, but she was very dependent on her mother. One morning a few weeks later, the mother found her daughter dead in her bed. It was just so sad. I had to come to terms with the fact that I was powerless to change their dynamic and had done the best job I could to help.

As opposed to this tragic situation, nurses should also be aware that some families are uncomfortable with the ill person being dependent and do not allow the necessary "down time" for recovery. For example, if a man who is very much in control in a family has a heart attack and is in the coronary care unit, family members may have difficulty seeing the usually strong father in a helpless position. They may continue to bring family problems to him. Other families may find it difficult to shift responsibilities back to the formerly ill member as he or she becomes able to resume role functions, thereby prolonging dependence.

The nurse needs to recognize the anxiety in the family and take steps to reduce it. Talking with family members, explaining what is happening and what to expect, and teaching them how to participate in their family member's care can be helpful. During hospitalizations, it may be helpful to allow family members to be present during invasive procedures such as central line placements and chest tube insertions. Their presence can comfort and support the patient and allay family members' anxiety about such procedures. Some family members of course cannot tolerate seeing procedures being done or hearing expressions of discomfort or pain and should feel free to leave the room. As in any case, the patient's safety comes first.

Some families find that becoming active in seeking information, such as through the Internet, helps them manage their anxieties. Support groups and chat rooms where family members can express their concerns and hear from others with similar issues are also helpful. Nurses can help family members use these adaptive coping activities effectively by assisting them to find credible websites and evaluate the information they find online. The Internet, however, can make things worse. Here is an example from a young man's experience of seeking information on the Internet about a severe birth defect that had been diagnosed in his expected child:

> *I wrote down the word "anencephaly" on a piece of paper and put it in my pocket. That night after my wife went to bed, I got the paper out and got on the Internet to see what I could find out. I saw pictures that I couldn't have imagined and I never want to see again. I got really upset about what my baby might look like. I felt like I had to hide what I had seen from my wife. I wish I hadn't looked.*

Nurses must be prepared to accept the anger and distrust that often is directed toward care providers who are unable to cure disease or relieve the negative consequences of illness. Understanding that anger expressed by patients and families is not personally directed can enable nurses to assess patients objectively and respond to feelings expressed in a nondefensive manner. Box 13.10 summarizes common examples of family feelings and behaviors that nurses need to

---

> **BOX 13.10 Potential Reactions to Illness in a Family Member**
>
> - Frightened
> - Resentful
> - Angry
> - Guilty
> - Exhausted
> - Feelings of uselessness
> - Feelings of hopelessness
> - Distrust of health care providers
> - Critical and demanding behavior
> - Withdrawal from the situation
> - Confusion
> - Denial of seriousness of patient's illness
> - Promotion of dependence by patient

recognize, acknowledge, and explore in a sensitive manner with the family.

Caregiver stress is common in families of patients with prolonged, progressive illnesses, such as Alzheimer's disease and amyotrophic lateral sclerosis (ALS). Caregiver stress looks very much other stressful responses—anxiety symptoms, sleeplessness, fatigue, irritability, and so on. Many associations and support networks are dedicated to the care of persons with progressive illnesses. Caregivers can often find support from people going through the same experience, or who have had the same experience in the past. Nurses who work with patients and families with progressive illnesses should be aware of which websites are useful and provide substantial support and information.

Despite the numerous stresses, role strains, and adjustments necessitated by illness of a family member, many families find that there are also positive experiences in illness. Finding new activities to share and working together to meet challenges can lead to feelings of closeness and affiliation that were not present before. Previously unrecognized individual strengths may be identified as new roles and responsibilities are assumed. New meanings for the entire family may emerge as values are reassessed, priorities are shifted, and roles become more flexible.

THE IMPACT OF CAREGIVING ON NURSES

Caring is the foundation of professional nursing practice. Caring meets the essential human need for love and belongingness and assists nurses to provide high-quality nursing care. A caring attitude toward patients, their families, and colleagues begins with the caregiver—the nurse. Most nurses are not accustomed to caring for themselves, tending to put the needs of others before their own. Finding a balance between caring for others and self-care can be a challenging, lifelong pursuit.

Caring for Self While Caring for Others

Nurses can experience compassion fatigue, a condition in which one experiences loss of physical energy, burn-out, accident proneness, emotional breakdowns, apathy, indifference, poor judgment, and disinterest in being introspective (Coetzee and Klopper, 2010). Nurses often report that the needs of patients and families, as well as their own spouses and children, take priority over their own needs. They are left feeling stretched, overwhelmed, frustrated, unappreciated, and resentful. Negative feelings interfere with the ability to maintain a caring attitude and drain caring out of our interactions with others. One nurse described his episode with compassion fatigue:

> I didn't realize how tired and disinterested I had become about my work until one day my wife noted that I never talked about work anymore. Actually, she said that I never really talked about anything anymore. I had no energy, and I felt like every time I walked into the emergency department where I worked that I would scream if I saw one more drop of blood or heard one more patient crying. But I just "turned it off" and quit caring. It was a bad time in my career.

Although the NANDA-I diagnosis "caregiver role strain" refers to family caregivers and not professional nurses, some of the defining characteristics of this diagnosis are the same for nurses: anger, stress, lack of sleep, increased nervousness, frustration, lack of time to meet personal needs, low work productivity, gastrointestinal upset, impatience, difficulty performing/completing required tasks, lack of support, and insufficient time (Doenges et al., 2004, p. 139). These descriptors could also be applied to nurses who feel overwhelmed with competing demands in their work and professional lives.

Nursing theorist Jean Watson described caring as the essence of nursing practice. Caregivers who are filled with stress and negativity cannot provide an atmosphere conducive to healing. We must learn to care for ourselves to truly care for others. Watson, who is mentioned elsewhere in this text, is founder of the Center

for Human Caring in Colorado and a renowned nurse theorist, speaker, and author. She has identified the consequences of caring and noncaring for nurses (Watson, 2005). The consequences of caring for nurses include the following:

- Emotional: spiritual sense of accomplishment, satisfaction, purpose, and gratification
- Preserved integrity, fulfillment, wholeness, and self-esteem
- Living own philosophy
- Respect for life and death
- Reflective; increased knowledge
- Love of nursing

The consequences of noncaring for nurses include the following:

- Hardened attitude
- Oblivious to needs of patients and co-workers
- Robotlike manner
- Depression
- Fear
- Fatigue; worn-down feeling

Watson's work also includes the consequences of caring and noncaring for patients. She identified the consequences of caring for patients as follows:

- Emotional-spiritual: well-being, dignity, self-control, personhood
- Physical: enhanced healing, saved lives, safety, energy, fewer costs, more comfort, less loss
- Trust relationships; decrease in alienation, closer family relationships

The consequences of noncaring for patients, according to Watson, include the following:

- Humiliation, fear, feeling out of control, despair
- Helplessness, alienation, vulnerability
- Lingering bad memories
- Decreased healing, lack of trust, detachment

Professional nurses must stay tuned to themselves to avoid the consequences of noncaring for themselves and their patients. This is a lifelong challenge. How does one go about maintaining the ability to be caring? Diann Uustal (2009), an early proponent of work-life balance, recommended "creating a balanced life rather than merely maintaining a balancing act" (p. 7). She uses the analogy of the announcement heard before every flight departure: "Put on your own oxygen mask first, before assisting others who may need it" (p. 13). That announcement has a lot of relevance to our lives as professional caregivers. Just as airline passengers in an emergency depressurization need oxygen before they can help others, nurses need to meet their own needs so that they will have the physical and emotional energy to care for others.

Choosing to work in a setting that supports caring and professional nursing practice is an important strategy to reduce the stress nurses feel while at work. Hospitals are very stressful working environments for nurses today. Because of the nursing shortage and the expense involved in hiring and orienting new staff, nursing leaders in hospitals are focusing on retention—that is, keeping the nurses that they have. They realize that the atmosphere can help nurses cope with stress in the workplace, thereby enhancing retention. One example can be seen in the initiatives designed to create a "Caring Practice Environment" at Hamilton Medical Center in Dalton, Georgia (Wisdom, 2008):

- Development of a caring vision, mission, and philosophy for the department of nursing, involving all the nurses through surveys, focus groups, and interviews.
- Implementation of Caring Groups, monthly meetings with trained facilitators to promote humor, stress reduction, conflict resolution, and focus on care for self and fellow nurses.
- A caring/healing room, open 24 hours a day, where nurses can get massage therapy, paraffin treatments for hands and feet, aromatherapy, and soothing music. These services are available on a rotating and as-needed basis.
- Incorporation of new graduate nurses into a mentoring program with veteran nurses to help them integrate both clinically and socially into the world of nursing and to the caring environment.

Other activities you as an individual can do to reduce compassion fatigue and facilitate self-renewal include finding a coach or a mentor. Refer to Chapter 5 for more information about how to select and use a mentor.

Magnet Recognition Program

Another program that supports nurses is the American Nurses Credentialing Center's (ANCC's) Magnet Recognition Program. This program formally recognizes health care organizations that have a proven level of excellence in nursing care. The Magnet program was developed by the ANCC "to recognize health care organizations that provide the very best in nursing care and uphold the tradition of professional nursing practice"

(ANCC, 2009). Achieving Magnet designation demonstrates the importance of nursing and nurses to the entire organization and signals the importance of quality care and a positive practice environment for nurses. It recognizes the caliber of the nursing staff, which validates nurses for their hard work and elevates the self-esteem of the entire nursing staff. These facilities strive to be "nurse friendly," have low turnover and vacancy rates, and provide opportunities for professional and personal growth. All these factors lead to better patient care and greater career satisfaction.

Developing and Maintaining a Life-Work Balance

Nurses who feel chronically exhausted and irritable at home and at work; who worry more than usual, cannot seem to complete tasks, lack concentration, and/or are forgetful; and who have diminished self-confidence should be aware that these symptoms indicate a need for more self-care. Keeping the balance between work and personal responsibilities takes conscious and continuous effort. To remain energized and fully engaged in your profession, however, you can learn strategies to help you develop and maintain a life-work balance. Just as nurses use treatment plans to organize how they care for patients, they can also identify how to create balance in their own lives. Taking time to be with your friends and colleagues outside of work is an important strategy to reenergize yourself and prepare for the demands at work (Fig. 13.4).

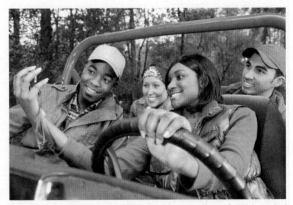

Fig. 13.4 By spending time having fun outside of the hospital, these nurses are taking care of themselves. Self-care is crucial in creating a long and healthy nursing career. (Photo used with permission from iStockphoto.)

Diann Uustal, in her book *Caring for Yourself, Caring for Others: The Ultimate Balance* (2009), recommended taking stock periodically using the guidelines listed in Box 13.11. Read these guidelines, and think about how you can begin now to apply them in your busy life. This can be the beginning of a lifelong effort to maintain balance so that you can continue to be the caring person you want to be in all aspects of your life.

BOX 13.11 Create a Balanced Life Care Plan for Yourself

Read the following ideas and reflect on their practical application in your life.

- Taking personal responsibility for your health—physically, emotionally, intellectually, socially, and spiritually—is not easy, but it is the first step. Like it or not, there is no one who can do a better job of taking care of yourself than you.
- Start today with the changes you know are healthful. Make your choices one meal at a time or one day at a time. Do not beat yourself up if you do not always stick to the care plan.
- Balance. Try to stay in balance from a holistic perspective. What this means is different to each of us and different at various stages in our own lives.
- Increase your happiness quotient. Identify the things that bring you happiness and joy and enhance your quality of life. Try to do something pleasurable or satisfying each day.
- Identify and decrease the stressors in your personal and professional life. Develop strategies for decreasing the overall level of stress in your life. Some situations and habits can be corrected easily; others will take a real commitment and time to change.
- Make sure your goals and expectations are realistic. Unrealistic goals are self-defeating. Make sure the goals are measurable, manageable, and meaningful to you, not to please somebody else.
- Give yourself permission to relax and take some time for yourself each day. Learn to take "mental health breaks," no matter how brief. Enjoy the time without thinking about what you should be doing, so you can return refreshed.
- Prioritize your commitments based on your values. Make sure you give appropriate time and attention to the relationships that have stability and meaning over time.
- Learn to say "no" if you are pressured and overcommitted. Learn to say no without feeling guilty. Practice thinking that every problem is not your sole responsibility.

- Treat yourself like you treat your best friend. Do something special and befriend yourself.
- Be a person of encouragement—to yourself. Be affirming to yourself. Do not criticize yourself harshly.
- Make your physical fitness a priority. Commit to a balanced fitness program that includes stretching, aerobic exercise, and strength exercises. Sneak exercise into your daily life and exercise with a friend.
- Nutrition. Eat a balanced diet, take a multivitamin, drink lots of water, and limit refined sugar intake. Practice portion control. If necessary, consult a dietitian.
- Sleep. Know how much you need and plan to get it. A pattern of too little sleep can injure your health. Avoid trying to be more productive by sleeping less. That can be counterproductive.
- Pay attention to your spiritual growth. Is your faith a first resort or a last resort when all else fails? What does it mean to be "spiritual"? Is being a part of a faith community important to you?
- Challenge yourself intellectually and develop your intellectual curiosity. Try to learn something new every day, no matter how small or insignificant it may seem.
- Stay connected with healthy people. Set time aside and plan for fun with people who can help you lighten up and enjoy some free time. Get out and do things you enjoy doing.
- Spend as little time as possible with people who affect you negatively.
- Make sure you get enough time alone. How much time alone each of us needs varies, so find out what is right for you. Most caregivers spend very little time alone. Check out your balance.
- Express your creativity through music, painting, needlework, sports, decorating, acting, or whatever lets you share yourself from the inside out.
- Don't be afraid to talk with a friend or a professional counselor to help you clarify your direction and put you back in balance again.

Reproduced from Uustal DB: *Caring for yourself, caring for others: the ultimate balance,* ed 2, East Greenwich, Educational Resources in Healthcare, Inc. *Orthopedic nursing,* 11(3), 11–15, 1992.

CONCEPTS AND CHALLENGES

- *Concept:* Illness is a highly personal experience and reactions to illness are affected by one's culture.

  Challenge: Culture is not always determinative of a person's responses to illness; explaining a response in terms of culture only can lead to stereotyping.

- *Concept:* Persons with illness may progress through stages of disbelief and denial, irritability and anger, attempting to gain control, depression, and acceptance and participation.

  Challenge: Stages of responses to illness are not encountered in a linear way. Patients will move back and forth between stages over time.

- *Concept:* Because of the stress and anxiety involved with illness, patients' abilities to cope may be tested.

  Challenge: Resourcefulness and resilience are characteristics of some persons who may cope with change and stress well, but coping skills can be taught to those who are not naturally as resourceful or resilient.

- *Concept:* Providing holistic care means that nurses must consider their patients' physical, mental, emotional, spiritual, social, cultural, and family strengths and challenges to personalize care.

  Challenge: Recognizing that family is a system in which a change in one member affects all the other members helps nurses anticipate ways in which a family may be affected by illness.

- *Concept:* Illness causes alterations in usual family functioning that results in emotional responses such as anger and guilt; old patterns such as fostering dependence can become very entrenched during illness.

  Challenge: The nurse needs to assess both how the family is influencing the patient and how the family is being influenced by the member who is ill.

- *Concept:* An understanding of the cultural factors that affect behaviors associated with illness can provide a better framework for the provision of nursing care that is both effective and satisfying to patients, families, and nurses.

  Challenge: Understanding that culture influences health behaviors and responses is not the same as understanding a particular culture. Effective nurses have cultural humility.

- *Concept and Challenge:* Creating a work-life balance, in which caring for self has a high priority, is the key to sustaining a caring approach to others.

IDEAS FOR FURTHER EXPLORATION

1. If you or someone close to you has been hospitalized, how did the nurses and family members encourage or discourage dependent behaviors? Independent behaviors?

2. Try to identify your own cultural group's response to illness. What are your family's characteristic responses to illness of a family member?

3. In a small group, discuss aspects of spiritual nursing care that you have been exposed to, feel comfortable using, or do not feel comfortable using. Appoint a group member to monitor those interventions or behaviors that primarily benefit the patient and those that primarily benefit the nurse. What stands out to you in terms of your response to providing spiritual care?

4. Identify the ways you show a caring attitude toward patients and toward yourself. Who do you treat better—your patients or yourself? In what ways can you provide better care for yourself?

5. Design a nurse-friendly work setting. What makes it nurse friendly? Does being nurse friendly affect the level of care your patients would receive?

REFERENCES

American Association of Colleges of Nursing: Cultural competency in baccalaureate nursing education (website), 2008. Available at: www.aacn.nche.edu/leading-initiatives/education-resources/competency.pdf.

American Nurses Credentialing Center (ANCC): ANCC magnet program: recognizing excellence in nursing services (website), 2009. Available at: www.nursecredentialing.org/Magnet/ProgramOverview.aspx.

Benson H, Klipper MZ: *The relaxation response, twenty-fifth anniversary update*, New York, 2000, HarperCollins.

Carey B: *Long-Awaited Medical Study Questions the Power of Prayer*, New York Times (website), 2006. Available at: www.nytimes.com/2006/03/31/health/31pray.html?ex-=;1145937600&en=3cd622f0fc1f109b&ei=5070.

Centers for Disease Control and Prevention: Chronic diseases: The leading causes of death and disability in the United State (website), 2015. Available at: www.cdc.gov/chronic-disease/overview/.

Coetzee SK, Klopper HC: Compassion fatigue within nursing practice: a concept analysis, *Nurs Heal Sci* 12:235–243, 2010.

Doenges ME, Moorhouse MF, Murr AC: *Nursing care plans: guidelines for individualizing client care across the life span*, Philadelphia, 2014, FA Davis.

Karademas EC, Karamvakalis N, Zarogiannos A: Life context and the experience of chronic illness: is the stress of life associated with illness perceptions and coping? *Stress Heal* 25:405–412, 2009.

Leininger M: *Personal communication*, 1999.

Massachusetts General Hospital Benson-Henry Institute for Mind Body Medicine (website), 2015. Available at: www.bensonhenryinstitute.org.

McEwen M: Spiritual nursing care: state of the art, *Holist Nurs Pract* 19(4):161–168, 2005.

Parsons T: *The social system*, New York, 1964, Free Press.

Roberts S: *A generation away, minorities may be the U.S. majority*, New York Times, 2008. pp A-1.

Selye H: *The stress of life*, New York, 1956, McGraw-Hill.

U.S. Department of Health and Human Services: *Office of Minority Health: National Standards for Culturally and Linguistically Appropriate Services in Health Care*, [Final report]. Washington, DC, 2001, U.S. Department of Health and Human Services.

Uustal DB: *Caring for yourself, caring for others: the ultimate balance*, ed 2, Jamestown, RI, 2009, Sea Spirit Press.

Watson J: *Caring science as sacred science: caritas/love and caring-healing*, King of Prussia, Penn, 2005, presentation at the American Holistic Nurses Association 25th Annual Conference.

Wisdom K: *Personal communication*, 2008.

14

Health Care in the United States

Kimberly Fenstermacher, PhD

To enhance your understanding of this chapter, try the Student Exercises on the Evolve site at http://evolve.elsevier.com/Black/professional.

LEARNING OUTCOMES

After studying this chapter, students will be able to:

- Describe the four basic categories of services provided by the health care delivery system.
- Describe the shared governance model, and explain its use in nursing.
- Relate two major mechanisms used to maintain quality in health care agencies.
- Explain how disparities in health care disproportionately affect minority and poor populations.

- Identify the key members of the interprofessional health care team, and explain what each contributes.
- Explain the economic principles of supply and demand, free-market economies, and price sensitivity, and discuss their relevance to health care costs.
- Describe current methods of payment for health care.
- Discuss the possibility of universal health care as an outcome of health care reform.

TODAY'S HEALTH CARE SYSTEM

Health care reform continues to be a hot topic in American life and across the political scene. Namely, how health care is delivered, how it is accessed, and how it is paid for have become polarizing issues. The complexities and detail cause misunderstanding and confusion. In a manner of speaking, this debate mirrors the system of health care in place in the United States today.

The term *health care system* as it is used in the United States is something of a misnomer. Rather than providing health care, the system has traditionally provided illness care, focusing on treating health problems once they have occurred rather than encouraging wellness through healthy habits. The complexity of the system has resulted in fragmentation that is difficult to understand and navigate. Although the United States has some of the most up-to-date health care technologies, highly sophisticated procedures, and well-educated health care

providers, many people do not have access to basic care and even fewer to care that is focused on wellness.

In 1979 the federal government initiated the *Healthy People* program, a science-based program that every 10 years sets forth national objectives focusing on health promotion and disease prevention. Every decade *Healthy People* sets new national health objectives and monitors the progress of these objectives, building on lessons learned in the previous decade. Input is sought from both experts and the general public through a collaborative process. The *Healthy People* campaign was instituted in the late 1990s to establish health benchmarks and monitor progress toward these benchmarks. The intention was to encourage collaborations across communities and sectors; empower persons to make informed health decisions; and measure the impact of prevention activities (www.healthypeople.gov). The main goals for *Healthy People 2020* are shown in Fig. 14.1. The Healthy

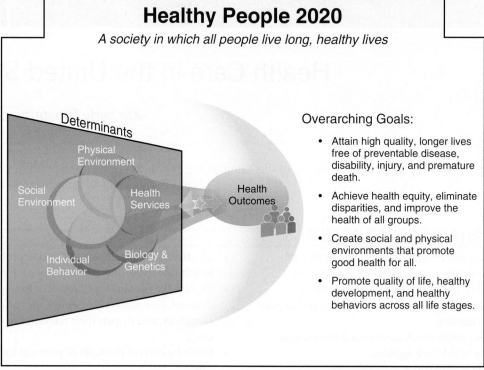

Fig. 14.1 Healthy People 2020 Framework. (From U.S. Department of Health and Human Services, Office of Disease Prevention and Health Promotion, 2018. Available at www.healthypeople.gov.)

People 2030 goals will be the fifth edition of Healthy People. These goals are being formulated upon a set of principles that include the belief that health is essential to a full-functioning, equitable society and that health and well-being for all is a shared responsibility.

The *Healthy People* initiative encourages individuals, agencies, communities, and states to participate in its programs, but it does not mandate change in the health care system. The passage of the State Children's Health Insurance Program (SCHIP) reauthorization legislation in 2009 and the Affordable Care Act (ACA) in 2010 were crucial steps in addressing systemic problems in the health care system, particularly with regard to the financing of health care by improving access to health insurance coverage for most Americans. The ACA, also known as "Obamacare," has withstood two significant challenges in the U.S. Supreme Court, one in 2012 and the other in 2015. Most recently, in 2017, an effort by Senate Republicans to repeal and replace the ACA failed because of a shortfall of support. Undoubtedly there will be challenges ahead to maintain affordable health care insurance coverage for Americans.

You are likely to enter the nursing workforce with much of the current system still recognizable. This chapter will give you basic information about the way health (and illness) care in the United States is delivered and nursing's role within this system; health care finance is also addressed.

Major Categories of Health Care Services

Four major categories of health services make up the current system: (1) health promotion and maintenance, including early detection; (2) illness prevention; (3) diagnosis and treatment; and (4) rehabilitation and long-term care. Even though these services are provided in a wide variety of settings, virtually all care falls into one of these four categories.

Health Promotion and Maintenance

Health promotion and maintenance services assist patients to remain healthy, prevent diseases and injuries, detect diseases early, and promote healthier lifestyles. These services require patients' active participation and cannot be performed solely by health care providers.

Health promotion and maintenance services are based on the assumption that patients who adopt healthy behaviors are more likely to avoid certain illnesses such as heart attacks, lung cancers, and certain infections than those whose behaviors are not as healthy.

An example of health promotion and maintenance services is prenatal classes. By adopting good nutritional and exercise habits, a pregnant woman may improve the likelihood that she will have a healthy infant born at full term. Other examples of health promotion and maintenance include education about safe driving, alcohol consumption, and responsible sexual activity.

Health promotion also includes the detection of warning signs indicating the presence of a disease in early stages. Early detection may mean minimal and less costly treatment and good patient outcomes. An example of early detection is breast self-examination and mammography, both aimed at detecting breast cancer in its early stages, thereby providing a better chance for successful treatment. There is significant disagreement among experts, however, about the necessity or wisdom of screening such as mammography or prostate-specific antigen (PSA) that may result in a high number of false-positive results and unnecessary distress and treatment. Recommendations about health screenings change as we gain new knowledge from ongoing research studies that are conducted. It is important for nurses to be aware of the latest recommendations for health promotion and maintenance.

Illness Prevention

With the increasing ability to identify risk factors, such as a family history of disease and genetic predispositions, illness prevention services are now better able to assist patients in reducing the impact of those risk factors on their health and well-being. These services require the patient's active participation.

Prevention services differ from health promotion services in that they address health problems after risk factors are identified, whereas health promotion services seek to prevent development of risk factors. For example, a health promotion program might teach the detrimental effects of alcohol and drugs on health to prevent individuals from using alcohol and drugs. Illness prevention services are used when the patient has been abusing alcohol or drugs and is at risk for developing conditions related to using these substances. The boundaries between health promotion and maintenance, early detection, and illness prevention are often

---

BOX 14.1 Examples of Health Promotion and Maintenance, Early Detection, and Illness Prevention Activities

Health Promotion/Maintenance
- Health education programs (e.g., prenatal classes)
- Exercise programs
- Health fairs
- Wellness programs (worksite/school)
- Nutrition education

Early Detection
- Mammograms
- Vision and hearing screening
- Cholesterol screening
- Periodic histories and physical examinations
- Blood glucose screening
- Osteoporosis screening

Illness Prevention
- Community health programs
- Promotion of healthy lifestyles to counteract risk factors
- Occupational safety programs (e.g., use of eye protection for work that endangers the eyes)
- Environmental safety programs (e.g., proper disposal of hazardous waste)
- Legislation that prevents injury or disease (e.g., seat belt/child restraint laws; motorcycle helmet laws).

---

blurred. Box 14.1 gives examples of activities in these three areas.

Diagnosis and Treatment

Traditionally, in the U.S. health care system, heavy emphasis has been put on diagnosis and treatment. Modern technology has enabled the medical profession to refine methods of diagnosing illnesses and disorders and to treat them more effectively than in the past. Scientific advances permit many noninvasive tests and treatments to be performed. For instance, imaging has become important in diagnosing and following the size and location of solid tumor cancers through sophisticated combinations of positron emission tomography (PET) and computed tomography (CT) images. In addition, three-dimensional (3-D) ultrasonography creates 3-D images of various organs and structures, including fetal development. Another example of advanced technology is called breast tomosynthesis, which is a special mammography technique that provides a 3-D picture that gives a clearer image and makes it easier to detect a breast mass. The future promises more noninvasive visual technologies that will aid in diagnosis and treatment.

Minimally invasive surgery techniques have transformed surgical procedures, allowing incisions of a half-inch or less. This technology has reduced postoperative pain; reduced hospital stays from days to hours, thereby reducing costs; and enabled patients to return to normal function much more rapidly. Procedures that reduce postoperative pain are especially favorable because of the national attention on the issue of addiction and the sense of urgency to reduce the use of prescription opioids.

Unfortunately, high-tech services can lead patients to feel dehumanized. This occurs when caregivers focus on machines and techniques rather than on patients. Even in high-tech settings, nurses must remember that patients benefit most when they understand their diagnoses and treatments and can be active participants in the development and implementation of their own treatment plans—in other words, when care is patient centered.

Rehabilitation and Long-Term Care

Rehabilitation services help restore the patient to the fullest possible level of function and independence after injury or illness. Rehabilitation programs also deal with conditions that leave patients with diminished functioning, such as strokes or severe burns. Both patients and their families must be active participants in this care if it is to be successful. Rehabilitation services should begin as soon as the patient's condition has stabilized after an injury or illness. These services may be provided in institutional settings such as hospitals, in special rehabilitation facilities, in long-term care facilities such as nursing homes, or in the home and the community. The objectives of rehabilitation are to assist patients to achieve the highest level of functioning possible so that they may have the best quality of life they can.

Rehabilitation services also include disease management services. Disease management services deal with chronic diseases, such as congestive heart failure and diabetes, and ongoing conditions, such as low back pain and hypertension, that contribute to higher health care costs and a reduced quality of life, particularly for aging populations. Disease management programs focus on helping participants understand and manage their chronic conditions more effectively through phone calls or e-mails, coaching and education, symptom prevention and management, and collaboration with their providers. These steps give providers information between office visits so that they can actively manage the participant's condition before emergency or hospital services are required, thus reducing health care costs and improving the quality of life for their patients.

Long-term care is provided in residential facilities such as assisted living, intermediate and skilled nursing facilities, and personal care homes. Personal care homes provide housing, food, and one or more personal services for two or more adults who are not related to the owner of the home. Long-term care is defined and regulated by states. Long-term care is tailored to provide services that the patient or family cannot provide but at levels that maintain the individual's independence as long as possible. The population is aging, and with more patients surviving serious trauma and living with illnesses that involve impairments in physical or mental functioning or both, long-term care facilities are expected to experience continuing growth.

Classifications of Health Care Agencies

There are many agencies involved in the total health care delivery system. Organizations that deliver care can be classified in three major ways: as governmental or voluntary agencies; as not-for-profit or for-profit agencies; or by the level of health care services they provide.

Governmental (Public) Agencies

Many governmental (public) agencies contribute to the health and well-being of U.S. citizens. All these public agencies are primarily supported by taxes, administered by elected or appointed officials, and tailored to the needs of the public.

Federal agencies. Federal agencies focus on the health of all U.S. citizens. They promote and conduct health and illness research, provide funding to train health care workers, and assist communities in planning and evaluating the outcomes of health care services. They also develop health programs and services and provide financial and personnel support to staff them. Federal agencies establish standards of practice and safety for health care workers and conduct national health education programs on subjects such as the benefits of not smoking, the prevention of acquired immunodeficiency syndrome (AIDS), and the need for prenatal care. Examples of federal agencies are the Centers for

Medicare & Medicaid Services (CMS), the National Institutes of Health, the U.S. Department of Health and Human Services, the Occupational Safety and Health Administration, and the Centers for Disease Control and Prevention (CDC). An example of a federally supported agency that provides care at the local level is the Federally Qualified Health Center (FQHC). According to the Health Resources and Services Administration (HRSA, 2018), an FQHC can provide primary care, dental services, and mental health services for underserved populations, such as migrant workers, the homeless, and residents of public housing.

State agencies. State health agencies oversee programs that affect the health of citizens within an individual state. Examples of state agencies include state departments of health and environment; departments of mental health; regulatory bodies that regulate and license health professionals, such as state boards of nursing; and agencies that administer Medicaid insurance programs for families and individuals in poverty. These agencies are not typically involved in providing direct patient care but license and support local agencies that do provide direct care.

Local agencies. Local agencies serve one community, one county, or a few adjacent counties. They provide services to both paying and nonpaying citizens. Public health departments are examples of local governmental agencies found in almost every county in the United States. All citizens, whether or not they can pay, are eligible for certain health care services through local public health departments. These services usually include immunizations, prenatal care and counseling, well-baby and well-child clinics, sexually transmitted infection clinics, tuberculosis clinics, and others. Community health nurses sometimes make home visits as well.

Voluntary (Private) Agencies and Nongovernmental Organizations

Citizens often voluntarily support agencies working to promote or restore health. When private volunteers support an agency providing health care, it is called a **voluntary (private) agency**. Support is generally through private donations, although many of these agencies apply for governmental grants to support some of their activities.

Voluntary agencies often begin when a group of individuals bands together to address a health problem.

Volunteers may initially perform all their services. Later they may obtain enough donations to hire personnel, staff an office, and expand services. They may be able to secure ongoing funding through grants or organizations such as the United Way. Examples of voluntary health agencies are the American Heart Association, the American Cancer Society, the American Red Cross, and the March of Dimes.

A nongovernmental organization (NGO) is an association of citizens that operates independently of the government with the goal to deliver resources or serve a social or political purpose. Much of the focus of health-related NGOs is international and involves the delivery of direct health care, providing drinkable water, mitigating endemic diseases such as malaria, and improving nutrition, among other highly significant causes. Médecins Sans Frontières (Doctors Without Borders) is a well-known NGO, as are the International Committee of the Red Cross, Oxfam, Project Hope, and Save the Children.

Not-for-Profit or For-Profit Agencies

The second major way to classify health service delivery agencies is by what is done with the income earned by the agency. A not-for-profit agency is one that uses profits to pay personnel, improve services, advertise services, provide educational programs, or otherwise contribute to the mission of the agency. A common misconception is that not-for-profit agencies do not ever make a profit. Actually, they may make profits, but the profits must be used to further the mission of the agency. Most voluntary agencies, such as the ones listed previously, are also not-for-profit agencies, as are many hospitals. The Joint Commission is an independent, not-for-profit organization that certifies health care organizations and programs in the United States.

For-profit agencies distribute profits earned to partners or shareholders. The growth in for-profit health care agencies has risen over the past several decades because of the potential for health care to be very profitable.

For-profit agencies include numerous home health care companies that send nurses and other health personnel to care for patients at home. Several large national chains of for-profit health care providers also exist and have demonstrated that it is possible to provide quality patient care and make a profit while doing so. Examples include national nursing home networks, specialty outpatient centers for ambulatory surgery, heart hospitals, urgent care clinics, and rehabilitation centers. A controversial issue related to for-profit health care organizations is the possibility that they might not treat nonpaying patients, meaning that these persons must go to publicly funded facilities that may be overburdened with patients who are unable to afford expensive health care.

Level of Health Care Services Provided

The third way in which health care services can be classified is by the level of health care services they provide. These levels have traditionally been termed *primary care, secondary care,* and *tertiary care.* A new level—*subacute care*—has emerged. These four levels are discussed next.

Primary care services. Care rendered at the point at which a patient first enters the health care system is considered primary care. This care may be provided in student health clinics, community health centers, emergency departments, physicians' offices, nurse practitioners' clinics, or health clinics at worksites. The major goals of the primary health care system are providing the following:

1. Entry into the system
2. Emergency care
3. Health maintenance
4. Management of long-term and chronic conditions
5. Treatment of temporary health problems that do not require hospitalization

In addition to treating common health problems, primary care centers are, for many citizens, where much of prevention and health promotion takes place. Access to primary care in the least costly setting is now mandated by third-party payers such as insurance companies, the government, and managed care organizations.

Secondary care services. Secondary care involves the management of a condition or illness by a specialist (e.g., endocrinologist, cardiologist, pulmonologist, oncologist) after having been referred by one's primary care provider. This includes management of patients with suspected or new diagnoses of a complex illness; evaluating patients with chronic illness who may need treatment changes; and providing counseling or other therapies that are not available in primary care settings.

Tertiary care services. Tertiary care services are those provided to acutely ill patients, to those requiring long-term care, to those needing rehabilitation services, and to terminally ill patients. Tertiary care usually involves many

health professionals working on interdisciplinary teams to design and implement treatment plans. Examples of tertiary agencies are specialized hospitals such as trauma centers, burn centers, and pediatric hospitals; long-term care facilities offering skilled nursing, intermediate care, and supportive care; rehabilitation centers; and hospices, where care is provided to the terminally ill and their families in the hospital, in the home, or in freestanding, independent hospice homes that provide a setting for terminally ill patients to die in comfort. An extension of tertiary care is even more specialized care sometimes referred to as quaternary care, such as at a research facility or very uncommon, highly specialized surgery requiring exceptional levels of training and expertise, such as fetal surgery.

Subacute care services. An additional segment of health care—subacute care services—emerged in the 1990s. Subacute care is goal-oriented, comprehensive inpatient care designed for an individual who has had an acute illness, injury, or exacerbation of a disease process. In general, the condition of an individual receiving subacute care is less complex than acute care and does not depend heavily on high-technology monitoring or complex diagnostic procedures. The goal of subacute services is to provide lower-cost health care and create a seamless transition for patients moving through the health care system.

Subacute care is generally more intensive than skilled nursing facility care and less intensive than acute inpatient care. It requires frequent patient assessment and review of the clinical course and treatment plan for a limited time ranging from several days to several months, until a condition is stabilized or a predetermined treatment course is completed.

In each of the types of health care services and agencies presented in this chapter, there is an important role for nurses to fulfill.

Organizational Structures within Health Care Agencies

The health care delivery system in the United States consists of a variety of agencies such as hospitals, clinics, associations, long-term care facilities, and home health services that provide any of the four major types of health services just discussed. Although the mission, category, and level of health care services provided vary, the organizational structures within them may be similar.

BOX 14.2 Board of Directors Responsibilities in Health Care Organizations

- Establish mission, visions, goals, and strategic plan
- Ensure the organization's financial health
- Ensure quality patient care
- Select and evaluate the CEO
- Board self-evaluation

From www.ache.org.

Organizational Structure

Organizational structure refers to how an agency is organized to accomplish its mission. The organizational structure of most agencies includes a governing body or board of directors, which may also be called a board of trustees.

Board of directors. In the past, board members were often chosen from two groups: community philanthropists, who were expected to donate generously to the facility; and physicians, who practiced in the institution. Boards were large, met infrequently, and had mainly ceremonial functions such as "rubber stamping" executive decisions or attending fundraising events.

As the health care environment has become more complex, board members are now chosen to represent various business and political interests of the community. They are expected to bring knowledge and expertise from the business world, as well as to have an appreciation and understanding of health care agencies and how they operate. Because nurses have particular expertise and perspectives about health care, they are often sought out to serve on boards.

Boards now carry significant responsibility and accountability for the mission of the organization, the quality of services provided, and the financial stability of the organization. Boards are not involved in the day-to-day running of the agency, but they are legally responsible for establishing policies governing operations and for ensuring that the policies are executed. They delegate responsibility for running the agency to the chief executive officer (CEO). Boards of directors may or may not be paid for their services. Box 14.2 is a list of the primary responsibilities of the board of directors of a health care organization. In Professional Profile Box 14.1, the editor of this text describes her role and activities as a director on the board of a large not-for-profit end-of-life care organization.

Chief executive officer. The chief executive officer (CEO) is the individual responsible for the overall daily operation and the strategic planning for the organization. He or she usually has a minimum of a master's degree in business or hospital administration. Responsibilities include making sure that the institution runs efficiently and is cost effective and carrying out policies established by the board. The CEO also has an important external role addressing health care issues in the community and usually sits on the board of directors, as well as reports to it. In larger organizations, a chief operating officer (COO) often assists the CEO to make decisions for the daily operations and leadership of the organization.

Nurses with advanced degrees and experience in administration, business, and health care policy increasingly occupy both CEO and COO positions. Boards, which are responsible for hiring CEOs, have found that the broad holistic education and clinical experience of nurses prepare them well for these positions.

Medical staff. A medical staff consists of physicians, who may be either employees of the health care organization or independent practitioners. In either case, they must be granted privileges by the board of directors to care for patients at that particular institution. They cannot simply decide to admit patients to an institution. A credentials committee, composed of members of the medical staff, performs the credentialing process. This committee is charged with the responsibility of assuring the board of directors that every physician admitted to the medical staff of that facility is a qualified and competent practitioner and that, over time, each one keeps his or her skills and knowledge updated.

In large medical centers associated with university schools of medicine, the medical staff may include house staff—that is, intern and resident physicians in their first years after completing medical school. Physician residencies are 3 to 4 years and are sometimes followed by fellowships that provide additional training in a specific field such as maternal-fetal medicine, neonatology, and pediatric surgery. Residents and fellows provide much of the hour-to-hour medical care of patients hospitalized in these settings; attending physicians make rounds with the residents and fellows usually once a day. Hospitalists—physicians who work in inpatient settings only—are becoming increasingly visible members of the health care team, managing patient care needs when a primary physician is unavailable or needs consultation. Likewise, nurse practitioners, particularly those with acute care certification, are increasingly filling a role in hospitals to provide care for hospitalized patients around the clock.

The medical staff, through its credentials committee, is also charged with the responsibility for credentialing providers such as advanced practice nurses, psychologists, optometrists, podiatrists, and others who admit or consult with patients.

Medical staff governance. In large organizations, medical staffs are usually organized by service (e.g., department of surgery, department of medicine, department of maternal-fetal medicine). The entire medical staff usually elects a chief of staff. The chief of staff and the chiefs of the various services work together with the CEO and other administrative representatives through the medical executive committee to make important decisions about medical policy and physician discipline for the institution. The rules and regulations that govern these activities are called bylaws. The board of directors, to which the physicians are responsible, must officially approve the credentialing and disciplinary actions of the medical staff.

Service on committees and leadership positions of the medical staff are time-consuming activities; therefore some institutions pay members of the medical staff a fee for special services or a stipend in recognition that time away from seeing patients reduces their income.

Nursing staff. The senior administrative nurse in an organization is known as the chief nurse executive (CNE) or chief nursing officer (CNO), vice president for nursing, or in smaller hospitals, director of nursing. Once excluded from broad institutional decision making, nurse executives today are often members of the board of directors. Progressive organizations now recognize that the CNE and the chief of the medical staff are of equal importance, and this is reflected in their organizational charts.

The educational preparation of CNEs typically requires a minimum of a master's degree in nursing, business, or health administration. Some nurse executives hold joint master of science in nursing and master of business administration (MSN/MBA) degrees or joint master of health administration and master of business administration (MHA/MBA) degrees. Many nurse executives are also choosing educational preparation at the doctoral level with a focus on leadership, such as the doctor of nursing practice (DNP) degree.

CNEs are responsible for overseeing all the nursing care provided in the institution and serve as clinical leaders and administrators. Because of the need to coordinate patient care and outcomes among all disciplines, the role may also include administrative responsibilities for departments other than nursing, such as surgery, pharmacy, respiratory therapy, and social services, among others.

The nursing staff consists of all the registered nurses (RNs), licensed practical nurses/licensed vocational nurses (LPNs/LVNs), unlicensed assistive personnel (UAP), and, in some settings, clerical and administrative assistants hired by the department of nursing. These staff members are usually organized according to the units on which they work.

Each patient care unit has its own budget and staff, for which the unit manager is responsible. The manager, who is usually a nurse, is also a communication link between the staff and the next level of management.

In large or networked organizations, there may be an additional level of management between the nurse executive and the manager of a unit. These are middle managers, known as clinical directors or supervisors. In most cases they are also nurses, but they may come from other clinical disciplines or from a business background. These directors are responsible for multiple units or for specific projects or programs. They ensure that nursing and all other services they manage are integrated with other hospital services. They also serve as the communication link between the unit managers and the executive staff.

Other nurses combine direct patient care responsibilities with research, education, and management responsibilities, such as nurse educators, nurse researchers, clinical nurse specialists, and infection control nurses. Nurses in these roles support direct care nurses and serve as expert resources to them in their areas of specialization. Examples of other specialty areas where nurses serve as experts include wound and ostomy care, case management, intravenous (IV) therapy, and quality improvement.

Nursing organization governance. In most health care agencies, nurses have a nursing staff organization. In some settings this organization serves mainly as a communication vehicle. In other more progressive settings, nurses govern themselves through the organization, much as the medical staff is expected to govern itself through the medical staff organization.

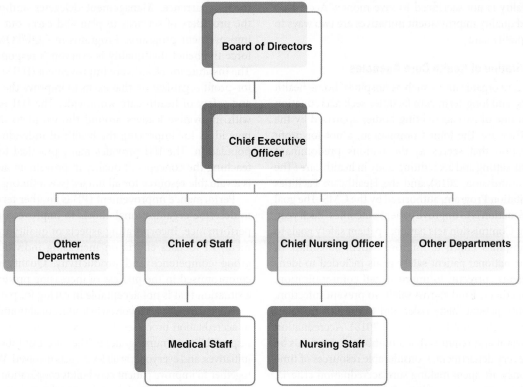

Fig. 14.2 This is a simple version of an organizational chart showing lines of responsibility in a large health care setting.

The concept of **shared governance** is founded on the philosophy that employees have both a right and a responsibility to govern their own work and time within a financially secure, patient-centered system. Shared governance promotes decentralization and participation at all levels of nursing. In shared governance, the role of the clinical nursing staff is to be responsible for the professional practice of their nursing unit by adhering to standards and benchmarks of quality care. The role of the nurse manager and other nurse leaders is to set expectations, facilitate, coordinate, support, and create partnerships with the staff in achieving the identified goals. The shared governance model promotes improved patient outcomes and enhanced nurse job satisfaction brought about by increased autonomy. Over the past several decades since the concept of shared governance was first introduced, our health care system has become more complex and nurses increasingly share in decisions and responsibilities. Experts have asserted that the time has come for nurses to replace the concept of shared governance with "professional governance" which includes

the core attributes of accountability, professional obligation, collateral relationships, and decision making (Clavelle et al., 2016). In a work environment that supports professional governance, nurses function as peers within the health care system and have the freedom to innovate and transform their practice, thereby contributing to the profession and the community.

Health care organizations are complex entities. The way they are organized may vary, but each has an organizational chart that shows its unique structure and explains lines of authority. When considering employment in a health care organization, you can learn a great deal by examining its organizational chart to see how nursing is governed and how it relates to senior management and the board of directors. Fig. 14.2 shows an example of a basic health care organizational chart.

Maintaining Quality in Health Care Agencies

Providing and maintaining high-quality services are goals of health care agencies. As pressure increases to control costs, it becomes even more important to ensure that quality is not sacrificed to save money. Accreditation and quality improvement initiatives are two ways to foster quality care.

Accreditation of Health Care Agencies

Health care organizations such as hospitals, home health agencies, and long-term care facilities seek accreditation through one of two accrediting bodies approved by the CMS. They are The Joint Commission, a not-for-profit organization that serves as the nation's predominant standard-setting and accrediting body in health care (The Joint Commission, 2018), and the Healthcare Facilities Accreditation Program, authorized by the CMS. The goal of accreditation is to improve patient outcomes. Each year, the Joint Commission sets national patient safety goals to guide hospitals' efforts to improve patient outcomes. In 2018 the national patient safety goals included to identify patients correctly, to improve staff communication, to use medicines and alarms safely, to prevent infection, to identify patient safety risks, and to prevent mistakes in surgery (The Joint Commission, 2018). Accreditation is important and requires that a number of standards be met in every department. Considerable resources of time and money are spent making sure accreditation criteria, set by these external accrediting bodies, are met.

Continuous Quality Improvement and Total Quality Management

An additional strategy through which most organizations choose to work internally toward improvement in patient outcomes is continuous quality improvement (CQI).

The concept of CQI was first developed by management expert W. Edwards Deming in the 1940s, when he suggested that managers in industry should rely on groups of employees, which he called quality circles, as they made decisions about how work was to be done. In today's health care systems, CQI, also called total quality management (TQM), is one of the most important concepts borrowed from industry. Rather than trying to identify mistakes after they have occurred, these systems focus on establishing procedures for ensuring high-quality patient care. Using quality improvement concepts, groups of employees from different departments decide how care will be provided. They decide what outcomes are desired, and they design systems and assign roles and activities to create those outcomes. Every effort is made to anticipate potential problems and prevent

their occurrence. Management delegates authority to the providers of services to plan and carry out quality improvement programs. Programs in CQI/TQM reinforce the belief that quality is everyone's responsibility. The Institute for Healthcare Improvement (IHI) is a not-for-profit organization that exists to improve the quality and safety of health care worldwide. The IHI partners with innovative leaders around the world to discover new ideas for improving the health of individuals and population. The IHI provides many practical tools for teaching the concepts of quality improvement and thus is a valuable resource for all nurses (www.ihi.org).

Performance improvement (PI) is another term used to describe organizational efforts to improve corporate performance. Incorporating aspects of quality management, PI focuses efforts on increasing individual and group competence and productivity. Quality can be compromised in the process of increasing productivity, a situation that is not acceptable in caring for patients.

Nurses are actively involved in leading quality and PI and in accreditation processes, but these activities are not the responsibility of nursing alone. They are institution-wide initiatives, and everyone, at all levels, gets involved. Working together to improve patient care builds cooperation among departments and clinical disciplines and, when done well, fosters an environment of collegiality and cooperation.

A Continuing Challenge: Health Care Disparities

The phrase *health care disparities* refers to the differences in access to and the quality of health care provided to different populations. Ethnic or racial disparities receive much attention among those examining health care delivery; however, differences also have been found to exist between the treatment and treatment outcomes of men and women, as well as younger and older people. Health care disparities may be due to race, ethnicity, gender, age, income, education, disability, sexual orientation, and rurality (Healthypeople.gov, 2018). Factors that influence health outcomes, such as the societal and economic influences that people have no power to control, are considered social determinants of health. Access to clean water, healthy food, and unpolluted air are examples of social determinants of health. Other examples include safe work places, quality education, and healthy relationships (Healthypeople.gov, 2018). The powerful influence of social determinants of health makes it difficult to reduce disparities despite increasing

CONSIDERING CULTURE BOX 14.1

The Ongoing Challenge of Disparities in Health Care

Office of Minority Health and Health Equity issued a report in 2013 listing key factors that influence health and lead to health disparity. Below are just a few of the findings from this report. For the entire report, visit www.cdc.gov/

Mortality

- The rates of premature death (death before age 75 years) from stroke and coronary heart disease were higher among non-Hispanic Blacks than among Whites.
- The infant mortality rate for non-Hispanic Black women was more than double that for non-Hispanic White women in both 2005 and 2008.

Morbidity

- Women, minority racial/ethnic groups (except Asian/Pacific Islanders), the less educated, those who spoke a language besides English at home, and those with a disability were more likely to report fair or poor self-rated health, more physically unhealthy days, and more mentally unhealthy days than others.
- Non-Asian racial/ethnic minorities continue to experience higher rates of human immunodeficiency virus (HIV) diagnoses than whites. Compared with Whites, a lower percentage of Blacks diagnosed with HIV were prescribed an antiretroviral therapy and a lower percentage of both Blacks and Hispanics had suppressed viral loads.

Health Care Access and Preventive Health Services

- During 2010, approximately two of five Hispanic adults and one of four non-Hispanic black adults were classified as uninsured. In 2010 the uninsured rate for adults aged 18 to 34 years was approximately double the uninsured rate for adults aged 45 to 64 years.

Behavioral Risk Factors

- Despite an 18% decrease in adolescent birth rates during 2007–2010, rates for non-Hispanic Black and Hispanic teenagers remain approximately double those for non-Hispanic Whites and Asian/ Pacific Islanders.

Environmental Hazards

- The likelihood of working in a high-risk occupation—an occupation with an elevated injury and illness rate—is greatest for those who are Hispanic, are low wage earners, were born outside of the United States, have no education beyond high school, or are male.

Social Determinants of Health

- The highest percentage of adults not completing high school were Hispanic, persons at <1.9% of the federal poverty level, those with a disability, or foreign born. The highest percentage of adults living below the federal poverty level were non-Hispanic Black or Hispanic, those with less than a high school education, those with a disability, or foreign born.

Modified from Office of Minority Health and Health Equity, Centers for Disease Control and Prevention. (2013): CDC Health Disparities and Health Inequalities Report, 2013 (website). Available at https://www.cdc.gov/healthequity/about/index.html

attention to their significant negative effect on large segments of the population.

You can read more in Considering Culture Box 14.1, which contains additional information about the latest trends in health disparities.

The Health Care Team

A wide array of providers deliver care across the variety and spectrum of health care settings presented in this chapter. At one time, physicians and nurses were the central members of the health care team, but as health care became complex and technology expanded, a number of other health disciplines developed. Today there are many different health care providers who come from a variety of educational backgrounds. Physicians, nurses, and all the other individuals who work with patients are called the health care team, or **multidisciplinary team.** *Multidisciplinary* refers to the presence of more than one discipline (e.g., nursing, medicine, social work) on the team working together. The team is supported in their work by a number of other departments, such as nutrition, environmental services, pharmacy, and laboratory services, among others. The decision about which of these various personnel should be involved in the care of a patient depends on the desired patient outcomes. You may also hear the term *interprofessional* used to refer to different disciplines working together to offer specialized knowledge and skills to collaboratively care for patients. Professional nurses must understand and appreciate the education and skills of all members of the health care team and strive to work effectively with them. One approach to help nurses understand how members from other health care disciplines are educated is called interprofessional education. Interprofessional education involves students from a variety of disciplines, such as nursing, medicine, and respiratory therapy, learning together during their professional training. Several of the key members who are most likely to be involved in the care of patients are discussed next.

Physicians

Physicians are responsible for assigning medical diagnoses and prescribing interventions designed to restore patient health. Although physicians have traditionally been involved mainly in restorative care and treatment of diseases and disorders, physicians now recognize the value of health promotion and maintenance, as well as illness and injury prevention. Some physicians are also integrating nontraditional or alternative treatment choices such as chiropractic medicine, acupuncture, herbal treatments, and massage therapy into their practices.

Physicians have completed college and 3 or 4 years of medical school and are licensed by a state board of medical examiners. Although a hospital residency is not required to practice medicine in all states, most physicians have completed one, and many do postgraduate work in a specialty area and then take examinations to become board certified in the specialty area.

Physician Assistants

Physician assistants (PAs) have emerged in the past 30 years as members of the health care team. According to the American Academy of Physician Assistants (2018), PAs practice medicine, including prescribing medications, as part of a health care team with physicians and other providers, working in all 50 states, the District of Columbia, and all U.S. territories except Puerto Rico.

Prerequisites for entering a PA program vary, depending on the degree offered. Virtually all programs require that applicants have health care experience before attending a PA program, which usually lasts approximately 26 months, or three academic years. Beyond graduation from this program, PAs must pass a national certifying examination and are required to be licensed by the state in which they practice. They are required to obtain continuing medical education and regularly be retested on their clinical skills. PAs may also choose to then complete a postgraduate PA program in a clinical specialty area.

Unlicensed Assistive Personnel

Unlicensed assistive personnel (UAP) are unlicensed workers who are key members of the nursing staff. UAP work under the supervision of nurses to assist with basic patient care. Certified nursing assistants (CNAs) are the most well known of UAP. Their responsibilities include the management of tasks such as assisting with personal hygiene; measuring and recording vital signs, height, weight, and intake and output (I&O); collecting and testing specimens; and reporting and recording patients condition and treatments. They also help patients meet their nutritional needs by checking and delivering food trays, assisting with feeding patients when necessary, and replenishing bedside water and ice. Additional duties include assisting patients with their mobility by turning and positioning, performing range-of-motion exercises, transferring patients to and from wheelchairs or bedside chairs, and assisting with ambulation.

To become a UAP, specialized training may be required in a vocational or technical school or a community or junior college. Individuals who become UAP sometimes pursue additional education to become LPNs/LVNs or RNs. Some other types of UAP include medical assistants, home health assistants, doulas (birth assistants), and surgical technologists. Some of these UAP have on-the-job training or short-term courses to learn a specific aspect of health care. UAP who are certified have had more in-depth training and have taken a state-sponsored certification examination; certification is not the same as being licensed, however. In some states, certain UAP such as CNAs are regulated by the nursing practice act.

Licensed Practical Nurses/Licensed Vocational Nurses

Licensed practical nurses/licensed vocational nurses (LPNs/LVNs) care for patients under the direction of physicians and RNs. (LPNs and LVNs are essentially the same—they take the same licensing examination; only Texas and California use the term *LVN*.) The supervision required varies by state and job setting. LPNs/LVNs provide basic bedside care. They measure and record patients' vital signs, such as height, weight, temperature, blood pressure, pulse, and respirations. They also prepare and give injections and enemas, monitor catheters, and perform uncomplicated wound care. They assist with bathing, dressing, personal hygiene, moving in bed, standing, and walking. They might also feed patients who need help eating. LPNs/LVNs collect samples for testing, perform routine laboratory tests, and record food and fluid I&O. They clean and monitor medical equipment. Sometimes they help physicians and RNs perform tests and procedures. Some LPNs/LVNs help care for and feed infants.

LPNs/LVNs monitor their patients and report adverse reactions to medications or treatments. They gather information from patients, including their health history and how they are currently feeling. They may use this information to complete insurance forms, preauthorizations, and referrals, and they share information with RNs and physicians to help determine the best course of care for a patient.

Most LPNs/LVNs are generalists and work in all areas of health care. However, some work in a specialized setting, such as nursing homes or doctors' offices, or in home health care. LPNs/LVNs in nursing home facilities help evaluate residents' needs, develop care plans, and supervise the care provided by nursing aides. In doctors' offices and clinics, they may be responsible for drawing blood, measuring vital signs, making appointments, keeping records, and performing other clinical and clerical duties. LPNs/LVNs who work in home health care may prepare meals and teach family members simple nursing tasks. In some states, LPNs/LVNs are permitted to administer prescribed medicines, start IV fluids, and provide care to ventilator-dependent patients (Bureau of Labor Statistics, 2018).

Training programs for LPNs/LVNs are offered in state-approved vocational or technical schools or community or junior colleges. The programs usually last 1 year. To become licensed, graduates must pass a national examination, the National Council Licensure Examination for Practical Nurses® (NCLEX-PN®), developed and administered by the National Council of State Boards of Nursing.

Dietitians

Many patients require management of their nutritional intake as part of the healing process. Others need to learn how to shop for and prepare food to maintain a healthy diet. Registered dietitians (RDs) understand how what one consumes, whether oral or IV, can affect a patient's recovery and promote and maintain health. They focus on the therapeutic value of foods and on teaching people about appropriate diets and healthy nutrition. Dietitians are especially helpful in assisting patients with specific dietary restrictions (patients with diabetes, patients seeking help with weight management) or those who need extra caloric support (high-risk neonates or people with cancer). Dietitians have bachelor's or higher degrees and may have completed internships in specialty areas, such as pediatrics. Only a person who is a nutritionist who becomes registered with the Commission on Dietetic Registration (CDR) may call him- or herself a dietitian or RD. Not all nutritionists are RDs, but all RDs are nutritionists.

Pharmacists

Pharmacists prepare and dispense medications, instruct patients and other health workers about medications, monitor the use of controlled substances such as narcotics, and work to reduce medication errors. Pharmacists require special education and training to safely and accurately prepare, dispense, and monitor the effects of complex medications on patients. Clinical pharmacists spend time on hospital units working closely with physicians and nursing case managers to coordinate complex drug administration, such as chemotherapy. They assist in monitoring and minimizing the drug interactions resulting from a patient taking multiple medications, and in outpatient settings they are involved in counseling patients about their medications (Fig. 14.3).

Pharmacists must obtain a doctor of pharmacy degree, also known as a PharmD, which takes 6 years to complete, and pass a state board of pharmacy's licensure examination (Bureau of Labor Statistics, 2018). Depending on state licensing requirements, they may also be required to complete an internship. Certified pharmacy technicians, who are certified by state licensing boards, assist them.

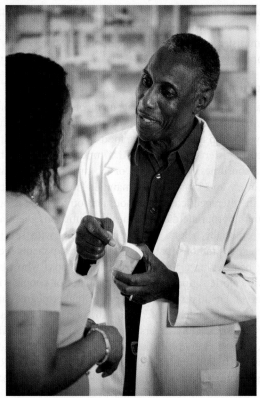

Fig. 14.3 An important part of the work of pharmacists is consulting with patients about their medications. (Photo used with permission from iStockphoto.)

Technologists

Technologists are personnel who assist in the diagnosis of patient problems.

Laboratory technologists handle patient specimens—such as blood, sputum, feces, urine, and body tissues—to be examined for abnormalities. They also manage blood banks (Fig. 14.4). Laboratory technologists carefully subject these body substances to various tests to determine deviations from normal ranges. Technologists have at least a bachelor's degree and are often assisted by laboratory technicians, who have 2-year associate degrees. Technologists must pass a state licensing examination to practice.

Radiology technologists (RTs) perform imaging procedures, assist physicians with procedures such as angioplasty, and administer therapeutic radiation. Although patients still need routine flat-plate radiography studies, technology in this field has become much more sophisticated. Subspecialties such as CT, magnetic

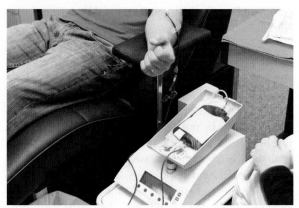

Fig. 14.4 Collection and safe management of blood are critical aspects of care in the hospital. (Photo used with permission from iStockphoto.)

resonance imaging (MRI), and PET have developed. All these techniques allow practitioners to see what is occurring inside the body without surgery. They also require specially educated technicians who operate multimillion-dollar equipment. RTs are educated in formal programs lasting from 1 to 4 years. Specific requirements, such as licensing and certification for working as an RT, vary from state to state (see www.arrt.org).

Respiratory Therapists

Acutely ill or injured patients often require assistance in breathing. Respiratory therapists operate equipment such as ventilators, oxygen therapy devices, and intermittent positive-pressure breathing machines. They also perform some diagnostic procedures, such as pulmonary function tests and blood gas analysis. With the increase in respiratory care in the home and community, these health care team members work closely with home health agencies and community health centers. Respiratory therapists must complete a 2- or 4-year educational program and obtain state licensure; in some states they must complete an internship. Respiratory therapists take a certification exam to become a certified respiratory therapist (CRT). Once credentialed as a CRT, the respiratory therapist can take an optional voluntary clinical simulation examination to earn the credential of registered respiratory therapist (www.aarc.org/careers/, 2018).

Social Workers

The social worker is specifically educated and trained to assist patients and their families as they face the impact of illness and injury. They serve as liaisons between hospitalized patients and the resources and services available in the community. They help patients and their families deal with financial problems caused by interruption of work or inadequate insurance benefits; they also direct them to the appropriate community support systems or facilities for home health care, long-term care, or rehabilitation. In addition to counseling patients and families, social workers are called on to assist other health care personnel to cope more effectively with the stresses associated with caring for patients in crisis. Social workers hold either a bachelor's or a master's degree and are licensed.

Therapists

Therapists help patients with special challenges. Physical therapists, known as physiotherapists in some countries, assist patients to regain maximum possible physical activity and strength. They focus on assessing preillness or preinjury function, current deficits, and potential for recovery. They then develop a long-term plan for gradual return to function through exercise, rest, heat, hydrotherapy, and other measures. The Commission on Accreditation in Physical Therapy Education (CAPTE) has mandated that attainment of the Doctor of Physical Therapy degree is the minimal professional educational qualification for physical therapists graduating from an accredited program in 2018 or after (www.apta.org, 2018). Physical therapists also supervise physical therapy assistants, who hold associate degrees.

Occupational therapists work with physical therapists to develop plans to assist patients in resuming the activities of daily living after illness or injury. They may help patients learn to cook, carry out their personal hygiene, or drive a specially equipped car. In addition, they assist patients to learn skills to return to their previous jobs or retrain patients for new employment options. The Accreditation Council for Occupational Therapy Education (ACOTE) has mandated that entry level into occupational therapy be at the doctoral level and programs offering the OT degree must transition to doctoral programs by 2027 (www.aota.org, 2018). Other types of therapists include recreational therapists, art and music therapists, speech therapists, and massage therapists.

Administrative Support Personnel

In all organizations, administrative support staff members are needed for clerical jobs such as admitting patients, answering phones, directing visitors, scheduling patient tests, filing insurance claims, filing forms, paying bills, facilitating payroll, and other support functions. These activities require considerable time. Hiring administrative staff members frees the clinical staff to concentrate on direct patient care.

The administrative staff ensures that the operations of the facility run smoothly and that clinicians have the resources necessary to meet patient needs. These staff members also educate the clinical staff on financial constraints and work with the staff to find ways to provide quality care at the lowest possible cost.

Keeping complete and accurate medical records is an extremely important administrative function that ensures proper insurance billing, eligibility for accreditation, and legal protection of the hospital and its staff. Registered records administrators are vital members of the administrative staff. These professionals staff the medical records department. Many organizations today now refer to the medical records departments as "health information services."

The Nurse's Role on the Health Care Team

Whatever the setting, nurses fulfill a number of roles on the health care team. As the health care delivery system changes, the evolving role of the RN requires new competencies and skills in each of the following roles.

Provider of Care

Nurses provide direct, hands-on care to patients in all health care agencies and settings. As providers, they take an active role in illness prevention and health promotion and maintenance. They offer health screenings, home health services, and an array of health care services in schools, workplaces, churches, clinics, physicians' offices, and other settings. They are instrumental in the high survival rates in trauma centers and newborn intensive care units, among others. Nurses with advanced nursing degrees are increasingly providing care at all levels of the health care system. Their breadth and depth of knowledge, their ability to care holistically for patients, and their natural partnership with physicians make nurses some of the most sought after and trusted care providers. A major role of the nurse is to ensure continuity in a patient's transition from inpatient to outpatient care through coordination of home-based services, community services, and discharge teaching.

Educator

As patient and family educators, nurses provide information about illnesses and teach about medications, treatments, and rehabilitation needs. They also help patients understand how to deal with the life changes necessitated by chronic illnesses and teach how to adapt care to the home or community setting. In the current health care climate, patients are being discharged from hospitals faster than ever before. Patients and their families must often manage complex treatments, such as central lines or feeding tubes, in the home setting.

Nurses also act as educators in community settings. The major focus of the nurse in the community setting is health promotion and injury and illness prevention. Often nurses teach classes jointly with other health care team members. For example, a nutritionist and a nurse may teach a group of expectant parents the benefits of breastfeeding their infants. Nurses also have a responsibility to understand and teach how a healthy or unhealthy environment may affect both the short- and long-term health of the community.

Nurses also serve as patient educators in disease management companies. By educating patients about their chronic diseases and coaching them in effective self-care behaviors, nurses work with the patient and the primary care provider to keep the patient healthier. Thus nurses as patient educators help reduce health care utilization and cost.

Nurses often teach other team members about the patient and family and why different interventions may have varying degrees of success. Nurses help other team members find cost-effective, quality interventions that are desired and needed by the patient rather than wasting resources on ineffective, inefficient, undesired, or unneeded services. Importantly, nurses also serve as teachers of the next generation of nurses.

The Internet plays a significant role in health education today, having transformed access to and dissemination of information for millions of Americans. Nurses functioning in the role of educator assist patients to use the Internet as an enhancement to traditional education by teaching them how to select reliable websites and evaluate the health information they find. Therefore nurse educators must keep up to date with technology advances as related to teaching patients.

Manager

In their daily work, all nurses are managers. The bedside staff nurse must manage the care of a group of patients,

> ### BOX 14.3 Key Elements of the Role of Nurse Administrator
>
> - Nursing practice issues
>   - Nursing autonomy
>   - Accountability for nursing practice
>   - Nursing control of nursing practice
>   - Promotion of evidence-based practice
> - Oversight of practice environment
>   - Safe and healthy workplace
>   - Evidence-based practice
>   - Adequate numbers of competent staff
> - Communication between staff and administration
> - Promotion of positive working relationships
> - Responsible stewardship of resources

Data from American Nurses Association (ANA): *Nursing administration: scope and standards of practice*, ed 2, Silver Spring, Md, 2016, ANA, p. 11.

prioritize how to accomplish patient care activities during an 8- or 12-hour period, and determine staff and patient assignments. Nurses are also involved in reviewing patient cases and coordinating services so that quality care can be achieved at the lowest cost.

In addition, nurses serve in the role of managers of patient care units, outpatient clinics, or home health agencies. The effective management of nursing resources is essential. With budgets ranging from hundreds of thousands to millions of dollars, nurse managers manage "businesses" larger than many small companies. Nurse managers must have clinical and administrative expertise, including leadership, human resources, finance, organizational behavior, system and program design, outcome research, and marketing.

Chief nursing officers, also known as chief nurse executives, may manage more than 1000 employees and multimillion-dollar budgets. They interact with other top executives and community leaders, often sitting on the health care organization's board of directors. CNEs must ensure the quality of nursing care within financial, regulatory, and legislative constraints. As noted earlier, nurses often serve as patient care executives, COOs, and CEOs. Key responsibilities of nurse administrators, both as managers and executives, are listed in Box 14.3.

Researcher

All nurses should be involved in nursing research whether or not research is a nurse's primary responsibility.

According to the ANA's *Scope and Standards of Practice 2015* (ANA, 2015), the RN integrates research findings into practice and engages in evidence-based practice. Nurse researchers investigate whether current or potential interventions work to achieve their expected outcomes, what options for care may be available, and how best to provide care. Nursing research is focused on many aspects of phenomena important to nursing, such as patient outcomes, the nursing process, nursing systems, aspects of patient care, and interventions, in addition to testing theory.

Outcomes research has become an integral part of the health care delivery system. Insurers and regulatory agencies require health care organizations to report outcome data related to quality of care, which requires research by nurses. Participation in research by all nurses is essential to the growth and development of the nursing profession. The increasing emphasis on evidence-based practice underscores the need for nurses at all levels to know how to evaluate and use research.

Collaborator

With so many health care workers involved in providing patient care, collaboration among the professions is increasingly important. The collaborator role is a vital one for nurses to ensure that everyone agrees on the same goals and plan to reach the best patient outcomes. Interprofessional teams require collaborative practice, and nurses play key roles as both team members and team leaders. Collaboration requires that nurses understand and appreciate what other health professionals have to offer. Nurses must also interpret to others the nursing needs of patients.

An often-overlooked collaborative function of nurses is collaboration with patients and families. Involving patients and their families in the plan of care from the beginning is the best way to ensure their cooperation, enthusiasm, and willingness to work toward the best patient outcomes. More in-depth information about collaboration can be found in Chapter 12.

Patient Advocate

The word *advocate* comes from Latin *advocare,* meaning "to call to one's aid." Some nursing experts believe that being a patient advocate is the most important of all the nursing roles. Rules and regulations designed to help a complex health care system run efficiently can sometimes get in the way of a patient's treatment, and an impersonal health care system may infringe on a patient's rights. This may occur when there is an unsafe patient load, a patient is being discharged too early, a treatment plan needs revision, or the patient's wishes are not being followed (Trossman, 2008). Advocacy is an important part of patient-centered care; therefore it is every nurse's constant responsibility to advocate for patients—that is, to "call to [their] aid" when they cannot do this for themselves.

Nurses who are advocating for patients must know how to cut through the levels of bureaucracy and red tape of health care organizations and stand up for the patient's rights, advocating for his or her best interests at all times. They must value patient self-determination—that is, the patient's right to autonomy and therefore independence in decision making.

Nurses advocate more effectively as they mature in their practice. As an advocate, nurses sometimes help patients bend the rules when it is in the patient's best interests and doing so will harm no one. The discussion on Benner's Stages of Nursing Proficiency in Chapter 5 underscores the ability of more experienced nurses to know when it is safe and appropriate to bend rules. Patient advocates are nurses who realize that policies are important and govern most situations well but occasionally can, and should, be stretched or even broken. For example, special care units may have restricted visiting hours. Family members may be allowed to see the patient for only 10 minutes each hour. If a patient's recovery appears to be impeded as a result of his or her separation from family, the nurse, as the patient's advocate, may allow them more generous visitation than the policy provides.

Well-prepared nurses participate both as leaders and as members of the interdisciplinary team, with the best interests of their patients always their first priority.

Nursing Care Delivery Models

Before World War I, nurses usually visited the sick in their homes to care for them. As hospital care improved and nursing education evolved, more sick people were treated in hospitals. Providing care to groups of patients rather than to individuals required nurses to be efficient and use their time effectively. Over the years, various types of care delivery models were designed to meet the goals of efficient and effective nursing care. Organizing patient care today often requires the professional nurse to work through other care providers, such as UAP and

BOX 14.4   Principles for Selecting a Care Delivery Model

The care delivery model should do all of the following:

- Facilitate meeting the organization's goals
- Be cost effective
- Contribute to meeting patients' outcomes
- Provide role satisfaction for nurses
- Allow implementation of the nursing process
- Provide adequate communication among all health care providers
- Support RNs' responsibility for the overall direction of nursing care
- Be designed to give RNs the responsibility, authority, and accountability for planning, organizing, and evaluating nursing care
- Ensure that the skills and knowledge of each care provider are used for the best patient outcomes
- Ensure that communication can occur
- Ensure that the model advances professional nursing practice
- Provide for care that is perceived by the patient as a coherent whole (unity of action by a team of RNs, LPNs/LVNs, or others)
- Provide the work groups of RNs, LPNs/LVNs, and other workers the appropriate knowledge required to meet the nursing care needs of the patient

From Rogers R: Adapting to the new workplace reality: maximizing the role of RNs within a collaborative nursing practice model, *Info Nurs* 39(1):18–20, 2008.

LPNs/LVNs, to achieve excellent patient outcomes. Delivery of high-quality patient care does not happen by chance. Each nurse manager, in collaboration with the staff, must select a care delivery model appropriate for the unit, the acuity of the patients, and the type and number of nursing staff members available. There are a number of principles for selecting a care delivery model. Box 14.4 lists 13 principles to consider when selecting a care delivery model.

Four patient care delivery models—team nursing, primary nursing, case management nursing, and patient-centered care—are reviewed in this chapter.

Team Nursing

In response to the frustration some nurses felt when using a functional approach to patient care, Lambertson (1953) designed **team nursing**. She envisioned nursing teams as democratic work groups with varying skill levels represented by different team members. They were assigned as a team to a defined group of patients.

Team nursing has been widely used in hospitals and long-term care facilities. The team usually consists of an RN, who serves as team leader; an LPN/LVN; and one or more UAP. The team leader, although ultimately responsible for all the care provided, **delegates** (assigns responsibility for) certain patients to each team member. Each member of the team provides the level of care for which he or she is best prepared. The least skilled and most inexperienced members care for the patients who require the least complex care, and the most skilled and experienced members care for the most seriously ill patients who require the most complex care.

In team nursing the RN team leader supervises and coordinates all care for a particular shift, makes assessments, and documents responses to care. The LPN/LVN team member provides direct care by performing treatments and procedures and reporting patient responses to the team leader. The UAP provides routine, direct personal care. Today, team nursing is still used, but the model is often modified. Many of the patient-focused care models use RNs as team leaders coordinating care for a group of patients and supervising multiskilled workers who have been trained to perform a variety of comfort measures such as positioning and technical procedures such as taking vital signs or drawing blood.

Team nursing has both advantages and disadvantages; these are presented in Box 14.5.

Primary Nursing

Developed in the 1970s as a result of the increased acuity (severity of illness) of hospitalized patients, **primary nursing** was designed to promote the concept of an identified nurse for every patient during the patient's stay on a particular unit. The goal of primary nursing is to deliver consistent, comprehensive care by identifying one nurse who is responsible, has authority, and is accountable for the patient's nursing care outcomes for the period during which the patient is in a unit.

In primary nursing, each newly admitted patient is assigned to a primary nurse. Primary nurses assess their patients, plan their care, and write the plan of care. While on duty, they care for their patients and delegate responsibility to associate nurses when they are off duty. Associate nurses may be other RNs or LPNs/LVNs.

BOX 14.5 Team Nursing Advantages and Disadvantages

Advantages
- Potential for building team identity
- Provides comprehensive care
- Each worker's abilities used to the fullest
- Promotes job satisfaction
- Decreases nonprofessional duties of RNs

Disadvantages
- Ongoing need for communication among team members requires commitment of time
- All team members must promote teamwork, or team nursing is unsuccessful
- Team composition varies from day to day, which can be confusing and disruptive and decreases continuity of care
- May result in blurred role boundaries, resulting in confusion and resentment

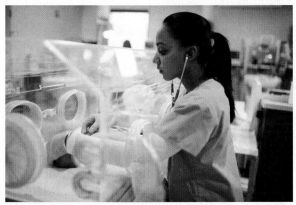

Fig. 14.5 Sick infants and those born prematurely commonly have long stays in neonatal intensive care units, where primary nursing is often practiced. (Photo used with permission from iStockphoto.)

Patients are divided among primary nurses in such a manner that each nurse is responsible for the care of a group of patients 24 hours a day. Unless there is a compelling reason to transfer a patient, the primary nurse cares for the patient in the unit from the time of admission to the time of discharge. The primary nurse may be assisted by other care providers (such as other nurses, aides, and technicians) but retains **accountability,** or responsibility, for care outcomes 24 hours a day while the patient is in the unit. The primary nurse communicates effectively with associate nurses caring for the patient on other shifts and with primary nurses in other units if the patient is transferred (e.g., to the operating room or intensive care unit). Fig. 14.5 shows a nurse caring for an infant in the neonatal intensive care unit, where the complex care and the prolonged hospital stays of their tiny patients is amenable to primary nursing.

Primary nursing is used in a variety of settings and is often modified from its original form. Advantages and disadvantages of primary nursing are listed in Box 14.6.

Case Management Nursing

A more recent evolution in nursing care delivery is case management nursing. Begun in the late 1980s as an attempt to improve the cost effectiveness of patient care, case management allows the nurse to oversee patient care and manage the delivery of services from all health care disciplines throughout a patient's illness. Nursing case management keeps costs down by striving to achieve predetermined daily patient outcomes within a specified period for patients within the same diagnostic group—for example, patients having total knee replacement. The desired daily outcomes are outlined in a plan of care called a care map or critical path. You may also hear these referred to as clinical care plans or tracks.

Two models of case management nursing have evolved over time. These are characterized by either an "internal" focus, in which the case manager works within a treatment facility, or an "external" approach, in which the case manager oversees patients and the delivery of services over the continuum of an illness or chronic disease, whether patients are in a treatment facility or at home. Although different in scope, these two models share the same principles of efficiency and cost effectiveness.

In the internal model of case management, nursing case managers serve as primary nurses for patients in an identified diagnostic group, such as spinal cord injury. They not only care for these patients while on their assigned units but also manage the plans of care from admission to discharge, crossing interdepartmental lines. Although nursing case managers do not physically provide care to the patient group on units other than their own, they actively collaborate with primary nurses assigned to the patients in those units. In this nursing model, critical paths are used for all patients. A **critical path** is an interdisciplinary agreement showing who will provide care in a given time frame to achieve agreed-on outcomes. The use of critical paths is

---

BOX 14.6   Primary Nursing Advantages and Disadvantages

Advantages
- High patient and family satisfaction
- Promotes RN responsibility, authority, autonomy, and accountability
- Nurse can care for entire patient—physically, emotionally, socially, and spiritually
- Patient knows nurse well, and nurse knows patient well
- Promotes patient-centered decision making
- Increases coordination and continuity of care
- Promotes professionalism
- Promotes job satisfaction and sense of accomplishment for nurses

Disadvantages
- Difficult to hire all RN staff
- Expensive to pay all RN staff
- Nurses are not familiar with other patients, making it difficult to "cover" for one another
- May create conflicts between primary and associate nurses
- Stress of around-the-clock responsibility
- Heavy responsibility, especially for new nurses

BOX 14.7   Case Management Nursing Advantages and Disadvantages

Advantages
- Promotes interdisciplinary collaboration
- Increases quality of care
- Is cost effective
- Eases patient's transition from hospital to community services
- Nurse has increased responsibility

Disadvantages
- Requires additional training
- Requires nurses to be off the unit for periods of time
- Is time consuming
- Is most useful only with high-risk patients and high-cost/high-volume conditions

---

intended to standardize patient care and allow hospitals to plan staffing levels, lengths of stay, and other factors that heretofore could not be anticipated. Patients whose progress varies from the path are quickly identified. Once the causes for the variation are identified, team members attempt to plan solutions to reduce variances and get the patient back on track. The goal is to treat each patient by using best practices to reduce the length of stay, thereby reducing costs.

In the external model of case management, nurse case managers are part of a large network consisting of, for example, hospitals, clinics, home health agencies, and long-term care settings. They may provide services anywhere in the system, as well as when the patient is at home. They partner with patients and their families to achieve the goal of preventing hospitalizations, thereby reducing costs and minimizing disruptions to the patient's life and family. Nurse case managers play an important role in assuring safe transitions of care as patients move through the health care system from hospital to home.

As can be seen from the type of activities in which they engage, case managers perform complex and challenging work. Nurses generally need about 5 years of clinical experience to fill this role effectively. Social workers, psychologists, rehabilitation counselors, or other professionals may also serve as case managers. All case managers, regardless of their discipline, work to reduce the cost of providing services through coordination of providers across the continuum of care. Advantages and disadvantages of case management nursing are shown in Box 14.7.

Patient-Centered Care

Patient-centered care is a contemporary care delivery model implemented by a multidisciplinary team of health professionals. This model of care is based on the patient's right to individualized care that takes his or her values and beliefs into consideration when planning and providing care. Nurses and other providers must be flexible, respect the patient's beliefs and wishes, and negotiate with the patient to meet patient expectations.

BOX 14.8 Patient-Centered Care Advantages and Disadvantages

Advantages
- Expedites care
- Promotes patient convenience
- Capitalizes on professional competence of team members
- Emphasizes continuum of care and reduces fragmentation of care
- Uses resources efficiently
- Fosters teamwork, collaboration, and communication

Disadvantages
- Requires "right staff at right time" to meet patient needs
- Difficult to explain; uses several models of care delivery
- Expensive, requires a high percentage of RNs with both clinical and management skills

Modified from Shirey MR: Nursing practice models for acute and critical care: overview of care delivery models, *Crit Care Nurs Clin North Am* 20:365–373, 2008.

Patient-centered care is more an attitude than a particular model of care, and traditional models, alone or in combination, may be used. The attitude of caregivers is that patients' needs have priority over the institution's needs. The model was pioneered by the Planetree Institute in 1978 after its founder experienced several "dehumanizing" hospitalizations. Patient-centered care brings together traditional and nontraditional components of care that work toward optimizing the healing environment. Such components as the architectural design of the facilities; educational programs for patients and families; emphasis on beauty, gardens, art, food, and nutrition; availability of complementary therapies such as massage and aromatherapy; emphasis on spirituality; and community interaction are the hallmarks of patient-centered care. These components are integrated with best medical practices to form a coherent continuum of care characterized by teamwork, communication, and collaboration among professionals and with patients and families. Advantages and disadvantages of patient-centered care are shown in Box 14.8.

FINANCING HEALTH CARE

The health care system in the United States is characterized by high costs and a large number of uninsured citizens, although those numbers have decreased substantially since the individual mandate provision of the ACA was upheld by the U.S. Supreme Court in 2012. The nation's dilemma remains: how to provide high-quality health care services to all citizens while keeping costs down.

Among developed nations, the United States has, by far, the largest percentage of its gross domestic product (GDP) spent on health care, yet has some of the worst health outcomes. Financial issues profoundly affect nurses and nursing practice. These issues affect nurses professionally, in their nursing practice, and personally, in the type of insurance and health services they and their families are able to afford. Therefore students of professional nursing need to understand the overall economic context in which nursing care is provided. In this section, several concepts necessary to understanding health care finance will be explored, including basic economic theory, the economics of nursing care, a brief historical review of the causes of health care cost escalation, cost-containment efforts, current methods of payment, and the role nurses can play in managing health care costs in their everyday work settings.

Basic Economic Theory

Nursing school curricula do not typically require undergraduates to take courses in economics, yet there is an urgent need for nurses to understand the economic context in which they practice.

Supply and Demand

A basic economic theory is the law of supply and demand. According to this theory, a normal economic system consists of two parts: suppliers, who provide goods and services, and consumers, who demand and use goods and services. In a monetary environment—that is, one in which money is used as a unit of exchange—consumers exchange money for desired goods and services.

In an efficient marketplace, the market price of goods and services serves to create an equilibrium in which supply roughly equals demand, and demand roughly equals supply. When demand exceeds supply, prices rise. When supply exceeds demand, prices fall.

Principles of the Free-Market Economy

In a free-market economy, consumption of any good or service is determined by an individual's ability to pay. In a pure free market, a portion of the population would be denied health care if they were unable to pay. People who support this position consider health care a privilege. Conversely, others believe that everyone should have access to basic health care and consider health care a right, to be administered at the federal and state levels of government. An example of this is the United Kingdom, where the National Health Service (NHS) provides access to basic health care to its citizens.

Despite the United States' general posture favoring a free-market economy, most Americans consider health care a right, not a privilege. Rather than allowing economically disadvantaged citizens to do without health services, the federal government has taken steps to ensure certain groups have access to health care services through publicly funded programs such as Medicare and Medicaid. Although this is generally considered an ethical policy, it is nevertheless a policy decision that is inconsistent with free-market principles.

Price Sensitivity in Health Care

In the days before health insurance existed, people paid their own medical bills; providers set their fees with some sensitivity to what patients could afford to pay; and many physicians used sliding-scale payment plans or accepted in-kind payments, for example, exchanging medical care for farm products or a service such as cobbler services. Health insurance created an indirect payment structure known as **third-party payment** that removed price sensitivity from the concern of most health care consumers because they pay only a small portion of the actual costs. A third party (the employer, insurance company, or government) pays the rest. If someone other than the consumer pays, demand can increase because the consumer may be insensitive to or unaware of costs.

Additional Influences on the Health Care Market

Economists have identified a number of other factors that affect the health care market in ways that violate the assumptions surrounding an effective free-market system. For example, consumers cannot always control demand for health care services. With ordinary products, a consumer can delay a purchase until there is a sale or forgo the purchase altogether. Health care is different because health care needs tend to be immediate. The consumer might suffer serious harm or even death by a delay in seeking services. Certainly in the case of severe traumatic injury, delay of care is not possible, and the costs of the intensive care using sophisticated

technologies are enormous in this circumstance. The leading cause of personal bankruptcy in the United States today is medical expenses.

Economics of Nursing Care

Until fairly recently, few efforts were made to determine the actual cost of nursing care. The average hospital bill simply included the cost of nursing services in the general category of "room rate," just as housekeeping services, linens, and food are included in the room rate. It was assumed that the cost of nurses contributed a major portion of overall hospital expenses. During difficult economic times, the first cost-reduction efforts were therefore aimed at reducing the number of nursing personnel, sometimes substituting lower-paid UAP. However, research did not support this prevailing view about the costs of nursing. Instead, research showed that determining the cost of nursing services and developing standardized reimbursements based on costs would enhance the ability of nurse managers to control nursing resources and negotiate for a fair share of hospital financial resources, and many efforts to determine the actual cost of nursing services were conducted.

Not knowing the exact costs of nursing services limits nursing management's ability to calculate the expense required to provide nursing care. Determining the best ratio of RNs to LPNs/LVNs and UAP in each unit is also impaired when the cost of nursing care is unknown. Different patients require different amounts of nursing time, depending in large part on how sick they are. **Patient classification systems** were developed to identify patients' needs for nursing care in quantitative terms to help hospitals determine the need for nursing resources. However, estimating the cost of nursing services remains an inexact science. Evidence-Based Practice Box 14.1 describes a major study to determine the economic value of professional nursing.

When the drive to provide high-quality nursing care meets the constraints of cost containment head-on, it can create a very difficult situation. What nurses hope, as both providers and consumers of health care, is that quality will not suffer because of the emphasis on "the bottom line." The financial realities that affect the institutions in which most nurses practice—hospitals—cannot be ignored. To stay in business, hospitals must make at least enough money to pay personnel, maintain buildings and equipment, and pay suppliers of goods and services.

EVIDENCE-BASED PRACTICE BOX 14.1
Demonstrating Nursing's Value

The ANA, with a coalition of other nursing associations, supported a study to improve the understanding of the economic value of the services of RNs. The objective was to quantify the economic value of professional nursing to help shape staffing decisions and policies in the nation's hospitals. A group of researchers from George Mason University in Virginia and a nearby health care policy research firm, the Lewin Group, conducted the study. They reviewed the research literature on the relationship between RN staffing levels and adverse patient outcomes for a number of nursing-sensitive *nosocomial* (hospital-acquired) complications. Examples of nursing-sensitive complications include urinary tract infections, pressure ulcers, blood infections, postoperative infections, patient falls, and adverse drug events, among others. They used data from a comprehensive literature review, as well as from the 2005 Nationwide Inpatient Sample of more than 1000 hospitals sponsored by the Agency for Healthcare Research and Quality.

The cost of complications—in increased length of stay, health care expenditures, and losses of national productivity—were subjected to statistical analyses to determine estimates of the economic value of nursing. The researchers reported that, as a result of increasing nurse staffing levels, patient risk of nurse-sensitive complications and hospital length of stay both decreased, "resulting in medical cost savings, improved national productivity, and lives saved" (p. 97). They concluded that only a portion of professional nurses' services "can be quantified in pecuniary terms, but the partial estimates of economic value presented illustrate the economic value to society of improved quality of care achieved" (p. 97) through higher RN staffing levels.

Modified from Dall T, Chen Y, Seifert R, et al.: The economic value of professional nursing, *Med Care* 47(1):97–104, 2009.

The leadership of the ANA has been repeatedly outspoken in their assertion that overzealous cost-containment efforts have led to lower-quality hospital care. A strong boost to their contention that the number and mix of nurses in a hospital make a difference in patient outcomes came early in the 21st century with research that showed an increased patient death rate with higher patient to nurse ratios (see Chapter 1). Peter Buerhaus, PhD, RN, FAAN, of Montana State University, a nurse and a health care economist, has developed a substantial body of work related to nurse-patient ratios and other matters related to the nursing workforce. As research continues to demonstrate the link between nursing and quality of care, the demand for nurses will continue to increase.

History of Health Care Finance

Before 1945, more than 90% of Americans either paid directly from their own pockets for health care or depended on charity care. Few had private health insurance. Public insurance programs, such as Medicare and Medicaid, did not exist. After World War II, most industrialized countries began publicly financed health care systems that provided care for all citizens. The United States, however, did not adopt a public, universal access system, choosing instead to continue the private, fee-for-service system.

The entire history of health care finance in this country is a fascinating study in unintended consequences. As each initiative to improve coverage, access, and quality was implemented, it opened up unforeseen loopholes that have driven costs skyward. Providers, such as hospitals, physicians, insurers, pharmaceutical companies, and others, have learned to "work the system," exploiting loopholes while protecting or enhancing their own bottom lines. All the while, population growth and increases in the number of elderly and chronically ill Americans have further complicated efforts to find solutions.

If you are interested in learning more about the complex history of health care finance, including cost-containment initiatives through the years and factors fueling increases in health care costs, refer to the Evolve website (http://evolve.elsevier.com/Black/professional).

Current Methods of Payment for Health Care

There are four major methods of payment for health care in use today: private insurance, Medicare, Medicaid, and personal payment, or self-pay. Workers' compensation is an additional mechanism for financing some health care services. Each of these is briefly explained in the following paragraphs.

Private Insurance

Private insurance, also called voluntary insurance, is a system wherein insurance premiums are paid by either insured individuals or their employers or are shared between individuals and employers. Periodic payments (**premiums**) are paid into the insurance plan, and certain health care benefits are covered as long as the premiums are paid. Early in the development of private insurance, many treatments were covered only if they were performed in an inpatient (hospital) setting. This feature drove up the cost of services. Today most insurers stipulate that costs of hospitalization are reimbursable only if treatment cannot be performed on an outpatient basis, where costs are typically lower. Most private insurers are heavily influenced by the federal insurance program, Medicare, in determining coverage and amount of reimbursements they will pay.

Medicare

Medicare, or Title XVIII of the Social Security Act, is a nationwide federal health insurance program established in 1965. Medicare is available to people aged 65 years and older, regardless of the recipient's income. It also covers certain disabled individuals and anyone with permanent kidney failure requiring dialysis or a kidney transplant. Medicare has four basic programs.

The first program, known as Part A (Hospital Insurance), helps cover inpatient hospitalization, part-time or intermittent skilled care in nursing facilities, hospice care, and some home health care. Long-term care or custodial care is not covered. Hospice care, available to people with a terminal illness who are expected to live 6 months or less as certified by a physician, is covered under Medicare. People who paid Medicare taxes while working do not pay a Part A premium, but they do pay a deductible, and certain restrictions apply to lengths of stay and benefit periods.

Part B (Medical Insurance) is a supplementary medical insurance program that covers visits to physicians' offices and other outpatient services. It also covers some preventive services. There is a 20% copay for medical and other services and a $183 yearly deductible. Mental health services are covered at 50%. Part B premiums are subject to means testing, meaning that individuals with higher incomes pay more in monthly premiums than do those with lower incomes. In 2018 the monthly premium ranged from $134.00 for individuals with a yearly income less than $85,000 to $428.60 for individuals with a yearly income more than $160,000 (CMS, 2018). The Internal Revenue Service provides tax return information to Medicare to assist in verifying income.

Part C (Medicare Advantage Plans) offers a variety of managed-care options instead of the fee-for-service

programs of Parts A and B. Part C plans are run by private companies approved by Medicare. Costs and services vary by plan.

Part D (Prescription Drug Coverage) is an additional supplementary insurance program that helps cover prescription drug costs. Part D has complex regulations including a "gap" period in coverage that many find difficult to understand. In addition to the four basic parts of Medicare, Medigap plans, or supplemental coverage, are available to Medicare-eligible individuals. They are sold by private insurance companies to help fill the "gap" between Medicare and out-of-pocket costs.

Originally intended to be a no-cost or low-cost program for the elderly, the cost of participating in Medicare has risen steadily. Although the program was originally designed to be all-inclusive, many elderly people now find they cannot afford to participate in Medicare. Ironically, some elderly are so poor that they qualify for Medicaid assistance (described next) in paying their Medicare premiums. Medicare regulations and costs change annually. For the most recent updates on Medicare, consult www.medicare.gov.

Medicaid

Medicaid, or Title XIX of the Social Security Act, is a group of jointly funded federal-state programs for low-income, elderly, blind, and disabled individuals. It, too, was established in 1965. There are broad federal guidelines, but states have some flexibility in how they administer the program. People must meet eligibility requirements determined by each state. Eligibility depends on income and varies from state to state. Rates of payment also vary, with some states providing far higher payments than others. The amount the federal government contributes to Medicaid varies from a minimum of 50% of total costs to a maximum of 76.8%.

The differences in eligibility and payment rates lead to wide variations in the level of care provided to the poor in different states and create disparities in care. In contrast to those on Medicare, people who receive Medicaid are not required to pay any fees to participate. Table 14.1 highlights the similarities and differences in the Medicare and Medicaid programs.

Personal (Out-of-Pocket) Payment

Personal payment for health care services is the least common method. Few people can afford **out-of-pocket payment** for more than the most basic health services. At

TABLE 14.1 Facts about Medicare and Medicaid

	Medicare	Medicaid and State Children's Health Insurance Plan (SCHIP)
Funding	Federal government	Federal and state governments
Administration	Federal government	State governments
Eligibility	≥65 years ≤65 with certain disabilities All ages with end-stage renal disease	*Mandatory eligibility groups:* 133% of the federal poverty level for all Americans ≤65 years based on modified adjusted gross income (MAGI) *SCHIP:* Varies by state, but many states have expanded coverage for children above the federal minimums
Level of benefits	National program with no variation in benefits across states	Varies from state to state
Payment by recipients	Some monthly premiums are required for different parts (A, B, C, D) but varies by plan	States can charge premiums and enrollment fees for certain groups
Coverage	Inpatient care, outpatient care, prescriptions	Comprehensive inpatient and outpatient care, prescriptions with lower copayments for use of generic versus brand-name drugs

Modified from data retrieved from www.medicare.gov and www.medicaid.gov, 2018.

today's prices, an illness or injury severe enough to require hospitalization can quickly exhaust a family's financial reserves, forcing them into bankruptcy. In general, only those people without access to some form of private group insurance or public insurance rely on personal payment. It can take years for a family to pay a single large medical bill.

Workers' Compensation

Workers' compensation constitutes a small proportion of insurance coverage. The program varies from state to state but generally covers only workers who are injured on the job. It usually covers treatment for injuries and weekly payments during the time the worker is absent from work for injury-related causes. In the case of accidental death, the worker's family receives compensation. Companies are required by law to contribute to a compensation fund from which money is withdrawn when accidental injuries or deaths occur at work.

In Fig. 14.6 you can see what health care dollars are spent on in the United States. Note the large percentage that is spent on physician/clinical and hospital care and that 10% is spent on prescription drugs.

Nurses' Role in Managing Health Care Costs

Staff nurses can play an important role in controlling health care costs. They have the most frequent and direct contact with patients and can have a positive impact by reducing unnecessary spending. Reducing spending does not have to mean sacrificing quality patient care. Many small economic changes can lead to large savings.

The first step is to become cost conscious. As a group, nurses tend to have limited awareness of costs. When they are made aware of costs, their supply use patterns can change. Such simple methods as posting the price of supplies on shelves, cutting down on "borrowing" between units, and transferring all patients' bedside equipment, medications, and supplies carefully can make dramatic changes in per-patient expenditures. Making staff nurses aware of less-expensive alternatives is only one way they can reduce costs. Starting or expanding a revenue-generating recycling program is another measure that all hospital employees can support.

Nurses are positioned to produce even more meaningful savings by providing excellent patient care and being advocates for their patients' personal finances. Nurses must recognize that no matter how well-insured patients may be, they will have to pay some portion of charges personally. Even a small percentage of a health care bill can be huge, given the high costs of care. A family's financial resources can be quickly overloaded.

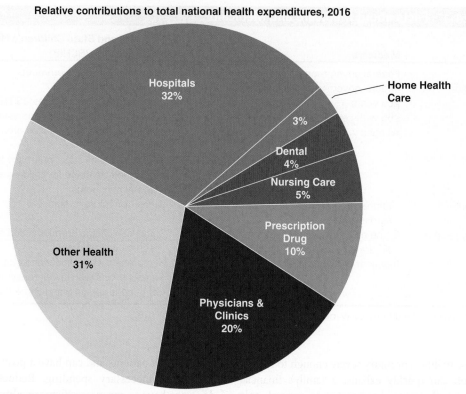

Fig. 14.6 Distribution of health spending: Hospital care and physician/clinical services account for slightly more than half of health care expenditures. (From Kaiser Family Foundation analysis of National Health Expenditure (NHE) data from Centers for Medicare and Medicaid Services, Office of the Actuary, National Health Statistics Group.)

Nurses who question unnecessary or repetitive tests, suggest generic drugs rather than name brands, and teach patients and their families how to monitor their health conditions and detect problems early to avoid repeated hospitalizations all contribute to cost management. Such nursing measures as meticulous handwashing to prevent infections, turning patients on schedule to avoid pressure ulcers, and vigilance to reduce the risk of falls are not usually thought of as cost-containment measures, yet they are. Medicare no longer reimburses facilities for the treatment of certain "reasonably preventable" hospital-acquired conditions ("never conditions") including pressure ulcers, catheter-associated urinary tract infections, falls with injury and burns, and vascular catheter–associated infections, among others, all of which are conditions that can be prevented by nurses. Every day a patient must be hospitalized beyond the length of stay authorized by the payer results in additional charges to the patient and costs to the hospital.

In both inpatient and outpatient settings, organizing and streamlining the flow of patients for maximum efficiency represents a huge savings for the facility and is under the control of nurses and nurse managers. Although nurses can and should look for ways to reduce costs, controlling costs must never take priority over patient care. Remembering the *Code of Ethics for Nurses* will help you maintain your ethical standards: "The nurse's primary commitment is to the patient, whether an individual, family, group, or community" (ANA, 2015).

HEALTH CARE REFORM AND UNIVERSAL ACCESS

The United States and South Africa are the only two industrialized nations that do not provide universal access to health care to all of their citizens. South Africa, however, is implementing a universal system that will be completely phased in by 2026. Despite the fact that U.S. health care expenditures by far exceed those of any other country in the world, the U.S. infant mortality rate was an alarming 5.8 in 2017, ranked 170 of 225 ranked nations (Central Intelligence Agency, 2018). Nations with similar rates include Cayman Islands (5.8), Serbia (5.8), and Gibraltar, (5.9); nations with the lowest rates include Monaco (1.80), Japan (2.00), and Iceland (2.10). The infant mortality rate is a sensitive indicator of a nation's health care practices. Furthermore, the premature birth rate, another sensitive indicator of a nation's health, remains stubbornly high at 10%, with a disparity in African American women, who experience a 14% preterm birth rate (CDC, 2018).

Recent History of Health Care Reform Efforts in the United States

Concerns about health care practices in the United States are not new. In the 1992 presidential campaign, candidates in both political parties, as well as nonpartisan groups, advocated some type of health care reform. These groups included nursing organizations, the American Association of Retired Persons (now called AARP), labor unions, the American College of Physicians, the National Leadership Coalition for Health Care Reform, and numerous members of the U.S. Congress. Most of these groups put forward specific plans for reform, including *Nursing's Agenda for Health Care Reform* by the ANA, which was endorsed by more than 60 nursing organizations and associations. Early in President Bill Clinton's first term, then–First Lady Hillary Clinton led a bipartisan effort to improve access to health care. For a time, it appeared that progress was being made.

Despite widespread public support for reform, however, the effort ultimately failed. Lobbying against health care reform was well funded by powerful interest groups such as the pharmaceutical, health insurance, and medical equipment industries, as well as the American Medical Association and the American Hospital Association—associations with two of the most powerful lobbies in Washington. These entities, as well as others, preferred to maintain the status quo because of the financial interests they had at stake.

During the 2008 presidential campaign, concerns about access to health care, the quality of care, and disparities in care fueled renewed debate about health care in this country. President Barack Obama's administration's commitment to reform health care within his first year in office

remained a priority. The economic recession, however, placed severe restrictions on what could be achieved, and partisan politics continues to create stalemates in Congress, where health care legislation must be conceived and approved. The same special interest groups that opposed change and defeated the Clinton plan again brought out their forces to oppose the Obama administration's efforts.

An encouraging early sign of President Obama's commitment to change, however, was the passage of the State Children's Health Insurance Program (SCHIP) only a few weeks after he took office. This legislation reauthorized and expanded CHIP coverage to include 4 million additional children. Many, including nursing organizations, applauded this action on behalf of uninsured children. In addition, on March 23, 2010, after very contentious congressional debates and political maneuvering, President Obama signed the ACA into law. This law included comprehensive reforms that improve access to affordable health coverage for everyone and that protect consumers from abusive insurance company practices, such as lifetime limits on coverage and denial of coverage for preexisting conditions. In addition, young people up to age 26 could be added to their parents' insurance policies. Challenges to certain provisions of the ACA, including the individual mandate, were brought before the U.S. Supreme Court. In 2012, in a 5-4 decision, the Supreme Court upheld these provisions. In 2015, in a 6-3 decision, the Supreme Court ruled that nationwide tax subsidies to help poor and middle-class citizens buy health insurance were not unconstitutional, and hence the ACA remained viable. Despite these positive steps, the issue of affordable health care in the United States remains a significant political and social problem.

Clearly, increasing the number of people covered would increase expenses unless drastic cost-management measures were put in place. In the future, we can expect to see state-by-state efforts to address the specific current issues of concern discussed earlier. Most experts agree that reform efforts must be projected to reduce, or at least not increase, the cost of health care if they are to be supported by Congress. Shortly after President Trump took office, he set about to overturn the ACA in favor of a newly designed plan. The proposed changes were not widely accepted, and the efforts to overturn the ACA failed in 2017. Despite wide-ranging differences of opinion about the specifics of health care reform proposals, some general questions should be asked in evaluating reform proposals:

1. Is there a uniform minimum set of benefits for all citizens, otherwise known as universal access?

2. Are coverage and benefits continuous and not dependent on where people live or work?

3. Are there mechanisms for controlling costs, especially administrative expenses?

4. Are provisions made for care to be provided by the most cost-effective personnel, taking quality issues and patient outcomes into consideration?

5. Are the issues of adequate facilities and personnel to ensure access for all addressed?

6. Is there an emphasis on quality care?

7. Are there incentives for healthy lifestyles and preventive care?

Further changes in nursing and health care delivery and finance are certain to be on the horizon. These changes will likely be gradual rather than revolutionary. It remains to be seen whether these changes will improve access to and quality of health care for all Americans.

PROFESSIONAL PROFILE BOX 14.1
A MEMBER OF THE BOARD: USING THE LESSONS OF NURSING

As a lifelong resident of the Triangle area of North Carolina (Raleigh-Durham–Chapel Hill), I had always known that Hospice of Wake County (HOWC) was the primary provider of end-of-life care in the area. Several close family members received expert care from this agency at the end of their lives. When I was nominated and then elected to serve a 3-year term on the 23-member Board of Directors (BOD), I was both humbled and pleased for the chance to give back something to HOWC. I was one of the few nurses ever to serve on the board in its 30-plus years of existence. Although I was a former hospice nurse, I will admit I was pretty intimidated by the collective wisdom and expertise of the other directors, who represented a host of other professions, including law, marketing, finance, medicine, clergy, and funeral home management. I couldn't imagine how much I was going to learn about organizational structure, health care finance, quality indicators, not-for-profit governance, and strategic planning.

At the start of my second year on the BOD, I made a plea at a board meeting to consider the development and implementation of a pediatric palliative and end-of-life care program. My faculty research and collaboration with local providers had demonstrated the profound need for this service. The development of the pediatric program was not the BOD's first priority because we were beginning the very difficult work of changing the organization's name, but the peds program was added to the strategic plan. Now known as Transitions LifeCare, we have five service lines—hospice, palliative care, grief counseling, a caregiver support service, and home health. And in September 2015 we opened our sixth service line—a pediatric palliative and end-of-life care service

In my second term, I was elected president of the board. As I reflect back on my long nursing career, I think that my work on the Board of Directors was among the most meaningful endeavors of my professional life. I am both honored and humbled to serve this organization, using the lessons that nursing taught me to improve the lives of families at their most difficult, vulnerable time.

Beth Perry Black, PhD, RN, FAAN

CONCEPTS AND CHALLENGES

- *Concept:* Health care in the United States is delivered in a complex system that provides health promotion, illness prevention, diagnosis and treatment, and rehabilitation and long-term care.

  Challenge: Streamlining the health care system and focusing on the promotion of health rather than on the treatment of illness can have significant positive effects on the health care economy and the health of individuals.

- *Concept:* Access to comprehensive treatment and positive treatment outcomes varies among populations, creating disparities that disadvantage certain groups such as minorities and poor people.

  Challenge: Correcting health care disparities has proved to be a complex task, with only modest progress reported.

- *Concept:* Historically, there have been a number of systems for the provision of nursing care, each of which has advantages and disadvantages.

  Challenge: Many variations and combinations of the major nursing care delivery systems are in use today, and the effectiveness of any one model depends a great deal on the patient population and setting of care.

- *Concept:* Medicare and Medicaid programs, begun in 1965, created financial strain on federal and state budgets that continues today. In response, cost-containment efforts were begun by the federal government in the 1970s and persist in various old and new forms.

Challenge: Regardless of the type of cost-containment efforts used, health care costs have continued to increase. Without serious health care reform, this will continue.

- **Concept:** The ACA, signed into law by President Obama in 2010, was a start in improving access to affordable health care coverage for all residents of the United States.

    Challenge: Until the severe problem with health disparities is addressed, the health of a large segment of the American population will continue to suffer.

IDEAS FOR FURTHER EXPLORATION

1. Obtain the organizational chart of a local health care facility. Examine it to see how nursing fits into the overall structure. Who reports to the CNE, and to whom does the CNE report? What other administrative staff members are on the same level with the nurse executive?
2. Consider the four types of nursing care delivery systems (team, primary, case management, and patient-centered care) from the viewpoint of the patient. If you were a patient, which system would you prefer? Why?
3. Look at the same issue from the standpoint of the nurse. Which system would you find most satisfying in terms of your practice? Which would you like least?
4. Determine what type of governance structure is used by the nursing staff. What do nurses see as the positive and negative aspects of their governance

structure? Do they feel that they are important contributors in this structure?

5. Consider this question: Is access to health care a basic human right or a privilege? Be able to defend your position.
6. What process should be used to determine how health care resources are allocated? List criteria you would suggest to determine whether or not a person should receive a kidney transplant, a hip replacement, or a bone marrow transplant.
7. Should people with healthy behaviors pay the same for care or insurance as those whose habits result in a greater likelihood of illness? How could such a differentiation be determined?
8. Consider some things you as an individual nurse can do to become more cost aware and participate in managing health care costs.

REFERENCES

American Academy of Physician Assistants: What is a PA? (website), 2018. Available at: www.aapa.org/what-is-a-pa/.

American Association for Respiratory Care (website), 2018. Available at: http://www.aarc.org./careers/.

American Nurses Association (ANA): *Code of ethics for nurses with interpretive statements*, Washington, DC, 2015, American Nurses Publishing.

American Nurses Association (ANA): *Nursing administration: scope and standards of practice*, ed 2, Silver Spring, MD, 2016. nursingworld.org.

American Nurses Association (ANA): *Nursing: scope and standards of practice*, ed 3, Washington, DC, 2015, American Nurses Association.

American occupational therapy association (website), 2018. Available at: www.aota.org.

American physical therapy association (website), 2018. Available at: www.apta.org.

American registry of radiologic technologists (website), 2018. Available at: www.arrt.org.

Bureau of Labor Statistics: US Department of Labor: Occupational outlook handbook (website), 2018. Available at: www.bls.gov/ooh/home.htm.

Centers for Disease Control and Prevention: Preterm birth (website), 2018. Available at: https://www.cdc.gov/reproductivehealth/maternalinfanthealth/pretermbirth.htm.

Centers for Medicare & Medicaid Services (CMS): Part B costs (website), 2018. Available at: www.medicare.gov/your-medicare-costs/part-b-costs/part-b-costs.html.

Central Intelligence Agency: The world factbook: rank order—infant mortality rate (website), 2018. Available at https://www.cia.gov/library/publications/resources/the-world-factbook/rankorder/2091rank.html.

Clavelle JT, Porter-O'Grady T, Weston MJ, Verran JA: Evolution of structural empowerment: moving from shared to professional governance, *J Nurs Adm* 46(6):308–312, 2016, https://doi.org/10.1097/NNA.0000000000000350.

Dall T, Chen Y, Seifert R, et al.: The economic value of professional nursing, *Med Care* 47(1):97–104, 2009.

Health Resources and Services Administration: Federally qualified 0020 centers. Available at: https://www.hrsa.gov/opa/eligibility-and-registration/health-centers/fqhc/index.html.

Healthy People 2020: Framework. U.S. *Department of Health and Human Services: Office of Disease Prevention and Health Promotion* (website), 2018. Available at: www.healthypeople.gov.

Healthy People 2030 Framework. *U.S. Department of Health and Human Services: Office of Disease Prevention and Health Promotion* (website), 2018. Available at: www.healthypeople.gov.

Institute for Healthcare Improvement: About us. (website) Available at: http://www.ihi.org/about/Pages/default.aspxhttp://www.ihi.org/about/Pages/defaultspx.

Joint Commission: The: facts about the Joint Commission (website), 2018. Available at: https://www.jointcommission.org/about_us/about_the_joint_commission_main.aspx.

Kaiser Family Foundation: Analysis of national health expenditure (NHE) data from Centers for Medicare and Medicaid Services, Office of the Actuary, *National Health Statistics Group* (website), 2018. Available at: https://www.healthsystemtracker.org/indicator/spending/national-spending-services/.

Lambertson E: *Nursing team organization and functioning*, New York, 1953, Columbia University.

Office of Minority Health and Health Equity: Centers for Disease Control and Prevention: *CDC health disparities and health inequalities report, 2013* (website), 2018. Available at: https://www.cdc.gov/healthequity/about/index.html.

Rogers R: Adapting to the new workplace reality: Maximizing the role of RNs within a collaborative nursing practice model, *Info Nurs* 39(1):18–20, 2008.

Shirey MR: Nursing practice models for acute and critical care: Overview of care delivery models, *Crit Care Nurs Clin North Am* 20:365–373, 2008.

Trossman S: Issues up close: The personal risks of advocating for patients, *Am Nurs Today* 3(8):38–39, 2008.

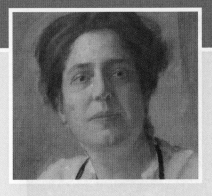

15

Political Activism in Nursing: Communities, Organizations, and Government

Kimberly Fenstermacher, PhD

ⓔ To enhance your understanding of this chapter, try the Student Exercises on the Evolve site at http://evolve.elsevier.com/Black/professional.

LEARNING OUTCOMES

After studying this chapter, students will be able to:

- Differentiate between politics and policy.
- Explain why professions have associations.
- Demonstrate an understanding of the complex role that associations play in the profession and in society.
- Recognize the opportunities that associations offer to increase the leadership capacity of nursing students and registered nurses.
- Explain the concept of personalizing the political process.

- Describe the debate in nursing regarding unionization.
- Cite examples of sources of both personal and professional power.
- Describe how nurses can become involved in politics and policy development at the levels of citizen, activist, and politician.
- Explain how organized nursing is involved in political activities designed to strengthen professional nursing and influence health policy.

The national policymaking stage is close at hand to the American public because of national media networks, 24-hour cable news coverage, and social media. Life "inside the Beltway" of Washington, D.C., is increasingly streamed into American living rooms and to our mobile phones, and thus it is under scrutiny. Interest and involvement of American citizens in governmental processes and accountability are good for democracy. Keeping abreast of events on the national and even the world stage is an important part of good citizenship (Fig. 15.1).

National politics and policy are of great interest; however, much of the politics and policy that affect our daily lives occurs at the state and local levels. The workings of government in your state legislature and local municipalities are likely to be much less familiar to you than what is occurring nationally. Even less conspicuous are the policymaking and policy-influencing activities that occur within the professional organizations that support and shape nursing practice. Yet our day-to-day lives, both professionally and personally, are shaped to a large degree by what happens at the local and organizational levels. This chapter will focus on politics and policymaking in several arenas of importance to nursing. This discussion will start with professional organizations and their roles in setting practice and policy, then will turn to politics and policy in government from both national and local perspectives.

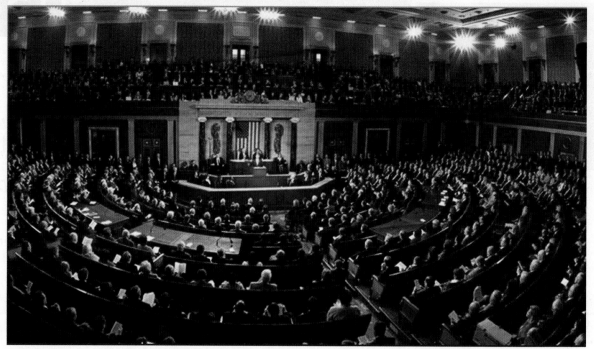

Fig. 15.1 The State of the Union address is delivered once a year by the President of the United States to a joint session of Congress, attended by the Supreme Court justices and the President's Cabinet. All three branches of government are represented at this important address to the nation.

Several chapters of this book cover material that is heavily influenced by government. The content of Chapter 1, the current status of nursing, will be the content of a future edition's Chapter 2, the history and social contexts of nursing. The content of both these chapters reflects policy and politics that affect who nurses are and what we do. Chapter 6 is directly concerned with policy that affects practice. Governmental regulation through licensure is an issue, but the influence of professional organizations to set standards and affect nursing practice acts demonstrates the two-way process that is required to keep nursing relevant and up to date within the health care arena. The focus on ethics in Chapter 7 describes issues of justice and autonomy, foundational principles in American jurisprudence, which shape how we understand and resolve ethical dilemmas.

Issues of nursing education (see Chapter 4) are directly shaped by governmental regulation to ensure that schools of nursing produce graduates who can be entrusted to provide safe care. In Chapter 10, you learned about the National Institutes of Health (NIH)

and specifically about the National Institute for Nursing Research (NINR), which are federally funded agencies of the U.S. Department of Health and Human Services. Research is key to the development of the knowledge base of nursing, which in turn protects its status as a profession and an academic discipline and its influence in both academic and policy arenas. The previous chapter, Chapter 14, addressed the complex issues surrounding how health care is delivered and financed. This is a heavily regulated endeavor with incredibly intricate implications affecting how and where nurses practice. This completes the circle, leading you back to Chapter 1, the current status of nursing, and where we are going.

Furthermore, you are beginning your practice at the time when health care reform continues to be a major focus of politicians throughout the United States. Nurses are poised to participate in decisions about health care reform. As the largest single group of health care providers in the country, nurses can have significant influence on future reforms to our health care system.

POLICY AND POLITICS: NOT JUST IN WASHINGTON, D.C.

Policy and politics are more than what is happening in Washington, D.C. They encompass what happens to us in our daily lives, in the workplace, and in our organizations, as well as in government. According to the Merriam-Webster dictionary (Merriam-Webster, 2018), the word **politics** has three meanings. Concise definitions are as follows:

a: the art or science of government

b: the art or science concerned with guiding or influencing governmental policy

c: the art or science concerned with winning and holding control over a government

We tend to think of politics in terms of the third definition, the one associated with political parties; campaigns; promises; and wrangling for votes, support, and position. However, the first and second definition have the more lasting impact on society. The government is the political body that has to do with the regulation and preservation of the nation. The politics of the third definition is the process by which we determine who will occupy the government in our representative democracy.

Policy, on the other hand, refers to "a definite course or method of action selected from among alternatives and in light of given conditions to guide and determine present and future decisions; a high-level overall plan embracing the general goals and acceptable procedures especially of a governmental body" (Merriam-Webster, 2018).

Policy is shaped to a great degree by those who are successful in the political arena (the second definition). These are the elected officials who describe their agenda before the election to receive support, endorsements, and, ultimately, enough votes to be elected into office. For instance, during the 2008 presidential campaign, the pros and cons of health care reform were discussed and debated at length, and as the nominee, Barack Obama took a stand in favor of health care reform. After his election, legislation known colloquially as the Affordable Care Act (ACA) was passed by Congress and signed into law on March 23, 2010. Health care reform was debated again in the 2012 campaign, and numerous challenges to the ACA have been unsuccessful, including more than 50 attempts by Congress to have the ACA repealed and two cases argued before the Supreme Court. The first (*National Federation of Independent Business v. Sebelius)* challenged the individual health insurance mandate; the second (*King v. Burwell)* challenged subsidies obtained through HealthCare.gov, claiming that they were illegal. In both cases the Court found for the government. (Sebelius and Burwell were secretaries of the U.S. Department of Health and Human Services when these cases were filed.)

It should have been no surprise to anyone paying attention that President Obama embarked on a complex and wide-ranging effort to make health care more affordable. The 24-hour cable news outlets both reported and argued the various merits of his health care campaign agenda throughout the two presidential campaigns. In other words, President Obama used politics as a process (the second definition) to achieve a goal of managing the government (first definition) so that he could influence change in health care policy with the expectation and hope of improving affordability. One of the first pieces of legislation signed by President Obama during his first term was the State Children's Health Insurance Program (SCHIP) reauthorization legislation that extended health insurance coverage to 8 million children whose parents cannot afford health insurance coverage (Fig. 15.2).

Power, Authority, and Influence

A review of the concepts of *power, authority,* and *influence* will help focus the discussion of policy and the

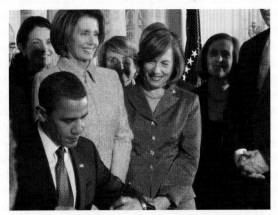

Fig. 15.2 President Barack Obama at a White House signing ceremony of the SCHIP legislation 2 weeks after taking office in January 2009. He said, "I refuse to accept that millions of our children fail to reach their full potential because we fail to meet their basic needs." (Used with permission from United Press International.)

remainder of this chapter. Power is strength or force that is exerted or capable of being exerted. Power in and of itself is latent.

A person who has authority has legitimacy to exert power—that is, to enforce laws, demand obedience, make commands and determinations, or judge the acts of others. People who have been vested with this power—for instance, through a fair and democratic process—are known as *authorities,* especially a government or body of government officials. Influence is a form of power that is not legitimated through official channels, such as elections or appointments by one in authority, but influence is the action or process of producing effects on the actions, behavior, and opinions of others. For example, the issue of lobbyists got much attention in the past two presidential elections. Lobbyists are people who try to influence government officials to act in a certain way that will benefit the constituency that hired the lobbyist to work on its behalf—that is, to exert influence.

A simple clinical example will clarify the difference among these three concepts.

Jane Wilson, RN, is an experienced labor and delivery nurse, and her patient is Ms. Foster. Ms. Foster has been in labor for several hours but is not making very much progress (in SBAR terms, "lack of progress in labor" would be her assessment). Jane believes that augmenting her labor with oxytocin would be appropriate (in SBAR terms, this would be her recommendation). Jane cannot begin this infusion because she does not have the authority to do so without Dr. Martin prescribing it. Dr. Martin has both the power and the authority to prescribe the infusion. Jane, because she is very experienced, understands that she can influence Dr. Martin's decision by giving Dr. Martin her expert opinion on the situation, and in fact SBAR provides her with an excellent structure to provide information necessary for Dr. Martin to make a safe judgment. Jane calls Dr. Martin, influences Dr. Martin to prescribe the oxytocin, and begins the infusion in a few minutes. Ms. Foster gives birth to a healthy baby girl 3 hours later. Note that Jane exerted power through influencing Dr. Martin's decision; Dr. Martin had latent power—that is, power that had not yet been used to prescribe the oxytocin; and Dr. Martin had the authority as a licensed physician to write the prescription.

This is a common scenario between nurses who need something for their patients and physicians who hold the authority to prescribe. You can also see in this example the interdisciplinary collaboration that includes both independent and interdependent actions on the part of Nurse Wilson.

Policy

Policy involves principles that govern actions directed toward given ends; policy statements set forth a plan, direction, or goal for action. Policies may result in laws, regulations, or guidelines that govern behavior in the public arena or in the private arena. *Health policy* refers to public or private rules, regulations, laws, or guidelines that relate to the pursuit of health and the delivery of health services. Policy reflects the choices that an entity (government or organization) makes regarding its goals and priorities and how it will allocate its resources.

Policy decisions (i.e., laws or regulations) reflect the values and beliefs of those making the decisions. As values and beliefs change, so do policy decisions. For instance, laws limiting smoking in public buildings or private restaurants were nonexistent 50 years ago because the harmful effects of smoking and secondhand smoke were not yet well known. As the public became more aware of the dangers of smoking, values about smoking changed. Changes in laws followed the change in values. Laws limiting smoking and the sale and use of tobacco products are common. Elected officials responded to the changing values of the public and recognized that the public supported the passage of laws limiting smoking. In a representative democracy, this is how policy is changed. Officials are elected to represent and then act on the interests of their constituents—that is, the people of their state, congressional district, or municipality.

In professional organizations, policy focuses on the rules and guidelines established by the governing body of the organization, usually a board of directors. Those guidelines or policies also reflect the values of the organization. For instance, one would expect a nursing organization such as the American Nurses Association (ANA) to focus on issues of health promotion, illness prevention, and nursing practice issues. That would be quite different from an organization such as the National Collegiate Athletic Association (NCAA), in which the values of its members would be reflected in policies and recommendations supporting and regulating athletics at the college level across the country.

Politics

Politics is a process that requires influencing the allocation of scarce resources. *Allocation* assumes that there are not enough resources for all who may want them. Those resources might be money, people, time, supplies, or equipment. Who gets what, or how those resources are allocated, is determined through the political process. Policies are the decisions; politics is influencing those decisions. There are always stakeholders—individuals with a vested interest—who try to influence those with the power to make the final decisions.

In organizations, stakeholders are the members, the larger community served by the work of the organization, and other groups or individuals affected by those decisions. For example, Patients Out of Time, an organization started by a nurse, works to educate the public and health care professionals about the therapeutic use of cannabis and to advocate for the medicinal use of marijuana (www.medicalcannabis.com). Founded in 1995, stakeholders for Patients Out of Time are patients and their families, health care providers, and those who make decisions about the laws and regulations about cannabis use. These include state and federal legislators, as well as the U.S. Food and Drug Administration (FDA), the Secretary of Health and Human Services (who oversees the policies of the FDA), and organizations such as the American Public Health Association, which issued a position statement in 1995 supporting patients' safe access to therapeutic marijuana (cannabis) (American Public Health Association, 1995); The ANA issued a position statement in 2016 calling for the development of prescribing standards and evidence-based guidelines for the use of medical marijuana (ANA, 2018).

Politics works similarly in the public arena. For example, to garner support from state legislators to increase funding for nursing scholarships, an organization or coalition of organizations must have a plan to mobilize stakeholders to lobby legislators. Such stakeholders would include administrators of nursing organizations, colleges of nursing, hospitals, nursing homes, and other health care organizations, as well as physician groups and others who know the necessity of having a competent and adequate nursing workforce. The more

stakeholder support that can be generated, the more likely it is that policymakers will note and respond positively to the broad constituent support for the issue; in this example, this means they would vote for increased funding for nursing education and scholarships.

Linking Practice, Policy, and Politics

Leaders in nursing, from Florence Nightingale to Lavinia Dock, saw and understood the connection between their work and the larger world in which policy decisions affected what they were able to do. Nightingale could not have been successful in the Crimea without the support of Sir Sidney Herbert, Secretary of War. Lavinia Dock joined with other nurses to found the ANA, pressure hospital administrators to improve working conditions for nurses, and galvanize support for nursing registration (Lewenson, 2007, p. 23). A more recent example of improving the working conditions for nurses can be found in the story of Karen Daley, a nurse who went public with her needlestick injury, from which she contracted human immunodeficiency virus (HIV) and hepatitis C infections (Daley, 2007). She went public to influence legislation requiring protective devices. In each instance, these leaders knew that nursing practice could be improved only through legislation, regulation, or unification to create a formidable national organization. Daley recognized the power in her story and the extent to which her experience could influence those with authority to make nursing practice safer. She testified before the House Committee on Education and the Workforce's Subcommittee on Workforce Protection, taking her experience to a large, influential national stage. The larger world of public policy and the work of organizations become the arena in which someone with a vision for improved health or working conditions can change the way health is delivered and improve the health of populations. With these examples in mind, we now turn our attention to professional organizations as a means of activism.

PROFESSIONAL ORGANIZATIONS: STRENGTH IN NUMBERS

Professionals in many domains create organizations to work together on issues that enhance their work and community involvement, to ensure continued learning and competence, and to use political action to influence policymakers to support the organization's mission. The collective strength of a large group of committed persons in a robust organization can be impressive. Professional organizations offer a supportive way to learn leadership skills, to test ideas, and to follow these ideas to completion. Nursing has a national organization open to all registered nurses (RNs), the ANA (www.nursingworld.org); a national student nurses organization, the National Student Nurses Association (NSNA, www.nsna.org); and many other specialty organizations developed around particular practice areas. Nursing organizations influence public policy in a variety of ways. The following section examines the role and function of organizations, explores why nurses do or do not join organizations, and discusses examples of collective action. Because organizations are often the catalyst for involvement in political action, we will also explore the broader area of political action in the public arena.

Joining a Professional Organization

Nurses join organizations to network with colleagues, to pursue continuing education and certification opportunities, to stay informed on professional issues, to develop leadership skills, to influence health policy, and to work collectively for job security. Yet less than 10% of the nation's RNs are members of the ANA and only about 20% of nurses belong to one of the many specialty nursing organizations. Nurses cite high cost of dues, lack of time, and lack of interest as reasons they do not join. In some states, complex relationships between the state nurses association, the ANA, and collective bargaining units restrict ANA membership. There are also different expectations and interests among generations of nurses. Although Baby Boomers and older members may accept traditional organizational structures and volunteer tasks, younger colleagues prefer short-term projects, using technology such as blogs and chat rooms rather than face-to-face meetings. Organizations are incorporating processes and products that reflect preferences of younger members. Professional Profile Box 15.1 contains comments from Megan Williams, MSN, RN, FNP, former President of the North Carolina Nurses Association, on how nurses make a difference through their state nurses associations and the ANA.

PROFESSIONAL PROFILE BOX 15.1
MAKING A DIFFERENCE THROUGH THE STATE NURSES ASSOCIATION AND THE ANA

If you have invested in nursing as your career, the next step is to invest in your profession, and joining a professional association such as the American Nurses Association (ANA) is a great start. As an undergraduate nursing student at the University of North Carolina at Wilmington, I was a member of my school chapter of the Association of Nursing Students (ANS). I attended the National Student Nurses Association (NSNA) annual convention in Atlanta, Georgia. Attending a national convention was a pivotal experience in my nursing career. I heard national leaders in nursing share their passion to improve patient care. I was inspired by those leaders to continue to invest in my career and in the nursing profession as a whole.

I joined the North Carolina Nurses Association (NCNA) and ANA as a new nurse graduate. As a member, I receive monthly publications with up-to-date "best practice" ideas that I can apply directly to my nursing practice, and I participate in continuing education programs with nurses from a variety of practice areas. Another valuable benefit of my membership has been creating professional relationships with nurses across the state and across the nation. I enjoy sharing ideas, asking for advice, and volunteering for leadership opportunities.

In the fall of 2013, I was elected as the 51st president of NCNA. In my role as president, I led the organization in developing a strategic plan to allocate the resources and align the many programs and services that are available to NCNA members with our organizational goals. As president, I provided outreach to the internal nursing community through a variety of communications and I represent NCNA in local, state, and national external venues. One of the most important external communities I communicated with were the state and national elected officials. I have advocated at the state and national level to increase access to care, positively influence the cost and quality of health care, and increase and advance the nursing workforce.

PROFESSIONAL PROFILE BOX 15.1
MAKING A DIFFERENCE THROUGH THE STATE NURSES ASSOCIATION AND THE ANA—cont'd

Nurses are in a unique position to share their expertise and knowledge when meeting with legislators. The ability to successfully exert influence in the various arenas where health care policy decisions are made and to present nursing's perspective on health care issues depends largely on being an engaged member of your professional association. The nursing profession has a rich history of legislative advocacy. Here in North Carolina, Mary Lewis Wyche, founder of NCNA, drafted the first Nurse Practice Act in 1893. In 2015 NCNA collaborated with all Advanced Practice Registered Nurse (APRN) groups and the North Carolina Board of Nursing to support legislation to modernize the Nursing Practice Act in North Carolina. This legislation is necessary to remove barriers to the utilization of nurses at all levels to practice to their full scope of knowledge and expertise in all settings and to receive just payment for their services rendered.

I really believe that the answers to major health care issues facing society today can come from a committed group of smart, thoughtful, and connected nursing professionals. It is time that nurses start leaning forward into every critical conversation at every intersection where health care decisions are made. Let's keep the conversations forward thinking and solution oriented. With so many benefits and opportunities awaiting you as a member of a professional nursing organization, what are you waiting for? Join today!

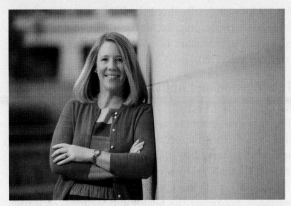

Megan P. Williams, MSN, RN, FNP
Former President, North Carolina Nurses Association

Courtesy Megan P. Williams.

Types of Organizations

There are more than 100 national nursing organizations and many more state and local groups. Nurses often express confusion about which group to join. In general, organizations (associations) can be classified as one of three main types:

1. Broad-purpose professional organizations
2. Specialty practice organizations
3. Special interest organizations

The ANA is an example of a broad-purpose organization. Individual nurses who belong to the ANA typically become members of their state's constituent member association. As the nursing profession's body of knowledge and research grows and diversifies, many nurses limit their practices to specialty practice areas such as maternal/infant care, school or community health, critical care, or perioperative or emergency/trauma nursing. They often join the specialty organization for their area of clinical interest. Members of specialty practice nursing associations also may choose to belong to the ANA or one of its constituent member associations (at the state level) to support the entire profession because specialty associations focus only on standards of practice or professional needs of the particular specialty. More than 60 specialty organizations and other nursing organizations are represented in the Nursing Organizations Alliance (the Alliance), a coalition of nursing organizations promoting the voice of nursing and cohesive action on issues of concern to nursing (Alliance, 2018).

Examples of special interest organizations include Sigma Theta Tau International (the Honor Society of Nursing), which one must be invited to join, and the American Association for the History of Nursing, which focuses on a particular area of study in nursing. Comprehensive and frequently updated lists of nursing organizations are available online at www.nurse.org/orgs.shtml. Nurses are connected internationally through the International Council of Nurses (ICN). The ICN is a federation of national nurse associations representing nurses in 118 countries. The ANA represents U.S. RNs in the ICN, and the NSNA represents U.S. nursing students in the ICN.

Founded in 1899, the ICN is the world's first and widest-reaching international organization for health professionals. Operated by nurses for nurses, the ICN works to ensure quality nursing care for all, sound health policies globally, the advancement of nursing knowledge, the presence worldwide of a respected nursing profession, and a competent and satisfied nursing workforce. For additional details about the ICN's activities in professional nursing practice, nursing regulation, and the socioeconomic welfare of nurses, visit the ICN home page (www.icn.ch).

The Mission and Activities of Organizations

An organization's activities reflect its mission statement. The mission statement is generated by the membership and defines the organization's purpose and goals and who is served by the organization. For instance, the ANA's goals are "fostering high standards of nursing practice, promoting a safe and ethical work environment, bolstering the health and wellness of nurses and advocating on health care issues that affect nurses and the public" (ANA, 2018a). These goals are reflected in their concise mission statement: "Nurses advancing our profession to improve health for all" (ANA, 2018a). These goals and mission define the association's areas of focus as practice standards, a code of ethical conduct, continuing education and conferences, and collective action around workplace issues.

Nurses and Unions

Unionization of nurses is a controversial topic. Nurses may choose to join unions to work collectively, to have control over their practice and workplace, and to work to equalize power between management and staff. This can be an effective approach if the health care organization is willing to work collaboratively with unions. Union affiliation is a highly complex process, one that is defined by rules and regulations under the National Labor Act and overseen by the National Labor Relations Board. There are limits on the issues for which unions can bargain; for instance, hours, pay, and benefits are included in all contracts for all unionized workers.

For nurses, additional issues are increasingly part of contract negotiations, such as staffing, work assignments, and shared governance responsibilities. The recent nursing shortage created an environment in which both management and nurses themselves aspired to develop work environments that decreased turnover and ensured a competent workforce.

National Nurses United (NNU) is an affiliation of collective bargaining organizations that work to improve working conditions for nurses because this in turn results in better care for patients. The NNU was formed in 2009 when United American Nurses (UAN), which represented only nurses, merged with the California Nurses Association (CNA), the National Nurses Organizing Committee, and the Massachusetts Nurses Association. Some non-nursing unions have nursing units: the Service Employees International Union (SEIU); the American Federation of Teachers (AFT); the Association of Federal, State, County, and Municipal Employees (AFSCME); and the United Mine Workers (UMW). These organizations all have nursing units but also represent larger, non-nursing constituencies.

Nurses wonder whether they should join unions. Much of that depends on where they work. If seeking a staff position in an institution in which a nursing union already exists, a nurse may be required to join the union as a condition of employment. This is called a "closed shop," meaning that management is required to bargain with the union, and union membership is required as a condition of employment. An "open shop" is one in which employees are not required to join but in which an individual's contract will be dependent on what union and management have negotiated. Most nurses work in nonunion facilities. Some states are more "union friendly" than others. States in which labor unions flourish, such as in the Northeast, Northwest, and Midwest, have the vast majority of nursing unions. Smaller states, particularly in the Southeast (other than Florida) and Southwest, have few or no nurse unions. These are known as "right to work states." Although unions have made numerous attempts to organize nurses in these states, the value system of the work culture is less supportive of union affiliation by nursing professionals. Fig. 15.3 shows nurses protesting during a 1-day strike in California in September 2011. In Professional Profile Box 15.2, you will read comments by Patricia Moyle Wright, PhD, RN, ACNS-BC, CNE, CHPN, who describes her views of the benefits of collective bargaining.

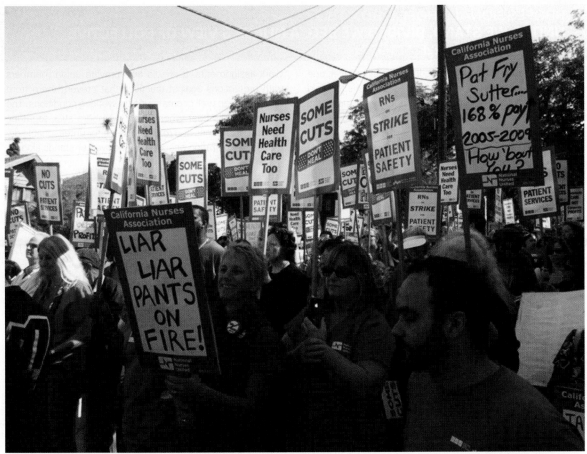

Fig. 15.3 "When nurses are on the outside, there's something wrong on the inside." So noted DeAnne McEwen, Co-President of the California Nurses Association (CNA), at a rally and 1-day RN strike on September 22, 2011. Approximately 23,000 RNs, members of the CNA/National Nurses United, were protesting proposed cuts in nurses' health care coverage and retiree benefits and widespread cuts in patient care services. Nurses carried signs that read, "Some cuts don't heal." (Courtesy California Nurses Association/National Nurses United.)

PROFESSIONAL PROFILE BOX 15.2
UNITED WE STAND, DIVIDED WE BEG: A NURSE'S VIEW OF COLLECTIVE BARGAINING

In my workplace, I serve as the chairperson for the faculty union. I am responsible for ensuring that the administration honors the union contract, which describes working conditions, job responsibilities, salaries, and benefits. A contract is negotiated through the bargaining process. Through my experience as a member of the union's bargaining team, I found that negotiating a contract is truly an "eye-opening" experience because bargaining team members get a glimpse of what administrators would do if they had free reign. Members of the negotiating team begin the process of preparing for negotiations long before the two teams ever meet at the bargaining table. Most unions survey their members to determine which issues are of greatest importance. The negotiating team is then empowered to bargain for the things that matter most to the people in their bargaining unit. At the bargaining table, the union's negotiating team works hard to secure gains for the membership, particularly in the areas cited by the members, which are usually related to salary, benefits, and working conditions. Many strategies are used throughout the negotiating process, and they

PROFESSIONAL PROFILE BOX 15.2
UNITED WE STAND, DIVIDED WE BEG: A NURSE'S VIEW OF COLLECTIVE
BARGAINING—cont'd

change from moment to moment. In general, however, one of the most important strategies the team uses is to avoid revealing which items are most important to their members because once the administration knows something is very important to the team, the cost of that item increases significantly. The cost of an item may be a concession in another area or an actual financial trade-off. Successfully negotiating a contract requires give-and-take. Sometimes the process goes smoothly and agreements are procured rather swiftly. Other times, it does not. If the bargaining process becomes stalled, particularly due to intransigence by the administration, union leadership will direct a campaign aimed at pressuring the administration into doing more to ensure that a fair contract is attained. Typically, the union takes actions such as instituting "work to rule," which means that the members do only the minimum required by the contract, or launching a public relations campaign. The contract itself determines what recourse members of the bargaining unit have if those measures are unsuccessful. A strike is an option of last resort and some contracts even include a "no strike/no lockout" clause that prevents union members from going on strike and administrators from locking employees out. The ultimate goal of contract negotiations is to develop a contract that provides fair remuneration, benefits, and

work assignments. It should also provide union members with protections against practices that prevent them from doing their job well or create unsafe working conditions. The process works best when union members stick together, support each other, and refuse to settle for unreasonable demands. Unionization ensures that no worker stands alone.

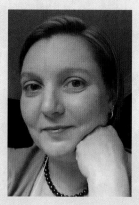

Patricia Moyle Wright, PhD, RN, ACNS-BC, CNE, CHPN
University of Scranton, Scranton, PA

Courtesy Patricia Moyle Wright.

BENEFITS OF JOINING A PROFESSIONAL ORGANIZATION

A variety of benefits result from membership in professional organizations. These range from certification and discounts on travel, products, and services, to opportunities to engage in research projects and learn political action strategies.

Developing Leadership Skills

Students who join the NSNA have opportunities to learn from and socialize with their peers in school and at the state and national levels. As NSNA members, they benefit from developing leadership and organizational skills that can be vital in their professional careers and personal lives. The NSNA embraces the following core values: Leadership and autonomy, quality education, advocacy, professionalism, care, and diversity (NSNA, 2018). From the school chapter level to the state and national levels, nursing students learn how to work in

shared governance and cooperative relationships with peers, faculty, students in other disciplines, community service organizations, and the public. In addition to preparing students to participate in professional organizations, practicing shared governance also prepares students to work in health care delivery settings that incorporate unit-based decision making, such as Magnet hospitals. For complete details about all of the NSNA's programs, visit their website (www.nsna.org).

Leadership skills are foundation blocks for nursing professional practice. Nurses have multiple opportunities to exercise leadership at the bedside, in clinical teams, and in management teams. The Nursing Alliance Leadership Academy (Nursing Organizations Alliance, 2018) was created to help nurses enhance leadership skills and focus on patients and care issues by inspiring and developing future nurse leaders. The academy also focuses on developing political skills and policy awareness (for more information, see www.nursing-alliance.org/dnn/Events/NALANursingAllianceLeadershipAcademy.aspx).

Professional associations offer a supportive environment in which members can practice the acquisition of important leadership skills. Speaking publicly, planning projects, managing resources, and developing resolutions and position papers are opportunities to practice skills essential to formal leadership roles. It is no coincidence that nurses who are active in associations also tend to be recognized leaders in their work settings.

Certification and Continuing Education

Practicing nurses want to be recognized, through both compensation and position, for their level of professional expertise. Toward those ends, they may pursue certification in a specialty area. Certification is granted through professional associations. As discussed in Chapter 4, certification is a formal but voluntary process of demonstrating expertise in a particular area of nursing. Certified nurses may receive salary supplements and special opportunities. For information about credentials in nursing, visit the website of the ANA's subsidiary, the American Nurses Credentialing Center, which offers a range of certification credentials (www.nursecredentialing.org).

Political Activism

Nurses depend on activism to protect their interests. For instance, nurses can obtain master's- or doctoral-level preparation to become nurse practitioners and practice independently. These nurses deserve direct reimbursement for their work and need state laws that mandate direct reimbursement. Others work in settings in which there are not enough RNs available to provide the quality of care the residents need. These nurses need laws that ensure appropriate RN staffing and control educational requirements for unlicensed assistive personnel.

In each of these instances, the ANA, labor unions, and specialty organizations are involved in political action with legislators and regulators in the government arena. There are those within these organizations who develop the positions that nursing organizations believe are in nursing's best interests. There are a number of people within these organizations whose responsibilities are to advocate for legislation to support nursing's position. The process of political action and policy recommendations involves both paid staff, usually in the government affairs department, and volunteer members of the organizations, usually practicing nurses. The legislative agenda—that is, the public policy issues the organization supports—is developed by members appointed by the board of directors, as well as by staff who are experts in political and policy issues. The board of directors approves the legislative agenda. Organizations with legislative agendas depend on members to lobby legislators. They provide members with background information and also create "talking points" to use when lobbying for the selected issue. You can read about the ANA's particular legislative interests online in the Policy and Advocacy section (www.nursingworld.org). As part of the process of encouraging nurses to lobby, information is given on the website about specific bills along with talking points for writing or speaking with congressional representatives. Association members can be very influential in lobbying legislators, particularly when the constituency is nationwide and representative of different stakeholders. Learning how to be politically active increases the power of both the individual and the organization represented.

Nursing organizations also work collaboratively through coalitions with other health professional and consumer groups. Such coalitions are focused on specific issues. For example, Health Care Without Harm is a group of hundreds of organizations in 52 countries whose mission is to "transform health care worldwide so that it reduces its environmental footprint, becomes a community anchor for sustainability and a leader in the global movement for environmental health and justice" (Health Care Without Harm, 2018). Hollie Shaner-McRae, DNP, RN, FAAN, founded this organization in 1996 when she became concerned about the waste created by disposable instruments in an operating room. The organization is now a significant national and international force advocating for a healthy climate, safer chemicals, healthy and sustainable food, zero waste from the health care sector (including pharmaceuticals), clean air and water, green buildings, and human rights, including access to health care for all (Health Care Without Harm, 2018).

Practice Guidelines and Position Statements

Organizations serve an important function by defining practice standards, taking positions on practice issues, and developing ethical guidelines. For example, the ANA has positions on bloodborne and airborne diseases that include statements about HIV infection and nursing students. These positions are consistent with the ANA's recommendation to require educational content about such infections by qualified faculty, mandating universal precautions, and providing postexposure support for students who may sustain a needlestick injury. These statements serve to guide the organization's work in both the practice and the policy arenas and to help individual nurses within workplaces implement the policy. Guidelines and position statements are based on evidence from research, as well as opinions of nurse experts in the field.

Another example is the most recent revision of the *Code of Ethics for Nurses* (ANA, 2015). A task force was appointed by the board of directors to review the previous Code and create revisions and recommendations. The revisions went through a process of approval by many entities within the ANA: the Congress of Nursing Practice, the Board of Directors, and the House of Delegates, which speaks on behalf of all the members. Approval from so many groups within an organization ensures "buy-in" by the membership. Buy-in is important because the Code serves as an ethical standard for all practicing nurses, whether they are ANA members or not, and is therefore of critical importance.

The NSNA also has a Code of Conduct (Box 15.1), which provides guidance for nursing students. This Code serves as the ethical foundation of student practice.

Other Benefits

There are many other benefits of membership, such as access to journals, newsletters, and action alerts about particular topics that need immediate response; eligibility for group health and life insurance; networking with peers; continuing education opportunities; and discounts on products and services, such as car rentals, computers, or books.

Deciding Which Associations to Join

As you decide whether to belong to an association, visit the group's website to find out more about its activities. Then ask yourself the following questions:

1. What is the mission and what are the purposes of this association?
2. Are the association's purposes compatible with my own?
3. How many members are there nationally, statewide, and locally?
4. What activities does the association undertake?
5. How active is the local chapter?
6. What opportunities does the association offer for involvement and leadership development?
7. What are the benefits of membership?
8. Does the association offer continuing education programs?
9. Does the organization lobby for improved health care legislation? How successful is it?
10. Is membership in this association cost effective?
11. Even if I am not active, what benefit will I derive from the legislative agenda and other activities that the association undertakes to advocate for nurses and patients?

Answering these questions and speaking with current association members should provide nurses with adequate information to make reasoned decisions.

BOX 15.1   National Student Nurses Association Code of Academic and Clinical Conduct

Preamble

Students of nursing have a responsibility to actively promote the highest level of moral and ethical principles and to embody the academic theory and clinical skills needed to continuously provide evidence-based nursing care given the resources available. Grounded in excellence, altruism and integrity, the clinical setting presents unique challenges and responsibilities while caring for people in a variety of health care environments. The Code of Academic and Clinical Conduct is based on an agreement to uphold the trust that society has placed in us while practicing as nursing students. The statements of the Code provide guidance for nursing students in the personal development of an ethical foundation for nursing practice. These moral and ethical principles are not limited to the academic or clinical environment and have relevance for the holistic professional development of all students studying to become registered nurses.

Code of Academic and Clinical Conduct

As students who are involved in the clinical and academic environments, we believe that ethical principles, in adherence with the NSNA Core Values, are a necessary guide to professional development.

Therefore within these environments we:

1. Advocate for the rights of all patients.
2. Diligently maintain patient confidentiality in all respects, regardless of method or medium of communication.

BOX 15.1 National Student Nurses Association Code of Academic and Clinical Conduct—cont'd

3. Take appropriate action to ensure the safety of patients, self, and others.
4. Provide care for the patient in a timely, compassionate, professional, and culturally sensitive and competent manner.
5. Are truthful, timely and accurate in all communications related to patient care.
6. Accept responsibility for our decisions and actions.
7. Promote excellence and leadership in nursing by encouraging lifelong learning, continuing education, and professional development.
8. Treat others with respect and promote an inclusive environment that values the diversity, rights, cultural practices and spiritual beliefs of all patients and fellow healthcare professionals.
9. Collaborate with academic faculty and clinical staff to ensure the highest quality of patient care and student education.
10. Use every opportunity to improve faculty and clinical staff understanding of the nursing student's learning needs.
11. Encourage mentorship among nursing students, faculty, clinical staff, and interprofessional peers.
12. Refrain from performing skills or procedures without adequate preparation, and seek supervision and assistance when necessary.
13. Refrain from any deliberate action or omission in academic or clinical settings that create unnecessary risk of injury to the patient, self, or others.
14. Assist the clinical nurse or preceptor in ensuring that adequate informed consent is obtained from patients for research participation, for certain treatments, or for invasive procedures.
15. Abstain from the use of any legal or illegal substances in academic and clinical settings that could impair judgment.
16. Strive to achieve and maintain an optimal level of personal health.
17. Support access to treatment and rehabilitation for students who are experiencing impairment related to substance abuse and mental or physical health issues.
18. Uphold school policies and regulations related to academic and clinical performance, reserving the right to challenge and critique rules and regulations as per school grievance policy.

First adopted by the 2001 House of Delegates, Nashville, TN.
Amended by the House of Delegates at the NSNA Annual Convention on April 7, 2017, in Dallas, TX.
From www.nsna.org.

POLITICAL ACTIVISM IN GOVERNMENT

Now that you understand how professional organizations use collective power to influence policy decisions, let us examine how policy influences the practice of nursing. The ability of the individual nurse to provide care is significantly affected by public policy decisions. Yet too few nurses are aware of the importance of their role in influencing such policy outcomes, because they miss the connection between their own practice and the world of public policy.

As discussed in Chapter 6, state licensure of an RN derives from legislation that defines the scope of nursing practice. The defined scope determines what a nurse legally can and cannot do. As a result of changes in education and clinical practice, nursing organizations influence legislators to change state nursing practice acts to reflect what nurses are qualified to do. For instance, at one time the administration of intravenous medications was not within the scope of nursing practice but instead was limited to medical practice. It is difficult to imagine how a hospital or other health care setting could function today if this were still the case. Regulations are developed to guide the implementation of legislation. They affect practicing nurses and their work environments. For example, the FDA, a regulatory agency of the federal government, sets the rules for administering and documenting the administration of narcotics. The FDA is a division of the Department of Health and Human Services. The way in which such regulations are written can greatly affect nursing practice.

The regulations in each state governing nursing practice are contained in the state's nursing practice act. When the regulations change—for example, adding a requirement for continuing education for license renewal—it affects all nurses in the state. For advanced practice nurses, there are a variety of regulations related to prescription writing and autonomy issues. These change from time to time, and if nurses do not actively participate in changes, new regulations can restrict rather than enhance nursing authority for regulated activities.

Broader issues affecting the nursing profession are also political in nature. Issues of pay equity, or equal pay for work of comparable value, are of concern to nurses because they have been chronically underpaid for their work. One of the earliest cases demonstrating the inequality of nursing salaries involved public health nurses in Colorado. These nurses brought a case against the city of Denver stating that they were paid considerably less than city tree trimmers and garbage collectors. The nurses demanded just compensation for their work by demonstrating that nursing requires more complex knowledge and is of greater value to society than the other occupations (although certainly the value of these other workers is not to be trivialized).

As a result of this suit, recognition of nursing's low pay was brought to public attention, which in turn mobilized public support for increasing nursing salaries. This is an example of political action by nurses that resulted in both policy outcomes (regulations that expanded comparable pay issues to other jobs) and professional outcomes (salary increases for the individual nurse). More recently, the issues of nurse-patient ratios and staffing increasingly have come under scrutiny. Nurses in California mobilized the public and other constituency groups to get the first legislation requiring specific nurse-to-patient ratios passed in 1999; however, the regulations were not implemented until 2004. As of 2018, only 14 states had implemented legislation or adopted regulations related to nurse staffing (California, Connecticut, Illinois, Massachusetts, Minnesota, Nevada, New Jersey, New York, Ohio, Oregon, Rhode Island, Texas, Vermont, Washington) (ANA, 2018b). You can find details of the ANA's principles of nurse staffing and a list of states with staffing laws at www.nursingworld.org/MainMenuCategories/Policy-Advocacy/State/Legislative-Agenda-Reports/State-StaffingPlansRatios. As of 2018, California was the only state requiring minimum nurse-patient ratios to be met at all times by unit. Massachusetts's law requires intensive care unit staffing at a 1:1 or 1:2 nurse-to-patient ratio, depending on how stable the patients are.

Becoming Active in Politics: "The Personal Is Political"

Women involved in the feminist movement in the 1960s coined the phrase "The personal is political." This statement recognized that each individual—woman or man—could use personal experience to understand and become involved in broader social and political issues. This concept enabled individuals who did not consider themselves political to gain insight into what needed to be changed in society and how they could help bring about the change. It gave power to each individual and resulted in people becoming involved in the political process—usually for the first time.

This premise of personalizing the political process has become a fundamental activity for organized nursing. Nurses at the grassroots level become involved in advocating for legislation and supporting candidates for elective office, because they understand the relationship between public policy and their professional and personal lives. Most associations, such as the ANA, American Association of Colleges of Nursing, American Hospital Association, and numerous specialty nursing organizations, actively engage in lobbying to advocate for the professional concerns of their members. Contemporary nursing leaders recognize that "being political," both through professional associations and as individuals, is a professional responsibility essential to the practice and promotion of the nursing profession.

This chapter started with a discussion about national politics because this was the source of a great deal of media coverage and public interest during the primary season and presidential elections of 2012 and 2016. However, remember that an important premise in the earlier discussion was that much of what affects our day-to-day lives occurs at the state and local levels. When you work in a practice setting, your scope of practice is set by state law in the nursing practice act and is enacted by your state board of nursing, which also is also the governmental agency that licenses you and certifies your ongoing safety for practice. You may be late for work today because of repairs being done on an old bridge, from funding through America Fast Forward bonds, an initiative to fund the improvement of state and local infrastructure. Because you are then in a hurry to get to work, you may be pulled over by your local police officer for speeding, and although she is sympathetic to your need to get to work, she cannot overlook the fact that you were both speeding and driving with an expired license, which you had been meaning to renew but had not gotten around to. You have been busy working extra shifts because your unit is short staffed, and the local economic conditions have required a hiring freeze, meaning that you are going to continue to be busy for a while. Each of these situations affecting your day-to-day life reflects the notion that you are always, one way or another, in some situation that involves legislation, regulation, or another form of government intervention. The personal is political, and the political is personal.

During the past 50 years of changing national and state health policies, nurses have increased their political astuteness. Through the well-orchestrated efforts of the ANA, other professional organizations, constituent member associations, and political action committees (PACs), nurses are now participating more effectively in both governmental and electoral politics than in the past. Nursing PACs raise and distribute money to candidates who support the profession's stand on certain issues. Nurses' endorsements of candidates have become a valued political asset for many local, state, and national candidates.

Nurses can make a difference in health policy outcomes. Through the political process, nurses influence policy in a variety of ways: by identifying health problems as policy problems; by formulating policy through drafting legislation in collaboration with legislators; by providing formal testimony; by lobbying governmental officials in the executive and legislative branches to make certain health policies a priority for action; and by filing suit as a party or as a friend of the court to implement health policy strategies on behalf of consumers. All major nursing professional associations engage in these activities. Because the ANA is the major organization that speaks for all nurses, specific examples of influencing public policy will be drawn largely from ANA's activities.

The ANA reports on the progress of nursing influence with the President, members of Congress and their staffs, and the regulatory agencies that set policy for health programs online on the Policy and Advocacy section of nursingworld.org. Such activity reflects the work of both ANA members and ANA staff. The ANA's political activity in Washington, D.C., is mirrored throughout the United States by other nursing organizations and by ANA constituent member associations conducting similar work with their state governments.

Recognizing the power behind the collective voice of nurses, the ANA declared 2018 as the Year of Advocacy for nurses to "inspire, innovate, and influence." Stories of how nurses have advocated at the bedside, in the boardroom, and even globally are shared through social media as means of inspiring others to action through advocacy. The ANA has created RNAction as a portal to provide the latest updates on health policy developments and advocacy opportunities through regular text messages to those who sign up to receive the notifications. By alerting RNAction members, ANA can rapidly mobilize nurses to lobby their federal representatives to support or oppose particular legislation or rules and regulations. Through the use of digital media and other resources, RNAction members can respond by sending well-timed, well-targeted messages to members of Congress. You can sign up for RNAction at http://p2a.co/Z5pXOHC. Organized activity identifying, financially supporting, and working for candidates who are committed to nursing and "nurse-friendly" issues has dramatically increased in the past two decades. The electoral process is an essential function of the professional association.

Individual nurses can make a difference in policy development and elections. Either by election or by appointment, nurses need to be making health policy decisions, not just influencing them. Getting elected or appointed requires visibility, expertise, energy, risk taking, and a belief that policy and politics are critically important in achieving nursing's goals.

GETTING INVOLVED

To get involved, a nurse must begin to understand the connections between individual practice and public policy. Once that happens, it is easy to get started. Three levels of political involvement in which nurses can participate are as nurse citizens, nurse activists, and nurse politicians.

Nurse Citizens

A nurse citizen brings the perspective of health care to the voting booth, to public forums that advocate for health and human services, and to involvement in community activities. For example, budget cuts to a school district might involve elimination of school nurses. At a school board meeting, nurses can effectively speak about the vital services that school nurses provide to children and the cost-effectiveness of maintaining the position.

Nurses tend to vote for candidates who advocate for improved health care. Here are some examples of how the nurse citizen can be politically active.
- Register to vote.
- Vote in every election.

- Keep informed about health care issues.
- Speak out when services or working conditions are inadequate.
- Participate in public forums.
- Know your local, state, and federal elected officials.
- Join politically active nursing organizations.
- Participate in community organizations that need health experts.

Once nurses make a decision to become involved politically, they need to learn how to get started. One of the best ways is to form a relationship with one or more policymakers, and clear communication is key in influencing them (Box 15.2).

Nurse Activists

The nurse activist takes a more active role than the nurse citizen and often does so because an issue arises that directly affects the nurse's professional life. The need to respond moves the nurse to a higher level of participation. An early nurse activist, Lillian Wald, whose picture opens this chapter, left a notable and lasting legacy after responding to the needs of vulnerable populations in New York City by establishing the Henry Street Settlement, which still is in operation more than a century later. Credited with establishing public health nursing,

---

BOX 15.2   Clear Communication: The Key to Influence

Cultivate a relationship with policymakers from your home district or state. Communicate by visits, phone, e-mail, and letters. When contacting policymakers, do all of the following:

- State who you are (a nursing student or RN and a voter in a specific district).
- Identify the issue by a file number, if possible.
- Be clear on where you stand and why.
- Be positive when possible.
- Be concise.
- Ask for a commitment. State precisely what action you want the policymaker to take.
- Give your return address, e-mail address, and phone number to urge dialogue.
- Be persistent. Follow up with calls or letters.
- If you plan to visit your policymaker, make your appointment in advance in writing and indicate what issue you are interested in discussing.
- Be quick to thank policymakers when they do something you support.

---

her tireless work on behalf of impoverished immigrants in New York City embodied her belief that the work of nurses was significant in improving the health of vulnerable people. Wald was also a member of the founding group of the National Association for the Advancement of Colored People (NAACP). Today's nurse activist may respond to a specific need not possibly envisioned in Wald's day. Several nurse activists are presented at various points in the chapter, some of whom became activists in response to a specific issue that became salient to their lives.

Nurse activists can make changes by doing the following:

- Joining politically active nursing organizations
- Contacting a public official through letters, e-mails, or phone calls
- Registering people to vote
- Contributing money to a political campaign
- Working in a campaign
- Lobbying decision makers by providing pertinent statistical and anecdotal information
- Forming or joining coalitions that support an issue of concern
- Writing letters to the editor of local newspapers
- Inviting legislators to visit the workplace
- Holding a media event to publicize an issue
- Providing or giving testimony to legislators and regulatory bodies

Box 15.3 includes guidance on how to affect health policy development.

Nurse Politicians

Once a nurse realizes and experiences the empowerment that can come from political activism, he or she may choose to run for office. No longer satisfied to help others get elected, the nurse politician desires to develop the legislation, not just influence it. Five nurses were elected in 2014 to the 114th Congress of the United States. Two of these nurses have been serving in the House of Representatives for 17 years or more. In 1992 Congresswoman Eddie Bernice Johnson (D-TX) (Fig. 15.4) was the first nurse elected to the U.S. House of Representatives and has been consistently reelected since. She received her bachelor of science in nursing (BSN) from Texas Christian University in 1967 and later earned her master's degree in public administration from Southern Methodist University. In 1998 Congresswoman Lois Capps (D-CA) (Fig. 15.5) became the third nurse to be elected

BOX 15.3 Key Questions for Nurses Who Want to Affect Health Policy

1. Know the system. Is it a federal, state, or local issue? Is it in the hands of the executive, legislative, or judicial branch of government?
2. Know the issue. What is wrong? What should happen? Why is it not happening? What is needed—leadership, a plan, pressure, or data?
3. Know the players. Who is on your side, and who is not? Who will make the decision? Who knows whom? Will a coalition be effective? Are you a member of the professional nursing organization?
4. Know the process. Is this a vote? Is this an appropriation? Is this a legislative procedure? Is this a committee or subcommittee report?
5. Know what to do. Should you write, call, arrange a lunch meeting, organize a petition, show up at the hearing, give testimony, demonstrate, or file a suit?

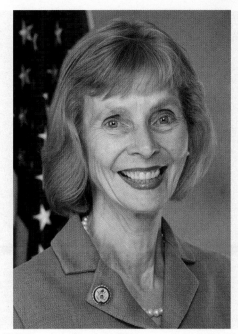

Fig. 15.5 Rep. Lois Capps (D-CA), a nurse who served in Congress.

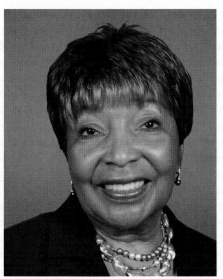

Fig. 15.4 Rep. Eddie Bernice Johnson (D-TX), a nurse in Congress.

to the House of Representatives. Congresswoman Capps was a longtime leader in health care and a school nurse. After her election to Congress, she drew on her extensive health care background to co-chair the House Democratic Task Force on Medicare Reform, and in 2003 she founded the Bipartisan Congressional Caucus on Nursing and the Bipartisan School Health and Safety Caucus. Capps founded and served as chair of the House

Nursing Caucus. She retired in 2017. Newer members of Congress include Congresswoman Karen Bass (D-CA), who was a nurse who became a physician assistant and participated in community organizing. She is the former speaker of the California Assembly and the first African American woman to lead the Assembly. Diane Black (R-TN), a former emergency department nurse and community organizer, previously served as a member of the Tennessee State House and Tennessee State Senate (ANA, 2018c).

Two other members of the U.S. Senate are high-profile "friends of nursing." Senator Richard Durbin (D-IL) (Fig. 15.6) introduced legislation (S. 497) in March 2009 backed by the American Organization of Nurse Executives and other nursing groups that would provide grants to nursing schools for faculty and other resources to increase enrollment. In mid-2015, Senator Durbin introduced a bill to expand a program to assist caregivers of veterans of Iraq and Afghanistan to include all veterans. Durbin was instrumental in the passage of legislation that created the Caregiver Program in the Caregivers and Veterans Omnibus Health Services Act of 2009. The program provides home health training, peer support, and financial stipends to the caregivers of veterans with severe injuries. Senator Barbara Mikulski (D-MD)

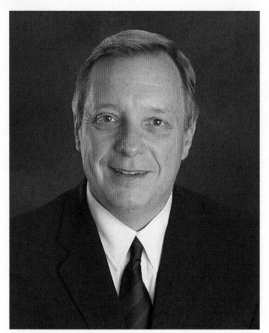

Fig. 15.6 Sen. Richard Durbin (D-IL), a friend of nursing.

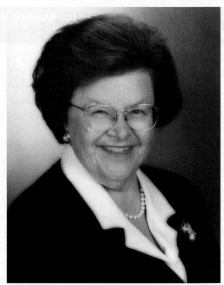

Fig. 15.7 Sen. Barbara Mikulski (D-MD), a friend of nursing.

(Fig. 15.7) was a member of the U.S. Senate from 1987 to 2017. As a senior member of the Senate Appropriations Committee, she announced the 2009 Omnibus Appropriations Act in March 2009, which contained several important health care–related measures. This bill provided $171 million for nursing programs for the Advanced Nursing Education Program, the Nurse Loan Repayment and Scholarship Program, and the Nurse Faculty Loan Program, all of which are dedicated to addressing the nationwide nursing and nursing faculty shortage. Before entering politics, Senator Mikulski was a social worker in Baltimore, where she worked with at-risk children and educated seniors about Medicare.

Nurses have shown that they can take on important and public roles in speaking for health care and for the profession of nursing. To be effective agents of change, nurses can do the following:

- Run for an elected office.
- Seek appointment to a regulatory agency.
- Be appointed to a governing board in the public or private sector.
- Use nursing expertise as a frontline policymaker who can enhance health care and the profession.

Nurses who have achieved success as leaders often started with no knowledge of the political process and no expectations of the greatness they would achieve. Instead, they became involved because some issue, injustice, or abuse of power affected their lives. Instead of complaining or feeling helpless, they responded by taking an active role in bringing about change. The story of nurse and retired Congresswoman Carolyn McCarthy (D-NY) is such an example. McCarthy was a licensed practical nurse who ran for office as a result of her stance on gun control. Her husband was killed and her son critically injured after a lone gunman with a 9-mm semiautomatic pistol walked through a train on the Long Island Railroad and killed 6 people and wounded 19 others. McCarthy was suddenly thrown into the national spotlight when she challenged the incumbent congressman running for office on his stand supporting a repeal on a ban for assault rifles. Her ability to speak passionately about the issue led to her campaign against the incumbent and her election to his seat. For 18 years, McCarthy was a leader in the House of Representatives on gun control, as well as on nursing issues. She retired in 2015.

The mark of a leader is the ability to identify a problem, have a goal, and know how to join others in reaching that goal. A leader must ask the right questions, analyze the positive and restraining forces toward meeting the goal, and know how to obtain and use power. A leader must know how to ask for help and how to give support to those who join the effort. These are the marks of nursing leaders who have become political experts.

NURSING NEEDS YOUR CONTRIBUTION

You no doubt hope to change the world (and you can), but at the same time you hope you pass your upcoming end-of-semester exams—a task that may seem daunting enough without your political aspirations intruding. You can do both. As mentioned throughout this book, mentors can help you become who you want to be. A mentor serves as a role model but also actively teaches, encourages, and critiques the process of growth and change in the learner. You might consider forming a relationship with a political mentor. All nurses who have become political leaders have found mentors along the way to guide and support their growth. Your mentor could be a faculty member, such as the adviser to the nursing student organization or honor society, who can teach you leadership skills. Ask for help in running for a class office or student council president. If elected office does not appeal to you, use your political skills to develop a school or community project with other nursing students. You might find a problem during a clinical experience that inhibits your ability to provide the level of care that you wish to provide. Seek a faculty member or nurse in a clinical facility who can guide you through the process of policy change within the agency or institution.

Seek the help and support of your friends and peers in your activity. The importance of grassroots organization that characterized the most recent election cycles has demonstrated the effectiveness of get-out-the-vote (GOTV) activities and becoming involved in politics at local, state, and national levels. In addition, no matter what your political leanings or positions on issues, it is important that, as a nurse and as a citizen of the democracy, you exercise your right to vote.

CONCEPTS AND CHALLENGES

- *Concept:* Professional associations are the vehicle through which nursing takes collective action to improve both the nursing profession and health care delivery.

  Challenge: There are many nursing associations from which to choose, offering a variety of benefits to the public, to the nursing profession, and to individual members. Selecting which associations to join can be a challenge.

- *Concept:* Professional organizations and professional nurses have much to offer in formulating policy

  decisions at federal, state, and local levels and in each branch of government.

  Challenge: Becoming politically active is as easy as signing your name in support of an issue, registering to vote, organizing a project, or speaking out on an issue.

- *Concept:* Today, organized nursing is involved in politics at many levels in promoting comprehensive health reform and creating a safer workplace.

  Challenge: Political involvement is empowering; one person can make a difference.

IDEAS FOR FURTHER EXPLORATION

1. Look in the media for articles, blog posts, or other communications about legislation that supports nursing's concerns, such as nurse-patient ratio legislation, or other nursing-related or patient-related legislation pending in your state. Contact your representative and/or senators with your opinion about the legislation.

2. Is there a student nurses association on your campus? If there is, consider joining. If there is not a student nurses association, consider establishing one. For resources, go to www.nsna.org.

3. As a student, attend a local or state nurses association meeting to gain a better sense of the issues in the profession so that you can be prepared for what lies ahead when you graduate. How is the association addressing these issues? Do they interest you? How can you get involved?

4. Consider the following hypothetical situation: You are near the end of your final clinical course, a capstone experience in which you have spent almost all of your senior year working with RNs on a medical unit. You have seen how working conditions

negatively affect patient care, and you are very concerned. You learn that the nurses in this hospital are unionized and are planning a 3-day strike in 2 weeks. You support their efforts very much and mention the planned strike to your clinical faculty, who, you discover, is very antiunion. She threatens to fail you for the course if you participate in the nurses' strike. How do you respond? What is at stake if you strike? What is at stake if you do not strike?

5. Consider registering to vote if you are not already registered, and find out what your state laws are regarding voter identification, early voting, absentee voting, and other issues that may affect your right to cast a ballot.

6. Because nurses have differing personal and political values, it has been a challenge to get them all united behind a single issue or candidate. If you were the president of the ANA, what techniques would you use to convince the 3.6 million American nurses to use the power of their numbers, their knowledge, and their commitment on behalf of their profession?

7. Find out whether the members of your state board of nursing are elected or appointed. What is the composition of the board (that is, how many RNs, licensed practical/vocational nurses, and consumers are there, for example)? Do nurses hold most of the seats on the state board? Are there any other health professionals, such as physicians, on the board of nursing? If so, are there any nurses on the state board of medicine?

REFERENCES

Alliance: *Nursing organizations alliance.* (website), 2018. Available at: www.nursing-alliance.org.

American Nurses Association (ANA): *About ANA.* (website), 2018a. Available at: http://www.nursingworld.org/FunctionalMenuCategories/AboutANA/.

American Nurses Association (ANA): *2016 Therapeutic use of marijuana and related cannabinoids.* (website), 2018. Available at: http://nursingworld.org/MainMenuCategories/EthicsStandards/Resources/Ethics-Position-Statements/Therapeutic-Use-of-Marijuana-and-Related-Cannabinoids.pdf.

American Nurses Association (ANA): *Nurse staffing plans and ratios.* (website), 2018b. Available at: www.nursingworld.org/MainMenuCategories/Policy-Advocacy/State/Legislative-Agenda-Reports/State-StaffingPlansRatios.

American Nurses Association (ANA): *Nurses currently serving in Congress.* (website), 2018c. Available at: www.nursingworld.org/MainMenuCategories/Policy-Advocacy/Federal/Nurses-in-Congress.

American Nurses Association (ANA): *Code of ethics for nurses with interpretive statements*, Washington, DC, 2015, American Nurses Publishing.

American Public Health Association: *Endorsement on medical marijuana access to therapeutic cannabis/marijuana.* (website), Nov 1995. Available at: www.drugpolicy.org/docUploads/APHAendorse.pdf.

Daley K: Needlestick injuries in the workplace: Implications for public policy. In Mason D, Leavitt J, Chaffee M, editors: *Policy and politics in nursing and health care*, ed 5, St. Louis, 2007, Saunders.

Health Care Without Harm: *What we do.* (website), 2018. Available at: https://noharm-uscanada.org/content/us-canada/mission-and-goals.

Lewenson S: An historical perspective on policy, politics and nursing. In Mason D, Leavitt J, Chaffee M, editors: *Policy and politics in nursing and health care*, ed 5, St. Louis, 2007, Saunders.

Merriam-Webster Dictionary. (website), 2018. Available at: https://www.merriam-webster.com/dictionary/politics.

National Organizations Alliance: *Educating leaders in nursing.* (website), 2018. Available at: http://www.nursing-alliance.org/dnn/Events/NALA-Nursing-Alliance-Leadership-Academy.

National Student Nurses' Association: *Code of academic and clinical conduct.* (website), 2018. Available at: http://www.nsna.org/nsna-code-of-ethics.html.

16

Nursing's Challenge: To Continue to Evolve

Heather Moulzolf, DNP, MA-N, BA-N, ARNP-BC, CNP-BC

(e) To enhance your understanding of this chapter, try the Student Exercises on the Evolve site at http://evolve.elsevier.com/Black/professional.

LEARNING OUTCOMES

After studying this chapter, students will be able to:

- Describe the major challenges facing the profession of nursing.
- List ways that nurses can protect the image of nursing.

- Describe how incivility escalates along a continuum.
- Explain how nursing's role in caring for the environment is related to health.
- Describe four major components of the American Nurses Association's Health System Reform Agenda.

Nursing is a profession steeped in tradition yet responsive to the changing world around us. Nurses Florence Nightingale, Lillian Wald, and Isabel Hampton Robb were heroes, and their legacies continue today. Yet the work of nursing today rarely feels heroic; sometimes it just feels like the hard work that it is. Often, nurses are referred to as "unsung heroes" of health care.

Photographer and filmmaker Carolyn Jones has produced a documentary *The American Nurse: Healing America* and a book *The American Nurse* published in 2012. This inspiring film and book chronicle the lives and work of nurses in many settings (Jones, 2015). The faces of the nurses capture America—male, female, Black, White, Asian, Latino—in a way that no pie chart or list of statistics can possibly illustrate. The faces of nursing today stand in stark contrast to those featured in the historical documentary *Sentimental Women Need Not Apply: A History of the American Nurse* (see Chapter 4). Nursing in America has come a long way in response to a world changed by war, social movements, and economics.

You have learned about several papers, books, and policy statements that call for nursing to evolve in response to the complex needs of today's world. Evolution means changing in ways that are specific and responsive to changes in the surrounding world. Author George Bernard Shaw once wrote, "Progress is impossible without change, and those who cannot change their minds cannot change anything." Progress is movement forward. In this short chapter, you will be presented with challenges for change and progress in nursing that move from the individual—you—to the global.

THE CHALLENGE: CARING FOR YOURSELF

Nurses have an obligation to care for self as highlighted in the American Nurses Association (ANA) *Code of Ethics for Nurses with Interpretive Statements, Provision 5* (2015). However, the challenge is that nursing is hard work—physically, mentally, and emotionally—and yet at the end of their workdays, many nurses go home to encounter other demands of adult life, including parenting, care of elderly parents, and economic stresses. Many younger nurses enter the profession at a time when they are of age to become parents. Older nurses face the common situation of the "sandwich" generation, referring to people at midlife who face both the challenges of parenting teens and increasing responsibilities for their own parents. Family is usually one's priority over work and career, although today's economic conditions require many nurses to continue to work even though the demands of their families are high. Balancing the responsibilities of work and family can be stressful, making concentrating on one's work difficult and leaving little time for self-care.

The hard work of nursing lies in the fact that nurses bear heavy responsibilities that they take very seriously. There is no question that nurses affect the lives of their patients in ways that cannot be quantified or fully appreciated. The works of Aiken and of Buerhaus, both mentioned at different points throughout this book, have shown consistently that registered nurses (RNs) make a profound difference in the quality of care of patients in hospitals. Projections show that the supply of nurses is increasing, but with the workforce aging and the demand for professional nurses, there likely will still be shortages of nurses in some states by 2030 (U.S. Department of Health and Human Services, Health Resources and Services Administration, National Center for Health Workforce Analysis, 2017).

These predictions, the hard work of nursing, the working environment, and the economic and family stresses that nurses often experience can lead to any number of responses, some healthier than others. Selye, who described the body's response to stress as the general adaptation syndrome, recognized that unresolved stress over time eventually changes one's body as it attempts to restore homeostasis. Selye noted, "Every stress leaves an indelible scar, and the organism pays for its survival after a stressful situation by becoming a little older" (Selye, n.d.).

You can probably describe the basis of nursing as caring, citing theorists, books, and papers that support this key concept in nursing. However, the caring work that nurses do can have consequences such as secondary traumatic stress or compassion fatigue discussed in Chapter 13.

Caring for yourself is foundational to being able to care for others, whether it is the professional caring characteristic of nursing or the personal caring for your friends and family. Seventeen years ago, Carolyn

Cooper, PhD, RN, published a unique book, *The Art of Nursing: A Practical Introduction* (2001), in which she claimed that foundational to caring for others is caring for oneself and her work is just as relevant today. Noting that "Nursing teaches hard lessons" (p. 250), Cooper identified the challenges to self-care for nurses: burnout, professional dynamics, and personal responses to nursing. Notably, what Cooper did not do is create a standard formula for those activities that you can read in most self-help books or websites: exercise, sleep, eat well—today's almost clichéd recipe for "taking care of yourself."

Importantly, what Cooper did do was challenge nurses to pay attention to "environmental challenges that may be depleting" (p. 256). By paying attention, you can name specifically what is depleting you, what can be done about it, and then act on it. *What* you do is not as important as doing *something*, thereby positioning yourself to take care of yourself (p. 256). By acting, you bring to the forefront those parts of your life over which you can take charge. You now are making informed choices—and are taking responsibility for those choices. Here is an example:

Alan is a nurse with 3 years' experience in critical care; he has developed excellent assessment skills and is known for being calm under pressure. He has taken advanced life support training, and at every opportunity attends continuing education courses, conferences, and has joined his professional organization. He has gotten the reputation for being a "superstar" on his unit. His dream job gets posted: there is an opening on the flight team. Alan applies and "aces" his interview. He is not hired for his dream job. He described his response: "I was really mad and took it out on my colleagues for a few days. I was going to quit, I was going to sue, you name it. Then a colleague told me to get over myself and go find out why I wasn't hired. So I did." What he learned was that despite his excellent credentials, he had one fatal flaw: he had developed the reputation for being somewhat arrogant and a "hothead." Alan took this feedback and wrestled with its implications. He could take charge of his responses to stressful circumstances, which he did. Although he has not yet completely "mellowed out," he has used this humbling experience to take responsibility for his actions. He still wants to be a flight nurse someday.

According to Cooper (p. 257), Alan used this situation to assess his vision of his career and what influenced

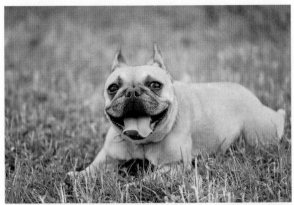

Fig. 16.1 Our pets have a good way of reminding us of the healthful simplicity of eating, sleeping, and playing. (Photo used with permission from iStockphoto.com.)

his career, and he acted accordingly. Knowledge of self is a form of self-care. This allows you to understand changes both in yourself and in the profession of nursing. Change can be difficult, and successful adaptation to change "entails abandoning the hope of always controlling work-related changes, accepting the reality that change is inevitable, tolerating the unpredictability of the future" (p. 257), which can lead to creative problem solving rather than being a victim of one's circumstances. Alan, in the previous example, refused to be a victim of his circumstances—not getting hired for his dream job—by taking specific steps to change in response to information that was both painful and helpful.

Using this larger view of self-care, exercising, sleeping, and eating well are healthful responses to true caring for one's self. There are other forms of self-care that you may find helpful, including volunteering, becoming involved in a hobby, honoring your spiritual tradition, having a pet, or other source of renewal that keeps you balanced and energetic (Fig. 16.1). Achieving balance through a variety of practices and activities is important to your health, which in turn will allow you to be more effective in all of the roles you fulfill in your life—as a student, nurse, spouse, parent, daughter or son, and friend.

THE CHALLENGE: CARING FOR THE PROFESSION

Nurses own nursing and nursing practice. Nursing has become a profession with a distinct body of knowledge and self-regulation, with a science that continues to be developed and a central role in the evolving health care system of today. This success reflects the tremendous work of nurses who have been relentless in their efforts on behalf of the profession, and ultimately on behalf of our patients. It remains a challenge for today's nurses—including students—to continue to be responsive to the changing landscape of health care and to move nursing into positions of power and influence in the health care system. Here are some suggestions.

Join Professional Organizations

You have been introduced in this text to some of the most pressing challenges to nursing today. One of the key problems, and one to which you can respond readily, is the lack of involvement of nurses in professional organizations and the ANA through your constituent state organization. Professional organizations such as the Association of Nurses in AIDS Care (ANAC), American Association of Critical-Care Nurses (AACN), and Association of Women's Health, Obstetric and Neonatal Nurses (AWHONN), among many others, provide up-to-date information about the state of the clinical practice area in which you work or are interested. These organizations provide many outlets for keeping your practice current with the latest developments and research through conferences, webcasts, position papers, websites for members only, and journals. Although there are annual dues, the work of these organizations pays off in keeping you involved and current in your practice, aware of developments in standards of care in your practice area, and advocating for policy change on the behalf of nursing.

The ANA and its constituent state members is the official voice of nursing. The code of ethics, scope and standards of care, and articulation of nursing's social policy are developed and advanced through the ANA. As the official voice for nurses, the ANA publishes position papers on a wide variety of issues and topics and has a political action committee that raises funds from constituent member association members and contributes to political candidates at the federal level whose views of health care legislation and regulation are consistent with those of the ANA. Sadly, only about 10% of RNs in the United States are members of the ANA's constituent organizations, meaning that nurses are silencing their own voices by not participating in the work of this organization dedicated to the profession.

Protecting the Image of Nursing

Care of the profession also means that as a nurse, you become aware of the image of nursing in the media and respond appropriately to both negative and positive portrayals of nurses. The Truth About Nursing is a non-profit organization with the mission to "increase public understanding of the central, front-line role nurses play in modern healthcare." The organization asks nurses to take responsibility for its public image by monitoring media images of nursing. Nurses can thereby advocate for accurate images by contacting the organizations/ companies with negative or inaccurate images, boycott programs, and applaud efforts of organizations that do portray an accurate image of nursing (www.truthabout-nursing.org). This watchdog organization keeps the image of nursing front and center in its mission, such as by advocating for the halt of a Netflix production called *Ratched*, a series that would negatively represent the nursing profession (Truth About Nursing, 2018). A past story included the coverage of the 2014 Ebola outbreak that eventually brought two American nurses into the spotlight: an RN from Texas who contracted Ebola from caring for a patient who eventually died from the virus and a nurse from Maine who was quarantined unnec-essarily in New Jersey after returning from her work in Africa with patients with Ebola (Truth About Nursing, 2014). Each nurse was referred to in the media as "Ebola nurse," a designation that trivialized their experiences and ignored their vital work. Truth About Nursing noted that the media consulted chief nurse Susan Mitch-ell Grant, MS, RN, NEA-BC, FAAN (Emory University Hospital), who explained why her facility accepted the first patients with Ebola brought into the United States. Truth About Nursing also pointed out that otherwise, physicians were heavily featured in accounts about car-ing for patients with Ebola.

The persistent underreporting or even disappearance of nurses from media coverage of health-related events poses a challenge in getting the media to pay attention to the expertise and work of nursing. Examples of min-imizing the value of the work nursing does is the use of the phrase "nursing secrets" in a magazine and on a popular TV show hosted by a physician. This trivializes nursing knowledge as a list of "tips" rather than substan-tive science that promotes wellness, prevents serious complications, and otherwise improves lives.

Another damaging problem for nurses is the highly sexualized images of nurses often portrayed in the

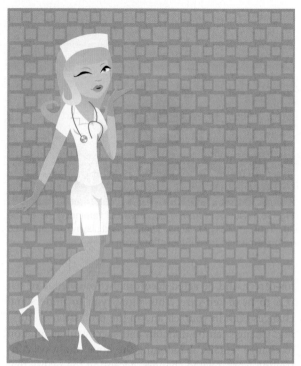

Fig. 16.2 Images that are meant to be humorous are still hurt-ful to nursing. This cartoon image diminishes the work and reputation of nurses. (Photo used with permission from iStock-photo.com.)

media and other venues. In 2012 nurses were outraged over the portrayal of nurses by the Dallas Mavericks of the National Basketball Association, whose dancers performed a halftime routine in revealing "naughty nurse" costumes complete with nursing caps to the tune of the old song that begins, "Doctor, doctor…" (Truth About Nursing, 2012). The image in Fig. 16.2 demon-strates the insidious message from even cartoon figures: a very slender White nurse with long blonde hair, a cap, a short white uniform, and heels is winking and blowing a kiss at some unknown recipient of her attention. This image is mild compared with the grotesquely sexualized images of nurses that are easy to find on the Internet and elsewhere. Nurses must protest the use of these images commercially and for entertainment.

Maximizing Your Education

Another way of caring for the profession is for nurses to become as educated as possible and to work at the upper limits of their education. From Chapter 4, you learned that nursing education is undergoing significant

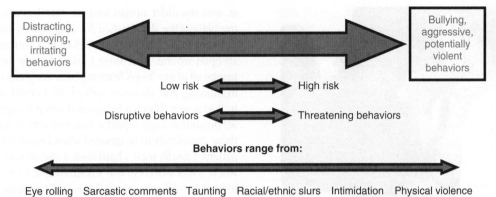

Fig. 16.3 The continuum of incivility goes from simple acts such as being distracting and eye-rolling to aggressive behaviors and bullying. (Courtesy Cynthia Clark.)

changes. With the increasing complexity of the health care system—and the society in which that system operates—the issue of the requirement of a bachelor of science in nursing (BSN) degree for entry into practice is likely to get significant traction over the next several years. Already, significant numbers of nurses with associate degrees are returning to college to complete their BSN. The doctor of nursing practice (DNP) degree may eventually replace the master of science in nursing (MSN) degree for advanced practice nurses, although the MSN will continue to be offered for other purposes.

The doctor of philosophy (PhD) degree will remain the degree for nurse scientists, with intense training in research methods and scholarship. PhD-prepared nurses will continue to be needed to advance the science of nursing, and DNP-prepared nurses will join the ranks of other health care providers for whom a doctorate is the degree for advanced clinical practice. Nurses have the opportunity at this transformational time in health care to assume their rightful place as leaders in primary care and other forms of practice for which they are well prepared.

Promoting Civility

Incivility in nursing is a troubling problem that is getting increasing attention, so much that in 2015 the ANA published a position statement on incivility, bullying, and workplace violence. In a profession dedicated to caring for strangers, the spiral of incivility is difficult to explain but crucial to address. In March 2011 Medscape Nurses, a widely read web-based source of information about nursing, featured an interview with Cynthia Clark, PhD, RN, and Sara Ahten, MSN, RN, who addressed several aspects of nursing incivility (Stokowski, 2011). They described a continuum of incivility (Fig. 16.3). Incivility in nursing is manifested as bullying between colleagues and between faculty and students in academic settings. The latter is particularly troubling because nursing school is a potent agent of professional socialization (Luparell, 2011).

The continuum of incivility starts with common behaviors that are distracting, annoying, or irritating to others. Examples of these behaviors are talking on one's phone in a restaurant or sending and reading text messages while someone is talking to you. These behaviors are a matter of poor manners in some cases but that leave the recipient of the behavior feeling annoyed. Increasingly disruptive behaviors include taunting, using ethnic slurs, and intimidation even without physical contact. At the most extreme of the continuum, bullying, aggression, and violence occur (Stokowski, 2011). Incivility in the workplace has implications for nurses, patients, and health care organizations, with poor communication and unprofessional behaviors negatively affecting patient outcomes and safety (Luparell, 2011).

Incivility occurs when people are stressed and feel powerless. Incivility can briefly give one a sense of control or power, even though it is misplaced and misguided. Furthermore, the widespread use of social media and faceless communication over e-mail, messaging, and so on keeps the other person's humanity at a distance. Talking to or about someone without face-to-face communication foments incivility. You are much more likely to express something in an aggressive manner if you are

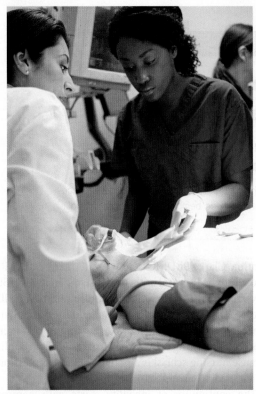

Fig. 16.4 When nurses treat each other with dignity and respect, patients benefit. (Photo used with permission from iStockphoto.)

not required to speak directly to the person, even if by phone. Hearing someone's voice is a reminder that you are indeed speaking to a real person.

Cooper's recommendations related to self-care are appropriate to the issue of incivility: you do not have to be victimized by a system that is uncaring and hurtful. You do not have to bully to claim power for yourself, and you do not have to acquiesce to bullying. Valuing others and treating each person with respect are core values in nursing (Fig. 16.4). The disconnection between what is taught and what we do is both alarming and tragic. You will be hearing more about incivility in the workplace as you continue your career in nursing. You do not have to be a part of this disturbing development in our profession. Here is one nurse's experience:

My stomach hurt every day before I got to work as a new graduate. Everything I suggested was at first just ignored, then later my suggestions were just laughed at, and the older nurses told me that I needed to learn my place. One day I asked for help with a complicated problem that I had not seen before in a patient who had an open wound. The nurse I asked to help me said that maybe all of my "book learning" was not going to help me in nursing, and then she walked off. I could not believe it. It was one thing to be ignored when I suggested that we do shift change report a different way. It was another thing completely to be ignored when I needed help with a patient. I finally took a hard look at myself and at the unit where I was working, and I realized that I was not going to be able to change much there. So I put in for a transfer as soon as I could. On my last day, one of the nurses told me that she knew I was not going to be able to make it there. It was her parting shot at me, but I was so relieved to be leaving that I did not even care anymore. By the way, I loved the new unit that I transferred to. I finally felt like I was going to be a good nurse.

Strategies exist to assist nurses to combat this ongoing issue. Cognitive rehearsal is one approach that can be helpful to nurses when managing situations that are not civil (Longo, 2017). The Passionate About Creating Environments of Respect and Civilities (PACERS) *Civility Tool Kit* developed by Robert Wood Johnson Fellows in 2012 is another source that offers resources including videos and cue cards on how to approach difficult conversations and tools to help increase awareness of bullying (http://stopbullyingtoolkit.org).

THE CHALLENGE: CARING FOR THE ENVIRONMENT

Environmental issues encompass almost every aspect of human life. In its broadest sense, the environment connotes the air, water, organisms, and other natural resources that surround us. It also connotes the social and cultural milieu in which people live. The previous section touched on the social and cultural milieu that has become the breeding ground for incivility—the environment of health care. On its largest scale, the environment is about the world and its resources over which humans are stewards.

The Natural Environment

Reports of the deterioration of the environment are daily occurrences. Catastrophic occurrences such as the earthquakes in Japan, Haiti, and Nepal will continue to affect those nations for decades, if not centuries. These occurrences overshadow the less dramatic but insidious gradual decline in the quality of the world's air, water, and plant and animal life.

Acute and chronic respiratory diseases are increasing, as are cancers of all types and debilitating allergic reactions to chemicals in the environment. Increasing evidence supporting climate change as a result of high carbon dioxide levels in the atmosphere; lead and mercury poisonings; toxic shellfish beds; oil spills in oceans; pesticides and other toxins spilling into streams and rivers; and accidental release of radioactive steam from nuclear power plants all occur with unsettling regularity. Meanwhile, deforestation, destruction of wetlands by development, and relaxing of standards for waste emissions by industries have become common business practices.

Scientists now overwhelmingly agree that climate change as a result of global warming is accelerating and is attributable to human activity (Fig. 16.5). Much debate continues in the popular media about whether the science of climate change is believable; however, according to scientists across the planet, the evidence demonstrating the relationship between human activity and the trapping of carbon dioxide in the atmosphere is irrefutable.

Failure to care for the environment has health implications beyond the most obvious ones such as lung diseases and the development of certain cancers. **Epidemiologists,** who study the origins and spread of diseases, believe that there is a relationship between environmental decline and increases in certain diseases, including animal-borne diseases. Emerging diseases and multidrug-resistant strains of organisms once under control, such as *Mycobacterium tuberculosis* and *Staphylococcus,* will increasingly challenge health care resources.

As of mid-January 2017, the world population was estimated to be 7.6 billion and is projected to increase to 8.6 billion by the year 2030 (United Nations, 2017). Feeding, immunizing, providing drinkable water, and caring for this many human beings threaten to overwhelm the environmental, economic, social, and medical systems of the world. In the United States alone, there is one birth every 8 seconds, one person emigrating every 29 seconds, and one death every 11 seconds—for a net gain of one person every 15 seconds (U.S. Census Bureau, n.d.).

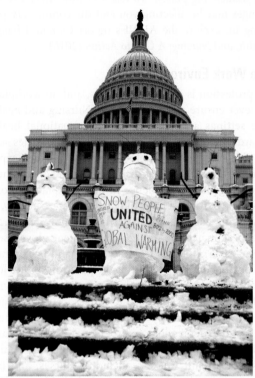

Fig. 16.5 The melting "snow people united against global warming" on the steps of the U.S. Capitol in Washington, D.C., was a humorous but very pointed protest against policies resulting in global warming that has resulted in climate change. (Photo used with permission from iStockphoto.)

At the Climate Change Conference held in Copenhagen, Denmark, in 2009, the metaphor of the overloaded lifeboat was often used. World overpopulation, overdevelopment, and overconsumption by wealthy nations threaten to deplete the resources and damage the environment of the entire world, not just overpopulated countries. The problems of climate change, the deterioration of the environment, and overpopulation are health care issues that nurses face now, and these issues will likely intensify in the future. These are immense problems with no easy solutions, and they often affect our most vulnerable populations; elderly, children, pregnant women, and those living in poverty. The Alliance of Nurses for Healthy Environments (AHNE) is dedicated to "promoting healthy people and healthy environments by educating and leading the nursing profession, advancing research, incorporating evidence practice and influencing policy." To discover how these climate changes may be affecting you and the community you living in, explore the AHNE's report *Climate Change, Health, and Nursing: A Call to Action* (2016).

The Work Environment

No profession is free from hazards, and no workplace can ever ensure absolute security. Nursing and health care settings are no exception. Occupational health hazards in nursing include needlestick injuries and possible infection with bloodborne pathogens; exposure to chemicals such as disinfectants and chemotherapeutic agents; and violence in the workplace, among others. Additional hazards include latex allergy, a continuing concern for nurses, with a prevalence rate of approximately 8% to 12% in frequent glove users (ANA, 2006). Injuries from accidents and back strain are not uncommon, resulting in pain, disability, lost income, absenteeism, and decreased productivity. Shift work itself is a hazard to nurses, causing a variety of physical and psychological problems, including exhaustion, depression, interpersonal problems, and accidents. Sleep deprivation is a significant source of stress in shift workers, including nurses, and has been associated with an increased risk of breast cancer, obesity, and mortality (Beccuti and Pannain, 2011; Davis and Mirick, 2006; Gallicchio and Kalesan, 2009). Stress from work overload, inadequate staffing, and the intense feelings generated by caring for acutely ill and dying patients add to the mix of workplace hazards faced by nurses.

Assuring nurses of a healthy work environment is a major challenge over which nurses have some control. Nurses must take positive, effective, united action to ensure the basic dignity and safety of practicing nurses everywhere. They must demand and use safe needlestick devices and disposal containers; high-efficiency ventilation systems; alternatives to latex gloves and products; adequate environmental services support; adequate lifting assistance with devices or additional personnel; reduction or elimination of shift rotation and double shifts; and appropriate occupational safety and health training. Many nurses are fortunate enough to work in settings where they can take these practices for granted; however, with the wide variety of settings where health care is provided in the United States, some nurses work without the advantages of up-to-date safety technologies or scheduling practices. The Occupational Safety and Health Administration (OSHA) regulates work environments and has a whistleblower protection program to protect from retribution those workers who believe that their workplace is dangerous.

Genetics and Genomics

Genes are minute nucleotide polymers with huge implications for nurses. The Human Genome Project was the initial mapping and sequencing of a composite set of human genes in 2003. An increasing number of genetic conditions can be identified prenatally, and parents can be aware of some of the genetic conditions of which they may be carriers. Providers can use genomic information to inform their care plan in the areas of screening, monitoring, and treatment decisions; allowing for personalized care. Pharmacogenetics is a developing field in which genetic variants that affect drug metabolism can help providers determine the correct dose of a particular drug and, possibly, whether a particular drug will work at all. As a nurse, it is an important responsibility for you to be able to explain pharmacogenetics and to assist your patients in understanding what these drugs can and cannot do.

Schools of nursing are increasingly offering courses in basic genetics and genomics to prepare graduates for the demands of this increasingly visible field in health care. Competence in genetics is becoming increasingly necessary for nurses.

THE FINAL CHALLENGE: UNITE AND ACT

The call to unite is a loud and constant one. Most of the crucial issues the nursing profession will face in the next decade cannot be resolved by any one group of nurses. These concerns will require the attention of the entire profession, working in a focused, united, active manner through nursing's professional associations. Although collective power is the only way nurses will effectively address and resolve issues affecting their practice, education, and the health care system in a time of reform, the lack of organization and involvement in professional organizations is an unfortunate commentary on the lack of priority most nurses place on this vital aspect of professionalism.

As the largest health care profession in the United States, nursing can and should have a powerful voice and presence in every setting where substantive health care issues are discussed, from the National Institutes of Health to the halls of Congress and the White House. Serious discussions occur in less lofty surroundings than the federal government, and nurses can have a strong presence in many venues where health care is central; however, nursing has let arguments regarding levels of education, political philosophies, and relative importance of practice settings be divisive. The tremendous clinical skills of critical care nurses are no better or worse than the insightful care of psychiatric nurses; the high energy of the emergency department nurse is no better or worse than the calming influence of the nursery nurse rocking a crying baby. Each has his or her own specific and important role. The diversity of skills among nurses should be honored and recognized as a sign of the strength of the profession (Fig. 16.6).

If you think for a moment about other groups to which you belong—for example, a political party, church, or parent-teacher association—you do not expect to agree with every position taken by the organization or its leaders. Nurses seem to have such an expectation of their professional association, though, and use that as a reason for not participating. This is naïve and unrealistic. With nursing and society becoming increasingly diverse, nurses of the future must become more tolerant of differences and work hard to find common ground with their colleagues in the profession. If we fail to do so, nursing will not prosper, nor will its practitioners. In preparing for our future, the four major principles of successful implementation of health care reform set forth by the ANA are noteworthy (ANA, 2017):

1. "Ensure universal access to a standardized package of essential healthcare services for all citizens and residents.
2. Optimize primary, community-based, and preventative services while supporting cost effective use of innovative, technology-driven, acute hospital-based services.
3. Encourage mechanisms to stimulate economic use of healthcare services while supporting those who do not have the means to share in costs.

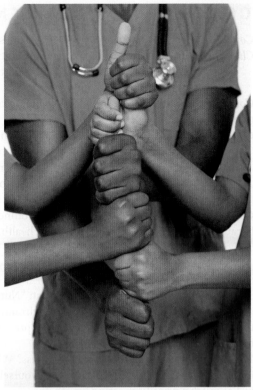

Fig. 16.6 Individual nurses can make positive changes; nurses working together can be even more powerful. (Photo used with permission from iStockphoto.)

4. Ensure a sufficient supply of a skilled workforce dedicated to providing high quality health care services."

This is a time of change in nursing, and you, the readers of this book, are the future of nursing. You represent our best hope for building nursing into an even more powerful force in improving the lives of those entrusted to our care, whether they are individuals, families, communities, or nations. Look around at the other members of your class, all 25 or 125 or 200 of you. You represent an amazing collection of energy and talent—combine those talents and harness that energy and you will accomplish more than you can imagine. So it is with nursing's future: we can accomplish far more by working collectively than alone. All nurses, individually and as a profession, will benefit from the results. Then, most important, so will our patients. In the words of anthropologist Margaret Mead, *"Never believe that a few caring people can't change the world. For, indeed, that's all who ever have."*

CONCEPTS AND CHALLENGES

- **Concept:** Care of the profession begins with care of self.
  Challenge: Working to the extent of your education and seeking to become more educated are important means of caring for the profession and yourself.
- **Concept:** Incivility reflects the lack of valuing and respect for others.
  Challenge: Acts of incivility can be small, such as rolling one's eyes—it is important to pay attention to your professional behavior to avoid even small gestures of incivility. Arm yourself with the tools to combat incivility and bullying behaviors.
- **Concept:** Nurses must care for the environment, because failure to do so is a direct threat to health.
  Challenge: Notice that your environment includes your home, workplace, and community. Challenges to your health may require attention to your local environment.
- **Concept:** You have a significant say in how the profession of nursing evolves. Join forces with those who think and believe like you do, and, collectively, you will make a big difference in the future of nursing.
  Challenge: Don't back down from challenges that seem insurmountable. Nurses are well positioned by their education, experience, creativity, and worldview to improve the health of populations in ways that you cannot yet imagine.

IDEAS FOR FURTHER EXPLORATION

1. Take a position on the following statement: "Nurses of the future will have an impact on the environment that exceeds that of the ordinary citizen." Be prepared to defend your position.
2. What strategies can you use to manage stress? What ideas do you have to ensure that caring for yourself is just as much a priority as caring for others?
3. How have you encountered incivility both in nursing school and in practice? How have you responded?
4. Identify two nursing organizations you are interested in joining. Read their websites, and determine whether they have reduced fees for students. If you can afford it, join one or both. If joining is not yet possible, consult the organizations' websites frequently. Most have some content that is accessible to nonmembers and will be useful to you.

REFERENCES

American Nurses Association (ANA): Healthcare reform. (website). 2017. Available at: http://ana.aristotle.com/SitePages/healthcarereform.aspx.

American Nurses Association (ANA): *code of ethics for nurses with interpretive statements*, Washington, DC, 2015a, 2015, American Nurses Publishing.

American Nurses Association (ANA): Position statement on incivility, bullying and workplace violence. (website). 2015. Available at: http://nursingworld.org/DocumentVault/Position-Statements/Practice/Position-Statement-on-Incivility-Bullying-and-Workplace-Violence.pdf.

American Nurses Association (ANA): Workplace issues: Occupational safety and health. (website). 2006. Available at: www.nursingworld.org/MainMenuCategories/ANAPoliticalPower/Federal/AGENCIES/OSHA/SHLATEX11704.aspx.

Beccuti G, Pannain S: Sleep and obesity, *Curr Opin Clin Nutr Metab Care* 14(4):402–412, 2011.

Cooper C: *The art of nursing: a practical introduction*, Philadelphia, 2001, Saunders.

Davis S, Mirick DK: Circadian disruption, shift work and the risk of cancer: a summary of the evidence and studies in Seattle, *Cancer Cause Cont* 17(4):539–545, 2006.

Department of Health and Human Services, Health Resources and Services Administration, National Center for Health Workforce Analysis. *National and regional supply and demand projections of the nursing workforce: 2014-2030*, Rockville, Maryland, 2017.

Gallicchio L, Kalesan B: Sleep duration and mortality a systematic review and metanalysis, *J Sleep Res* 18(2):148–158, 2009.

Jones C: American nurse project. (website). 2015. Available at: www.americannurseproject.com/landing-book.

Longo J: Cognitive rehearsal, *American Nurse Today* 12(8):41–42, 51, 2017. Available at: https://www.americannurseto-day.com/wp-content/uploads/2017/08/cognitive-rehearsal-american-nurses-association-journal.pdf.

Luparell S: Incivility in nursing: the connection between academia and clinical settings, *Crit Care Nurs* 31(2):92–95, 2011.

Passionate About Creating Environments of Respects and Civilities (PACERS): Civility Tool Kit. (website). 2012. Available at: http://stopbullyingtoolkit.org/Mnemonic-BE-AWARE...and-Care.pdf.

Selye, H: *General adaptation syndrome.* n.d. (website). Available at: www.essenceofstressrelief.com/general-adaptation-syndrome.html.

Stokowski LA: The downward spiral: incivility in nursing. (website). 2011. Available at: www.medscape.com/viewarticle/739328_3.

The Alliance of Nurses for Healthy Environments (ANHE): *Climate change, health and nursing: a call to action,* (website). 2016. Available at: https://envirn.org/climate-change/.

Truth About Nursing: Ratched or Wretched?. (website). 2018. Available at: http://blog.truthaboutnursing.org/2018/01/marysue-heilemann-on-nurse-ratched/.

Truth About Nursing: You can smile with your eyes: Ebola and nursing in the news media. (website). 2014. Available at: www.truthaboutnursing.org/news/2014/dec/ebola.html.

Truth About Nursing: A bad case of loving nurses. (website). 2012. Available at: http://www.truthaboutnursing.org/news/2012/feb/mavericks.html.

United Nations, Department of Economic and Social Affairs, Population Division: World population prospects: the 2017 revision, data booklet. 2017. Available at: https://www.un.org/development/desa/publications/world-population-prospects-the-2017-revision.html.

U.S. Census Bureau: *US world and population clock.* (website). Available at: https://www.census.gov/popclock/, n.d.

Epilogue

You are inheriting a rich legacy of achievement and progress in the profession of nursing. Some of you will be the names and faces of your generation of nurses, like Lillian Wald (my nursing hero) or Isabel Hampton Robb or Jessie Sleet Scales, persons whose energy and persistence moved not just nursing but the world forward. Change and evolution are necessary for progress, and although much has been accomplished, there remains much work to be done to transform nursing in ways that make sense in today's complex world. As professional nurses—and as citizens of world—you will be challenged to be leaders in solving the injustice of health disparities, improving access to health care for the disenfranchised, containing health care costs, and finding solutions for problems that we cannot possibly imagine at the moment. No doubt this seems like a long way in the future. It is not.

I hope that through using this book you have been inspired to develop values and beliefs consistent with professional nursing; that you are eager for more knowledge; that you aspire to a high degree of professionalism; and that you understand your potential as a nursing leader of the future and as a positive force for change in the nursing profession and in the world.

You can begin to exert your influence to improve the profession by evaluating this book. Please feel free to e-mail me with any observations you would like to share about this current edition. With your generous help, I will work to improve this book to meet the needs of students in the future.

— **BPB**
beth_black@unc.edu

A

Acceptance An accepting attitude that conveys neither approval nor disapproval (nonjudgment) of patients or their personal beliefs, habits, expressions of feelings, or chosen lifestyles.

Accountability Responsibility for one's behavior.

Accreditation A voluntary review process of educational programs or service agencies by professional organizations.

Active collaborator One who is engaged as a participant with another person.

Active listening A method of communicating interest and attention using such signals as maintaining eye contact, nodding, and encouraging the speaker.

Acuity Degree of illness.

Acute illness Sudden, steadily progressing symptoms that subside quickly, with or without treatment, such as influenza.

Adaptation A change or coping response to stress of any kind.

Adaptation model A conceptual model that focuses on the patient as an adaptive system; that is, one that strives to cope with both internal demands and external demands of the environment.

Adjudicate To decide or sit in judgment, as in a legal case.

Administrative law Law created by a governmental agency to meet the intent of statutory law.

Advance directives Written instructions recognized by state law that describe individuals' preferences in regard to medical intervention should they become incapacitated.

Advanced degrees Degrees beyond the bachelor's degree; master's and doctoral degrees.

Advanced practice Nursing roles that require either a master's degree or specialized education in a specific area.

Advanced practice nurse A registered nurse who has met advanced educational and practice requirements beyond basic nursing education.

Aesthetics Branch of philosophy that studies the nature of beauty.

Affective domain Field of activity dealing with a person's mood, feelings, values, or belief system.

Alternative therapies Treatments other than traditional Western medical treatments.

Altruism Unselfish concern for the welfare of others.

Ambulatory care Health services provided to those who visit a clinic or hospital as outpatients and depart after treatment on the same day.

American Assembly for Men in Nursing (AAMN) Professional organization that seeks to encourage, support, and advocate for men in nursing.

American Association of Colleges of Nursing (AACN) A national organization devoted to advancing nursing education at the baccalaureate and graduate levels.

American Nurses Association (ANA) Nursing's major professional organization made up of constituent state associations. Addresses issues of policy, ethics, standards of care, and the economic and general welfare of nurses. Membership is limited to nurses.

American Nurses Credentialing Center (ANCC) The organization that deals with certification of individual nurses, and approval of organizations as continuing education providers.

American Organization of Nurse Executives (AONE) An organization for high-level nursing managers, such as chief nurses. Leaders in nursing education can be associate members.

Analysis The second step in the nursing process during which various pieces of patient data are analyzed. The outcome is one or more nursing diagnoses.

Anxiety A diffuse, vague feeling of apprehension and uncertainty. Also a psychiatric condition.

Applied science Use of scientific theory and laws in a practical way that has immediate application.

Appropriateness A criterion for successful communication in which the reply fits the circumstances and matches the message, and the amount is neither too great nor too little.

Articulation An educational mobility system providing for direct movement from a program at one level of nursing education to another without significant loss of credit.

Assault A threat or an attempt to make bodily contact with another person without the person's consent.

Assessment The first step in the nursing process involving the collection of information about the patient.

Assisted suicide Suicide by a person with help from another person, such as a health care provider.

Associate degree in nursing program A form of basic nursing education program, leading to the associate degree in nursing (ADN), consisting of 3 or fewer years, and usually offered in technical or community colleges.

Association An organization of members with common interests.

Authority Possessing both the responsibility for making decisions and the accountability for the outcome of those decisions.

Autonomy Self-determination. Control over one's own professional practice.

B

Bachelor of science in nursing (BSN) Degree offered by programs that combine nursing courses with general education courses in a 4- or 5-year curriculum in a college or university.

Balance of power A distribution of forces among the branches of government so that no one branch is strong enough to dominate the others.

Basic program Any nursing education program preparing beginning practitioners.

Battery The impermissible, unprivileged touching of one person by another.

Belief The intellectual acceptance of something as true or correct.

Belief system Organization of an individual's beliefs into a rational whole.

Beneficence   The ethical principle of doing good.

Biases   Prejudices, often outside the individual's awareness.

Bioethics   An area of ethical inquiry focusing on the dilemmas inherent in modern health care.

Biomedical technology   Complex machines or implantable devices used in patient care settings.

Birthrate   The number of births in a particular place during a specific time period, usually expressed as a quantity per 1000 people in 1 year.

Burnout   A state of emotional exhaustion attributable to cumulative stress.

C

Cadet Corps   A government-created entity designed during World War II to rapidly increase the number of registered nurses being educated so they could assist in the war effort.

Caregiver stress   A condition affecting individuals responsible for meeting the needs of others, often a family member, with a chronic condition such as Alzheimer's disease. Consists of feeling overwhelmed and a variety of other emotional and physical symptoms of stress.

Caring   A theoretical framework central to nursing that results in a professional form of relating to, attending to, and providing for the needs of others.

Case management   Systematic collaboration with patients, their significant others, and their health care providers to coordinate high-quality health care services in a cost-effective manner with positive patient outcomes.

Case management nursing   A growing field within nursing in which nurses are responsible for coordinating services provided to patients in a cost-effective manner.

Case manager   An individual responsible for coordinating services provided to a group of patients.

CCNE   Commission on Collegiate Nursing Education, the accrediting arm of the American Association of Colleges of Nursing.

Centers for Medicare and Medicaid Services (CMS)   Federal cost-containment program that establishes standards and monitors care in the Medicare and Medicaid programs.

Certification   Validation of specific qualifications demonstrated by a registered nurse in a defined area of practice.

Certified nurse-midwife (CNM)   A nationally certified nurse with advanced specialized education who assists women and couples during uncomplicated pregnancies, deliveries, and postdelivery periods.

Certified registered nurse anesthetist (CRNA)   A nationally certified nurse with advanced education who specializes in the administration of anesthesia.

Change agent   An individual who recognizes the need for organizational change and facilitates that process.

Chief executive officer (CEO)   The senior administrator of an organization.

Chief nurse executive (CNE)   The senior nursing administrator of an organization. Also chief nurse officer (CNO).

Chief nurse officer (CNO)   The senior nursing administrator of an organization. Also chief nurse executive (CNE).

Chief of staff   A physician in a health care facility, generally elected by the medical staff for a specified term, who is responsible for overseeing the activities of the medical staff organization.

Chronic illness   Ongoing health problems of a generally incurable nature, such as diabetes.

Civil law   Law involving disputes between individuals.

Clarification   A therapeutic communication technique in which the nurse seeks to understand a patient's message more clearly.

Cliché   An often-repeated expression that conveys little real meaning, such as "Have a nice day."

Clinical director   Middle management nurse who has responsibility for multiple units in a health care agency. Also known as a clinical coordinator.

Clinical judgment   The ability to make consistently effective clinical decisions based on theoretical knowledge, research findings, informed opinions, and prior experience.

Clinical ladder   Programs allowing nurses to progress in the organizational hierarchy while staying in direct patient care roles.

Clinical nurse leader   A nurse with an advanced degree who is a clinical expert in the care of a distinct group of patients and who may provide direct patient care.

Clinical nurse specialist   An advanced practice nurse with an advanced degree who serves as a resource person to other nurses and often provides direct care to patients or families with particularly difficult or complex problems.

Closed system   A system that does not interact with other systems or with the surrounding environment.

Code of ethics   A statement of professional standards used to guide behavior and as a framework for decision making.

Code of Ethics for Nurses   A formal statement by the ANA of the nursing profession's code of ethics.

Cognitive   Pertaining to intellectual activities requiring knowledge.

Cognitive domain   Area of activity that affects an individual's knowledge level.

Cognitive rebellion   A stage in the educational process wherein students begin to free themselves from external controls and to rely on their own judgment.

Collaboration   Working closely with another person in the spirit of cooperation.

Collective action   Activities undertaken by or on behalf of a group of people who have common interests.

Collective bargaining   Negotiating as a group for improved salary and work conditions.

Collective identity   The connection and feeling of similarity individuals in a particular group feel with one another; group identification.

Collegiality   The promotion of collaboration, cooperation, and recognition of interdependence among members of a profession.

Commission on Collegiate Nursing Education (CCNE)   The accrediting arm of the American Association of Colleges of Nursing.

Common law   Law that develops as a result of decisions made by judges in legal cases.

Communication   The exchange of thoughts, ideas, or information; a dynamic process that is a primary instrument through which change occurs in nursing situations.

Community-based nursing   Nursing care provided for individuals, families, and groups in a variety of settings, including homes, workplaces, and schools.

Community health nursing   Formerly known as public health nursing; a nursing specialty that systematically uses a process of delivering nursing care to improve the health of an entire community.

Compassion fatigue A state experienced by those helping people in distress; an extreme state of tension and preoccupation with the suffering of those being helped to the degree that it is traumatizing for the helper.

Competency Refers to the capability of a particular patient to understand the information given and to make an informed choice about treatment options.

Complementary therapies Those treatments intended to augment Western medical treatments such as massage therapy or acupuncture.

Concept An abstract classification of data; for example, "temperature" is a concept.

Conceptual model or framework A group of concepts that are broadly defined and systematically organized to provide a focus, a rationale, and a tool for the integration and interpretation of information.

Confidentiality Ensuring the privacy of individuals participating in research studies or being treated in health care settings.

Congruent A characteristic of communication that occurs when the verbal and nonverbal elements of a message match.

Constituent members Organizational members of the American Nurses Association, such as state nurses associations or specialty nursing organizations.

Consultation The process of conferring with patients, families, or other health professionals.

Contact hour A measurement used to recognize participation in continuing education offerings, usually equivalent to 50 minutes.

Context An essential element of communication consisting of the setting in which an interaction occurs, the mood, the relationship between sender and receiver, and other factors.

Continuing education (CE) Workshops, conferences, and short courses, in which nurses maintain competence during their professional careers.

Continuous quality improvement (CQI) A management concept focusing on excellence and employee involvement at all levels of an organization.

Contracts Documents agreed on by workers and management that include provisions about staffing levels, salary, work conditions, and other issues of concern to either party.

Copayment The portion of a provider's charges that an insured patient is responsible for paying.

Coping The methods a person uses to assess and manage demands.

Coping mechanisms Psychological devices used by individuals when a threat is perceived.

Cost containment An attempt to keep health care costs stable or increasing only slowly.

Criminal law Law involving public concerns against unlawful behavior that threatens society.

Criteria Standards by which something is judged or measured.

Critical paths Multidisciplinary care plans outlining a patient's treatments and expected outcomes, day by day.

Cross-training Preparing a single worker for multiple tasks that formerly were performed by multiple specialized workers.

Cultural assessment The process of determining a patient's cultural practices and preferences in order to render culturally competent care.

Cultural care, theory of A nursing theory focusing on the importance of incorporating a patient's culturally determined health beliefs and practices into care.

Cultural competence The integration of knowledge, attitudes, and skills that enhance cross-cultural communication and appropriate interactions with others.

Cultural diversity Social, ethnic, racial, and religious differences in a group.

Culturally competent education Nursing education that incorporates knowledge, attitudes, and skills that enhance cross-cultural communication and appropriate interactions with others.

Culturally congruent nursing care Care that incorporates knowledge, attitudes, and skills that enhance cross-cultural communication and appropriate interactions with others.

Culture The attitudes, beliefs, and behaviors of social and ethnic groups that have been perpetuated through generations.

Culture of nursing The rites, rituals, and valued behaviors of the nursing profession.

D

Data Information or facts collected for analysis.

Deaconess Institute A large hospital and planned training program for deaconesses established in 1836 by Pastor Theodor Fliedner at Kaiserswerth, Germany.

Decentralization An organizational structure in which decision-making authority is shared with employees most affected by the decisions rather than being retained by top executives.

Deductible The out-of-pocket amount individuals must pay before their health insurance begins to pay for health care.

Deductive reasoning A process through which conclusions are drawn by logical inference from given premises; proceeds from the general case to the specific.

Defining characteristics Signs and symptoms of disease.

Delegate To refer a task to another.

Delegation The practice of assigning tasks or responsibilities to other persons.

Demographics The study of vital statistics and social trends.

Demography The science that studies vital statistics and social trends.

Deontology The ethical theory that the rightness or wrongness of an action depends on the inherent moral significance of the action.

Dependency The degree to which individuals adopt passive attitudes and rely on others to take care of them.

Dependent intervention Nursing actions on behalf of patients that require knowledge and skill on the part of the nurse but may not be done without explicit directions from another health professional, usually a physician, dentist, or nurse practitioner.

Developmental theory A theory in which growth is defined as an increase in physical size and shape toward a point of optimal maturity.

Diagnosis Identification of a disease or condition.

Dietitian Bachelor's or master's degree–prepared nutrition expert who specializes in therapeutic diet preparation and nutrition education. Also known as a registered dietitian (RD).

Diploma program The earliest form of formal nursing education in the United States; usually based in hospitals, requires 3 years of study, and leads to a diploma in nursing.

Disaster An event or situation that is of greater magnitude than an emergency; disrupts essential services such as housing, transportation, communications, sanitation, water, and health care; and requires the response of people outside the community affected.

Disease A pathologic alteration at the tissue or organ level.

Disease management A process of helping patients understand and manage their chronic conditions effectively through coaching and education, symptom recognition and management, and collaboration with the patient's health care provider.

Disenfranchised The state of having no power or voice in a political system.

Disseminate Publish or widely distribute scientific information, such as the findings of a research study.

Dissonance Lack of harmony.

Distance learning The process of taking classes and earning academic credit through technological means such as televised or online classes. The teacher and student may be many miles apart.

Documentation Written communication about a patient's condition, care, and reactions to treatments; found in the patient record/chart.

Dominant culture Mainstream culture that contains one or more subcultures.

Double effect Ethical concept encompassing the belief that there are some situations in which it is necessary to inflict potential harm in an effort to achieve a greater good.

Duty of care The responsibility of a nurse or other health professional for the care of a patient.

Duty to report The requirement, according to state law, for health professionals to report certain illnesses, injuries, and actions of patients.

E

Efficiency A criterion for successful communication that consists of using simple, clear words timed at a pace suitable to participants.

Electoral process The procedures that must be followed to select someone to fill an elected position.

Empathy Awareness of, sensitivity to, and identification with the feelings of another person.

End-of-life care Care aimed at comfort and dignity for patients who are nearing death and for their families and other significant persons in their lives.

Entrepreneur A person who envisions, organizes, manages, and assumes responsibility for a new enterprise or business.

Environment All of the many external and internal factors, such as physical and psychological, that influence life and survival.

Epistemology The branch of philosophy dealing with the theory of knowledge.

Ethical decision making The process of choosing between actions based on a system of beliefs and values.

Ethics The branch of philosophy that studies the propriety of certain courses of action.

Ethnocentrism The belief that one's own culture is the most desirable.

Ethnographic research A type of qualitative research focusing on culture and the phenomena associated with a culture.

Euthanasia The act of painlessly ending the life of a terminally ill individual for whom cure is not possible.

Evaluation Measuring the success or failure of the results or "outputs," and consequently the effectiveness, of a system. It is the final step in the nursing process wherein the nurse examines the patient's progress to determine whether a problem is solved, is in the process of being solved, or is unsolved. In communication theory, it is the analysis of information received.

Evidence-based practice The use of research findings, clinical expertise, and patient preference as the three-pronged basis for practice rather than trial and error, intuition, or traditional methods, such as problem solving.

Exacerbation Reemergence or worsening of the symptoms of a chronic illness.

Executive branch The branch of government responsible for administering the laws of the land.

Experimental design Research design that provides evidence of a cause-and-effect relationship between actions.

Expert witness An individual called on to testify in court because of special skill or knowledge in a certain field, such as nursing.

Extended care Medical, nursing, or custodial care provided to an individual over a prolonged period.

Extended family A term used to describe nonnuclear family members such as grandparents, aunts, and uncles.

External factors Values, beliefs, and behaviors of significant others that have an impact on an individual.

F

Faith community The members of a church, synagogue, mosque, or other entity who worship together and share common beliefs about religion.

Faith community nurse A specialized nurse who focuses on the promotion of health within the context of the values, beliefs, and practices of a church, synagogue, mosque, or other faith community. May also be known as a *parish nurse*.

False reassurance A nontherapeutic form of communication that seeks to reassure that everything will turn out well.

Family system The group of individuals who comprise the basic unit of family living and their interactions with one another and the larger society.

Feedback The information given back into a system to determine whether or not the purpose of the system has been achieved. A major element in the communication process.

Fidelity An ethical principle that values faithfulness to one's responsibilities.

Flexibility A criterion for successful communication that occurs when messages are based on the immediate situation rather than preconceived expectations.

Flexible staffing A mechanism whereby nurses may work at times other than the traditional hospital shifts.

Flexner Report A 1910 study of medical education that provided the impetus for much-needed reform.

Formal socialization The process by which individuals learn a new role from the direct instruction of others.

For-profit agency A health care agency established to make a profit for the owners or shareholders.

Frontier Nursing Service Founded in Kentucky in 1925; it provided the first organized midwifery service in the United States.

G

General election An election in which all registered voters may vote and may choose a candidate from any party on the ballot.

Generalizable Research findings that are transferable to other situations.

General systems theory A theory promulgated by Ludwig von Bertalanffy in the late 1930s to explain the relationship of a whole to its parts.

Generic master's degree An accelerated master's degree in nursing for people with nonnursing bachelor's degrees.

Genetic counseling Health and reproductive advice given to individuals based on their genetic composition.

Goldmark Report A major study of nursing education published in 1923 and named *The Study of Nursing and Nursing Education in the United States.*

Governmental (public) agency An agency primarily supported by taxes, administered by elected or appointed officials, and tailored to the needs of the communities served.

Grand theory A very broad conceptualization of nursing phenomena.

Grassroots activism The involvement of a large number of people, generally widely dispersed, who are concerned about a particular issue.

Growth An increase in physical size and shape toward a point of optimal maturity.

H

Health An individual's physical, mental, spiritual, and social well-being; a continuum, not a constant state.

Health behaviors Choices and habitual actions that promote or diminish health.

Health beliefs Culturally determined beliefs about the nature of health and illness.

Health care network A corporation with a consolidated set of facilities and services for comprehensive health care.

Health Insurance Portability and Accountability Act (HIPAA) Federal law, passed in 1996, designed to protect health insurance coverage for workers and their families when they change or lose their jobs.

Health maintenance Preventing illness and maintaining maximal function.

Health maintenance organization (HMO) A network or group of providers who agree to provide certain basic health care services for a single predetermined yearly fee.

Health promotion Encouraging a condition of maximum physical, mental, and social well-being.

Health promotion model A theoretical nursing model that uses illness prevention and health promotion as a basic framework.

Helping professions Professions such as social work, teaching, and nursing that emphasize meeting the needs of clients.

Henry Street Settlement A clinic for the poor founded by Lillian Wald and her colleague Mary Brewster on New York's Lower East Side.

Heterogeneous Composed of parts of differing kinds.

High-level wellness Functioning at maximum potential in an integrated way within the environment.

High-tech nursing Nursing care that involves the use of technologies such as monitors, pumps, and ventilators. This is not a nursing specialty, however.

Holism A school of health care thought that espouses treating the whole patient—body, mind, and spirit.

Holistic nursing care Nursing care that nourishes the whole person—body, mind, and spirit.

Holistic values The approach to nursing practice that takes the physical, emotional, social, economic, and spiritual needs of the person into consideration.

Home health agency An organization that delivers various health services to patients in their homes.

Home health nursing Field of nursing in which care is provided to patients in their own homes.

Homeostasis A relative constancy in the internal environment of the body.

Homogeneous Composed of parts of the same or similar kinds.

Hospice An agency providing end-of-life care to terminally ill patients and their families.

Hospice and palliative care nursing Specialized nursing care provided at the end of life to patients and their families in homes and residential facilities. Aimed at a comfortable and dignified death that honors the wishes of patients and loved ones.

Hospitalist Hospital-based physicians who care for patients only while patients are hospitalized.

Human Genome Project A scientific project designed to map the genetic structure of composite human DNA, the initial phase of which was completed in 2003.

Human motivation Abraham Maslow's conceptualization of human needs and their relationship to the stimulation of purposeful behavior.

Human needs theory Theory proposed by Abraham Maslow that human motivation is determined by the drive to meet intrinsic human needs.

Hypothesis A statement predicting the relationship among concepts or variables.

I

Illness An abnormal process in which an individual's physical, emotional, social, or intellectual functioning is impaired.

Illness prevention All activities aimed at diminishing the likelihood that an individual's physical, emotional, social, and intellectual functions become impaired.

Implementation A stage of the nursing process during which the plan of care is carried out.

Incongruent Describes a confusing form of communication that occurs when the verbal and nonverbal elements of a message do not match.

Independent intervention Actions on behalf of patients for which the nurse requires no supervision or direction.

Individualized care plan A plan of care designed to meet the needs of a specific person.

Inductive reasoning The process of reasoning from the specific to the general. Repeated observations of an experiment or event enable the observer to draw general conclusions.

Inertia Disinclination to change.

Infant mortality The number of deaths of infants (1 year of age or younger) per 1000 live births.

Informal socialization The process through which individuals learn a new role by observing how others behave.

Informatics nurse A nurse who combines nursing science with information management science and computer science to manage and make accessible the information that nurses need.

Information technology (IT) Hardware and software used to manage and process information.

Informed consent process The process of informing individuals who are scheduled to undergo diagnostic procedures or surgery or who are potential research participants of the procedures and risks. Their consent is indicated by signing a consent form voluntarily once any questions they have are answered and their privacy has been ensured.

Infrastructure Basic support mechanisms needed to ensure that an activity can be conducted.

Input The information, energy, or matter that enters a system.

Institutional review board (IRB) A committee protecting the rights of human participants in the research. Any research involving human participants must have approval of the IRB or the IRB's determination that a study is not human subjects research.

Institutional structure The way in which the workers within an agency are organized to carry out the functions of the agency.

Integrative care Care that combines the best of both standard and nontraditional treatments, for example, pain control through both prescription medication and acupuncture.

Interdependent intervention Actions on behalf of patients in which the nurse must collaborate or consult with another health professional before or while carrying out the action.

Interdisciplinary team Group composed of individuals representing various disciplines who work together toward a common end, blending their expertise in the development of a common goal.

Internal factors Personal feelings and beliefs that influence an individual.

Internalize The process of taking in knowledge, skills, attitudes, beliefs, norms, values, and ethical standards and making them a part of one's own self-image and behavior.

International Council of Nurses (ICN) The federation of national nurses associations, currently representing nurses in more than 100 countries.

Internship An apprenticeship under supervision.

Interpreter A professional who is fluent in a second language or is bilingual who translates the spoken words.

Interprofessional education (IPE) Students across health care disciplines such as nursing, social work, and medicine learning together to address complex health problems collaboratively.

Interprofessionality Teamwork and practice across disciplines using competencies that are central to all health care professions.

J

Jargon Specialized vocabulary used by those in the same line of work to communicate about work-related matters.

Judicial branch The branch of government that decides cases or controversies on particular matters.

Justice An ethical principle stating that equals should be treated the same and that unequals should be treated differently.

K

Knowledge-based power Authority or control based on the way information is used to effect an outcome.

Knowledge technology The use of computer systems to transform information into knowledge and to generate new knowledge; expert systems.

L

Latent power Untapped strength.

Law All the rules of conduct established by a government and applicable to the people, whether in the form of legislation or custom.

Learned resourcefulness An acquired ability to use available resources in one's behalf.

Legal authority A group of people in whom power is vested by law, such as the powers vested in state boards of nursing by nurse practice acts.

Legislative branch The branch of government consisting of elected officials who are responsible for enacting the laws of the land.

Licensure The process by which an agency of government grants permission to qualified persons to engage in a given profession or occupation.

Licensure by endorsement A system whereby registered nurses or licensed practical/vocational nurses can, by submitting proof of licensure in another state and paying a licensure fee, receive licensure from the new state without sitting for a licensing examination.

Lifelong learning Continuing education and increasing knowledge throughout an individual's professional life.

Lobby An attempt to influence the vote of legislators.

Locus of control The place where an individual believes the power in his or her life resides, either within or outside of himself or herself.

Logic The field of philosophy that studies correct and incorrect reasoning.

Long-term care Care provided to individuals, such as people with Alzheimer's disease, who require ongoing assistance in the maintenance of activities of daily living.

Long-term goals Major changes that may take months or even years to accomplish.

Lysaught Report A 1970 report titled *An Abstract for Action* that made recommendations concerning the supply and demand for nurses, nursing roles and functions, and nursing education.

M

Magnet Recognition Program An initiative of the American Nurses Credentialing Center (ANCC) that recognizes excellent patient outcomes, a high level of job satisfaction among nurses, low staff nurse turnover rate, and appropriate grievance resolution, among other factors.

Malpractice An act resulting in injury that occurs when a professional fails to act as a reasonably prudent professional would under similar circumstances.

Managed care A process in which an individual, often a nurse, is assigned to review patients' cases and coordinate services so that quality care can be achieved at the lowest cost.

Managed care organization (MCO) Any of a number of organizations that attempt to coordinate subscriber services to ensure quality care at the lowest cost.

Mandatory continuing education The requirement that nurses complete a certain number of hours of continuing education as a prerequisite for relicensure.

Medicaid A jointly funded federal and state public health insurance that covers citizens below the poverty level and those with certain disabling conditions; established in 1965.

Medically indigent Individuals and families who do not qualify for Medicaid or Medicare but cannot afford health insurance or medical care.

Medicare A federally funded form of public health insurance for citizens 65 years of age and older; established in 1965.

Mentor An experienced nurse who shares knowledge with less experienced nurses to help advance their careers.

Message An essential element of communication consisting of the spoken word and/or nonverbal communication.

Metaparadigm The most abstract aspect of the structure of knowledge; the global concepts that identify the phenomena of interest for a discipline.

Metaphysics The branch of philosophy that considers the ultimate nature of existence, reality, and experience.

Middle-range theory Theory that makes connections between grand theories and nursing practice.

Milieu Surroundings or environment.

Mission The special task(s) to which an organization devotes itself.

Model A symbolic representation of a concept or reality.

Modeling An informal type of socialization that occurs when an individual chooses an admired person to emulate.

Moonlighting The practice of working a second job in addition to the regular one.

Moral development The ways in which a person learns to deal with moral dilemmas from childhood through adulthood.

Moral distress Pain or anguish of a person who unwillingly participates in perceived moral wrongdoing.

Morals Established rules or standards that guide behavior in situations in which a decision about right and wrong must be made.

Mortality rate The number of deaths in a particular population during a specific period of time; usually expressed as a quantity per 1000 people in a specific year.

Mutuality Sharing jointly with others.

Mutual recognition model A system whereby a registered nurse may be licensed in the state of residency yet practice in other states, after being recognized by them, without additional licenses.

N

NANDA International Group working since 1970 to establish a comprehensive list of nursing diagnoses.

National Council Licensure Examination for Practical Nurses (NCLEX-PN®) The examination that graduates of practical nursing programs must take to practice as licensed practical nurses (LPNs) or licensed vocational nurses (LVNs).

National Council Licensure Examination for Registered Nurses (NCLEX-RN®) The examination that graduates of basic nursing programs must take to become licensed to practice as registered nurses (RNs).

National League for Nursing (NLN) National organization that seeks to advance the profession of nursing through advocacy and improving educational standards for nurses. Nonnurses may be members.

National League for Nursing Accrediting Commission (NLNAC) The arm of the National League for Nursing that accredits schools' associate degree, diploma, baccalaureate, and master's programs in nursing.

National Student Nurses Association (NSNA) National organization devoted to developing leadership skills in nursing students.

Negligence The failure to act as a reasonably prudent person would have acted in specific circumstances.

Network A system of interconnected individuals; useful to develop contacts or exchange information to further a career.

Nonexperimental design Research with the intent to describe or clarify a phenomenon. Not intended to test a hypothesis.

Nonjudgmental Describes an attitude that conveys neither approval nor disapproval of patients' beliefs and respects each person's right to his or her own beliefs.

Nonmaleficence The duty to inflict no harm or evil.

Nonverbal communication Communication without words; consists of gestures, posture, facial expressions, tone and loudness of voice, actions, grooming, and clothing, among other things.

Nosocomial Hospital-acquired, as a nosocomial infection.

Not-for-profit agency An organization that does not attempt to make a profit for distribution to owners or stockholders. Any profit made by such organizations is used to operate and improve the organization itself or to extend its services.

Nuclear family Term used to describe a couple, parent, or parents and their children; as opposed to *extended family*.

Nurse activist A nurse who works actively on behalf of a political candidate or certain legislation.

Nurse anesthetist A nurse with specialized advanced education who administers anesthetic agents to patients undergoing operative procedures.

Nurse-based practice A clinic, office, or home practice in which nurses carry their own caseloads of patients with physical and/or psychiatric needs.

Nurse citizen A nurse who exercises all the political rights accorded citizens, such as registering to vote and voting in all elections.

Nurse entrepreneur A nurse who engages in a business undertaking related to health care or nursing, such as owning a traveling nurse agency.

Nurse executive The top nurse in the administrative structure of a health care organization.

Nurse Licensure Compact An agreement among certain states, authorized by legislation, that they will honor licenses issued to registered nurses by other states in the compact.

Nurse manager A nurse who is in charge of all activities in a unit, including patient care, continuous quality improvement, personnel selection and evaluation, and resource (supplies and money) management. Formerly known as a head nurse.

Nurse-midwife A nurse with advanced specialized education who assists women and couples during uncomplicated pregnancies, deliveries, and postdelivery periods.

Nurse-patient relationship The mode of connection between a nurse and patient.

Nurse politician A nurse who runs for political office.

Nurse practitioner A nurse with advanced education who specializes in the health care of a particular group, such as children, pregnant women, or the elderly.

Nursing The provision of health care services, focusing on the maintenance, promotion, and restoration of health.

Nursing diagnosis A process of describing a patient's response to health problems that either already exist or may occur in the future.

Nursing goal A statement of the desired long-term or short-term outcome as a result of one or more nursing interventions.

Nursing informatics The branch of nursing that manages knowledge and data through technology with the goal of improving patient care.

Nursing information system A software system that automates the nursing process.

Nursing Outcomes Classification (NOC) A classification system describing patient outcomes sensitive to nursing interventions.

Nursing practice act Law defining the scope of nursing practice in a given state.

Nursing process A cognitive activity that requires both critical and creative thinking and serves as the basis for providing nursing care. A method used by nurses in dealing with patient problems in professional practice.

Nursing research The systematic investigation of events or circumstances related to improving patient outcomes.

Nursing theory A formal statement of related concepts used to explain, predict, control, and understand commonly occurring phenomena of interest to nurses.

O

Obesity A body mass index (BMI) of 30 or more.

Objective data Factual information obtained through observation and examination of the patient or through consultation with other health care providers.

Occupation A person's principal work or business.

Occupational and environmental health nurse A nurse specializing in the care of a specific group of workers in a given occupational setting.

Open-ended question An inquiry that causes the patient to answer fully, giving more than a "yes" or "no" answer.

Open posture Body position, such as squarely facing another person with arms in a relaxed position.

Open system A system that promotes the exchange of matter, energy, and information with other systems and the environment.

Organizational structure How an agency is organized to accomplish its mission.

Orientation phase The beginning phase of a nurse-patient relationship in which the parties are getting acquainted with one another.

Outcome criteria Expected results of nursing intervention.

Out-of-pocket payment Direct payment for health services from individuals' personal funds.

Output The end result or product of a system.

P

Palliative care nursing A rapidly developing specialty in nursing dedicated to management of symptoms and improving the quality of life of seriously, chronically ill patients, patients at the end of their lives, and their families.

Parental modeling A type of socialization that occurs when parents' behavior and responses to various stimuli influence a child's future behaviors and responses.

Participants The individuals who are studied in a research project. Formerly referred to as "subjects."

Patient acuity The degree of illness of a particular patient or group of patients; used to determine staffing needs.

Patient advocate One who promotes the interest of patients. A nursing role.

Patient care technician (PCT) A health technician working under the supervision of a registered nurse, physician, or other health professional to provide basic patient care.

Patient-centered care A system that emphasizes coordinating patient care to maximize patient comfort, convenience, and security.

Patient classification system (PCS) Identification of patients' needs for nursing care in quantitative terms.

Patient interview A face-to-face interaction with the patient in which an interviewer elicits pertinent information.

Patient Self-Determination Act Effective December 1, 1991, this law encourages patients to consider which life-prolonging treatment options they desire and to document their preferences in case they should later become incapable of participating in the decision-making process.

Patients' rights Responsibilities that a hospital and its staff have toward patients and their families during hospitalization.

Pay equity Equal pay for work of comparable value.

Peer review The process of submitting one's work for examination and comment by colleagues in the same profession to ensure scientific and scholarly value.

Perception The selection, organization, and interpretation of incoming signals into meaningful messages.

Performance improvement (PI) Organizational efforts to improve corporate performance, incorporating aspects of quality management.

Person An individual—man, woman, or child.

Personal payment Direct payment for health services from an individual's personal funds.

Personal space The amount of space surrounding individuals in which they feel comfortable interacting with others; usually culturally determined.

Personal value system The social principles, ideals, or standards held by an individual that form the basis for meaning, direction, and decision making in life.

Phenomena Occurrences or circumstances that are observable. The singular form of the word is phenomenon.

Phenomenological inquiry/research A qualitative research approach focusing on what people experience in regard to a particular phenomenon, such as grief, and how they interpret those experiences.

Philosophy The study of the truths and principles of being, knowledge, conduct, or nature of the universe.

Planning The third step in the nursing process, which begins with the identification of patient goals.

Policy The principles and values that govern actions directed toward given ends. Policy sets forth a plan, direction, or goal for action.

Policy development The generation of principles and procedures that guide governmental or organizational action.

Policy outcome The result of decisions made by governmental or organizational leaders who choose a certain course of action.

Political action committees (PACs) Groups that raise and distribute money to candidates who support their organization's stand on certain issues.

Politics The area of philosophy that deals with the regulation and control of people living in society; in government, it includes the allocation of scarce resources such as health care resources.

Population The entire group of people possessing a given characteristic; for example, all brown-eyed people older than age 65.

Position paper Statement pertaining to the stance a group or organization takes on an issue; for example, the American Nurses Association's 1965 Position Paper advocated the baccalaureate degree as the entry level into the practice of registered nursing.

Posttraumatic stress disorder (PTSD) An anxiety disorder characterized by an acute emotional response to a traumatic event or situation.

Powers of appointment The authority to select the people who serve in positions such as judges, ambassadors, and cabinet officials.

Practical nurse (LPN/LVN) program A 1-year educational program preparing individuals for direct patient care roles under the supervision of a physician or registered nurse.

Preceptor A teacher; in nursing, usually an experienced nurse who assumes responsibility for teaching a new nurse (novice).

Preferred provider organization (PPO) A form of HMO that contracts with independent providers such as physicians and hospitals for a negotiated discount for services provided to its members.

Premium The amount paid for an insurance policy, usually in installments.

Primary care Basic health care, including promotion of health, early diagnosis of disease, and prevention of disease.

Primary election An election in which voters who are declared members of a political party choose among several candidates of that same party for a particular office.

Primary nursing A system of nursing care delivery in which one nurse has responsibility for the planning, implementation, and evaluation of the care of one or more clients 24 hours a day for the duration of the hospital stay.

Primary source The patient is considered the primary source of data about himself or herself; in a literature review, a primary source is the original writing of a theorist or author.

Principalism Use of multiple ethical principles, such as beneficence, autonomy, nonmaleficence, veracity, justice, and fidelity, in the resolution of ethical conflicts rather than a single principle.

Private insurance Insurance obtained from a privately owned company, as opposed to public or governmental insurance.

Private practice Nursing practice engaged in by some nurses with advanced education; usually provided on a fee-for-service basis, as in most medical practices.

Privileged communications The principle that information given to certain professionals (e.g., attorneys, clergy) is protected and is not to be disclosed even in court.

Problem solving A method of finding solutions to difficulties specific to a given situation and designed for immediate action.

Profession Work requiring advanced training and usually involving mental rather than manual effort. Usually has a code of ethics and a professional organization.

Professional A person who engages in a specific profession, such as law, medicine, or nursing.

Professional accountabilities In the shared governance model, a basic set of responsibilities of all professional nurses regardless of practice setting.

Professional association An organization consisting of people belonging to the same profession and thereby having many common interests.

Professional boundary The dividing line between the activities of two professions. The area in which a professional person functions to avoid both underinvolvement and overinvolvement, maintaining the patient's needs as the focus of the relationship.

Professional outcomes The impact on a profession from political action by its practitioners.

Professional practice advocacy Includes activities such as education, lobbying, and advocating individually and collectively to advance a profession's agenda.

Professional review organization (PRO) Organizations that review Medicare hospital admissions and Medicare patients' lengths of stay.

Professional socialization The process of developing an occupational identity.

Professionalism Professional behavior, appearance, and conduct.

Professionalization A process through which an occupation evolves to professional status.

Proposition A statement about how two or more concepts are related.

Protocol A written plan specifying the procedure to be followed.

Provider A deliverer of health care services—hospital, clinic, nurse, or physician.

Proximate cause Action occurring immediately before an injury, thereby assumed to be the reason for the injury.

Psychomotor domain Area of activity referring to motor skills or actions by an individual; for example, learning to dance is in the psychomotor domain.

Pure science Information that summarizes and explains the universe without regard for whether the information is immediately useful; also known as "basic science."

Q

Qualitative research A type of inquiry that is characterized by studying phenomena in their natural setting using interviews, observations, and other techniques; includes ethnography, grounded theory, and phenomenology.

Quantitative research Research that uses data-gathering techniques that can be repeated by others and verified. Data collected are quantifiable—that is, they can be counted, measured with standardized instruments, or observed with a high degree of agreement among observers.

Quaternary care Extremely specialized care that may be available in a very few locations, such as a research medical center; a form of very advanced care.

R

Reality shock The feelings of powerlessness and ineffectiveness often experienced by new nursing graduates; usually occurs as a result of the transition from the educational setting to the "real world" of nursing in an actual health care setting.

Receiver An essential element of communication; the person receiving the message.

Reengineering Radical redesign of business processes and thinking to improve performance.

Referendum An election resulting from registered voters being asked by a legislative body to express a preference on a policy issue.

Reflection A communication technique that consists of directing questions back to patients, thereby encouraging patients to think through problems for themselves.

Reflective practice A method of focusing on one's practice, both in the moment and after an event, with an open and curious mind, drawing on all the senses to know oneself more fully.

Reflective thinking The process of evaluating one's thinking processes during a situation that has already occurred, as opposed to evaluating one's thinking during the situation as it occurs.

Registered nurse (RN) An individual who has completed a basic program for registered nurses and successfully passed the NCLEX-RN®.

Rehabilitation services Those activities designed to restore an individual or a body part to normal or near-normal function after a debilitating disease or an accident.

Reliable Yielding the same values dependably each time an instrument is used to measure the same thing.

Remission A period of chronic illness during which symptoms subside.

Replication The process of repeating a research study as closely as possible to the original.

Research process Prescribed steps that must be taken to plan and conduct meaningful research properly.

Research question A statement, question, or hypothesis that a research study is designed to answer.

Resilience A pattern of successful adaptation despite challenging or threatening circumstances.

Resocialized The outcome of a transitional process of giving up part or all of one set of professional values and learning new ones.

Resolution A written position on an issue presented to the voting members of an association for their consideration, discussion, and vote.

Respondeat superior Legal theory that attributes the acts of employees to their employer (Latin term).

Retrospective reimbursement Insurance payment made after services are delivered.

Risk management A program that seeks to identify and eliminate potential safety hazards, thereby reducing patient injuries.

RN-to-BSN in nursing Programs enabling registered nurses who hold associate degrees or diplomas in nursing to acquire baccalaureate degrees in nursing.

Role A goal-directed pattern of behavior learned within a cultural setting.

Role model An individual who serves as an example of desirable behavior for another person.

Role strain Stress created by difficulty experienced in adjusting to a life or occupational role.

S

Salary compression A phenomenon in which pay increases are limited during an individual's career, so that the salary of an experienced nurse may be little higher than that of a recently hired novice nurse.

Sample A subset of an entire population that reflects the characteristics of the population.

School nurse Nurse specializing in the care of school-age children or adolescents and practicing in school settings.

Scientific discipline A branch of instruction or field of learning based on the study of a body of facts about the physical or material world.

Scientific method A systematic, orderly approach to the gathering of data and the solving of problems.

Scope of practice The boundaries of a practice profession's activities as defined by law.

Secondary care An intermediate level of health care performed in a hospital having specialized equipment and laboratory facilities.

Secondary source Sources of data such as the nurse's own observations or perceptions of family and friends of the patient.

Self-actualization A process of realizing one's maximum potential and using one's capabilities to the fullest extent possible.

Self-awareness Understanding of one's own needs, biases, and impact on others.

Self-care The ability to care for oneself—that is, engage in activities of daily living without assistance.

Self-care model Nursing theoretical model based on the concept of ability to care for oneself.

Self-efficacy A belief in self as possessing the ability to perform an activity, such as administering daily insulin.

Sender An essential element of communication; the person sending a message.

Separation of powers Under the U.S. Constitution, each branch of the federal government has separate and distinct functions and powers.

Set A group of circumstances or situations joined and treated as a whole.

Shared governance Incorporation of unit-based decision making in nursing practice models. Generic term used to describe any organization in which decision making is shared throughout.

Short-term goals Specific, small steps leading to the achievement of broader, long-term goals.

Sigma Theta Tau International (STTI) The international honor society for nursing.

Sign Outward evidence of illness visible to others—for example, a rash or bleeding.

Socialization The process whereby values and expectations are transmitted from generation to generation.

Social services Services designed to assist individuals and families in obtaining basic needs, such as housing, food, and medical care.

Somatic language Language used by infants to signal their needs to caretakers—for example, crying; reddening of the skin; fast, shallow breathing; facial expressions; and jerking of the limbs.

Spelman Seminary Site of the first nursing program for Blacks; founded in Atlanta, Georgia, in 1886.

Spirituality Belief in and sense of connectedness with a higher power.

Spiritual nursing care Care that recognizes, respects, and, if appropriate, facilitates the practice of a patient's spiritual beliefs.

Staff nurse The bedside nurse who cares for a group of patients but has no management responsibilities for the nursing unit.

Stage theory A theory that views human development as a series of identifiable stages through which individuals and families pass.

Stakeholders Individuals with an interest in an outcome or process.

Standard of care A guideline stating what the reasonably prudent nurse, under similar circumstances, would have done.

Standards of practice Formal statements by a profession of the accountability of its practitioners.

State board of nursing The regulatory body in each state that regulates and enforces the scope of practice and discipline of the members of the nursing profession.

Statutory law Law established through formal legislative processes.

Stereotypes Simplistic and preconceived image about a person or group.

Stereotyping Erroneous belief that all people of a certain group are alike.

Stress Any emotional, physical, social, economic, or other type of factor that requires a response or change.

Stressors Stimuli that tend to disturb equilibrium.

Subjective data Information obtained from patients as they describe their needs, feelings, and strengths, as well as their perceptions of the problem.

Subsystems The parts that make up a system.

Supervision The initial direction and periodic inspection of the actual accomplishment of a task.

Suprasystem The larger environment outside a system.

Symptom An indication of illness felt by the individual but not observable to others, such as pain and nausea.

Synergy Combined action that is greater than that of the individual parts.

System A set of interrelated parts that come together to form a whole.

Systems theory See *General systems theory*.

T

Taxonomy A framework for classifying and organizing information.

Team nursing A system of nursing care delivery in which a group of nurses and ancillary workers are responsible for the care of a group of patients during a specified period, usually 8 to 12 hours.

Technologists Personnel, such as laboratory technologists or radiologic technologists, who assist in the diagnosis of patient problems.

Telehealth The practice of providing health care by means of telecommunication devices, such as telephone lines or televisions; the removal of time and distance barriers for the delivery of health care services and related health care activities through telecommunication technologies such as telephones.

Telehealth nursing The delivery of nursing care services and related health care activities through telecommunication technology, such as telephones, video conferencing, and others.

Termination phase The final phase of the nurse-patient relationship wherein a mutual evaluation of progress is conducted.

Tertiary care Specialized, highly technical level of health care provided in sophisticated research and teaching hospitals.

Tertiary source Sources of data including the medical records and health care providers, such as physical therapists, physicians, or dietitians.

Theory A general explanation scholars use to explain, predict, control, and understand commonly occurring events.

Therapeutic milieu An environment created to foster healing.

Therapist Any of several health care workers with differing educational backgrounds who work with patients with specific deficits; examples include physical therapists and occupational therapists.

Third-party payment Payment for health services by an entity other than the patient or the provider of services, such as the government or insurance companies.

Throughput The processes a system uses to convert raw materials into a form that can be used, either by the system itself or by the environment.

Tort A civil wrong against a person; may be intentional or unintentional.

Total quality management (TQM) Management philosophy and activities directed toward achieving excellence and employee participation in all aspects of that goal.

Transcultural nursing Nursing care that is based on the patient's culturally determined health values, beliefs, and practices.

Transmission In communication theory, the expression of information verbally or nonverbally.

U

Universal health care Provision of health care to all people.

Unlicensed assistive personnel (UAP) Health care personnel, such as nursing assistants and home care aides, who are not licensed but are supervised by licensed individuals, such as nurses or physicians.

Urbanization The process of population migration to cities.

Utilitarianism An ethical theory asserting that it is right to maximize the greatest good for the greatest number of people.

V

Valid Measuring what it is intended to measure, as in a valid test question or research instrument.

Value ethics Ethical beliefs and behaviors that arise from the character of the decision maker.

Value statement A statement regarding the desirability of something.

Values The social principles, ideals, or standards held by an individual, class, or group that give meaning and direction to behavior.

Veracity Truthfulness.

Verbal communication All language, whether written or spoken; represents only a small part of communication.

Virtue ethics The system of ethics based on a person's natural tendency to act, feel, and judge but developed through training; ethics based on the natural traits of the decision maker.

Voluntariness The degree to which an action is brought about by an individual's own free choice.

Voluntary (private) agency An agency supported entirely through voluntary contributions of time and/or money.

Vulnerable populations Groups who are at risk and unable to advocate for themselves, such as young children, persons with mental illness, developmentally challenged individuals, the frail elderly, or the socially marginalized, such as prisoners.

W

Whistle-blower A person who speaks out against unfair, dishonest, or dangerous practices by a company or agency. Usually an employee of that company or agency.

Woodhull Study on Nurses and the Media A comprehensive 1997 study of nursing in the print media.

Workers' compensation A federally mandated insurance system covering workers injured on the job.

Work ethic A belief on the part of an employee or group in the importance of work; an appreciation for the characteristics employers desire in employees and a commitment to exhibiting them.

Working phase The middle phase of the nurse-patient relationship, wherein goals are achieved.

Working poor Those who, although employed, are unable to earn enough to live at more than a very modest level.

Work-life balance The equilibrium between the amount of time and effort a person devotes to work and that given to other aspects of life.

Workplace advocacy Action ensuring that workers have a voice in the issues that concern them, either through collective action or through other effective means.

Yale School of Nursing The first school of nursing in the world to be established as a separate university department with an independent budget and its own dean, Annie W. Goodrich.

INDEX

Note: Page numbers followed by "f" indicate figures, "t" indicate tables, and "b" indicate boxes.

Digitized by
Google
from the library of
Stanford University